Health Care
Economics

To Anna

Health Care Economics

Sixth Edition

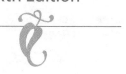

Paul J. Feldstein, Ph.D.
Professor
Robert Gumbiner Chair in Health Care Management
Graduate School of Management
University of California
Irvine California

THOMSON

DELMAR LEARNING

Australia Canada Mexico Singapore Spain United Kingdom United States

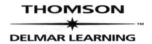

THOMSON
DELMAR LEARNING

Health Care Economics, 6th Edition
by Paul J. Feldstein

Vice President,
Health Care Business Unit:
William Brottmiller

Editorial Director:
Cathy L. Esperti

Acquisitions Editor:
Maureen Rosener

Developmental Editor:
Laurie Traver

Editorial Assistant:
Elizabeth Howe

Marketing Director:
Jennifer McAvey

Marketing Coordinator:
Kip Summerlin

Production Director
Karen Leet

Production Editor
Jack Pendleton

For permission to use material from this text or product, contact us by
Tel (800) 730-2214
Fax (800) 730-2215
www.thomsonrights.com

Library of Congress Cataloging-in-Publication Data

Feldstein, Paul J.
    Health care economics / Paul J. Feldstein.—6th ed.
        p. cm. — (Delmar series in health services administration)
    Includes index.
    ISBN-13: 978-1-4018-5979-4
    ISBN-10: 1-4018-5979-8
    1. Medical economics. 2. Medical economics—United States. I. Title. II. Series.
    RA410.F44 2005
    338.4'73621'0973—dc22   2004049793

NOTICE TO THE READER

THOMSON DELMAR LEARNING SERIES IN HEALTH SERVICES ADMINISTRATION

Stephen J. Williams, Sc.D., Series Editor

Ambulatory Care Management, third edition
Austin Ross, Stephen J. Williams, and Ernest J. Pavlock, Editors

The Continuum of Long-Term Care, second edition
Connie J. Evashwick, Editor

Essentials of Health Care Management
Stephen M. Shortell and Arnold D. Kaluzny, Editors

Essentials of Health Services, second edition
Stephen J. Williams

Essentials of Human Resources Management in Health Services Organizations
Myron D. Fottler, S. Robert Hernandez, and Charles L. Joiner, Editors

Financial Management in Health Care Organizations, second edition
Robert McLean

Health Care Economics, sixth edition
Paul J. Feldstein

Health Care Management: Organization Design and Behavior, fourth edition
Stephen M. Shortell and Arnold D. Kaluzny, Editors

Health Politics and Policy, third edition
Theodor J. Litman and Leonard S. Robins, Editors

The Hospital Medical Staff
Charles H. White

Introduction to Health Services, sixth edition
Stephen J. Williams and Paul R. Torrens, Editors

Motivating Health Behavior
John P. Elder, E. Scott Geller, Melbourne F. Hovell, and Joni A. Mayer, Editors

Really Governing: How Health System and Hospital Boards Can Make More of a Difference
Dennis D. Pointer and Charles M. Ewell

Strategic Management of Human Resources in Health Services Organizations, second edition
Myron D. Fottler, S. Robert Hernandez, and Charles L. Joiner, Editors

Health Services Research Methods
Leiyu Shi

BRIEF CONTENTS

DETAILED CONTENTS

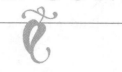

PREFACE

This book is an introductory text that provides an analytical approach to the study of medical services, and through the use of numerous applications, to illustrate the usefulness of economics to the understanding of public policy issues affecting this sector. The material in this book presumes some familiarity with some of the economic concepts presented in a microeconomics course. Several of these concepts are, however, reviewed when the applicability of economics to medical issues is discussed. (A new section reviewing supply, demand, and price elasticity has been included as an Appendix to Chapter 1). Since the institutional knowledge of medical care issues is generally not uniform among students, descriptive information and definitions are also provided.

Audience/Author's Approach

While those outside of academia's walls will find this book to be a useful resource, the intended use in the classroom is for a one-semester course in health economics. Realizing that instructor's preferences for topics to include in such a course may differ, more material is included than would normally be covered in one semester. For the interested student, both recent and historical references are provided should the student wish to pursue a particular subject in greater depth.

In writing this book I have tried to clarify those subjects that my students found most difficult and inadequately explained in the classroom. For example, as a result of student comments I became aware of the need to make explicit the relationship between economic analysis and the value judgments underlying different public policies. For this reason I have tried to stress these issues in the various subjects discussed.

The emphasis of this book is on the financing and delivery of personal medical services, rather than on the broader issues of health and health services. This narrower focus reflects the extensive emphasis of federal and state legislation and of current policy issues, such as financing medical services and concern with efficiency in the delivery of services, on personal medical services rather than health or health services, which might well be more appropriate. The relationship of personal medical services to health is discussed in an early chapter; thereafter, the text emphasizes the definition, measurement, and selection of public policies to achieve economic efficiency and equity in the financing and delivery of personal medical services.

Changes in the Industry

Since the time the first edition appeared, in 1979, the medical sector has undergone dramatic changes. Health policy is constantly changing. The emphasis on national health insurance, once high, declined, and may once again be rising; initial concerns over a shortage of physicians changed to a concern over a possible surplus of physicians, and currently to whether a shortage may again occur. From being reimbursed on the basis of their costs, hospitals now face prospective, fixed, prices, and physician payment under Medicare has similarly undergone dramatic changes. The structure of the medical services sector has also been changing, from independent community hospitals to multi-hospital systems. Managed care, which includes delivery systems such as HMOs and PPOs and cost containment methods such as demand management, was virtually non-existent before the 1980s, became the predominant method of delivering medical services during the 1990s. In more recent times interest in "Consumer Driven" health care (greater reliance on consumer decision making combined with catastrophic coverage) has been increasing.

New to this Edition

This latest edition includes a new chapter on the Pharmaceutical Industry which has had, and continues to have, a significant influence on the medical sector. Also new to this edition is the Appendix to Chapter One. This appendix covers supply, demand and price elasticity, thereby providing both new learners and those with some knowledge of the field with a review of the basic economic principles. Readers will appreciate the recent data on the medical sector, the latest information on legislative changes affecting the industry, and incorporation of recent literature, all while providing an historical perspective within which these changes are occurring. Also worth mentioning is the addition of Learning Objectives at the beginning of the chapters, where readers will find the Key Terms and Concepts as well. These elements will provide the reader with a preview of what they can expect to find in each chapter; many of the chapters have been extensively revised.

New for the Instructor

Available to educators as a companion to the textbook, is a new Online Companion, found exclusively online at Thomson Delmar Learning's website. Created with the intention of saving educators valuable class preparation time, the Online Companion not only provides an Instructor's Manual, but also includes all figures and tables from the book, available in PowerPoint format. Educators who use PowerPoint in their lectures should find having the images made available to them in this format to be especially helpful. The instructor's manual will include such elements as additional questions for the students, web links to additional resources, expanded comments on figures and tables, chapter overviews, and "In the News" features which will help illustrate the "real world" applications of the ideas presented in the chapters.

In writing this book and in teaching my course, I have greatly benefited from the work of other health economists. Some measure of that debt is indicated by the numerous references found throughout this book. Since this edition is a continuation of previous editions, I also wish to acknowledge some of my previous research assistants, Elzbieta Kozlowski, Courtand Reichman, John Goddeeris, Thomas Wickizer, Robert Miller, and Darrell Graham. A number of my colleagues also provided helpful comments on the various editions, and I have acknowledged them, along with the sixth edition reviewers—Richard Dwore, Mary Helen McSweeney, Ronald Vogel, Glenn Melnick, Carolyn Watts, and Peter Buerhaus—on the next page.

Paul J. Feldstein
Irvine, California

ACKNOWLEDGEMENTS

Peter Buerhaus, Ph.D., R.N., F.A.A.N.
Valere Potter Distinguished Professor, School of Nursing
Associate Dean for Research
Vanderbilt University
Nashville, Tennessee

Robert J. Caswell, Ph.D.
Associate Professor, Health Services Management and Policy
Dean for Graduate and Professional Studies
School of Public Health
Ohio State University
Columbus, Ohio

Richard Dwore, Ph.D.
Associate Professor, College of Health
Clinical Associate Professor,
Family and Preventative Medicine, College of Medicine
University of Utah
Salt Lake City, Utah

Jeremiah German, Ph.D.
Professor Emeritus, Department of Economics
Towson University
Towson, Maryland

John Kuder, Ph.D.
Associate Professor, Department of Policy Analysis and
    Management
College of Human Ecology
Cornell University
Ithaca, New York

Judith R. Lave, Ph.D.
Professor, Graduate School of Public Health
Department Chair, Health Policy and Management
University of Pittsburgh
Pittsburgh, Pennsylvania

Mary Helen McSweeney, Ph.D.
Assistant Professor, Department of Health Care Programs
Iona College
New Rochelle, New York

Glenn Melnick, Ph.D.
Professor, School of Policy, Planning and Development
University of Southern California
Los Angeles, California

Ronald J. Vogel, Ph.D.
Professor, College of Pharmacy
University of Arizona
Tucson, Arizona

Carolyn Watts, Ph.D.
Professor, Department of Health Services
Adjunct Professor in Economics, Evans School of Public Affairs
University of Washington
Seattle, Washington

Jack Wheeler, Ph.D.
Professor, Health Management and Policy
Professor, Pediatrics and Communicable Diseases
Faculty Associate, Institute for Social Research
School of Public Health
University of Michigan
Ann Arbor, Michigan

LIST OF FIGURES

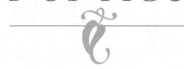

Chapter 5

Chapter 6

Chapter 11

Chapter 12

Chapter 13

Chapter 14

Chapter 15

Chapter 16

LIST OF TABLES

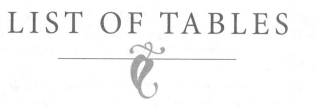

Chapter 5

Chapter 6

Chapter 9

Chapter 19

CHAPTER

1

An Introduction to the Economics of Medical Care

KEY TERMS AND CONCEPTS

- Economic efficiency
- Technical efficiency
- Redistribution
- Two tools of economics
- Marginal analysis (optimization technique)
- Supply and demand
- Interrelationship of two tools of economics
- Criteria for cost minimization
- Definition of rational choice
- Criteria for maximizing consumer satisfaction
- Opportunity cost
- Production possibilities curve

Learning Objectives

Upon completing this chapter, the reader should be able to:

- Understand the historical trends in medical expenditures.
- Apply the basic tools of economics used in this book.
- Explain the different choices that must be made with regard to how much is spent on medical services, the best methods for producing medical services, and how medical services should be distributed.
- Describe how the tools of economics are useful in clarifying the above choices.

TRENDS IN MEDICAL EXPENDITURES

Expenditures on personal medical services have risen more rapidly than expenditures on most other goods and services in the economy. Annual expenditures on personal medical services have increased from $35 billion in 1965 to $1.34 trillion in 2002. In 1965, 5 percent of the gross national product (GNP) was being spent on *personal* medical services (see Table 1-1). By 2002, 12.8 percent of the GNP was being allocated to *personal* medical services. Total medical expenditures were approximately $1.553 trillion in 2002 and comprised 14.8 percent of GNP. The difference between personal and total medical expenditures, about $213 billion, are expenses for prepayment and administration ($105 billion), government public health activities ($51 billion), and research and construction of medical facilities ($57 billion).

Managed care's cost containment programs slowed the rate of increase in personal medical expenditures during the 1990s (as shown in Table 1-1). However, the backlash against managed care's tight restrictions on access to care, together with medical advances and an aging population, led to a more rapid rate of increase in medical expenditures in recent years. Medical expenditures account for an increasing portion of all goods and services produced in the United States. Rising medical expenditures are also a hardship to many who cannot afford higher health insurance premiums and out-of-pocket costs of care.

The main components of medical care expenditure increases have been population increases, higher prices, and increased quantity of medical services consumed. The population, however, has been growing at less than 1 percent (0.9) per year. Thus when expenditures are adjusted for population increases by examining expenditures on a per capita basis, the annual percentage increase in per capita medical expenditures over the past 25 years is still very close to the annual percentage increase in total personal medical expenditures. Further, simply adjusting for population does not consider the aging of the population, and the aged are large consumers of medical services.

Increased prices and quantity of medical services have been important contributors to expenditure increases. Medical care prices, as measured by the medical care component of the consumer price index, have increased rapidly over time, but again medical prices and quantities do not accurately adjust for the changing product that is medical care. Vast improvements in medicine have changed treatments and outcomes for hospital and medical care. Thus, simply observing the rapid rise in medical prices and quantities, hence expenditures, obscures the many underlying forces that are affecting each of these components of expenditures.

To better understand the changes that have occurred in medical care, it is important to have an historical perspective of this industry. In addition to demographic shifts and technological advances, important economic and legislative developments have changed demands for care, the costs of providing that care, and patient and provider incentives.

The start of Medicare and Medicaid in 1966 produced dramatic changes in the medical sector. Medicare is a federal program for financing the medical services of the aged; Medicaid is a federal-state financing program for the medically indigent. With the enactment of these two programs, the aged and the poor had increased access to medical care. Hospitals were paid according to their costs, and physicians received their usual and customary fees. Increased demand by the aged and poor, together with a lack of efficiency incentives by either the beneficiaries or the providers, led to rapid increases in use of services and in the price of medical care. Government's role as a payer of medical services increased dramatically, from paying 20 percent of medical expenditures before 1966 to 45 percent currently, with the federal government paying three-fourths of that amount.

The rapid growth in private medical insurance also lessened private patients' concern with the cost of their care. High economy-wide inflation rates and high federal marginal tax brackets (up to 70 percent) were an incentive for employees to substitute their taxable wages for non-taxable fringe benefits. Consequently, the aged (Medicare), the poor (Medicaid), and middle- and high-income employees (tax-exempt employer paid health insurance) increased their use of medical services and became less concerned with the price of those services.

Table 1-1.   Trends in Personal Medical Care Expenditures, 1950–2002

Calendar Year	Total (Billions)	Average Annual % Inc. Total	% of GNP	Annual % Inc. Per Capita Total	Annual % Inc. in CPI Medical Care	Private Expend. (Billions)	Average Annual % Inc. Private	% of Total	Public Expend.	Average Annual % Inc. Public	% of Total	Federal Expend. (Billions)	Average Annual % Inc. Federal	State and Local Expend. (Billions)	Average Annual % Inc. State
1950	$10.9		3.8			$8.5		78.0	$2.4		22.0	$1.1		$1.3	
1955	15.7	8.8	3.8	6.4	4.1	12.1	8.5	77.1	3.6	10.0	22.9	1.6	9.1	2.0	10.8
1960	23.4	9.8	4.4	7.6	4.5	18.4	10.4	78.6	5.0	7.8	21.4	2.1	6.3	3.0	10.0
1965	34.7	9.7	4.8	7.6	2.6	27.7	10.1	79.8	7.1	8.4	20.5	2.8	6.7	4.3	8.7
1970	63.2	16.4	6.0	14.5	7.0	41.0	9.6	64.9	22.3	42.8	35.3	14.5	83.6	7.8	16.3
1975	113.0	15.8	6.9	13.9	7.9	68.0	13.2	60.2	45.0	20.4	39.8	30.6	22.2	14.4	16.9
1980	214.6	18.0	7.6	16.0	11.5	128.0	17.6	59.6	86.6	18.5	40.4	62.8	21.0	23.8	13.1
1985	372.3	14.7	8.8	13.1	10.3	225.6	15.3	60.6	146.7	13.9	39.4	109.7	14.9	37.1	11.2
1990	609.4	12.7	10.4	11.2	8.7	371.5	12.9	61.0	237.9	12.4	39.0	174.2	11.8	63.8	14.4
1995	865.7	8.4	11.7	7.0	7.1	478.5	5.8	55.3	387.3	12.6	44.7	296.5	14.0	90.8	8.5
2000	1,135.3	6.2	11.6	4.6	3.7	645.5	7.0	56.9	489.8	5.3	43.0	372.0	5.1	117.8	6.0
2002	1,340.2	9.0	12.8	8.2	5.1	748.1	7.9	55.8	592.2	10.5	44.2	450.5	10.6	141.7	10.1

Source: Centers for Medicare & Medicaid Services, Office of the Actuary: National Health Statistics Group, http://www.cms.gov/statistics/nhe/ (accessed on January 8, 2004); U.S. Bureau of the Census, *Statistical Abstract of the United States*, (Washington, D.C.: U.S. Department of Commerce), various editions: 1985, 105th ed., table 714; 2001, 121st ed., table 2, 646, 694; U.S. Bureau of Economic Analysis, http://www.bea.gov/bea/dn/nipaweb/TableView.asp#Mid (accessed on January 8, 2004).

Note: "Personal medical care expenditures" is equal to total health care expenditures less expenditures for prepayment and administration, government public health activities, and research and construction of medical facilities.

Average Annual % Increase is calculated from prior year shown.

As private insurance and government payments lessened the financial burden on the patient, there were few constraints remaining to hold down the use of services and prices charged by providers. Hospital and physician prices rapidly increased, as did expenditures on medical services. This acceleration in medical prices continued until the early 1970s, when federal price controls (the Economic Stabilization Program) were imposed on the economy in 1971. Although the economy-wide price controls were removed after one year, they remained in place for the medical sector until 1974. With the removal of price controls, medical prices rose rapidly. As the economy-wide rate of inflation continued to increase in the late 1970s, so did medical prices.

The federal and state governments became alarmed as they saw their expenditures under Medicare and Medicaid exceed their budget projections for these two programs. As Medicare expenditures (funded by a special payroll tax) exceeded those tax revenues, the federal government raised the Medicare payroll tax and sought ways to reduce Medicare hospital expenditures. State governments, unable to run budget deficits, attempted to reduce their Medicaid expenditures by reducing Medicaid eligibility, paying hospitals and physicians less, and enacting regulatory approaches, such as controls on hospital capital investment, to hold down the rise in medical expenditures. Several states instituted controls on hospital rate increases. By the late 1970s, however, it was clear that the regulatory programs were not working.

A deep recession in the early 1980s, which reduced the double-digit inflation rates of the late 1970s, together with strong import competition, led business and labor to explore new ways to reduce the rapid increases in employees' health insurance premiums. And then by the mid-1980s, to the surprise of most health care experts, the medical care market became price competitive.

In the mid-1980s, Medicare instituted a new hospital payment system (Diagnostic Related Groupings, or DRGs) that paid hospitals a fixed price per admission; consequently, hospitals reduced the lengths of stay of their Medicare patients. Utilization management by managed care organizations also reduced use of the hospital, contributing to the growing excess capacity among hospitals. As a result of federal subsidies to expand the number of medical school spaces in the 1960s, an increased supply of physicians led to excess capacity among physicians by the 1980s.

The structure and dynamics of the medical care market changed as managed care firms became the dominant type of health insurer and were able to negotiate steep price discounts from hospitals and physicians for them to be included in their provider network. The growth of managed care and intense price competition among both insurers and providers led to a lower rate of increase in health insurance premiums during the 1990s. In California, one of the most competitive managed care markets in the country, premiums actually declined for several years.

By the start of 2000, health insurance premiums began to increase more rapidly. Managed care's cost containment approaches—lower hospital utilization, reduced access to specialists, and provider price discounts, had run its course. With the growth in incomes in the late 1990s, employees wanted greater access to specialists and broader provider networks, the threat of lawsuits and legislation limited insurers' willingness to deny experimental treatments, and hospital mergers reduced the number of competitors in their market, thereby enabling them to raise their prices. The balance of power, which had enabled large managed care firms to dictate hospital and physician prices, shifted from managed care firms back to providers.

Once again, health care public policy is concerned with approaches for limiting the rise in health insurance premiums and second, how to provide for the large number of uninsured. Efficiency and redistribution issues continue to dominate the policy agenda.

THE CONTRIBUTION OF ECONOMICS TO HEALTH POLICY

Government policy should be concerned with achieving two objectives: improving market efficiency and, based upon society's values, redistribution of resources or services. Market efficiency is typically concerned with improving the performance of an industry, such as eliminating anti-competitive elements so that an industry is price competitive and that both purchasers and sellers have sufficient information to make informed choices. Market efficiency is also concerned with "externalities" as when an industry produces pollution in the process of producing its product, in which case the cost of that product does not reflect all its costs, including pollution.

Redistribution is based on society's value judgment that those with higher incomes should be taxed to provide for those with lower incomes. The extent of redistribution is highly controversial. The economists' role with regard to redistribution policy is not to substitute their values for those of others, but to evaluate which redistributive approach is more efficient (less costly) for achieving a given set of values.

"Positive" economic analysis attempts to determine the *consequences* of a particular policy and which groups benefit and which groups bear the burden of that policy. "Normative" analysis states what policies *should* be implemented. The contribution of economics is with respect to positive analysis, which this book emphasizes.

The basic premise underlying all economic analysis is the concept of rational choice. Consumers and producers are assumed to weigh the costs and benefits of different courses of action and choose the most preferred alternative. Choice is necessary because there are inadequate resources to fulfill all of our wants. At times the scarce resource is time itself, which forces one to choose among alternative uses of their time. Since resources and time can be used in alternative ways, it becomes necessary to choose among alternative uses of those scarce resources. Implicit in the discussion of choice is that individuals, on average, are assumed to act rationally.

Problems of scarcity and, consequently, choice, are the basis for the development and use of the economist's two basic tools and a set of criteria with which to analyze issues of efficiency and redistribution.

The first tool is marginal analysis, which underlies all optimization problems. Optimization techniques specify the appropriate criteria to be used when allocating scarce resources so as to minimize the cost of producing a given output or similarly, maximize output, subject to a budget constraint. Techniques of optimization can be used, for example, to determine which set of health manpower, given their relative productivity and wages, are least costly for producing a given medical service or whether one combination of institutional settings is less costly than another for treating particular types of patients. Similarly, marginal analysis can be used by government agencies and managed care organizations to determine the most efficient allocation of medical and non-medical resources to achieve a given objective, such as an increase in a defined population's health status.

The second economic tool is supply and demand analysis necessary for predicting new equilibrium situations; for example, predicting the effect of a change in demand for a service or in its cost of production on the price and quantity of that service. Supply and demand analysis makes it possible to understand the reasons for the rapid increases in medical care prices and expenditures; it also enables us to forecast future prices and expenditures. Supply and demand analysis can also estimate the consequences, in price, quantity of service, and total expenditure, of redistributive policies to increase medical services in the population, such as through national health insurance.

The previously mentioned two tools, marginal analysis (optimization techniques) and supply and demand analysis (predicting new equilibrium situations), are inter-related. Demand analysis is based on the assumption that in allocating their resources, consumers try to maximize their satisfaction subject to a budget constraint (their income and prices, including time prices). By choosing how to allocate their scarce resources (income and time) across different goods and services given their prices, the consumer is attempting to "optimize." If the consumer's income or prices change, this will cause a change in the demand for particular services. Similarly, the supply of a service is based on the assumption that producers attempt to maximize their profit and, subject to an overall budget constraint, have to minimize the cost of producing their output by choosing among using different inputs, each having different prices. A change in any aspect of the consumers' or producers' budget constraint will, because each is assumed to optimize, cause changes in the demand for and supply of different goods and services. A change in consumer preferences or in the productivity of different inputs, will, through the optimization process, also result in changes in demand and supply. (For a more complete discussion of supply and demand analysis, see the Appendix: "Review of Supply, Demand, Equilibrium Price, Elasticity, and Competitive and Monopoly Analysis.")

Implicit in the use of the foregoing analytical tools is a set of criteria for evaluating economic welfare. These welfare criteria are used to determine whether someone is made better or worse off (whether their benefits exceed their costs) as a result of a particular action or policy. (Redistribution occurs whenever a group's benefits are not equal to their costs.) These welfare criteria also make it possible to evaluate the performance of an industry. For example, when the (marginal) costs of producing the output approximate the (marginal) benefits to consumers from purchasing that output, the industry output is greater than under different market structures. Public policy is based on the values held by individuals and their perception of the most efficient method for achieving the given set of values. A specific set of welfare criteria provides the means by which differences in values and differences in methods for achieving a set of values can be separately evaluated.

BASIC CHOICES THAT MUST BE MADE REGARDING MEDICAL SERVICES

The economist's skill in using marginal analysis (optimization techniques) and supply and demand analysis and the economists' criteria for evaluating economic performance is useful and necessary regardless of how medical care is organized and provided in a country. Given that resources are scarce, three basic decisions must be made in any medical system, regardless of whether they are made by consumers or by government.

Every country must decide how much it wants to spend on medical services (and the composition of those services), the best methods for producing medical services, and, third, the method for distributing medical services among the population. The first two choices are concerned with issues of economic efficiency (in consumption and in production), the third with equity in use of health services.

A discussion of the possible choices for each of the above decisions should clarify whether disagreements over the choice to be selected is based on differences in values or a disagreement over the method of achieving an agreed-on set of values. In the following discussion of these three sets of medical care decisions, the economic tools discussed above will be used to illustrate the usefulness of economics both in clarifying and in making choices.

Determining the Output of Medical Services

The first set of medical care decisions is referred to as the determination of output: How much should be allocated to, and what should be the composition of, medical services? In a medical system that relies upon a price system for resource allocation, consumer and physician decisions determine the quantity and quality of medical services. Theoretically, the consumer selects those services which, given his or her income and the prices of different services, maximize satisfaction. It is assumed that consumers make such choices rationally (they consider the costs and benefits of their choices), and they have information on both the benefits derived from different services and the prices of those services. If these assumptions are correct, consumers will allocate their scarce resources (both time and income) to those services and activities that provide them with the greatest amount of benefits. The accuracy of these assumptions with respect to medical services is discussed herein.

To understand the allocation process used by consumers when selecting among various goods and services and to be able to predict changes in consumer allocation, it is necessary to understand marginal analysis, which is the basis of the optimization technique. Consumers' purchases provide them with benefits, or utility; additional purchases of those same services provide additional (marginal) benefits, but these additional benefits decline as more units are purchased. The benefits derived from consuming the first unit of a commodity are high; subsequent units of that same commodity provide smaller benefits. *Although total benefits increase with additional units of the same commodity, the marginal benefit of additional units declines.* This relationship between marginal benefits and additional units of a service is shown in Figure 1-1A. The marginal benefit (MB) from consuming *OA* units of the particular commodity represented in Figure 1-1A is MB_1. If additional units are consumed, the marginal benefit received from those additional units declines, from MB_1 to MB_2.

The consumer receives benefits from many different commodities. To maximize the total benefits from all commodities purchased, the consumer will allocate his or her limited resources to ensure that the marginal benefits received from all commodities purchased are equal.[1] This optimization rule for equating the marginal benefits of the last units of different commodities does not mean that the same number of units of each commodity will be consumed. It is more likely that when the marginal benefits of different commodities are equal, the buyer will consume differing quantities of the commodities purchased. The reason is that the marginal benefits decline at different rates for different commodities. The consumer is likely to purchase more units of those commodities

with a gradual decline in marginal benefits than of those with a very sharp decline. As shown in Figure 1-1B, the marginal benefits are equal at MB_0 for different commodities when the consumer is purchasing OA units, OB units, and OC units of three different commodities. Any other allocation process would result in a lower *total* level of benefits. The consumer, therefore, maximizes the amount of benefits for a given income by allocating it across commodities to ensure that the marginal benefits from the last units are equal.

(The previous discussion also illustrates the concept of "opportunity cost." When the consumer makes a particular choice, the value they would have received from the next best choice is the opportunity cost of the choice they made. Opportunity cost includes both explicit, i.e., out-of-pocket costs, as well as implicit, i.e., use of one's time, costs. Given scarcity of resources, including time, the real cost of making a choice is the opportunity cost of that decision, namely, the value that would have been received from the next best choice.)

To allow for differences in commodity prices, the consumer must compare not only the marginal

---

1. For the sake of simplicity, it is here assumed that the prices of the different commodities are equal.

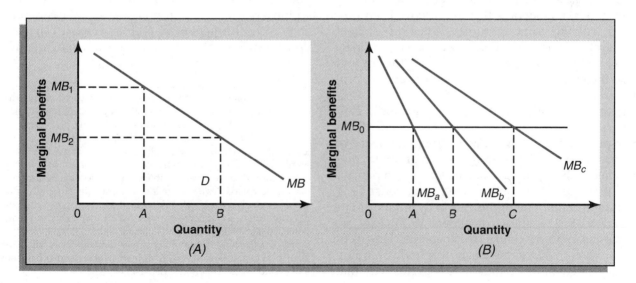

Figure 1-1.   Marginal benefit curves of (A) a single commodity, (B) different commodities.

benefits of different commodities but also the ratio of the marginal benefit to the price of each commodity (MB/P). When this is done, *the marginal benefit per dollar spent will be equal for all commodities.* (It should be noted that the marginal benefits received from the purchase of a commodity vary among consumers. These differences may be illustrated with reference to Figure 1-1B. The marginal benefit curves of Figure 1-1B in this case represent the marginal benefits received from the same commodity by different consumers.)

The consumer evaluates the marginal benefits of a purchase in relation to its price, or stated differently, the consumer compares the ratio of marginal benefit to marginal cost for each purchase with the ratio of every other purchase. The marginal cost to the consumer is the price he or she must pay for that commodity. When the consumer has equated the marginal benefits and the marginal costs of each purchase, his or her scarce resources have been allocated to maximize total benefits. In an equilibrium situation, the quantity demanded equals the quantity supplied; the equilibrium price reflects the value placed on the last units purchased by all consumers since all consumers face the same price in a given market. In a competitive market, prices represent the costs of production (which includes a normal profit). In turn, the costs of production reflect the value of other goods and services that might have been produced with the same resources. When an efficient price system is used for allocating resources, the marginal benefits to consumers of purchasing the last unit equal the marginal costs of the resources used to produce it.

Changes in any of the factors affecting consumers' allocation decisions will cause a change in their purchasing behavior: a change in the price of one commodity relative to the prices of other commodities, a change in income, or a change in perception of the benefits to be derived from consuming additional units. The optimization technique (marginal analysis) enables consumers to allocate resources so as to maximize their benefits. This technique also provides the basis for understanding changes in consumer demand. It is in this way that the two tools of economics—optimization techniques and the determination of equilibrium situations—are related.[2]

The previous description of the consumer choice process in a market system illustrates the importance of price in making choices. A non-market approach toward determining the amount of resources to be allocated to medical care requires a substitute mechanism that will perform the price function—that is, that will provide an incentive to consumers to limit their use of services to the point at which the cost of those services equals their value. Such a mechanism must also ration the available quantity of services among consumers and provide information of changes in consumer demand to providers. Although the functions that prices perform must still be performed in a non-price system, alternative mechanisms to perform these functions have been found to be unsatisfactory.

How Best to Produce Medical Services

The second set of decisions that must be made in any health system is selection of the best method for producing the amount of medical services (of constant quality) to be provided. Medical services can be provided in different institutional settings, such as a hospital, outpatient facility, or physician's office. Even within a particular institutional setting, the combinations of health personnel and equipment can vary. When providers of medical services have an incentive

---

2. This discussion of marginal analysis is not meant to imply that *every* consumer continuously undertakes an exact system of calculation for purchasing all commodities. Consumers, on average, do consider such factors as marginal benefits, relative prices, and their level of income when making their purchase decisions. While economic models also include non-economic variables, such as psychological and sociological variables, as predictors of consumer behavior, these variables do not change as frequently or rapidly as do the economic variables. Therefore, to the extent that consumers have information and act to maximize their total benefits, predictions based on changes in relative prices and income will result in more accurate predictions of consumer demand than will other (e.g., psychological or sociological) models of consumer behavior that exclude such economic variables.

to minimize their costs, they will use the various inputs—health personnel and capital—according to their relative costs and productivity. The optimization approach used by providers for determining the mix of institutional settings and the combination of resources used within each setting will be similar to that used by the consumer of medical services. In place of marginal benefits and relative prices on the consumer side, marginal productivity of inputs and their relative costs will be used by providers to determine the least costly method of providing a service. The decision rule will be the same. When the ratio of the marginal productivity of an input to its wage is equal to that of other inputs, the firm is minimizing its costs of providing medical services.

When the provider's costs are minimized, the combination of services (hospital, physician services, and outpatient care) and the inputs (types of health personnel and capital) used to provide medical care will be both technically and economically efficient. *Technical efficiency means that the combination of inputs used will produce the maximum quantity of medical services.* However, several different combinations of inputs may be technically efficient. To minimize the cost of providing medical services, it is necessary to be not only technically but also economically efficient. The decision-maker must choose among the several combinations of inputs, each of which is technically efficient, to determine which combination is also economically efficient—that is, least costly. To do so, the decision-maker must consider the relative costs of the different inputs as well as their productivities.

When the economist applies the optimization tools to the set of choices governing the production of medical services, several problems of medical services delivery are brought into sharper focus. Some medical professionals have proposed the use of standards in the delivery of medical services: four hospital beds per 1,000 population was one such standard; specified lengths of stay, by diagnosis, for hospitalized patients is another example; and ratios of the number of registered nurses per hospitalized patient is a third. Standards such as these imply that medical services can or should be produced by only one method. If the provision of medical services were actually subject to

such fixed proportions, no choice of production methods would exist, and the effectiveness of the economist's tools for minimizing medical care costs would be very limited. It is, however, unlikely that the choices for producing medical care are so limited.

Depending upon the illness being treated, ambulatory care and nursing home services can be substituted for hospital care with no decrease in the quality of treatment. Lengths of stay can be varied depending upon the availability of other facilities in the community and someone to care for the patient at home. To some extent, other kinds of nursing personnel can substitute for registered nurses in the care of the hospitalized patient. Presently, wide variations exist across communities in lengths of stay by diagnosis, in use of registered nurses, and in number of hospital beds per 1,000 population. Substituting medical services and personnel without a decrease in overall quality is more possible than some would have us believe.

Using specific standards as previously described, when substitution is possible, will hinder economic efficiency in providing medical care. Using inputs without regard to their relative costs is unlikely to result in the least-cost combination. As the relative costs (and productivities) of inputs change over time, it is to be expected that the combination of inputs that is least costly for providing medical services will change also. The economist's tools of optimization can determine which combination of services and inputs is most efficient for providing medical care. Similarly, the concepts embodied in these tools provide a decision-maker with vital information about the costs of different choices, which can then be used to decide how best to deliver medical services.

The second of the economist's tools, the prediction of new equilibrium levels of prices and quantities (supply and demand analysis), flows from the optimization technique and can be used to anticipate changes in the production of medical services. A change in the price of an input will, as previously discussed, result in a change in the combination of inputs that is least costly to use in producing medical care. It is also possible to analyze the new equilibrium situation that will result from that change. An increase in the price of an input (e.g., an increase in registered nurses' wages) will cause a reduction in the quantity demanded of it and an increase in demand for those inputs whose prices have not changed. If the higher-priced inputs are used mainly in the provision of one type of service, such as hospital care, we would then expect to observe a reduction in the quantity demanded of that service because its price has risen as its inputs have become more costly (supply will shift up or to the left along the demand curve for hospital care). As the cost of medical services increase, the supply curve of medical care will shift to the left. Assuming no change in the demand for medical services, the price of medical care will increase and the quantity demanded will decrease. The extent of the actual change in prices and quantities of medical care will depend upon the elasticities of supply and demand.

The tools of demand and supply can be used to trace the consequences of a change in input prices throughout the medical system. They can also be used to anticipate the effects of changes in medical technology on productivity, medical prices, and quantities of services. Such equilibrium analyses are particularly helpful in anticipating future expenditures for medical care to be borne either by patients or by the government, such as those that would occur under a system of national health insurance.

Relying on a price system whereby providers and health insurers compete for patients and enrollees provides providers and insurers with an incentive to minimize the cost of care and the insurance premium. A non-price system, such as the use of fixed input ratios or specified hospital days per 1,000, will not achieve the least cost combination for a given level of quality.

The Distribution of Medical Services

The third set of decisions that must be made in any medical system govern the distribution of the system's output. Medical services can be provided free of charge to all persons, or it can be distributed in accordance with consumers' willingness to spend their incomes for it (consumer sovereignty). With the latter approach, subsidies can be provided to those persons whose incomes are insufficient to purchase the amount of medical care society deems appropriate and necessary.

These alternative approaches for determining the distribution of medical services, free to all or consumer sovereignty, require rationing of medical services. No country will supply (and fund) all the medical services demanded at zero prices. Similarly, prices and income limit consumer demand for medical services. An important decision society must make is which of these two approaches will be used for determining the distribution of medical services. Elimination of money prices results in other mechanisms being used to ration services, such as "time" prices or patients' willingness to wait. Whenever the consumer cannot use money prices to make their allocation decisions between medical care and nonmedical services as well as between different types of medical services, then, as discussed earlier, the consumer is less able to maximize their satisfaction.

Two value judgments govern the distribution of medical services. The first is whether or not consumers should determine the amount they wish to spend on medical services. The second concerns the method and size of subsidy to be extended to low-income consumers whose use of medical services is below what society believes it should be. The economist cannot decide which set of values is preferable; however, economics can help make the process of choosing more rational by providing information on the costs and the implications of different sets of values, and also by providing criteria for determining the most efficient method for achieving a given set of values.

A more complete discussion of the different values underlying the subsidies designed to redistribute medical services is discussed in the chapter on National Health Insurance. That chapter also contains an analysis of the economic efficiency of existing methods of financing medical services, as well as of those proposed under alternative approaches to national health insurance.

THE APPLICABILITY OF ECONOMICS TO THE STUDY OF MEDICAL CARE

Critics have questioned the applicability of economics to the study of medical services on two levels: first, the accuracy of assumptions underlying the economic behavior of consumers and medical providers, and second, the implicit values, such as consumer sovereignty, that influence the goal to be achieved (i.e., consumer satisfaction). For example, critics have claimed that it is inaccurate to assume that the consumer of health services is rational and that he or she has sufficient information when deciding on use of services. Such critics also claim that the purchaser of medical services is not the consumer as in non-medical markets, but the physician, who also has a financial interest in the services purchased (which may place the physician's financial interest in conflict with that of the patient). And unlike other markets, consumers do not pay the full price of medical care; employer-paid health insurance is tax exempt, and government programs (Medicare and Medicaid) similarly affect consumer incentives to be concerned with prices.

With regard to economists' traditional assumptions about providers of medical services, critics claim that these providers are organized as nonprofit organizations and, therefore, do not have the same motivations as for-profit firms in other industries. Further, since consumers may be irreparably harmed by incompetent providers, more stringent controls must be exercised over the provision of medical services than over non-medical goods and services. Finally, such critics claim that access to medical services is considered a right by society, and its distribution cannot be left solely to the marketplace.

It is important to distinguish between criticism directed at the validity of economic assumptions and criticism of the use of economic criteria for evaluating medical system performance. If economic analyses are undertaken, they will be based upon a given set of assumptions which will lead us to predict a certain outcome. If the observed behavior is different from what would be expected in a competitive market, the assumptions are re-examined to determine whether a different assumption could explain the divergence between the expected and observed behavior.

For example, an important assumption affecting industry performance is entry of new firms (providers). An economic analysis would initially assume that there are no barriers to entry in a market, such as home health care services. Based on the as-sumption of no entry barriers, we expect to observe certain measures of market performance; an increase in demand for home health agencies would lead to high profits which, over time, would result in increased entry by new home health agencies until profits are similar to what could be earned in other industries. If, instead, market performance (long-term profitability) is different from what was predicted, then the free-entry assumption is re-examined. Thus economic analysis isolates those assumptions to be re-examined when a divergence occurs between expected and observed behavior. Market performance can be improved by making those structural changes, e.g., reduce entry barriers, that will bring an industry's performance into greater conformity with its expected performance.

For each medical sector to be analyzed in this book, the expected performance of consumers and providers in a competitive market is contrasted to observed performance. When a divergence exists, the underlying assumptions are re-examined to account for the observed behavior. Specific assumptions regarding consumer information, efficiency incentives, and barriers to entry are examined to determine their effect on economic performance when they differ from what is assumed in a competitive market.

Medical care is different from other markets primarily because of consumers' lack of information on their diagnosis and methods of treatment, their consequent need to rely on health professionals, the uncertainty of illness, treatment outcomes, and provider competence, all of which give rise to a greater demand for consumer protection. Different approaches to providing consumer protection are, however, available and are analyzed with respect to their impact on the performance of the medical care sector. Differences in information between consumers and health insurers regarding consumers' health status also have affected the market for insurance, such as leading to adverse selection. *Instances of market failure do not necessarily justify government intervention, since government intervention may not improve the situation;* this is discussed more completely in the chapter on "Health Policy and the Legislative Marketplace."

Medical care is also different in that society is more concerned with the redistribution issue, that everyone has access to medical care. A competitive market will not provide free care to those who cannot afford it; similar to other markets providing necessities such as food and housing, it is the role of government to provide such subsidies, and these subsidies can be efficiently distributed within a competitive market.

Criticisms of the values underlying the use of economic criteria for evaluating medical system performance are more difficult to resolve. Given a scarcity in the availability of resources for providing medical services, what criteria should society use for making the three basic medical care decisions? A medical system that values economic efficiency in consumption and production will base its choice of the amount to spend on medical services on the criterion of satisfying consumer preferences; it will base its method of providing services on the criterion of least-cost method of production; and it will base its choice of the amount and method of medical services redistribution on the criterion of consumer preference. Under this value system, medical service benefits are defined by consumer preference rather than by government or health agency perception of consumer preference.

If decision-makers reject the above criteria, new criteria must be specified. The criterion of efficiency in production is more likely to be acceptable than is the criterion of satisfying consumer preferences. Some prefer a "needs" approach to the allocation of medical services which relies on centrally determined resource allocations. However, because resources are insufficient to satisfy all medical needs, an additional decision rule must be developed that will enable decision-makers to choose which needs and which population groups will be given highest priority.

The replacement of one set of values by another does not diminish the usefulness of economics in the decision-making process; its value lies in its ability to make that process more explicit by showing what the costs of different choices are. To the extent that economic analysis can clarify the costs of alternatives and make the values underlying those alternatives explicit, it is a useful approach to the study of medical care.

THE TRADE-OFF BETWEEN QUANTITY AND QUALITY IN THE PROVISION OF MEDICAL SERVICES

The three basic choices that must be made regarding medical services can be illustrated in Figure 1-2, which represents a production possibilities curve. This curve shows the trade-off between two different goods or outputs, e.g., quantity and quality of medical services. The curve is shaped as it is (concave to the origin) because the resources used in producing quantity and quality (each of which is a different output) are not completely substitutable for one another. As more of one combination of services is produced (as represented by Point A or Point B), the resources are shifted from producing one type of service to the other. The released resources are more specialized, hence more efficient, in producing their previous output. Moving those same resources into the production of a different good or service will cause them to be less efficient in the production of that new service. Therefore, the costs of producing more of the new output are increased.

The first choice that must be made in any medical system concerns the types of medical services to be produced, namely, for a given budget, which combination of quantity and quality of medical services to select? If health professional training times are very long and if the equipment and facilities used are the most technically advanced, fewer services will be available to the entire population. Point A represents a combination where quality (which actually refers to the level of training of health professionals—a process measure, not an outcome measure, of quality) is relatively high and is received by a small percentage of the population. Point B represents a different combination: a large percent of the population receives medical services while the quality of those services is relatively low. If society desires more of one type of output, it must give up some of the other output. Thus the opportunity cost of using scarce resources to expand quality of care (Point A) is the foregone use of those resources to provide a greater number of people with medical care (Point B).

What criterion should determine the combination of quality and quantity of medical services that a society

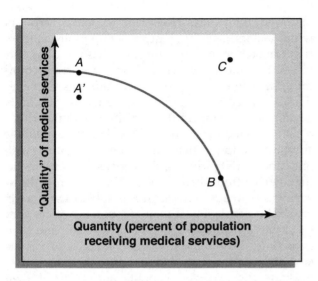

Figure 1-2. The quantity-quality trade-off in medical care.

should choose? If the criterion were the maximization of consumer preferences, then, assuming adequate information and proper safeguards, consumers would be the appropriate group to select the quantity-quality combination that should prevail.[3] Alternatively, health professionals can select the quantity-quality trade-off, as they have in the United States. For example, health professionals establish the educational requirements and determine the number of educational institutions through their accreditation policies. Less emphasis on process requirements and greater emphasis on outcomes and testing would provide greater assurance of quality at lower cost, hence greater quantity.

The quantity-quality trade-off can also be used to illustrate the second set of choices that must be made in any medical care system—namely, how best to produce medical services. Any quantity-quality combination on the production possibilities curve is assumed to be produced in the least costly manner. The

area under the curve represents the amount of resources devoted to medical services. If, owing to the placement of restrictions on the least costly manner of production or the use of a method of provider reimbursement that removes efficiency incentives, the providers of medical services are not as efficient as they might be, then fewer medical services will be produced for the same amount of resources. This situation is shown in Figure 1-2 where A' represents the same amount of resources as used at Point A but the output is less than that achieved at Point A. A' is obviously inefficient in that resources are being wasted; either more medical services or medical services of higher quality could be produced with the same quantity of resources. It is important to determine whether the current medical care system is at Point A or A' and, if so, the reasons why.

The third set of choices concerning distribution of medical services can be illustrated by an analysis of the statement, "All Americans should receive the highest quality of medical care." The highest quality of medical care to all would be represented by point C in Figure 1-2, which is equivalent to 100 percent of the population (farthest to the right on the horizontal axis), and by the highest point on the quality axis. To achieve such a goal, additional resources equivalent to the distance between Point C and the current production possibilities curve would be required. These additional resources would be financed either by an increase in taxes or by decreased expenditures on other programs. These choices provide differing marginal benefits. Who is to decide their relative benefits? Health professionals attach greater benefits to medical as opposed to other services; however, they do not bear the costs of their decisions. Consumers, who *will* bear the costs, may not share professional estimates of the relative benefits.

SUMMARY

Economics employs the optimization technique based on marginal analysis for the allocation of scarce resources to achieve a given objective. Supply and demand analysis, the second tool of economics,

---

3. The resultant quantity-quality combination would maximize consumer satisfaction because the marginal benefits of those services (to the consumer) would equal the marginal cost of resources used in their production.

enables economists to predict new equilibrium situations, such as increased prices, quantities, and expenditures. Optimization underlies both demand and supply, thus the two tools are interrelated. The welfare criteria used by economists, again based on marginal analysis, provides a means to judge whether people are made better or worse off as a result of a policy change and which type of industry structure performs better.

The economist's tools and welfare criteria clarify the consequences of how society responds to three basic decisions: how much to spend on medical services, how best to produce those services, and how to distribute them. People differ in their values as to how those choices should be made. To evaluate how the medical system performs with respect to each of those choices, it is necessary to establish criteria for what is considered good performance.

The performance criteria used by economists is based upon a set of values incorporated into their definition of economic efficiency—namely, maximizing consumer satisfaction and using the least costly method of production. If decision-makers disagree over these values, it is necessary to explicitly state an alternative set of values. People can then decide whether they prefer one set of values compared to another. For any alternative set of values, it is also necessary to state the criteria to be used for evaluating the performance of the medical system. The debate over appropriate public policy in medical care is often confused because a clear distinction is not made between differences in values and differences in the best way to achieve a particular set of values. Clarification of these differences should sharpen the debate over the most appropriate public policies for medical care.

APPENDIX: REVIEW OF DEMAND, SUPPLY, EQUILIBRIUM PRICE, PRICE ELASTICITY, AND COMPETITIVE AND MONOPOLY ANALYSIS

Assumptions Underlying Supply and Demand Analysis

Economics is concerned with being able to *explain* and *predict* observed outcomes. Innumerable factors affect observed outcomes. However, to make sense of which factors are on average most important, a theory is needed based on some simplified assumptions. The test of any theory is the accuracy of its predictions rather than the realism of its assumptions. A theory does not need to be perfect to be useful; it simply needs to be more accurate than alternative theories.

The demand for goods and services starts with the simple assumption that consumers attempt to maximize their utility; that is, the satisfaction or benefits they derive from their choices. The consumer, however, has scarce resources; (s)he is subject to a budget constraint consisting of their income, the prices they must pay for different goods and services, and their own time. In making choices, the consumer is assumed to be rational; that is, he or she attempts to evaluate the expected benefits and costs of their choices. And it is further assumed that consumers have information on the marginal benefits derived from their different choices and the marginal costs incurred for each of those choices, namely prices and time involved. Based on these assumptions, it is possible to predict the effect on the consumer's choices when changes occur in the relative prices to be paid for different goods and services, in their time costs, and in their incomes.

The supply side similarly assumes that the firm, the supplier of goods and services, has an objective, namely to maximize their profits, subject to a budget constraint consisting of the prices they must pay for their inputs, labor and capital, and the price the firm receives for its output. The firm is also assumed to be knowledgeable regarding the most efficient method for producing its output (the most technically efficient production process), the prices it must pay for the various inputs used in the production process, and the price it receives for its output. Based on these assumptions it becomes possible to explain how firms choose the combination of inputs used in production and the amount of output they produce.

The above assumptions regarding consumer and producer behavior are not always fulfilled, particularly with respect to medical care; consumers have little knowledge of their illnesses and treatment needs and physicians, non-profit hospitals, and medical schools may have objectives other than maximizing their profits. When assumptions and objectives are different from those hypothesized, it becomes possible to predict its consequences on consumer and producer behavior. The economic theory described below, when used at an aggregate level—not for individual consumers or particular physicians—is a powerful tool for explaining and predicting consumers' and firms' responses to changes in their budget constraints.

Factors Affecting Demand

Price:

A change in the *price of the service*, such as a physician office visit, would result in a *movement* up or down the consumer's demand curve for physician visits, *all other factors affecting demand being held constant*. As shown in Figure 1-3, a decrease in price from P_1 to P_2 would cause an increase in the quantity demanded of physician visits from Q_1 to Q_2. The demand curve pertains to a particular time period, such as quantity per month or per year. The negative (inverse) relationship between price and quantity is referred to as *The Law of Demand*.

There are two reasons for this inverse relationship. The downward sloping demand curve represents the declining marginal benefit to the consumer of purchasing additional units; the first unit offers the highest marginal benefit, the second somewhat less, and so on.

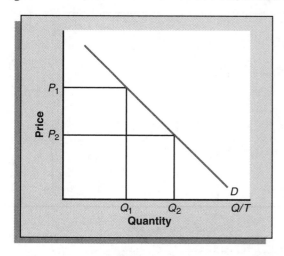

Figure 1-3.   A downward sloping demand curve.

The quantity demanded by the consumer will depend on the price they must pay (which is the consumer's marginal cost). When the price equals the marginal benefit they receive from consuming an additional unit, then the marginal cost to the consumer equals the marginal utility/benefit received from that last unit. If the price declines, the consumer would be willing to buy an additional unit whose marginal benefit is lower than the previous unit; at that point the marginal cost of the last unit again equals the marginal benefit of the last unit purchased. Along the demand curve the consumer is making a trade-off between the marginal benefit of consuming an additional unit versus the marginal cost (price) of buying that additional unit.

The second reason for the downward sloping demand curve is that as the price falls, consumers who previously did not buy that item now enter the market. For the new consumers, the previously higher price exceeded the marginal benefit they would have gained from consuming that item (their marginal cost exceeded their marginal benefit). As the price falls, the declining marginal cost equals their marginal benefit.

The downward sloping demand curve may be thought of as the consumer's continual trade-off between their marginal benefit of buying additional units and the price (marginal cost) they must pay for each unit.

Although the consumer would be willing to pay a high price for the first unit and a lower price for the next unit (and so on), when there is a single market price, the consumer only pays one price for all the units purchased. The difference between what the consumer is willing to pay for each unit and the amount they have to pay is called *Consumer Surplus*, graphically shown in Figure 1-4. At a price of $10 per unit, the consumer would be willing to buy one unit; at a lower price of $9, the consumer would be willing to buy a second unit, and so on. The consumer would have been willing to spend $40 for 5 units ($10 + $9 + $8 + $7 + $6), which is the total value to the consumer of those 5 units. However, at a market price of $6, the consumer can buy 5 units for $30. The difference, $10, is consumer surplus. (As will be discussed in Chapter 10, The Physician Services Market, a price-discriminating monopolist attempts to price their service so as to capture the entire consumer surplus.)

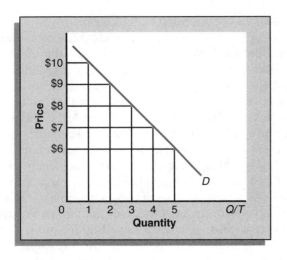

Figure 1-4. Consumer surplus.

Price of Substitute Products:

A *shift* in the consumer's demand curve for physician office visits will occur if there is a change in the *price of a substitute* to physician office visits (substitutes can partially replace the other service). A decrease in the price of chiropractic visits, a substitute to some extent for physician visits, will cause the demand curve for physician visits to shift to the left. As shown in Figure 1-5, with the price of physician visits unchanged, a decrease in the price of a substitute from P_1 to P_2 will

cause the demand curve for physician visits to shift to the left, from D_1 to D_2, with a consequent decrease in demand for physician visits from Q_1 to Q_2. All other factors affecting the demand for physician services are assumed to be unchanged.

The relationship between changes in the price of a substitute and physician visits is *positive*, meaning that as the price of the substitute decreases, so does the demand for physician visits, or an increase in the price of a substitute leads to an increase in demand for physician services.

Price of Complementary Products:

Complements are goods or services that are used together. Thus, an increase in the *price of a complement* will have a *negative* effect on the demand for physician visits; the demand for physician visits will shift to the left (right) if the price of a complement is increased (decreased). For example, as shown in Figure 1-6, a decrease in the price of diagnostic tests from P_1 to P_2 will not only increase the quantity demanded of diagnostic tests (a movement along its demand curve) but should result in an increase in the demand for physician visits to interpret those test results, from Q_1 to Q_2.

When the price of a service increases and it leads to a decrease in demand for another service, then those two services are complements. When the price in-

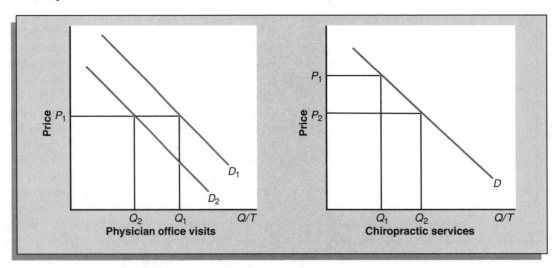

Figure 1-5. The effect on the demand for physician office visits of a decrease in the price of a substitute.

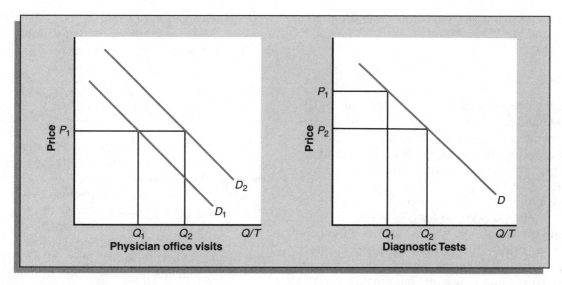

Figure 1-6.   The effect on demand for physician office visits of a decrease in the price of a complement.

crease leads to an increase in demand for another service, then the two services are substitutes.

Income:

An increase in a family's income relaxes their budget constraint and enables them to purchase more goods and services. Other factors affecting demand being held constant, an increase in *income will cause the demand curve to shift* to the right, resulting in an increase in demand for that service. See Figure 1-7. The positive relationship between income and demand is characteristic of a "normal" good. An "inferior" good is one where an increase in income results in a decrease in demand, or a negative relationship. Medical care is considered to be a normal good, meaning as incomes rise, people prefer to spend a portion of their increased income on additional medical services.

Tastes and Preferences:

There are a number of other, non-economic, factors, in addition to the economic factors described previously that will cause the demand curve to shift either to the right or left. Thus per-capita use of medical services will differ even if different groups have the same incomes and face the same prices. These non-economic factors are usually included under the category of *Tastes and*

Preferences. For example, an aging population will cause the demand for medical care to shift to the right; older males will have a greater demand for medical care (shift to the right) than older females. Differences in educational level and attitudes toward seeking care will cause shifts in the demand for different medical services. Economists include both economic and non-economic factors affecting demand. (A more complete discussion

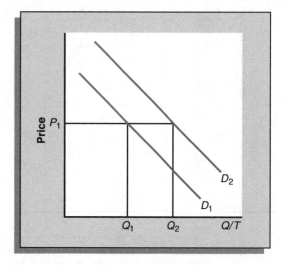

Figure 1-7.   The effect on demand of an increase in income.

of these non-economic factors is included in Chapter 5, "The Demand For Medical Care.")

Population:

Once all the economic and non-economic factors affecting demand have been specified, the *size of the population* becomes important. The more individuals there are in a community, the greater the demand for medical care; the demand curve shifts to the right, as shown in Figure 1-8.

Not everyone has to be responsive to changes in price for a demand curve to have its negative slope. Even though some people will not change their consumption as prices change (their demand curve is vertical), others will. When all the individual demand curves are summed up, it is the marginal buyer, the ones that are responsive to price changes, that result in an aggregate downward sloping demand curve.

Demand Equation:

A useful method for distinguishing between movements along a demand curve and shifts in demand, as well as the direction of those shifts, is the following equation. The signs in front of each variable indicate the direction of the variable's effect on demand.

$$Q_{da} = f(-Price_a, +Price_{sub}, -Price_{compl}, +Income, +Tastes) \times POP$$

This equation states that the quantity demanded of a good or service is functionally related to (dependent upon) its Price; changes in price are a movement along the demand curve, and the negative sign indicates that price is inversely related to quantity demanded. All of the remaining variables represent shifts in the demand for the service. An increase in the price of a substitute (positive sign) will cause the demand for A to increase, namely shift to the right. An increase in the price of a complement (negative sign) will cause the demand for A to decrease, shift left. An increase in income (positive sign), assuming it is a normal good, will cause the demand for A to shift right. Tastes represent non-economic factors that will cause shifts in the demand for A. The total demand for A is then equal to the sum of all the consumers' demand in the market.

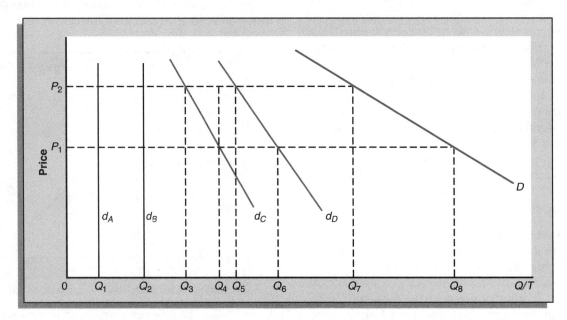

Figure 1-8. Summing individual demand curves to obtain market demand.

Factors Affecting Supply

Price:

The supply of a good or service is positively related to the *price paid for that service.* Higher product prices represent a movement along a supply curve. The producer is making a trade-off between the marginal cost of producing an additional unit versus the marginal benefit (price) offered for that unit. As shown in Figure 1-9, the higher the price, from P_1 to P_2, the greater the willingness of the supplier to increase output; the firm can hire more employees and buy additional supplies to increase production. Along a given supply curve, the prices of labor and non-labor inputs are assumed to be unchanged.

(The firm's supply curve in the short run is its marginal cost curve (MC). Marginal cost is equal to the input price, e.g., the wage rate, divided by the input's marginal productivity (MP). For example, assuming the wage rate is $10 and MP is 5 units, then MC equals $2 per unit. The reason the firm's supply curve is upward sloping is because of the *Law of Diminishing Returns.* In the short run, meaning that time period in which there is some fixed input that cannot be expanded such as the size of the building, as more labor is hired then, at some point, continually adding labor to work in that facility will result in a decrease in labor's productivity. As the MP of an additional employee declines and is lower than the previous employee hired, marginal cost increases. Thus MC = W/MP = $10/5 = $2 per unit, with another employee MC = $10/4 = $2.50 per unit.)

The firm will produce to the point where its marginal cost equals the price received for each unit of output. When the firm is producing at the point where its marginal costs equal its marginal revenue (the additional revenue received for each unit sold, which in this example is the price of the product), then the firm is maximizing its profits. The only way the firm can increase its output as its marginal costs increase is to be paid a higher price for its output. It is important to note that included in marginal cost are all the relevant costs to the firm, including *opportunity* costs, which are the sum of explicit (dollar) and implicit (value of the resource in its best alternative use, e.g., the highest wage the owner could have earned elsewhere)

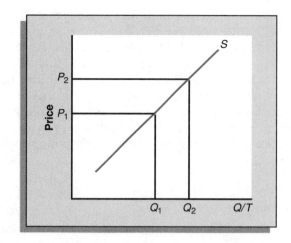

Figure 1-9. A movement along a supply curve.

costs. Thus economic costs are different from accounting costs, which only include explicit costs.

Input Prices:

The firm's supply curve will shift because of a change in the *price of either labor or non-labor inputs.* An increase in the wage rate will shift the supply curve upward (left), from S_1 to S_2. With the price of the product remaining unchanged at P_1, an increase in the wage rate will decrease supply from Q_1 to Q_2, as shown in Figure 1-10. An example illustrates the shift left in supply as the wage increases. Assume that P_2 in

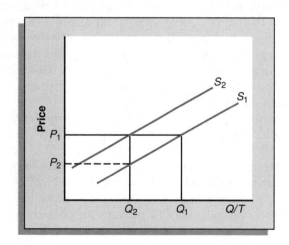

Figure 1-10. A shift in supply.

Figure 1-10 is $2 per unit, and assume that MC = W/MP = $10/5 = $2 per unit. With both price and MC equal to $2 per unit, the firm will produce Q_2 units. If the wage rate increases from $10 to $20, then MC = $20/5 = $4 per unit. The supply curve has shifted up; to produce the same rate of output, Q_2, the price of the product, would have to increase to $4 per unit. At a price of $4 per unit, the firm would have been able to produce a greater output with the previous supply curve, Q_1.

Technology:

Figure 1-10 can also be used to illustrate another reason for a shift in supply. *Technological improvements* that increase labor's productivity increase each employee's marginal product, thereby shifting the supply curve to the right or down, from S_2 to S_1. Again, assuming MC = W/MP = $10/5 $2 per unit, introducing a new technology that increases productivity would result in a decrease in marginal cost per unit; MC = $10/10 = $1 per unit. Thus the same output, Q_2, can be produced for less (on the new supply curve S_1), or a greater rate of output, Q_1 (on supply curve S_1), could be produced for the same price.

The following equation describes the factors affecting supply and the direction of each factor's effect. The price at which the output is sold is positively related to the quantity supplied; changes in price represent a movement along a given supply curve. Changes in the price of labor and non-labor inputs cause the supply curve to shift. Input price changes are inversely related to supply where an increase in input prices causes a decrease in supply, and the supply curve shifts left. Technology that increases input productivity is positively related to supply, and the supply curve shifts right.

In addition to the price at which the product may be sold (the price of inputs and technology), there may be other supply factors that are relevant to a particular industry, such as weather affecting the supply of agricultural products. However, the determinants of supply previously described (price, input prices, and technology), affect all industry supply curves.

Number of Suppliers:

In addition to these factors, the total supply of a product or service depends on the *number of suppliers*. Therefore, (similar to an increase in population on the demand side) an increase in the number of suppliers will cause the supply curve to shift to the right; each supplier's supply curve (their marginal cost curve) is summed horizontally to equal the industry supply curve for that product.

Supply Equation:

The following equation summarizes those factors affecting the supply of a product common to all industry supply curves. The quantity supplied is positively related to the price paid for the product; the supply curve will shift left (decrease) with an increase in the price of inputs; and supply will shift to the right (increase) with technological improvements that increase input productivity. An increase in the number of suppliers will also shift the supply curve to the right.

$$Q_{sa} = f(+\text{Price}_a, -\text{Price}_{inputs}, +\text{Technology}) \times N_s$$

Market Equilibrium

The interaction of supply and demand curves result in market equilibrium; a situation where, at the prevailing price, the quantity demanded equals the quantity supplied. The equilibrium price will not change unless there are changes in demand or supply. Equilibrium is assumed to occur instantaneously, even though in reality neither demanders nor suppliers have perfect information when prices change.

Market forces cause price to move toward equilibrium. Assume that the initial supply and demand curves are D_1 and S_1 in Figure 1-11A. The initial equilibrium price is P_1 and output is Q_1. Further assume that consumer incomes increase, and that the service is a normal good. With an increase in incomes, demand shifts to D_2. If equilibrium occurred immediately, price would rise to P_2 and output would increase to

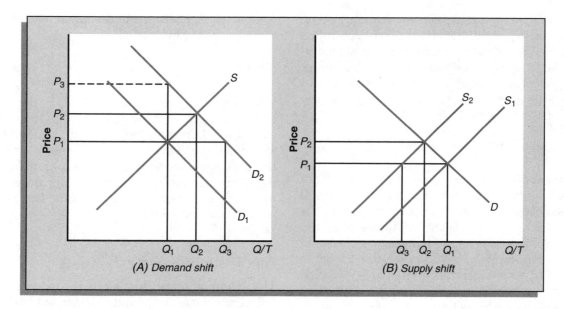

Figure 1-11.   Market equilibrium.

Q_2. (Note, the shift in demand results in a movement along the supply curve.) If consumers do not have perfect information, then with a shift in demand, consumers would demand Q_3 output at the original price P_1. Since the consumers would not be able to buy that amount of output at price P_1, they would start to bid up the price. As the market price increases, suppliers are willing to increase the quantity supplied (a movement along their supply curve) and consumers realizing they have to pay a higher price move up their new demand curve, D_2. When the price reaches P_2, the market is again in equilibrium.

Market Disequilibrium: Regulation

When the government regulates the price of the product and does not permit the price to rise as demand increases, a shortage will develop. At price P_1 and demand curve D_2 in Figure 1-11A, demand exceeds supply and there is a shortage equal to $Q_3 - Q_1$. Shortages are resolved in one of several ways. Suppliers might ration the available supply, OQ_1, according to who is willing to wait to receive the service; criteria other than waiting times might be used, such as favoritism,

race, religion, etc. In health care markets, examples of non-price rationing are admissions to medical schools and access to medical services when Medicare pays physicians' fees that are lower than the market price. The Canadian health care system also uses waiting times as a rationing mechanism. Alternatively, a black market might develop in which consumers are willing to pay suppliers an amount that is greater than the regulated price. Physicians in regulated Eastern European health care systems have used this approach. (The marginal value to consumers of output Q_1 is P_3, which is the height of the demand curve at that point. Consumers would be willing to pay P_3 but are unable to do so, consequently there will be a shift to the right in the demand for substitutes.)

Figure 1-11B illustrates market equilibrium when there is a shift in supply. Supply will shift up or to the left with an increase in the wage rate. (The shift in supply is a movement along the demand curve.) The higher price will result in a decrease in the quantity demanded of the product, from Q_1 to Q_2. If, however, prices are regulated and not permitted to increase as input costs rise, there will be a shortage, $Q_3 - Q_1$, similar to the earlier example. An example of input costs rising faster than regulated prices are rent controls on housing. Consequently, the quality of rent-controlled housing has deteriorated, leading to the abandonment of large numbers of rent-controlled buildings. (One might consider what hospitals' response would be if Medicare payments to hospitals rose less rapidly than hospital input costs.)

Market Equilibrium in Multiple Markets

A shift in supply (or demand) in one market will not only affect market equilibrium in that market, but will also cause changes in equilibrium prices and quantities in markets whose products are substitutes and complements. As shown in Figure 1-12, wage increases in the market for hospital care lead to a shift to the left in the supply of hospital services from S_1 to S_2. Hospital prices increase from P_1 to P_2 and there is a decrease in the quantity demanded of hospital care from Q_1 to Q_2. Outpatient surgery centers are a substitute for certain inpatient surgeries. Thus the higher price for hospital care leads to a shift to the right in the demand for outpatient surgery centers (which is a movement along the supply curve for outpatient surgery). Similarly, higher hospital prices will lead to a shift to the left in the demand for complements to hospital care.

Therefore, a change in any of the factors affecting demand or supply in one market will also lead to new equilibriums in markets that provide substitute and complementary services to the initial market experiencing a change in price.

Elasticity

When there are price movements along the demand and supply curves as well as shifts in demand and supply, it is important for forecasting and public policy initiatives to have an estimate of the magnitude of those changes. Economists use the concept of elasticity, which standardizes the units of measurement, to indicate the quantitative impact of the factors affecting demand and supply.

Price Elasticity of Demand:

The definition of the price elasticity of demand is the "percent change in quantity demanded divided by the percent change in price." Price elasticity of demand is negative because of the inverse relationship between price and quantity demanded.

The formula for price elasticity is:

$$\frac{\Delta Q/Q}{\Delta P/P} = \frac{\%\Delta Q}{\%\Delta P} = -Pe$$

(Change is denoted by the symbol Δ and percent change by $\%\Delta$). For example, if price is decreased by

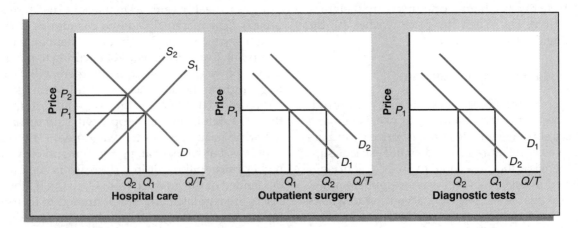

Figure 1-12. Market equilibrium in multiple markets.

10 percent and quantity demanded increases by 20 percent, then the Pe equals –2.

$$\frac{+20\%}{-10\%} = -2$$

Similarly, if the quantity demanded changes by only 5 percent with a 10 percent decrease in price, then Pe equals –0.5.

When the percent change in quantity demanded is greater (less) than the percent change in price, then the demand curve (at that point) is "price elastic" ("price inelastic"). Unit price elasticity is when the percent changes in price and quantity demanded are equal.

The better (or closer) the substitutes to a product, the greater the price elasticity of demand. How the product is defined, either broadly or narrowly, will determine the closeness of substitutes. The aggregate demand for hospital care in an area is typically price inelastic since there are no close substitutes to hospital care. However, the demand for a particular hospital in a market with several hospitals is typically price elastic since the other hospitals are substitutes to that hospital. The same occurs for all anesthesia services (price inelastic) in a market versus a single anesthesiologist (price elastic).

Applications of Price Elasticity:

The concept of price elasticity is useful for understanding pricing strategies, anti-competitive behavior and anti-trust, and public policies, such as national health insurance.

A hospital that raises its price when it has a price elastic demand curve (close substitutes) will suffer a loss in total revenue since the percent change in quantity demanded will exceed the percent increase in price. For example, if a hospital raises its price to a health insurer and nearby hospitals are considered to be very good substitutes, the health insurer is likely to shift more of its enrollees to those hospitals not raising their prices. With good substitutes, the hospital raising its price will have a high price elasticity of demand and suffer a greater-than-proportionate decrease in the quantity demanded of its services; its total revenue will decrease. Conversely, if the hospital is the only one in the area and the closest substitute is 100 miles away, then the hospital is likely to have a price inelastic demand curve; increasing its price will result in an increase in its total revenue.

If all the anesthesiologists in a market formed one group, their demand curve would be price inelastic because there are no close substitutes to all anesthesiologists; increasing their prices would increase their total revenue. Eliminating competition by becoming a single firm monopolizes the market for anesthesia services. This type of behavior is anti-competitive.

If the government subsidized the price of medical services to the uninsured, the cost of the program will be determined by whether the demand for medical services is price elastic or inelastic. Total expenditures (consequently the taxes required to finance the program) will be much higher if demand were price elastic than if it were price inelastic. (Assuming a price elasticity of –4.0 and the price is reduced from $100 to $50, quantity demanded would increase from 1,000 to 3,000 visits; the total cost of the subsidy will be $50 x 3,000 = $150,000. If, instead, the price elasticity were –0.5, a 50 percent reduction in price would lead to an increase in quantity demanded of only 250 visits; the total subsidy cost would then be $50 x 1,250 = $62,500.)

Cross Price Elasticity:

The concept of elasticity is also used to indicate the closeness of substitutes and the effect on complementary services of a change in price. For example, if the price of physician office visits increased, not only would there be a movement down the demand curve for physician visits, but there would be an increase (a shift to the right) in the demand for substitutes, such as chiropractic services. (See Figure 1-5.) Patient perceptions of how good a substitute chiropractic services are to physician services would determine how large a shift occurs in the demand for chiropractic services. The formula for cross price elasticity is the percent change in the demand for a substitute (chiropractic services) divided by the percent change in price of physician services. If the price of physician office visits increased by 10 percent, the demand for chiropractic services might increase by 2 percent, resulting in an estimate of +0.2.

$$\frac{\%\Delta Qchiro}{\%\Delta Pmd} = \frac{+2\%}{+10\%} = +0.2$$

If the price of physician office visits increased by 10 percent, there would also be a decrease in demand (shift to the left) for complementary services such as lab tests. (See Figure 1-6.) Thus if the demand for lab tests decreased by 5 percent, then the cross price elasticity would be –0.5.

$$\frac{\%\Delta Qlab\ tests}{\%\Delta Pmd} = \frac{-5\%}{+10\%} = -0.5$$

Price elasticity and cross price elasticity estimates are important for determining whether adding a new service as part of an insurer's benefits will increase or decrease the total cost of that insurance. For example, if a health insurer includes a lower-priced substitute (such as home health care) to an expensive service (such as hospital care), there will be an increase in the quantity demanded of that new service and a shift to the left in the demand for hospital care. Depending on the price elasticity of demand for the new service and the cross price elasticity of demand for hospital care, together with their respective prices, it can be determined whether the decrease in cost of hospital care more than offsets the increased cost of the new service. (For an illustrative calculation of including lower-priced substitutes to decrease the use of more expensive facilities, see Chapter 6, Appendix 3: "The Effect on the Insurance Premium of Extending Coverage to Include Additional Benefits.")

Income Elasticity of Demand:

Income elasticity of demand is the percent change in demand for a given percent change in income. (See Figure 1-5.) If income elasticity is positive (a normal good) and the income elasticity is 1.5, then a 10 percent increase in income will increase (shift to the right) demand by 15 percent.

$$\frac{\%\Delta QMd\ visits}{\%\Delta Income} = \frac{+15\%}{+10\%} = +1.5$$

Supply Elasticity:

The responsiveness of supply to changes in price of the service is given by the elasticity of supply. As price increases, so does the quantity supplied—a movement along the supply curve. If a 10 percent increase in price leads to a 20 percent increase in the quantity supplied, then the elasticity of supply is +2.0.

$$\frac{\%\Delta QMd\ visits}{\%\Delta PMD\ visits} = \frac{+20\%}{+10\%} = +2.0$$

Competitive Industry Analysis

Competitive markets serve as the basis for evaluating other types of markets, for understanding the reasons for the existence of price differences, and for predicting the consequences of changes in demand and supply. Although the assumptions of competitive markets, such as a homogeneous product, many buyers and sellers, and free entry and exit, are rarely fulfilled in the real world, the competitive model provides a basis for predicting the effect on prices and output if a particular assumption was violated. Further, as long as there are no entry barriers, competitive markets are an important predictive tool.

In the long run, after entry and exit from the industry has occurred and a new equilibrium is established, competitive prices will reflect the costs of production, including explicit as well as implicit costs. When prices equal their production costs, then the output of the industry is considered to be optimal since the marginal benefits to consumers of those last units equal the marginal costs of producing those units. In other, less competitive market structures, price exceeds marginal cost; the greater the price over marginal cost, the lower the output, hence the greater the divergence from a competitive market.

When markets are reasonably competitive, then competitive models provide an explanation for observed differences in prices between regions (and within the same region over time). In the long run, price differences are the result of cost differences; otherwise firms would enter the industry to compete away excess profits (prices greater than costs).

Competitive models make it possible to predict the effects on prices and output (and prices and output of related industries) of changes in any of the factors affecting demand or supply of that product. Also, the consequences of regulated prices or barriers to entry can be predicted and evaluated using competitive market models. Further, mergers (such as between hospitals) can be evaluated for anti-trust purposes based upon whether the merger lessens competition in a market.

(Chapter 7, "The Supply of Medical Care," provides a more complete discussion of competitive markets, as well as the theory of production, different types of cost curves, determinants of market structure, and different types of markets.)

The following example illustrates the use of the competitive model. As shown in Figure 1-13A, the demand and supply curves represent the industry supply and demand curves, together with the resulting equilibrium price and quantity, P_1 and Q_1. The industry supply curve is the sum of each firm's marginal cost curve (above variable cost). Figure 1-13B shows

the typical firm within the industry. The firm has a horizontal demand curve; it can sell all it wants at the prevailing price. The other firms in the industry are perfect substitutes, thus if the firm raised its price above the industry price it will be unable to sell anything. Each firm's output is hypothesized to be so small that no firm is able to affect the prevailing price. The prevailing price is also the firm's marginal revenue curve (MR); the firm can sell each additional unit at the market price. (Each firm has an incentive to minimize its costs, otherwise its average total cost curve (ATC) would exceed the market price and it could not survive.)

Included in the average total cost curve (ATC) is a normal profit (in contrast to an accountant's definition of costs which only considers explicit costs and excludes opportunity costs). When the ATC is tangent to the horizontal demand curve, price equals ATC (as shown in Figure 1-13B) and the firm is earning a normal profit. When firms are earning a normal profit, the industry is in equilibrium; firms have no incentive to enter or exit the industry. The firm's marginal cost curve (MC) intersects the ATC at its minimum point and in equilibrium, the MC of additional units equal the marginal benefit received by consumers from purchasing those additional units (recall from Figure 1-1

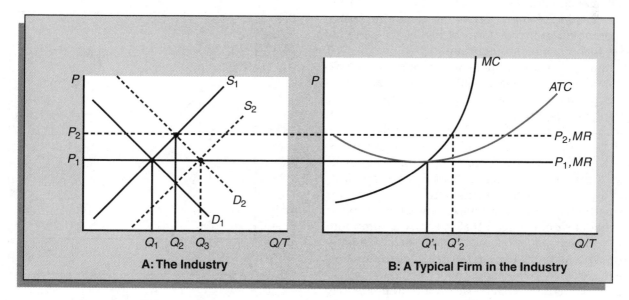

Figure 1-13.   The Competitive Model.

the equilibrium price reflects the value placed on the last units purchased by all consumers since all consumers face the same price in a given market).

Assume, as shown in Figure 1-13 that, as a result of an increase in consumer incomes, the market demand curve shifts to D_2. In the short run (that period of time before entry and exit of firms occur), the market price increases to P_2. As demand increases, each firm increases its output (Figure 1-13B). The higher price provides each firm with an incentive to expand its production to the new profit maximizing point where its MC equals MR (which is also P_2); the firm moves along its MC curve and increases its output to Q_2.' Consequently, the industry output expands to Q_2 (as a result of increases in output from *existing* firms). With the increase in demand, price exceeds each firm's ATC; each firm is making excess profits (the difference between P_2 and its ATC).

The existence of excess profits causes new firms to enter the industry. As they enter, the industry supply curve shifts right to S_2 (since the industry supply curve is the sum of a larger number of the firm's MC curves). As supply shifts right, the equilibrium price declines until once again the market price equals the minimum point on each firm's ATC. A new equilibrium is established with a greater output (Q_3) as a result of an increase in the number of firms. (If the industry has increasing, constant, or decreasing costs, the new equilibrium point may be higher, the same, or lower than the initial equilibrium).

Although the assumptions underlying a competitive model, such as perfect information, a homogeneous product, and many competing firms are important, the ability of firms to enter and exit the industry is often the most violated assumption.

In the previous example, if, with an increase in demand, existing firms received excess profits and over time those excess profits continued, an economist would examine whether firms were entering the industry. If there was no or limited entry, the competitive model would suggest that the entry assumption was violated. An economist would then examine what types of entry barriers, such as government licensing, existed in that industry.

The competitive model is an important predictive tool; it enables one to predict the effect of changes in demand or costs on prices and output, to infer that differences in prices (in the long run) reflect differences in costs (P = ATC), otherwise there would be entry to compete away excess profits, and which assumptions are violated when the long-run predictions of the competitive model do not occur (such as no excess profits).

Monopoly Analysis

When a perfect substitute does not exist for a firm's product or service, then the firm has a downward sloping demand curve; it has some monopoly power. Although there may be a number of firms in an industry, if there are real or perceived differences in their services, then their demand curves will not be perfectly elastic.

With a downward-sloping demand curve, as shown in Figure 1-14, the firm's marginal revenue curve (MR) will be to the left of the demand curve. To sell an additional unit, the firm would have to reduce its price on all its units. Thus the additional revenue (MR) a firm receives from selling the last unit is not the price it receives from that unit but is instead that price less the reduction in price for all the previous units.

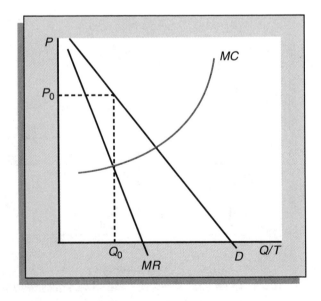

Figure 1-14. A Monopoly Model.

For example, assume a firm's demand curve is such that it sells one unit at $10, two units at $9, three at $8, and four at $7. If the firm moves down its demand curve and lowers its price from $9 to $8, the MR it receives for the third unit is $8 less the $1 reduction in price for each of the two units it could have sold at $9 if it did not reduce its price to sell the additional unit; its MR is therefore $8 – $2 = $6. Similarly, if the price were reduced to $7, MR would be $7 – $3 = $4 (subtracted from the price of $7 would be the reduction in price for three units from $8 to $7). Another way of calculating MR at any price on the demand curve is as follows: at a price of $9, two units are sold for a total revenue of $18; lowering the price to $8 and selling three units yields a total revenue of $24, the difference between $24 less $18 (equals $6) is the marginal revenue of that last unit. MR is the change in total revenue from selling one additional unit.

The firm will maximize its profits by setting price at that point on the demand curve where MC equals MR. As shown in Figure 1-14, if the firm lowered price beyond the point, where MC = MR, then MC would exceed MR and the firm would be less profitable. If the firm set price to the left of MR = MC, then the firm would be foregoing additional profit since MR exceeds MC.

Monopoly analysis emphasizes pricing behavior according to the price elasticity of a firm's demand curve. When very good substitutes are available to a firm's service, then the firm's demand curve will be very price elastic; its MR curve will be closer to its demand curve compared to a firm with a less price elastic demand curve. See Figure 1-15. Assuming both firms have the same MC curve, firms with more price elastic demand curves will charge lower prices. The price-to-cost ratio (the price markup over MC) will be higher for the firm with the less price elastic demand curve.

An important use of the monopoly model is to explain differences in prices. When price differences cannot be explained by differences in costs (the competitive model explanation), then an economist seeks to explain those price differences by determining whether there are differences in price elasticity of demand, which is the monopoly explanation. Firms that have less price elastic demand curves will be able to charge higher prices than firms that have more price elastic demand curves. For example, assume the fee charged by an orthopedic surgeon in one county is higher than the fee charged by an orthopedic surgeon in another county for the same procedure. The competitive model would suggest that the higher fees could result from higher costs, such as higher nurse wages. If, after examination, there were no cost differences between the two surgeons, then the monopoly model would be used to determine whether the surgeons differed in the price elasticity of demand for their services. Perhaps the first surgeon is the only

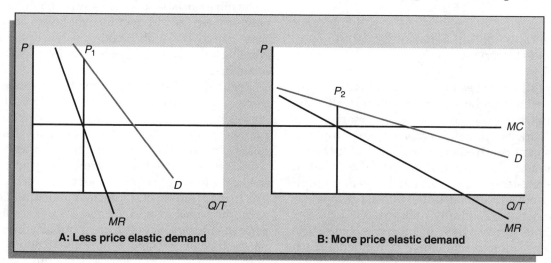

Figure 1-15.   Different firm price elasticities of demand.

surgeon in that community (fewer good substitutes), therefore their demand curve is less price elastic while in the other community ten surgeons must compete among themselves to be included in the insurer's provider network. The surgeon with the less price elastic demand curve is able to charge a higher profit maximizing fee.

Firms that are able to segregate their purchasers according to their price elasticity of demand will be able to further increase their profits. Those with less price elastic demands will be charged higher prices (Figure 1-15A compared to Figure 1-15B). (The ability of a firm to price discriminate requires two conditions. First, the firm must be able to separate purchasers with different demand elasticities and, second, keep the different markets separate preventing those in the low-priced market from re-selling to the higher priced market. The issue of re-importation of prescription drugs, discussed in Chapter 12, discusses this issue.)

Price discrimination has been and continues to be important to suppliers of health care services, such as physicians, hospitals, and pharmaceutical companies. The political position taken by health associations regarding government payment for their member's services is often based on maintaining the ability to price discriminate. (Monopoly pricing is reviewed more completely in Chapter 10, "The Physician Services Market.")

Understanding Political Behavior By Using Supply and Demand Analysis

Political positions of health interest groups can be understood using an economic framework. Health care firms compete in two markets, economic markets and political markets. Although firms, such as hospitals, compete against each other for patients and for insurance contracts, these same firms are allies when it comes to regulations and legislation affecting hospitals. The same is true for all health interest groups and trade associations. Politically, health associations seek legislation to increase their members' incomes. The types of legislation (or regulation) demanded by each health association are: to increase the demand for their members' services, subsidies to lower their

costs, increase the cost of their competitors' services, and to erect entry barriers. (A more complete discussion of these types of legislation, together with examples from different health associations, is in Chapter 18, "Health Policy and The Legislative Marketplace.")

The economic motivation behind health associations' legislative proposals can be illustrated using supply and demand analysis.

Every health association wants the demand for their members' services increased. For example, there would be an increase in the quantity demanded of physician services if a greater number of people had private insurance coverage for physician services. With insurance, the out-of-pocket price of physician services would be reduced, resulting in a *movement down the demand curve* for physician services (see Figure 1-3). The quantity demanded of physician services would increase. (Insurance pays the difference between the out-of-pocket price and the provider's fees, thus in aggregate an increase in insurance represents a shift to the right in the demand curve; see the Appendix to Chapter 5 on "The Effect of Co-insurance on the Demand for Medical Care.") Thus all health associations favor continuation of the tax-exempt status for employer-paid health insurance, which is a subsidy for the purchase of health insurance, and oppose any legislative attempts to reduce or limit the size of this tax exemption. Similarly, all health associations favor mandated employer coverage which would require employers to provide their employees with health insurance, thereby increasing the number of persons with private health insurance.

Regulations that increase the costs, consequently prices, of substitutes are an effective demand-increasing strategy; often these cost-increasing legislative proposals are in the guise of increasing quality of care. For example, physician associations have opposed legislation permitting Medicare and Medicaid to cover substitute services, such as chiropractors. Including chiropractors under public insurance programs would decrease the out-of-pocket price of chiropractic services for publicly insured patients, thereby causing a movement down the demand curve for chiropractic services and a shift to the left in the demand for physician services (see Figure

1-5). Similarly, for-profit health insurers favored legislation that would increase the costs of their non-profit substitute, Blue Cross. Removing Blue Cross' federal tax exemption would cause Blue Cross to increase its price, thereby shifting for-profit insurers' demand curves to the right.

An association would experience an increase in demand for their services (their demand curve would shift to the right) if the price of complementary services were decreased. For example, physicians favor including diagnostic and imaging services as an insured benefit.

Health associations favor several supply-side legislative policies. Legislative subsidies that reduce the cost of inputs to the services provided by an association's members would shift their members' supply curve down (or to the right). For example, medical associations favor legislation that would limit increases in physicians' malpractice premiums. Similarly, hospital associations favor subsidies to increase the supply of registered nurses. The price of hospital care would be reduced, resulting in an increase in the quantity demanded of hospital care.

Perhaps the most important legislative supply-side policy favored by associations is preventing entry by new competitors. Referring to Figure 1-11A, an increase in demand along a given supply curve results in higher prices. Existing suppliers benefit from these higher prices and incomes. Over time, however, other suppliers will be attracted to this market. As new suppliers enter the market, the supply curve will shift to the right (a movement down the new demand curve), and prices will decline. If existing suppliers are able to limit entry of new suppliers, the supply curve will not shift to the right, and prices will remain higher than they would have been with free entry. Maintaining higher prices and incomes is a strong financial incentive for suppliers to seek legislation imposing entry barriers (usually justified on the basis of maintaining quality of care).

Examples of entry barriers in health care are numerous. Medical associations have long favored limits on medical school capacity to restrict the number of new physicians. Hospitals—and even home health agencies—have favored Certificate of Need legislation that makes it difficult for new competitors to enter their market. The American Nurses Association favors immigration limits on foreign-trained RNs, otherwise an increased supply of RNs would result in a decrease in RN wages. All professional health associations favor increased educational requirements before a health professional can practice; these requirements increase the cost of entering the profession, thereby reducing supply and, consequently, increasing prices and incomes for existing practitioners. Process measures for increasing quality are favored by every health profession instead of using outcome or testing procedures, which can be accomplished in a shorter training time. When standards are increased for new entrants, currently practicing professionals are always exempt from the new, more rigorous standards.

REVIEW QUESTIONS

1. Every economy, as well as the medical care sector, must decide the following: what should be produced, how it should be produced, how it should be distributed, and how to allow for growth and innovation. With respect to the medical care sector, how are these choices currently made? How have they changed over time? What are the assumptions and value judgments underlying each of these choices?

2. What are the two basic tools of economics? Give an example of each with respect to health, medical services, and hospitals.

3. Explain how the two tools of economics are inter-related.

4. Prices serve various purposes. For each purpose, give an application of the use of prices, or its lack thereof, in the medical care industry.

5. What is the economic criteria for an optimal rate of output? How well is this criteria met with respect to the medical care sector?

CHAPTER

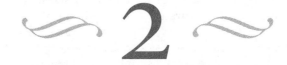

2

The Production of Health: The Impact of Medical Services on Health

KEY TERMS AND CONCEPTS

- 🐚 Health production function
- 🐚 Relationship between inputs and output
- 🐚 Declining marginal benefits of health inputs
- 🐚 Marginal, average, and total output effects
- 🐚 Allocation criterion
- 🐚 Marginal costs/marginal benefits
- 🐚 Marginal contribution of medical care to health
- 🐚 Macro and micro production function studies
- 🐚 Cost-effectiveness analysis

Learning Objectives

Upon completing this chapter, the reader should be able to:

- Understand that medical care is but one input into the production of health.
- Use marginal analysis when comparing alternative inputs for producing health.
- Explain the decision rule for maximizing the level of health for a given budget.
- Interpret the results of empirical studies regarding the marginal contribution of medical services to producing health.
- Apply the concept of a production function for health.

MEDICAL CARE AS AN OUTPUT OF THE MEDICAL SERVICES INDUSTRY AND AS AN INPUT TO HEALTH

There are two ways of analyzing medical care. The first is to regard it as the "output" of the medical care industry, produced by physicians, hospitals, and other providers. When viewing medical care as an output, it is important to determine how efficiently it is produced. The combination of resources that can produce these services at least cost for a given level of quality should be used. Efficiency depends not only on the mix of inputs, but also on the structure of the industry. A structural change might affect the productivity of certain inputs or their cost. For example, reorganizing physicians from solo practice into organized medical groups might make it possible to increase the productivity of physicians, thereby producing more services with the same amount of labor. Changing the requirements for entering a health profession would affect the cost of that manpower input. Industry analyses of the factors affecting the supply of and demand for physician services, hospital care, and the various manpower markets enables us to infer the performance of the medical care industry; that is, the price and output of the industry as it now exists can be compared to the price and quantity (as well as quality) that might exist if the medical care industry underwent a structural change. When medical care is viewed as the output of the medical services industry, our understanding of the structure of that industry (and of its component industries) enables us to evaluate its performance.

The second way of looking at medical care is to view it not as a final output, but rather as one input among many, all of which contribute to an output referred to as "good health." Improvements in health status (e.g., increased life expectancy or decreased morbidity) may be achieved by providing medical services, undertaking medical research, instituting environmental health programs (such as those which control air pollution), and by conducting health education programs aimed at changing the lifestyle of consumers.

The efficiency criterion is also important for determining the amount of resources to be allocated to the medical services sector if the objective is to increase health. It may be less costly to increase health levels by spending less on medical care and more on health education to improve diets and exercise. Viewing health levels as the output enables us to determine how resources should be allocated among different programs in order to improve health. The allocation problem for improving health levels is different from determining the efficient allocation of resources for producing medical care itself.

These two approaches for analyzing medical care should be recognized explicitly since each is useful for different public policies. To determine whether medical care is being produced efficiently, one must examine it as a final output; to determine the most efficient way to allocate resources to increase health, one must view medical services as one of several inputs for achieving that goal.

The second, or input, view is used in the remainder of this chapter. A theoretical approach for determining the allocation of medical versus other resources for improving health will be presented; second, empirical estimates of medical care's marginal contribution to increased health will be reviewed; and third, applications and implications of those findings will be discussed.

The concept of a health production function has become more relevant with the growth of managed care. As managed care organizations (MCOs) seek to reduce the medical costs of their enrolled population, they have an incentive to seek the least expensive way to care for their enrollees. For example, to reduce the use of costly neonatal intensive care units for caring for low birth weight infants, MCOs have an incentive to provide prenatal care so that fewer low birth weight infants are born. Similarly, providing family planning services to their enrollees' teenagers is likely to reduce the number of pregnancies among a risk group likely to give birth to low birth weight infants.

Further, as large employers attempt to reduce rising employee health insurance premiums, they are providing incentives to their employees to change their lifestyles (such as smoking cessation programs) in the hope that these preventive programs will, by improving health status, decrease medical expenditures. Medical services are only one input to produce health outcomes, and not necessarily the least costly way of doing so.

DETERMINING THE ALLOCATION OF RESOURCES TO MEDICAL CARE USING A HEALTH PRODUCTION FUNCTION

To determine the least costly input combination for achieving an increase in health levels, it is necessary to understand the concept of a "health production function." A production function describes *the technical relationship between combinations of inputs and the resulting output*. It is to be distinguished from a production possibility curve, which describes the trade-off between *different outputs from a given set of resources*. Health can be produced using different combinations of inputs. (It is assumed in empirical studies of health production functions that the estimated relationships are technically efficient; that is, the inputs produce the maximum possible output.) The economist (and the policy maker), however, is interested in more than technical efficiency; they want to determine which combination of inputs is *economically efficient*—that is, least costly, for producing the output, health.

Before the least costly combination of inputs for producing a given level of health can be determined, a specific health objective and its production function must be specified. Once specified and estimates have been developed for the marginal effects of each of the inputs on health, comparisons can then be made between increasing expenditures on different inputs. The process of allocating resources to increase health can be improved once information becomes available on each program's (input's) effect on health status and on the relative cost of expanding each program.

Often, the real intent of a program's expenditures may be inferred by determining the effect of its resources.

The first step in using a health production function for making allocation decisions is to state a specific function—that is, to define the output (or objective) to be achieved. Unless the desired output is explicitly defined, it will not be possible to state the alternative approaches for achieving that output, which is the second step. For example, if the objective is increased health of the population, the alternatives will also be fairly general: a better environment, improved nutrition, greater emphasis on preventive care, improved

access to medical services, and better personal health habits. For policymakers and MCO managers, however, these alternative policies are not sufficiently specific to indicate which environmental, preventive, or medical care programs to undertake in order to have an impact on the health levels of specified population groups. Unless the health objective is defined by age and sex groupings (and most likely location), it will not be possible to determine which project—a cancer screening program or a maternal and child health project—will have the greatest impact on health status.

Health professionals and others knowledgeable about health programs are best able to specify which programs are alternatives for increasing the health status of a particular age-sex population group. By using optimization tools, the third step, the economist can determine how to allocate limited health funds among alternative programs to achieve the largest possible increase in health status.

The following discussion illustrates the approach that should be used to allocate expenditures among alternative programs to achieve the maximum possible increase in the health objective.

Assume that the health objective is to decrease the infant mortality rate. On which programs should additional funds be spent? For illustrative purposes, assume that there are only two programs for reducing infant mortality rates: one is to establish additional intensive care units in selected hospitals for infants of high risk; the other is to increase funding for prenatal care to low-income expectant mothers. The following approach demonstrates the type of information and analysis required to determine how best to allocate limited funds between these two programs (1).

The relationship between spending additional funds on each program and their impact on infant mortality rates is assumed to be as shown in Figure 2-1A and Figure 2-1B. The curve in Figure 2-1A represents the relationship between increased program expenditures or size of that program (on the horizontal axis) and the total effect (output) of those program inputs. When a program is relatively small, additional inputs devoted to that program are likely to result in relatively large increases in the program's output (decreased infant mortality rates). As additional resources are allocated to that program, total output will continue to increase, but at a more gradual rate. Finally, increases in output will become negligible even though the program's inputs continue to increase. The relationship between program inputs and program output is *curvilinear* because as additional intensive care units (ICUs) are established, there are an insufficient number of high-risk infants to fill them. (Similar to the Law of Variable Proportions or Diminishing Returns, the number of high-risk infants in a community are assumed to be the fixed factor.) Thus, with additional ICU units either the number of high-risk infants per ICU unit declines or lower-risk infants will be admitted. In either case, improvements in infant mortality rates become smaller.

With prenatal care programs, initial programs are likely to provide care for those patients most likely to benefit from them. As more resources are devoted to prenatal care, it either becomes more costly to find recipients who will benefit most from these programs, or the program begins to include recipients whose need is not as great. In either case, the additional health improvement per unit of input begins to decline as the size of the program is increased.

It is, therefore, inappropriate to assume that there is a constant (i.e., linear) relationship between a program's inputs and its output. Additional resources spent on health programs are unlikely to produce the same increase in output as did previous increases in the program's expenditures.

Since the relationship between total program output and program input is curvilinear (as shown in Figure 2-1A), it must be determined at which point on that total output curve a particular program is operating. If the size of the program is relatively large, as shown by point A_3, then adding resources equivalent to A_3–A_4 will result in an increase in total output of the magnitude Q_3–Q_4. If the program is smaller—for example, at size A_1—the same increase in program resources will result in a larger increase in total program output, from Q_1 to Q_2. (For simplicity, it is assumed that both programs have the same curve as shown in Figure 2-1A. In reality, each program will have a different curve, although each curve will be curvilinear.)

Figure 2-1B is another way of showing the relationship between a program's inputs and output as

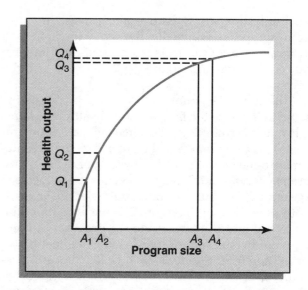

Figure 2-1A. The relationship between total output and program size.

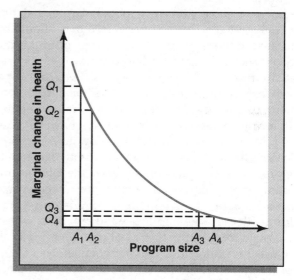

Figure 2-1B. Marginal effects on health with a change in program size.

the size of the program is increased. The curve shown in Figure 2-1B is the *slope* of the total output curve shown in Figure 2-1A, thus it shows the *marginal change in output* as inputs are increased. These marginal relationships, which reflect the change in total output resulting from a unit increase in a program's inputs, eventually decline with increased program size for the same reason that the total output curve shown in Figure 2-1A increases at a decreasing rate.

Still using the simplified example, if it costs the same to increase the inputs in two health programs, but one program (e.g., the intensive care unit program) is at size A_3 while the other (i.e., the prenatal care program) is at size A_1, to which of the two programs should additional resources be allocated? Assuming the output and input relationships for both are as shown in Figure 2-1, the allocation of a given amount of resources to the program at point A_1 would result in the largest change in health output. Therefore, the decision rule for allocating resources between the two programs (when the cost of changing both programs is the same) is to select that program whose change in total output would be greatest.

An alternative (incorrect) decision rule that has been suggested is that additional resources should be allocated to those programs whose total output is the largest. Such a decision rule, however, would not necessarily result in the largest increase in output for a given expenditure. Allocating additional resources among programs does not mean that those receiving little or no increase in their resources have to close down, thereby losing their entire output. Allocation decisions are based not on the total output of competing programs, but rather on *changes* in the total output of competing programs. The total output achievable from all programs will be at its maximum only when additional resources are allocated to programs whose increase in total output (marginal change) is greatest.

Once it is understood that marginal analysis is the tool for maximizing total output, the implications of allocation decisions based on a need criterion become clear. If additional resources were devoted to intensive care units, an increase in infant health levels from Q_3 to Q_4 would result. Advocates of the "need" approach would likely favor still additional resources to expand their program beyond Q_4, since further increases in output are possible. Scarce resources, however, have a "cost." The additional resources required to increase the ICU program beyond size A_4 could be spent on programs whose change in total output would have been greater. The real cost of the resources devoted to increasing the size of the ICU program is the benefit (output) that could have been achieved if those resources had been spent on alternative programs.

Resources will be allocated in an optimal manner when the additional output produced by resources in one program equals the forgone benefits of using those same resources on alternative programs. This approach toward allocating resources differs from that of health professionals, who generally see only the unmet needs that could be eliminated by devoting still more resources to their own programs.

Since empirical studies on the relationship between total program output and program inputs are not always available, it is difficult to develop estimates of the marginal effect of increased program resources. Data are more likely to be available on the program's total output and total expenditures. Analysts are therefore able to calculate the *average* benefits of the program (total output/total inputs). Because of the greater availability of average measures, they are often used as the basis for comparing the benefits of and allocating resources to competing programs. The use of such average measures, however, can result in an incorrect allocation of resources among health programs.

The average and marginal benefits of two programs are shown in Figure 2-2. At point Z (equivalent to a certain program size) the two programs could appear to be identical because their average benefits are equal. However, at point Z the marginal benefits of Program B are greater than those of Program A. Since resource allocations made on the basis of marginal benefits result in the greatest increases in total output, using average benefits (perhaps as a proxy for marginal benefits) can result in error, as this example illustrates.

In Figure 2-1 it was assumed for the sake of simplicity that the cost of increasing the size of the two programs was the same. This is generally not the

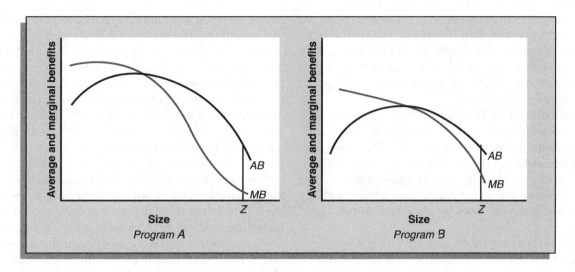

Figure 2-2.   Average and marginal benefits from alternative health programs.

case. When the costs of increasing a program's size are not equal, the comparison cannot simply be made between the changes in the output of the two programs. The relevant criterion for allocating resources to programs having different benefits and costs is to *select those programs whose marginal benefit per dollar spent is greatest*. For example, assume that an increase in Program A would result in a decrease in infant mortality of thirty infants. The marginal costs of achieving that increased benefit is $300,000. An increase in Program B yields, as a marginal benefit, a decrease in infant mortality of twenty infants at a marginal cost of $100,000. Dividing the cost by the benefit (MC/MB) yields a cost of $10,000 per life saved in Program A and $5,000 per life saved in Program B. It is clear from such an analysis that additional dollars should be spent to increase Program B.

If additional resources become available to further decrease infant mortality rates, then spending those additional resources on Program A might yield a lower cost per life saved. The cost of saving a life in Program A was $10,000, while further expanding Program B might result in only five infants saved per additional $100,000, resulting in a cost of $20,000 per

life saved. (The marginal benefit of each program declines as the size of the program is increased.)[1]

Based upon the foregoing discussion, the type of information needed to allocate scarce resources among alternative health programs can be summarized. First, the particular population group whose health is to be affected must be specified. Second, the disease category for that given population group

---

1. For simplicity, this discussion assumes that the input-output relationship for each program is independent of changes in scale in the other programs when, in fact, these inter-relationships exist. For example, an increase in resources for prevention is likely to affect the productivity of programs emphasizing acute care services. These interrelationships between health programs may cause the input-output curve of particular programs to shift either to the left or to the right; that is, the marginal benefits of the affected program may be increased or decreased without changing expenditures for that program. In some cases, acute care programs may become more productive, as for example after an increase in knowledge or technology (perhaps resulting from increased expenditures on research programs). An increase in knowledge or technology may enable a provider to see more patients or to have a more favorable effect on the outcome of the treatment provided. Alternatively, an increase in preventive programs may decrease the need for acute treatment, thereby lowering the number of patients treated in existing acute care programs. The productivity of existing programs would therefore be lessened.

must also be specified in order to be able to form a health production function. Third, the marginal effect on health of each of the health programs should be empirically estimated. And last, resources should be allocated to those programs whose marginal benefit per dollar spent is greatest.

Unfortunately, very little information exists among health professionals or economists about the marginal impacts of alternative health programs. Therefore, allocation decisions are currently being made with little or no information about the marginal effect that specific medical and other health programs have on disease-specific illness rates for particular population groups.[2]

If decision-makers are to allocate scarce resources to produce the maximum possible increase in health levels, they must understand the economic concepts underlying their allocation; they must also generate the information needed to enable appropriate analyses to be undertaken. Program managers often avoid generating useful information because they do not want their program to be compared with competing health programs. They believe that the uncertainty of their program's effects will enhance their bargaining position.

EMPIRICAL STUDIES OF A HEALTH PRODUCTION FUNCTION

The justification often given for government intervention to provide more medical services to the population in general and to underserved population groups in particular is the desire to improve health status. If the objective of government expenditures is to increase health levels, it is important to derive empirical estimates of the net impact that medical care has on health.

Empirical studies attempting to estimate the marginal contribution of medical services to increased health have been conducted at two levels of aggregation. At the more aggregate level, counties, states, and even countries were used as the unit of observation, and each of the factors affecting health, including the measure of health itself, were based on population averages. The less aggregate studies of health production, "microanalyses," used individuals as the unit of measurement. These studies attempted to estimate the independent effect that each of the various factors, including medical services, has had on health levels.

An important distinction between the macro and micro studies of health production lies in the variables used to measure health status. No single measure of health can adequately represent the concept of health status; health has many dimensions. In addition to physical health, there is mental health, and these two measures are interrelated. A person's mental health can affect their physical health and physical health, for example a stroke can affect a person's mental well being. Lack of data often results in defining health by certain of its quantifiable aspects. It is always implicitly assumed that these quantifiable measures are closely related to other aspects of health. On an aggregate level, available health measures are those collected by government agencies as part of vital statistics. These measures, such as births and deaths, also tend to be more accurate than others. Morbidity and disability measures of health are generally unavailable on an aggregate level, and they are not likely to be as reliable as mortality data. When mortality rates are used as the measure of health, the simplest such index is the crude death rate, which is the number of deaths per 1,000 population. More useful health indices are those that are age-sex specific. Such population-specific death rates, unlike the crude death rate, would not be affected by changes in the overall composition of the population (2).

When studies of health production use individuals as the unit of observation, mortality rates cannot be used meaningfully unless a longitudinal analysis is used. Instead, measures of health such as the number

---

2. Given the very limited data on the marginal effects of alternative health programs, only the grossest comparisons can be made. When more appropriate data become available, additional refinements can be incorporated into the comparisons. For example, differences over time in both the stream of benefits and costs of alternative programs should be discounted. However, before too great an emphasis is placed on such refinements, improvements must be made in the basic data used in the analysis. The large variability in estimates of a program's effects as a result of poor data often outweigh the consequences of these refinements.

of work-loss days, the individual's own evaluation of health status, and the number of chronic conditions are used.[3] The unavailability of data needed to measure health status adequately has led to the practice of measuring health by the use of its reciprocal, such as mortality rates. These measures are obviously incomplete in their assessment of what is believed to constitute good health.

Additional outcome measures have been used in health production functions, such as survival probabilities, which is the probability that a person in a particular treatment program will survive over a number of years. A survival curve is estimated that shows the survival experience of the group receiving a particular treatment. Thus, the average survival time of those receiving the particular treatment can be compared to the average survival time of those receiving a different treatment.

An outcome measure that has been used in cost-effectiveness studies is quality-adjusted life years (QALYs), which is the time spent in a health state (for a particular disease with specific symptom severity) multiplied by the utility score of that state. Thus, spending a year in perfect health is one QALY. As used in cost-effectiveness studies, a health program that enables patients to spend five years in a health state with a utility score of 0.8 is equivalent to one that allows patients to spend four years in perfect health (four QALYs) (3). When used in cost-effectiveness studies, minimizing the cost per QALY is a criterion for allocating a health budget.

Regarding the input side of the health production function, factors affecting age-sex specific health status/mortality rates include, in addition to medical services, lifestyle variables (such as income, occupation, cigarette smoking, and alcohol consumption); environmental variables (such as the quality of housing and urbanization which, in addition to capturing the effect of pollution, might also represent such offsetting factors as increased access to medical care); and an efficiency factor, measured by the number of years of formal education which assumes that persons who are more efficient at producing health can do so at a lower cost. The better-educated person may not only be able to recognize symptoms and seek treatment earlier than others, but may also be more likely to use preventive services.

Health production studies generally measure the contribution of medical services to health in several ways: by quantities of the individual components of medical services, such as the number of physicians and hospital beds per thousand population; by the utilization of medical services, such as the number of physician visits or hospital patient days; by aggregate expenditures on medical services, which include changes in prices, utilization of services, and differences in quality of services. When outcomes of specific diseases (such as the mortality rate from heart disease) are analyzed, then different treatment and prevention measures are included.

In an early study of an aggregate health production function, the authors analyzed interstate differences in age-sex adjusted mortality rates for 1960 (4). Their principal purpose was to estimate the elasticity of health with respect to medical services, which is the percentage change in mortality rates that would occur as a result of a 1 percent change in medical services. The authors used multivariate analysis and included measures of medical services as well as a number of environmental factors, believed to affect health.[4] The

---

3. Silver found that work loss was positively correlated with income but negatively correlated with the earnings rate (a weekly wage measure). Although Silver acknowledges that this finding may be caused by a combination of incentives and causations— higher earnings make work loss more expensive, while higher income may carry with it some health risks—he claims that recovery at home is a "superior" good. Therefore, the positive association of income with work loss represents normal economic behavior rather than a health risk. Silver therefore concludes that work loss may be an unreliable measure of true health status because it is too greatly affected by economic behavior. Morris Silver, "An Economic Analysis of Variations in Medical Expenses and Work-Loss Rates," in Klarman, ed., *Empirical Studies in Health Economics,* (Baltimore: Johns Hopkins University Press, 1970), 121–140.

---

4. An important assumption in such cross-sectional studies, of which the authors are well aware, is that the mortality rate is related only to the quantity of medical services used in the particular year for which the study was undertaken. In reality, it is likely that medical services and environmental factors will affect the population's health status over the lifetime of the population, rather than just during the current period.

medical services input was measured in two ways: as expenditures on medical services and as a separate production function for medical services (which included as inputs into that production function the number of physicians per capita, the number of paramedical persons per capita, and so on).

The statistical results of the study, which accounted for more than 50 percent of the interstate differences in mortality rates, indicated that environmental and personal factors had a greater effect on mortality rates than did medical services. The specific findings for some of the more important factors affecting interstate differences in mortality rates were: (a) expenditures on medical care had an elasticity of approximately –0.1, meaning that a 10 percent increase in medical expenditures would lead to a 1 percent decrease in age-sex adjusted mortality rates; (b) the elasticity of mortality rates with respect to education was almost twice as large as for medical services, –0.2; and (c) cigarette consumption per capita resulted in a positive increase in mortality rates (i.e., the elasticity estimate was +0.1, meaning that a 10 percent increase in cigarette consumption per capita results in a 1 percent increase in mortality rates). The total effect of environmental and personal factors (e.g., education and cigarette consumption) outweighed the marginal contribution of medical services to health status.[5]

Hadley estimated the impact (elasticity) of medical care, education, and income on both general and disease-specific mortality rates (5). Separate production functions were estimated for twelve age-race-sex cohorts; eight for adults 45 years of age and over, and four for infants. The data were from 1968 to 1972 and

were based on counties with a minimum population size. Although the results differed somewhat from cohort to cohort, Hadley found that the elasticity of the mortality rate from all causes with respect to medical care expenditures was approximately –0.15; that is, a 10 percent increase in medical care expenditures would lead to a 1.5 percent decrease in the mortality rate. The effect was much greater for white males than for African-American males. Income and education were also found to have a negative effect on mortality rates.

Using individuals as the unit of measurement, Michael Grossman estimated the individual's demand for healthy time. Good health, or healthy time, in Grossman's model is demanded both because it enters the individual's utility function directly for its consumption value, and because as an investment, it increases the time available for other activities. Grossman found that education increases efficiency in producing health, and that the elasticity of health with respect to medical services varies between 0.1 and 0.3. Grossman also found that the income elasticity of health is negative in spite of a positive income elasticity with respect to medical services (6).

A problem with cross-sectional studies that attempt to measure the effect of medical services on health status is that at any point in time, greater use of medical services may represent increased use by those whose health is poor. Further, increased use of medical services may have an effect on health status over a period longer than that in which they are used. To correct for these problems in interpreting the effect of increased use of medical services on health status, Lee Benham and Alexandra Benham studied the change in health status of groups of individuals during the period 1963 to 1970 (7). Using data from two different surveys, the authors classified individuals into twenty-eight education-age categories (consisting of four education and seven age groupings) and attempted to determine the impact that increased use of medical services had on the health status of each education-age category between 1963 and 1970. (Education was considered as a proxy measure for permanent income.)

During the period studied, 1963 to 1970, two large government programs were started (Medicare and

---

5. Believing that many changes have occurred in the health production function since Auster, et al., first conducted their study, Thornton estimated a similar production function using 1990 state-level data. The results were similar, namely lifestyle factors had a greater impact on mortality than medical care expenditures per capita. Specifically, he found that medical care expenditures per capita had a negative but statistically insignificant effect on mortality, while the effects of education (–0.2), income (–0.18), cigarette consumption (0.077), and crime (0.38) were statistically significant. James Thornton, "Estimating A Health Production Function for the U.S.: Some New Evidence," *Applied Economics*, Jan. 10, 2002, 34(11) 59–65.

Medicaid) to finance increased use of medical services for the poor and elderly. The measures of health status used were: health status reported, the number of symptoms reported, and disability days reported during the previous year. The contribution of medical services was measured by the number of non-obstetric physician visits and non-obstetric hospital utilization.

The authors' statistical analysis related the (average) health status of each education-age group in 1970 to the (average) health status of that same group in 1963 and to changes in that group's utilization of medical services between 1963 and 1970. The authors assumed that increased utilization of medical services between 1963 and 1970 was primarily the result of an increase in government financing of medical services to the poor and elderly rather than a response to changes in that group's health status. Increased use of medical services did not result in an improvement in health status during the period studied.

In another example of studies that have used individuals as the unit of analysis, Newhouse and Friedlander estimated the effect of medical resources on physiological measurements of health status (8). Believing it is difficult to isolate the contribution of medical care resources when mortality rates from all causes are aggregated, the authors instead focused on specific medical problems to develop a clearer impact of medical care inputs.

Using data from the U.S. Health Examination Survey which gave screening examinations to a random sample of the U.S. population from 1959 to 1962, the authors estimated the effect that medical resources in an area, together with demographic and socio-economic characteristics of the persons sampled, had on six physiological measures of health, three of which (blood pressure, cholesterol level, and electrocardiogram examination) are associated with heart disease).

The authors conclude that, similar to other studies, the impact of additional medical resources on the physiological measures appears to be minimal. A person's behavioral factors are probably more important than the quantity of medical resources in their area of residence.

Results from the RAND Health Insurance Experiment provide more evidence regarding the effect of an increase in medical care on health outcomes (9). Participants were assigned to alternative health insurance plans for a period of three to five years. The plans varied in the amount that the participant had to pay out of pocket for their medical care. Participants in plans with less cost sharing had higher utilization, with the highest utilization of medical services occurring in the insurance plan where the participant did not have to pay anything out of pocket. In addition to studying the effect that out-of-pocket payment has on medical use and expenditures, the study also analyzed the effect of greater use of medical services on the participants' health status.

The health of adults was compared according to whether they were in a plan in which utilization was greater (i.e., no out-of-pocket payment) or smaller (those plans where the patients paid various amounts for their medical services). General health measures, such as physical and role functioning, mental health, social contacts, and health perceptions were used, as well as measures of physiologic health, such as diastolic blood pressure and functional far vision. Of the numerous health status measures used, the health benefits of increased use of medical services were quite limited; greater use of medical services resulted in lower diastolic blood pressure for those initially diagnosed as hypertensive and improved far vision for those with initial far-vision problems. Further, increased medical use had no statistically significant impact on the general health of subgroups, which differed according to their incomes and their initial health status. The researchers concluded that, for the average participant, greater medical care use had no statistically significant effect on health habits associated with cardiovascular disease and certain kinds of cancer, nor on five general measures of health. However, "people with specific conditions that physicians have been trained to diagnose and treat (myopia, hypertension) benefit from free care."

Perhaps more persuasive than these statistical attempts to determine the contribution of additional medical services to increased health is Victor Fuchs's excellent discussion of causes of death by age (10).

Fuchs examined the contribution of living standards, lifestyle, and medical services to the decline in infant mortality rates since 1900 and to causes of adult deaths. The large decline in infant mortality rates from 1900 to the present has been due largely to rising living standards, the spread of literacy and education, a large decline in the birthrate, possibly chlorination of the water supply and pasteurization of milk, and the introduction of anti-microbial drugs in the 1930s.[6] "It is important to realize that medical care played almost no role in this decline" (11). It was not until the late 1960s that maternal and infant services were extended to underserved families and, subsequently, intensive care units became available for premature infants who were at high risk.

Fuchs also points out that in other developed countries with fewer medical services than the United States and a large proportion of home births delivered by a midwife, infant mortality rates are lower than in the United States. Specific medical service programs targeted to high-risk pregnancies are likely to make a larger contribution to decreases in infant mortality rates than merely making more medical services generally available to the entire population. For example, in countries where medical services are provided free, as in Great Britain, the infant mortality rate is still not as low as that achieved in other developed countries. The lowest infant mortality rates in 2002 (between 3.4 and 3.9 per 1,000 live births) were those of Sweden, Iceland, Finland, Japan, and Norway. When Fuchs examined mortality rates by cause of death for different age groups—adolescents and young adults (15 to 24 years of age), middle-aged persons (35 to 44), and late-middle-aged persons (55 to 64)—he again concluded that *increased use of medical services has a smaller impact on health than the way in which people live*. In the younger age groups, accidents (particularly from use of automobiles), suicides, and homicides are the major causes of death. In middle age, heart disease is the leading cause of death; accidents, suicides, cirrhosis of the liver (caused by alcoholism), and lung cancer are the other major contributors. Among nonwhites, homicides are the second leading cause of death.

Again, the major causes of death may be attributed to behavioral factors. For persons in their late middle age, heart disease is again the leading cause of death; neoplasms are second.[7]

Fuchs compares causes of death by age group in the United States and Sweden, with interesting results. The major factors explaining the lower Swedish mortality rates in each of the various age groups are again determined to be behavioral (Swedes are less violent and have fewer accidents) and attributed to lifestyle (diet, exercise, smoking, and stress). "At present . . . the greatest potential for reducing coronary disease, cancer, and the other major killers still lies in altering personal behavior." Fuchs further notes: "Given our present state of knowledge, even the most lavish use of medical care would not bring the U.S. rate more than a small step closer to the Swedish rate" (12).

The studies employing statistical techniques to estimate a health production function and the discussion by Fuchs on the leading causes of death both suggest that health status is more importantly related to lifestyle factors than to increments of medical services. Although the total benefit of medical services may be large, allocation decisions are rarely all-or-nothing decisions; instead, they are incremental. If policymakers have as their objective an increase in health status, increased provision of medical services is likely to have a relatively smaller impact on health than will alternative policies. Further, these additional expenditures on medical services are not without a cost; greater increases in health status could be achieved if these same funds were spent on other programs.

EXAMINING THE DECLINE IN MORTALITY FOR TWO CAUSES OF DEATH

The decline in mortality over the last 30 years is generally attributed to two components: declines in deaths from heart disease and in infant mortality rates.

---

6. For example, the U.S. infant mortality rate declined from 162 per 1,000 live births in 1900 to 26 per 1,000 in 1960. By 2001, the mortality rate had declined to 6.8 per 1,000 live births.

7. The data presented by Fuchs represents average relationships and does not indicate the relative marginal costs of achieving changes in health status. For policy purposes, it would be desirable to know the marginal effects of each of the variables on health status.

Cardiovascular Disease

The leading cause of death in the United States is cardiovascular disease. Between 1970 and 2002, the mortality rate from "Diseases of the Heart" declined more rapidly than any other cause of death, from 362 per 100,000 to 241 per 100,000. See Table 2-1. An important question concerns the reasons for this decline.

Several studies have analyzed the main contributing factors to the decline in heart disease and in its mortality. Goldman and Cook attempted to quantify the relative contribution of lifestyle changes and medical interventions in explaining the 21 percent decline in ischemic heart disease mortality that occurred between 1968 and 1976. They concluded that lifestyle changes accounted for 54 percent of the decline (reduced serum cholesterol levels contributed 30 percent, and reduced cigarette smoking 24 percent). Over the 9-year period studied, medical interventions accounted for less than 40 percent of the decline. The authors note that while the medical interventions (such as coronary care units) are expensive innovations, lifestyle changes, aside from government-financed publicity, are relatively costless and contributed more to the decline in ischemic heart disease mortality. Decreases in heart disease, however, are not uniform across the population. White males have done better than African-Americans, salaried workers better than hourly workers, and those with more education have

benefited more, since they have reduced by greater percentages their smoking and consumption of highly saturated fats (13).

The decline in the age-adjusted mortality rate from coronary heart disease (CHD) in the Twin Cities area of Minnesota has been similar to national trends. Starting in the late 1960s, the mortality rate declined by about 3.5 percent per year, and by the late 1980s it accelerated, declining about 25 percent between 1985 and 1990. McGovern, et al., examined the decline in mortality rates for the period 1985 to 1990 in the Twin Cities area for both out-of-hospital deaths from CHD, which reflect primary prevention measures, and in-hospital mortality, which reflect advances in acute medical treatment (14).

The authors found that there was a decline in the incidence of acute myocardial infarction in the population, which is consistent with improvements in the risk profile associated with CHD, such as declines in cigarette smoking and cholesterol levels. Second, patients hospitalized for acute myocardial infarction had a higher survival rate. The improved survival rate was likely attributable to greater use of diagnostic and therapeutic procedures, as well as secondary preventive measures after hospital discharge such as thrombolytic medications, changes in lifestyle, and aspirin. Between 1985 and 1990, in-hospital CHD mortality declined more rapidly than previously (1978 to 1985) and was greater than the decline in out-

Table 2-1.   Major Causes of Death, United States, 1970–2002

	Death Rates (per 100,000 population)			
	1970	1980	1990	2002
All causes	945.3	878.3	863.8	848.9
Diseases of heart	362.0	336.0	289.5	241.3
Cancer	162.8	183.9	203.2	193.8
Strokes (cerebrovascular diseases)	101.9	75.1	57.9	56.5
Chronic lower respiratory diseases	15.2	24.7	34.9	43.5
Accidents	56.4	46.7	37.0	35.5
Diabetes mellitus	18.9	15.4	19.2	25.4
Pulmonary diseases (influenza and pneumonia)	30.9	24.1	32.0	22.9

Sources: National Center for Health Statistics, *Deaths: Preliminary Data for 2002,* http://www.cdc.gov/nchs/data/nvsr/nvsr52/nvsr52_13.pdf (accessed on February 20, 2004); *Statistical Abstract of the United States: 1995,* table 125, http://www.census.gov/prod/1/gen/95statab/vitlstat.pdf (accessed on October 14, 2003).

of-hospital CHD mortality for men, but similar for women.

Cutler and Kadiyala also examined the large decline over time in deaths from cardiovascular disease (15). In the past 30 years, important advances have occurred in the treatment of heart disease. Cardiac catheterization was developed in the late 1950s, coronary bypass surgery was introduced in 1968, cardiac intensive care units with their specialized monitoring equipment started in the 1970s, and angioplasty was developed in 1978. In addition, new drugs were used in treatment to dissolve blood clots, such as beta-blockers introduced in the 1960s and thrombolytics in the late 1980s. The adoption of these treatment techniques and prescribing of new drugs among the medical profession occurred slowly over time. For example, the use of beta-blockers was 21 percent in the early 1970s and increased to 50 percent by the mid-1990s.

The authors estimate that the development of new treatment techniques and their increased use over time decreased cardiovascular disease deaths by about one-third.

The second major contributor to the decrease in heart disease deaths has been prevention, which may occur in two ways. First are behavioral changes in a person's lifestyle, such as quitting smoking, overweight people reducing their weight, and high-risk people limiting their intake of foods high in fat and cholesterol. Second are the use of innovative drugs to reduce high cholesterol and hypertension.

Preventive measures, both behavioral measures and drugs to reduce the risk from heart disease, occurred over time and were not uniform among all population groups. Preventive drugs were not consistently provided to all persons of similar risk. Nor were persons equally informed regarding behavioral changes to reduce their risk level. Nevertheless, diets, smoking habits, and the medical profession's prescribing of drugs changed over time. The authors attribute the remaining two-thirds of the reduction in deaths from heart disease to improved control of hypertension, high cholesterol, and smoking cessation.

The above studies, as well as many others that have examined the reduction in heart disease deaths over time, reach similar conclusions, the majority of the reduction in deaths has been the result of a reduction in risk factors through prevention, including new drugs to control high cholesterol and hypertension.

Neonatal Infant Mortality

During the period 1970 to 1988, very large declines occurred in infant mortality rates. The most important portion of the decline in infant mortality (77 percent) was the decline in the neonatal rate (i.e., infant deaths within the first 27 days of life per 1,000 live births), which is twice as large as and fell more rapidly than the postneonatal mortality rate (i.e., infant deaths occurring between 28 and 364 days). Attempts to explain the decline in infant mortality must therefore understand the reasons for the decline in the neonatal rate. As shown in Figure 2-3, neonatal infant mortality rates declined slowly from 1950 to 1970 (19.4 to 13.8 per 1,000 live births) and then declined rapidly from 1970 to 1990 (13.8 to 4.8 per 1,000 live births); the decline was greater for whites than for African-American infants, which declined from 22.8 in 1970 to 11.6 per 1,000 live births in 1990. It has been suggested that this more rapid decline in neonatal infant mortality rates resulted, for the most part, from factors other than increased medical care expenditures, particularly liberalized abortion laws.

Grossman and others conducted several studies to determine the causes of the decline in neonatal mortality rates. In one study, using county-level aggregate data, Corman and Grossman examined the determinants of neonatal mortality rates for a three-year period centered on 1977 (16). Specifically, the authors examined the impact on neonatal mortality of the availability of neonatal intensive care units, the legalization of abortion, subsidized family planning services for low-income women, community health centers, maternal and infant nutrition programs, and Medicaid. Separate analyses were conducted for white and African-American women to determine the effects of each of the above on the neonatal mortality rate. The various factors affecting neonatal mortality differed in their effects on white and African-American women.

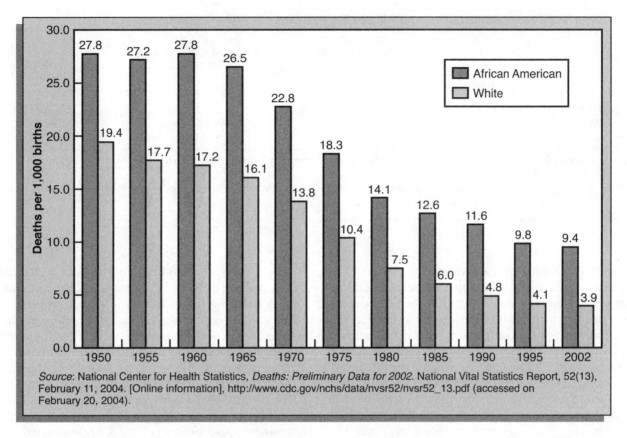

Figure 2-3.   Neonatal Mortality Rates, by Race, 1950–2002

The authors then used their estimates of a health production function to determine which programs were more cost-effective in reducing the neonatal mortality rate (17). For illustrative purposes, three of the programs analyzed are presented in Table 2-2, teenage family planning programs, neonatal intensive care units (NICUs), and prenatal care. Based on an empirical analysis, an estimate was derived of the number of lives saved per 1,000 additional participants for each of the above programs, which were respectively, 0.6, 2.8, and 4.5. The respective costs of these programs per 1,000 additional participants (in 1984 dollars) were $122,000, $13,616,000, and $176,000. Dividing the cost by the estimate of lives saved (e.g., $176,000/4.5) results in the following cost per life saved from each of these programs: $203,000

for teenage family planning, $4,778,000 for intensive care, and $39,000 for prenatal care. According to these results, prenatal care is the most cost-effective input for reducing neonatal mortality.

Policies such as teen family planning and prenatal care reduce the infant mortality rate by decreasing the number of births that are likely to be high risk (low birth weight), which is a less expensive approach than expanding the number of ICUs that increase the survival of the high-risk infant.

The authors also used the results of their analysis to explain the decline in infant mortality between the years 1964 and 1977. During that time, the white neonatal mortality rate declined from 16.2 to 8.7 per 1,000 live births, whereas the African-American neonatal rate declined from 27.6 to 16.1. The authors

Table 2-2.   Cost per Life Saved Among Three Programs to Reduce Neonatal Mortality

	Number of Lives Saved per 1,000 Additional Participants	Cost of Each Program per 1,000 Additional Participants	Cost per Life Saved
Teenage Family Planning*(a)*	0.6	$122,000	$203,000
Neonatal ICUs*(b)*	2.8	$13,616,000	$4,778,000
Prenatal Care*(c)*	4.5	$176,000	$39,000

Source: Theodore Joyce, Hope Corman, and Michael Grossman, "A Cost-Effectiveness Analysis of Strategies to Reduce Infant Mortality," *Medical Care,* 26 (4), April 1988, pp. 348–360, Table 3.

(a) Percentage of women, aged 15–19 with family income less than 200% of the poverty level in 1975 who used organized family planning services in 1975.

(b) Total hospital days in neonatal intensive care units in 1979 per average number of low birthweight births.

(c) Percentage of live births for which prenatal care began in the first three months of pregnancy.

determined that for African-Americans the most important factor causing a reduction in the neonatal rate was the availability of abortion; its effect, 1.2 deaths per 1,000 live births, was almost twice as large as the next most important contributor. Next in importance was availability of neonatal intensive care units and the increase in schooling, each reducing the rate by 0.7 deaths per 1,000 live births. Medicaid expenditures were fourth at 0.5 deaths per 1,000 live births. For whites, schooling was most important, followed by subsidized nutrition programs, Medicaid, and the availability of neonatal intensive care units; the availability of abortion was fifth. The abortion effect on African-Americans was four times greater than on whites, and the effect of neonatal intensive care units was twice as large.

The authors did not undertake a cost/benefit analysis of averting deaths because of the problems involved in valuing a human life. However, they were able to estimate the benefit/cost ratio of decreasing low birth weight infants. Considering just the hospitalization costs of caring for a low birth weight infant (which would be reduced) and dividing that cost by the program costs of decreasing low birth weight infants, the authors concluded that programs that decrease low birth weight, such as prenatal care, have very favorable benefit/cost ratios. The authors conclude that to continue to achieve declines in the neonatal mortality rate, attention must be focused on reducing the number of low birth weight infants.

The above studies indicate that decreasing the risk of having low birth weight infants is very cost effective in reducing infant mortality. Although prenatal care is more cost effective than neonatal care, advances in medical technology to care for low birth weight and premature infants, such as neonatal intensive care units, has also contributed to reductions in neonatal mortality. Cutler and Meara calculated the costs of caring for low birth weight infants (in-hospital medical services) and the resultant benefits (improved survival and quality of life converted into dollars using an average value of life per year) over the period 1960 to 1990. Although the rate of return is lower than for prenatal care interventions, the authors conclude that the benefits of technology for caring for low birth weight infants has been worth the additional cost (18).

THE RELATIONSHIP OF MEDICAL CARE TO HEALTH OVER TIME

The above studies have shown that lifestyle factors and secondary prevention have been major determinants of improved health. Similarly, health production function studies find that the marginal contribution of medical care to improved health is relatively small. Improvements in health status can be achieved less costly through increased spending on lifestyle factors. Over time, however, there have been major technological advances in medical care, such as new drugs to lower cholesterol and hypertension, diagnostic imaging, less invasive surgery, transplants, and treatment for previously untreatable diseases. Few would deny that these technological advances have reduced mortality rates and increased life expectancy.

Cutler and Richardson reconcile these seemingly conflicting findings of medical care's relatively low marginal contribution to health and technological advances that have clearly increased life expectancy; they separate medical care's effect at a point in time versus its technological contribution over time (20). The authors illustrate the relationship between the total contribution of medical care to health and greater quantities of medical care using Figure 2-4. Comprehensive health insurance combined with fee-for-service physician payment reduces both the patient's and physician's incentive to be concerned with the cost of care, resulting in the medical care system moving to Point A in Figure 2-4, where the marginal contribution of medical care to health is very small. Additional medical care expenditures increase health, but at a decreasing rate.

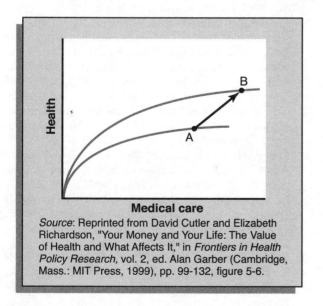

Medical care

Source: Reprinted from David Cutler and Elizabeth Richardson, "Your Money and Your Life: The Value of Health and What Affects It," in *Frontiers in Health Policy Research*, vol. 2, ed. Alan Garber (Cambridge, Mass.: MIT Press, 1999), pp. 99–132, figure 5-6.

Figure 2-4. The relation between medical care and health.

Over time, however, medical advances shift the production function for health upward. The same expenditure on medical care can produce better health outcomes. However, the number of patients being treated as a consequence of the new technology being available increases. The level of health has increased as have the number of patients treated, but the marginal contribution of medical care is still low, Point B. Too many patients whose need for treatment is doubtful are treated with the new technology and/or excess capacity occurs as too much of the new technology is made available.

Thus, although the public believes the medical care they receive today is much more valuable than treatments received 30 years ago, the medical care system remains inefficient; the marginal benefit of additional medical care expenditures is low.

SUMMARY

The explanation of the decline in mortality rates from cardiovascular disease over time and the cost-effectiveness analysis of decreasing neonatal infant mortality illustrate the types of analyses that can be undertaken based on knowledge of a health production function. To be useful for decision-makers, specific information on health production functions by disease categories and for different population groups is required. Before more precise estimates of health production functions can be derived, however, it is necessary for policy analysts to understand the types of data that need to be collected and how they will be useful for decision making.

A question that arises from the finding that the marginal contribution of additional medical expenditures on health is relatively small: Why have government medical expenditures increased so rapidly, particularly on some population groups (the aged) rather than others (the poor and young)? One possible explanation is that the government's objective has never really been to increase the health of the nation by allocating resources among alternative inputs. Instead, government medical expenditures are a means of redistributing wealth among different population groups. Further, that the criteria for such redistribution has not been medical or economic need, but has instead been to provide net benefits to those groups who are more politically powerful (19).

The remainder of this book examines the efficiency with which medical care is produced by the medical care industry and its distribution. Even though the marginal impact of medical services on health may be relatively small, the increase in private and governmental financing of medical services has been large. The contribution of medical expenditures to improved health will be reduced even further if inefficiency increases prices of medical services, thereby absorbing most of the increase in expenditures. The efficiency of medical services and the equity of their distribution are addressed in the remaining chapters.

REVIEW QUESTIONS

1. Explain why one would or would not use the total contribution of health services as compared to the marginal contribution of health services for decision making if the objective were to determine how to allocate a limited budget for increasing health levels.

2. Assume you are a consultant to an HMO that is being evaluated on how well it improves the health status of its enrolled population. What information would you need, and how would you use it to advise the HMO on how to allocate its resources?

3. What is a production function for health? How would you use it to explain changes in health status over time?

4. You have been hired by Medicaid to advise the Director on how to reduce infant mortality among women eligible for Medicaid. What are the various alternative programs you would suggest, and how would you allocate funds between them to achieve the greatest reduction in infant mortality for a given budget?

5. How can employers use the concept of a health production function for decreasing their employees' medical expenditures?

6. Describe a health production function for decreasing deaths of young adults.

REFERENCES

1. Peter Muennig, eds., *Designing and Conducting Cost-Effectiveness Analyses in Medicine and Health Care*, (San Francisco: Jossey-Bass, 2002).

2. For a more complete review of health measures, their definitions, and attendant difficulties, see "Advances in Health Status Assessment: Conference Proceedings," *Medical Care*, 27(3) Supplement, March 1989.

3. Alan M. Garber, "Advances in CE Analysis," in *Handbook of Health Economics*, vol. 1A, eds. A. J. Culyer and J. P. Newhouse, (New York: North-Holland Press, 2000), 181–222.

4. Richard Auster, Irving Leveson, and Deborah Sarachek, "The Production of Health, an Exploratory Study," *Journal of Human Resources*, IV, Fall 1969: 411–436.

5. Jack Hadley, *More Medical Care, Better Health?* (Washington, D.C.: The Urban Institute, 1982).

6. Michael Grossman, "On the Concept of Health Capital and the Demand for Health," *Journal of Political Economy*, 80(2) March–April 1972, 223–55.

7. Lee Benham and Alexandra Benham, "The Impact of Incremental Medical Services on Health Status, 1963 to 1970," in R. Andersen, J. Kravitz, and O. Anderson, eds., *Equity in Health Services: Empirical Analysis of Social Policy*, (Cambridge, Mass.: Ballinger, 1975).

8. Joseph P. Newhouse and Lindy J. Friedlander, "The Relationship Between Medical Resources and Measures of Health: Some Additional Evidence," *Journal of Human Resources*, 15(2), Spring 1980, 200–218.

9. Robert H. Brook et al., "Does Free Care Improve Adults' Health? Results from a Randomized Controlled Trial," *New England Journal of Medicine*, 309(23), December 1983: 1426–1434 and Emmett B. Keeler, et.al., "Effects of Cost Sharing on Physiological Health, Health Practices, and Worry," *Health Services Research*, 22(3) August 1987: 297–306.

10. Victor R. Fuchs, *Who Shall Live?* (New York: Basic Books, 1974), 30–55.

11. Ibid., p. 32.

12. Ibid., p. 46.

13. Lee Goldman and Francis Cook, "The Decline in Ischemic Heart Disease Mortality Rates: An Analysis of the Comparative Effects of Medical Interventions and

Changes in Lifestyle," *Annals of Internal Medicine,* 101(6), December 1984: 825–836.

14. Paul G. McGovern, et.al., "Recent Trends In Acute Coronary Heart Disease," *The New England Journal of Medicine,* April 4, 1996, 334(14)884–890.

15. David M. Cutler and Srikanth Kadiyala, "The Return to Biomedical Research: Treatment and Behavioral Effects," in *Measuring the Gains from Medical Research: An Economic Approach,* edited by Kevin M. Murphy and Robert H. Topel, (The University of Chicago Press: Chicago, Ill.) 2003, 110–162.

16. Hope Corman and Michael Grossman, "Determinants of Neonatal Mortality Rates in the U.S.: A Reduced Form Model," *Journal of Health Economics,* 4(3), September 1985: 213–236. For additional discussion of the reasons for the decline in infant mortality, see Jeffrey E. Harris, "Prenatal Medical Care and Infant Mortality," and Mark R. Rosenzweig and T. Paul Schultz, "The Behavior of Mothers as Inputs to Child Health: The Determinants of Birth Weight, Gestation and Rate of Fetal Growth," in Victor R. Fuchs, ed., *Economic Aspects of Health* (Chicago: University of Chicago Press, 1982).

17. Theodore Joyce, Hope Corman, and Michael Grossman, "A Cost-Effectiveness Analysis of Strategies to Reduce Infant Mortality," *Medical Care,* April 1988, 26(4): 348–360.

18. David M. Cutler and Ellen Meara, "The Technology of Birth: Is It Worth It?," in *Frontiers in Health Policy Research,* vol. 3, ed. Alan Garber (Cambridge, Mass: MIT Press, 2000), 33–67.

19. David Cutler and Elizabeth Richardson, "Your Money and Your Life: The Value of Health and What Affects It," in *Frontiers in Health Policy Research,* vol.2, ed. Alan Garber (Cambridge, Mass: MIT Press, 1999), 99–132.

20. For a more complete discussion of the redistributive aspects of government health policy see, Paul J. Feldstein, *The Politics of Health Legislation: An Economic Perspective,* (Chicago: Health Administration Press), 2nd ed. revised, 2001.

CHAPTER
3

An Overview of the Medical Care Sector

KEY TERMS AND CONCEPTS

- Health education markets
- Health manpower markets
- Institutional markets
- Demand subsidy effects
- Determinants of demand in each market
- Determinants of supply in each market
- Interrelationship of each type of market
- Outcomes of each market
- Supply subsidy effects

Learning Objectives

Upon completing this chapter, the reader should be able to:

- Understand how the different medical markets are interrelated.
- Trace through the effect of a change in demand on each of the medical markets.
- Trace through a change in supply on each of the medical markets.
- Illustrate how a change in supply or demand will affect the distribution of medical services.

DESCRIPTION OF THE MEDICAL CARE MARKETS

Expenditures on the Major Components of Medical Care

As an introduction to the medical care sector, let us examine the magnitude and changing composition of expenditures on the major components of medical care. As shown in Table 3-1, the two largest components of medical care, hospital and physician services, accounted for 36.3 and 25.3 percent of the $1.340 trillion of total personal medical expenditures in calendar year 2002. Hospital expenditures, $486 billion, are the largest component of medical expenditures and are about 50 percent greater than physician services, $339 billion. (Personal health care expenditures were approximately $213 billion less than total health care expenditures, which were $1.553 trillion—14.8 percent of GNP. The difference between the two, in billions, were expenses for prepayment and administration, $105, government public health activities, $51, and research and construction of medical facilities, $57).

The relative proportions of expenditures on hospital, physician, and other medical services have been changing over time. In 1965, hospital expenditures represented 40 percent of total personal medical expenditures, while physician services were 23 percent. By 1980, the hospital portion exceeded 47 percent and then declined to 36 percent by 2002. After the enactment of Medicare and Medicaid and the growth in private health insurance, out-of-pocket payments for hospital care dropped sharply, on average to 3 percent of the bill in 2002. And, as shown in Table 3-2, the remainder was paid primarily by government (59 percent) and private insurance (34 percent). Direct patient payments were smaller for hospital care than for any other medical service. On average, patients are responsible for 10 percent of expenditures for physician services and 30 percent of drug expenditures.

As the portion of the hospital bill paid for directly by the patient declined, so did the patient's and physician's incentive to question the prices charged by hospitals. The patient's use of the hospital is less responsive to the price charged than is the use of most other medical services. The declining portion of the hospital bill for which the patient is responsible, together with the small effect that price has on hospital use, removed patient and physician incentives to be concerned with how rapidly hospital prices increased or with the relative costs of hospitals. Under these circumstances, a more rapid increase in hospital expen-

Table 3-1. Total Private and Public Expenditures for Personal Health Care Services by Type of Expenditure and Source of Funds, Calendar Years 1965, 1980, and 2002

	1965			1980			2002		
	Total (Billions)	Percent Distribution(a)	Private Percentage	Total (Billions)	Percent Distribution	Private Percentage	Total (Billions)	Percent Distribution(a)	Private Percentage
Hospital care	$13.8	39.8%	63.0%	$101.5	47.3%	45.7%	$486.5	36.3%	41.1%
Physician and clinical services	8.3	23.9	94.0	47.1	21.9	69.4	339.5	25.3	66.2
Dental services	2.8	8.1	100.0	13.3	6.2	95.5	70.3	5.2	93.6
Prescription drugs	3.7	10.7	97.3	12.0	5.6	86.7	162.4	12.1	77.7
Other(b)	6.1	17.6	78.7	40.7	19.0	89.2	281.5	21.0	46.6
Total	34.7	100.1	79.8	214.6	100.0	59.7	1,340.2	100.0	55.8

Source: Centers for Medicare and Medicaid Services, Office of the Actuary, National Health Statistics Group, Internet site http://www.cms.gov/statistics/nhe/ (accessed on January 8, 2004).

(a) The percentages do not add up to 100 because of rounding.

(b) "Other" includes: other professional services, home health care, other medical products, nursing home care, and other personal health care.

Table 3-2. Amount and Percent Distribution of Personal Health Care Expenditures, by Source of Funds and Type of Expenditure, 2002

Type of Expenditure	Total	Out of Pocket	Third-Party Payments			Government Expenditures				
			Total	Private Health Insurance	Other Private Funds(a)	Total	Federal			State(c)
							Medicare	Medicaid	Other(b)	
Amount (Billions)										
Total	1,340.2	212.5	1,127.7	479.3	56.2	592.2	259.1	137.0	54.3	141.7
Hospital care	486.5	14.7	471.8	165.0	20.3	286.4	149.2	49.8	30.9	56.5
Physician services	339.5	34.3	305.3	166.9	23.6	114.8	68.8	14.5	11.5	20.1
Dental services	70.3	30.9	39.4	34.8	0.1	4.5	0.1	2.1	0.5	1.8
Prescription drugs	162.4	48.6	113.8	77.6	—	36.2	2.6	16.5	1.8	15.4
Nursing home care	103.2	25.9	77.3	7.7	3.5	66.1	12.9	30.5	2.0	20.5
All other services(d)	178.3	58.1	120.1	27.3	8.7	84.2	25.5	23.6	7.6	27.4
Percent Distribution										
Total	100.0	15.9	84.1	35.8	4.2	44.2	19.3	10.2	4.1	10.6
Hospital care	100.0	3.0	97.0	33.9	4.2	58.9	30.7	10.2	6.4	11.6
Physician services	100.0	10.1	89.9	49.2	7.0	33.8	20.3	4.3	3.4	5.9
Dental services	100.0	44.0	56.0	49.5	0.1	6.4	—	3.0	0.7	2.6
Prescription drugs	100.0	29.9	70.1	47.8	—	22.3	—	10.2	1.1	9.5
Nursing home care	100.0	25.1	74.9	7.5	3.4	64.1	12.5	29.6	1.9	19.9
All other services(d)	100.0	32.6	67.4	15.3	4.9	47.2	14.3	13.2	4.3	15.4

Source: Centers for Medicare and Medicaid Services, Office of the Actuary, National Health Statistics Group, Internet site http://www.cms.gov/statistics/nhe (accessed on January 8, 2004).

Note: Numbers and percent may not add to totals because of rounding.

(a) "Other Private Funds" includes: Philanthropy, interest and dividend income, income from rental of office space, and other nonpatient income.

(b) Includes expenditures for maternal and child health programs, vocational rehabilitation programs, Public Health Service activities, Indian Health Service programs, workers' compensation programs, Veterans' Administration Services, Alcohol, Drug Abuse and Mental Health Administration programs, and Defense Department programs.

(c) Includes state and local Medicaid payments.

(d) Includes other professional services, other non-durable medical products, durable medical equipment, other personal care, and home health care.

ditures would be expected. Conversely, a slower rate of increase in expenditures would be expected for those medical services for which patients paid a larger fraction of the bill and whose use is more affected by higher prices. These factors are important for understanding the changing composition of medical expenditures.

Before managed care, hospital use and expenditures increased more rapidly than the other components of medical services, where consumers had to pay a larger portion of the bill. Since the mid-1980s, the introduction of Medicare limits on hospital payments, the growth of managed care and utilization management, together with growing competitive pressures, resulted in hospital expenditures increasing less rapidly than other components of medical care. Hospitals' share of personal medical expenditures consequently decreased.

In 1965, before the introduction of Medicare and Medicaid, government expenditures represented 21 percent of personal medical expenditures. By 2002, the government share of personal medical expenditures climbed to 44 percent, with the greatest increases occurring in those sectors covered by Medicare and Medicaid, namely hospital and physician services.

Over time, as shown in Table 3-3, direct patient payments for all medical services declined from 52 percent in 1965 to 16 percent in 2002. As government and private insurance paid more of the bill for medical services, the importance of price on the patients' use of services and choice of a provider from whom to purchase that service diminished. The lessening of patients' price incentives enabled providers to more easily pass on higher prices and had important implications for the performance of the medical care market.

The government's financing of medical services has not been uniform for each of the components of medical care; it has been most concerned with cost containment in those areas to which it is financially committed. Higher prices for hospital services were of greater financial consequence, and therefore, of greater concern to the government than similar price increases for dental services, whose financing is predominantly private.

Table 3-3. Percentage Distribution of Personal Health Expenditures by Source in the United States, 1965, 1975, 1985, and 2002

Source	1965	1975	1985	2002
	Amount (Billions)			
	$34.7	113.0	372.4	1,340.2
	Percent Distribution(a)			
Private(b)	79.6%	60.2	60.6	55.8
Out of pocket	52.3	33.1	25.7	15.9
Insurance benefits	25.1	24.4	29.9	35.8
All other	2.2	2.7	5.1	4.1
Public	20.4	39.8	39.4	44.2
Federal	8.1	27.1	29.4	33.6
State and Local	12.3	12.7	10.0	10.6

Source: Centers for Medicare and Medicaid Services, Office of the Actuary, National Health Statistics Group, Internet site http://www.cms.gov/statistics/nhe/ (accessed January 8, 2004).

(a) Percent may not add to totals because of rounding.

(b) After 1980 the category "All other" was expanded to include a greater percentage of what was formerly "Direct payments." "All other" now includes: philanthropy, interest and dividend income, income from rental of office space, etc., all considered nonpatient revenue.

The sharp expenditure increases and changes in the composition of medical care expenditures indicate a need for a set of economic tools to predict equilibrium situations. To understand why expenditures have increased so rapidly, it is necessary to determine why prices and quantities of medical care have been changing. Understanding the reasons for such changes is essential for forecasting and for anticipating the effects of public policy on prices, quantities, and expenditures in each of the medical markets.

The Interrelationship of the Different Medical Care Markets

Medical care, which is the output of the overall medical care market, is in fact the outcome of several interrelated markets. These include the markets for registered nurses, hospital services, physician services, and even the market for health professional education. Within each market there is a demand and a supply side, which, when they interact, result in price, quantity, and total expenditures (price multiplied by quantity) on that service. The resulting price and quantity in one sub-market affect other sub-markets and are the links that tie these markets together. To be able to forecast the effects of a change in government policy on the medical care sector or to determine the effects of a natural change such as an increase in the aged population, it is necessary to have a model of the medical care sector that describes the relationship of various sub-markets and components of medical care to each other.

The following model describes the various sub-markets that comprise the medical care sector, demonstrates the way in which these different sectors are interrelated, and illustrates the usefulness of such a framework for forecasting and policy analysis (1). This overview of the medical care sector will also indicate the various subject areas to be covered in this book.

Three types of markets are present in the medical care sector, as shown in Figure 3-1. The patient's demand for a medical treatment (for a particular diagnostic category) is expressed by going to a physician whose determination of how to treat the patient is based on both economic and non-economic factors. The physician's selection of one or more of several institutional settings—hospitals, outpatient facilities, nursing homes, the physician's office, or even home care—is based on the relative prices (net of the patient's insurance) of each of those settings, the relative cost of each to the physician, and the efficacy of each in treatment. The demand for institutional care will depend on patient demand factors, physician considerations, and the relative price and efficacy of treatment in the different institutional settings. These institutional settings may thus be seen both as complements to and substitutes for one another.

(Under the traditional fee-for-service system, the physician is assumed to act as the patient's agent in determining which set of institutional settings would be used for providing care to the patient. Under traditional insurance coverage, each provider is paid separately. As managed care systems have developed, such as health maintenance organizations (HMOs), the HMO receives an annual capitation fee and is responsible for providing all the medical services the patient may require. In both cases, the physician continues to determine the combination of institutional settings that would be used in patient treatment. The incentives facing the physician, patient, and the HMO, however, may differ. This issue will be discussed in greater depth; nevertheless, the model described is relevant for understanding and forecasting change under each of these different delivery systems.)

A change in the demand for different institutional settings that is the result of, for example, a change in the age of the population, will be reflected in institutional demands for manpower and other factor inputs (e.g., capital and supplies). These comprise the second set of markets to be analyzed. Such institutional demands for manpower and other inputs represent the demand side of the health manpower (and input) markets. The demand for a particular health manpower category, for example, will depend upon factors relating to the patient's (and/or their physicians') demand for the institutional settings in which that manpower group is employed and the wages of the group, holding constant the relationship of their wages to those of other health workers and their relative marginal productivities.

The demand for an education by prospective health professionals will depend upon the demand for health professionals in the market just described. The demand for a health professional education, which is the amount that a person is willing to pay in terms of tuition and forgone income, is determined by the expected income and wages that might be earned (as determined in the manpower market) and by non-economic motivating factors.

The supply side of each of these markets works as follows. The supply of health professional educational institutions (in terms, for example, of institutional capacity and faculty) and the demands for such education determine the number of graduates

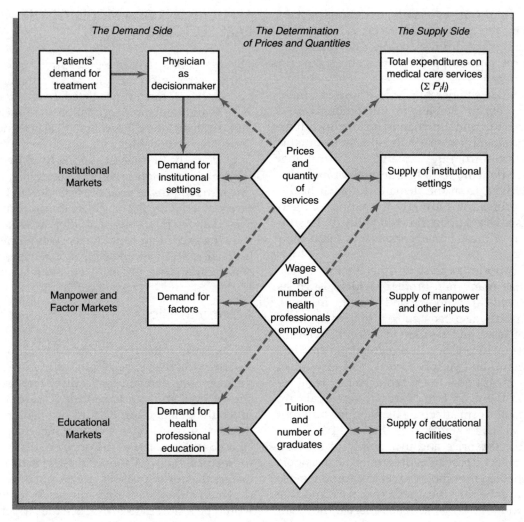

Figure 3-1. An overview of the medical care sector.

and the tuition rate to be charged. The supply of health manpower at any given time is determined by the number of graduates (the time required to educate each category of health manpower varies) plus the existing stock of health manpower (less deaths and retirements). The supply of each category of health manpower in conjunction with the demands for such manpower determines incomes and wages as well as employment (the participation rate). The outcomes of the health manpower (and other input) markets (wages and employment) affect the supply of services offered in different institutional settings. The cost of providing care in a given institutional setting rise as the wages for a given manpower group increase and as more members of that manpower category are used to provide care. In each institutional setting, the costs of providing care together with the demands for care will determine how much care is provided; this is the outcome of the institutional markets. Total expenditures for personal medical care consist, then, of the prices of each institutional setting multiplied by the quantity of care provided in each setting. (Total expenditures may be categorized according to the portion paid by the insurer, government, or patient.)

To summarize the demand side of each of these separate markets, the demand for institutional care is derived from the initial demands for medical treatments. The demand for health manpower (inputs) is similarly derived from the demand for institutional care, and the demand for a health professional education is derived from the demand for each health manpower profession. Similarly, the supply of medical services is based upon the availability of the supplies in each of these other markets and upon their costs.

Medical care, in contrast to other sectors of the economy, has many non-profit providers, such as hospitals, medical schools, and health insurers. Medical care has also been subject to a great many government laws and regulations. Provider incentives, government policies, and regulations, in addition to demand and supply factors, will also affect market prices and quantities. For example, legal restrictions on the tasks that health professionals are permitted to perform affect the demand for different health professionals, the wages they are paid, and consequently, the price and availability of medical services. Similarly, past subsidies to medical schools that have enabled the schools to set low tuition levels and fix the number of educational spaces irrespective of the demand for those spaces has affected the availability of physicians, their incomes, and the fees they charge.

To forecast the consequences of a change in the demand or supply side of any part of this model, it is necessary to understand how well the markets in each of the sectors perform. The performance of each of the separate markets—the different institutional markets, manpower markets, and educational markets—influences each of the other markets and the final prices and expenditures for medical care. A market in which price is higher and output lower than if it were functioning properly is subject to proposals for improving its performance.

APPLICATIONS OF A MODEL OF THE MEDICAL CARE SECTOR

The effects of alternative public policies on the final market—that is, on the price and availability of medical services—can be predicted (using the tools of supply and demand analysis) on the basis of an understanding of the different medical care markets and their interrelationships.

Our ability to forecast the likely consequences of changes in demand or supply conditions in medical care also requires an accurate overview of the medical care sector. Figure 3-2 describes the same markets discussed above by means of a different set of diagrams showing each of the separate markets within the institutional, manpower, and educational markets in terms of a traditional supply-and-demand relationship.

A Demand Policy

An increase in the population covered by health insurance would be expected to result in an increase in the aggregate demand for medical care (as would be shown by a shift in demand in Figure 3-2A). How much the demand for medical care will increase will depend, in part, on the importance of price to increased utilization (i.e., the price elasticity of demand for medical care). (While an increase in insurance that lowers the out-of-pocket price would be a movement down an individual's demand curve, in aggregate it would be a shift in demand. See the Appendix in the Chapter on The Demand for Medical Care.)

As a result of an increase in demand, both an increase in price and an increase in medical care utilization would be expected. To forecast the effect on prices and utilization for each component of medical care, one would have to analyze how this increase in medical care demand is transmitted to each of the other markets. As a result of lower out-of-pocket prices to consumers for medical care, following greater insurance coverage, the demand for different institutional settings will increase; certain institutional settings will experience a larger increase in demand than others depending, in part, upon which

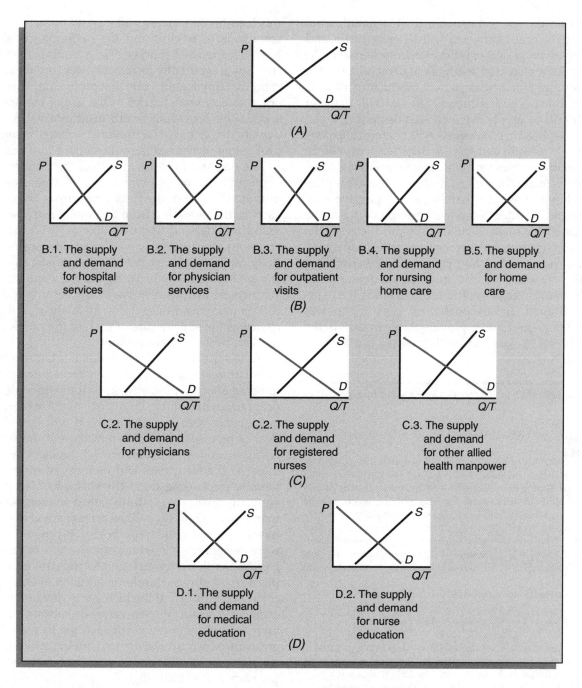

Figure 3-2.   An econometric model of the medical care sector: (A) the market for medical care services; (B) the markets for institutional services; (C) the markets for health manpower; (D) the markets for health professional education.

population groups will increase their demand, what types of medical treatments will be demanded, and how important price is to utilization in each market. As a result of the increased institutional demand, prices in these settings will increase, as will the quantity of services provided. The institutions affected will demand more inputs to supply that increased demand.

Various health professions will therefore experience an increase in demand for their services. Within each health manpower market, the employing institution's demand for a given health profession will be affected by the wages it would have to pay, the relative wages of other manpower groups that may be substituted for them, their relative productivity, the price of the output, and any legal restrictions that may prevent the use of certain personnel in performing specified tasks. With the increase in demand for health manpower given the existing stock (i.e., currently trained professionals) of that manpower group, wages and the employment rate in each of the health manpower markets will increase.[1] Exactly how

---

1. For example, the hospital demand for RNs may be expressed as follows:

$$Q_{DRNs} = f\ (-P_{RNs},\ +MP_{RNs},\ +P_{HOSP},\ +P_C,\ +Q_{HOSP})$$

Where the quantity of RNs demanded by hospitals (Q_{DRNs}) is functionally related to the price of RNs ($-P_{RNs}$) which represents the downward sloping demand curve for RNs; the remaining factors represent shifts in the demand for RNs; $+MP_{RNs}$ represents the marginal productivity of RNs, $+P_{HOSP}$ represents the price of hospital care (both the MP_{RNs} and P_{HOSP} represent the value marginal product of RNs in a competitive market), $+P_C$ represents substitutes to RNs, and $+Q_{HOSP}$ represents the quantity of hospital days since the demand for RNs is derived from the demand for hospital care.

The equation for the supply of RNs is:

$$Q_{SRNs} = f\ (+W_{RNs},\ -W_{LPNs},\ +Q_{GRAD},\ +Q_{STOCK}).$$

Where the quantity of RNs supplied (Q_{SRNs}) is positively related to RN wages (W_{RNs}), negatively related to the price of substitutes (W_{LPNs}), positively to the number of new RN graduates (Q_{GRAD}), and to the existing stock of RNs (Q_{STOCK}). The interaction of the demand and supply of RNs results in the wage and number of RNs employed. In turn, the RN wage becomes one of the input prices in the supply of hospital care equation.

much each will increase will depend upon the supply conditions (elasticity) and the performance of each health manpower market. The resulting higher incomes will eventually increase the demand for an education leading to entry into that profession. Thus, lowering an economic barrier to the use of medical care services by providing health insurance will increase demand for different institutional settings, manpower professions, and a health professional education.

The demand increase in each of the different markets will be followed by increases in prices as well as output. The size of the price and output increases in each market resulting from that initial increase in demand will depend upon the size of the demand increase and the responsiveness of supply (supply elasticity) within each market. The less elastic supply is, the greater the price increase and the smaller will be the increase in output. It is precisely because of this effect on prices and output that an analysis of the efficiency of the supply side of each of the medical care markets becomes so important.

If the supply side of the market is relatively inelastic—that is, if it takes a relatively large price increase to bring about an increase in output—then demand programs will result in large price increases and small output increases. Consequently, it will cost a great deal of money to achieve an increase in output. For example, according to Figure 3-3, an increase in demand will affect prices and quantity of services differently depending upon the elasticity of supply. If supply is relatively elastic (S_2), then an increase in demand, from D_1 to D_2, will be accompanied by a price increase, but it will be much less (P_2) than if supply were inelastic (S_1), in which case the new price would be (P_1). Similarly, a much greater increase in services provided will occur under conditions of elastic supply (Q_2 versus Q_1). If the increase in demand were to occur as a result of a government subsidy program and if supply were inelastic (S_1), the increased government expenditures for that program would pay for higher prices (P_1) and less output (Q_1) than if supply were more elastic (S_2).

It is therefore important to understand what the supply elasticity is for each of the medical care markets. If markets with relatively inelastic supply can be

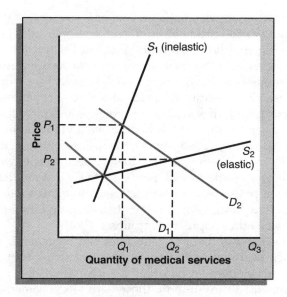

Figure 3-3. The effect on prices and medical services of an increase in demand when there are different supply elasticities.

made more elastic, the potential benefits in terms of lower prices and increased output can be very great. Therefore, each of the medical care markets will be examined in terms of economic efficiency to determine how well each performs. How do each of these markets respond to changes in demand? Could their prices be lower and outputs greater if changes were made in their structure? By examining each of the medical care markets in terms of structure and performance, the efficiency of those markets can be determined and, if they need to be improved, which policies will be most useful for improving economic performance.

Other demand policies will also be examined using the framework noted above. For example, one way in which the government can reduce its expenditures on hospital services to the aged is to provide coverage for care in a less costly setting. Providing insurance coverage to the aged for services provided by a hospice would, assuming that the hospice is a substitute for fewer hospital admissions, decrease the demand for hospital care (a shift to the left in the demand for hos-

pitals). As the demand for hospital services decrease, the hospital's derived demand for its inputs and staff would similarly decrease. As the out-of-pocket price to the aged for hospice services was reduced as a result of the government insurance coverage, there would be an increase in the quantity demanded of hospice services, with a consequent increase in the derived demand for inputs used by the hospice. Whether or not covering a lower-cost substitute to hospitals reduces the overall expenditure on services for that medical treatment depends on the relative cost and changes in use of each of those services. (Appendix 3, in the chapter "The Demand For Health Insurance" provides a detailed example of how to determine the savings of insuring a lower-cost substitute.)

A Supply Policy

A model of the medical care sector as described above is also useful for explaining how a supply subsidy might work. Typical governmental supply subsidies provide funds to educational institutions for increasing the number of health professionals. Such programs cause a shift to the right in the supply of the educational institutions and increase the schools' enrollment capacity. The effect is to increase the number of graduates in the educational market. As the number of graduates (e.g., physicians or nurses) increases and the supply of those particular health professionals in the health manpower market shifts to the right, the wages or incomes of the subsidized health professionals become lower than they might otherwise have been. The larger number of health professionals (those that were subsidized) and their relatively lower wages will result in an increase in the quantity demanded for them in the institutional market (a movement down the institutions' demand for such personnel) since they will be substituted for other health professionals whose wages and numbers were not affected by supply subsidies.

The effect on the institutional sector of the supply subsidy will be a shift to the right in the institution's supply curve since they can presumably produce the same quantity of services at a lower price (or a greater quantity of services at the same price). This is because the price of one of their inputs has been reduced as a result of the subsidy. The effect of a supply subsidy will affect each type of institution differently since some institutions use relatively more of the subsidized input (e.g., hospitals use relatively more registered nurses) than others. The subsidy program's overall effect on the final price and quantity of medical care will vary depending upon how much of an increase in the input occurs as a result of that supply subsidy, how much of a decrease in the price of that input occurs, how much of that subsidized input is used in the production of medical care, and so on.

A completely specified model of the medical care sector should enable us to trace the effects of a supply subsidy program throughout each of the different medical care markets. Different supply subsidy programs can be compared on the basis of what each program costs to achieve a change in the final price and quantity of medical care services. Thus the model of the medical care sector presented above enables the comparison of alternative government supply subsidies, each of which is designed to increase the availability of medical care. Such subsidy programs need not be directed solely at a manpower category; they may be directed at any number of inputs, such as less-trained personnel who increase the productivity of more highly trained professionals, or they may provide subsidies for hospital construction. Therefore, overall model of medical care allows any number of supply subsidy programs to be evaluated on the basis of the cost of the subsidy and its final effect on the price and availability of medical care.

ALTERNATIVE REDISTRIBUTIVE POLICIES

The model of medical care presented above will also be used to discuss alternative approaches to its redistribution. Even though inefficiencies continue to exist in the medical care market, society may decide to increase the consumption of medical care to the population or to selected population groups. Such an overview suggests that it is possible to achieve an increase in consumption of medical care services either by shifting the demands for care or by increasing the quantity of a particular input on the supply side (i.e., shifting supply). Each of these policies will result in an increase in the quantity of medical care services consumed, as shown in Figure 3-4. For example, to increase the quantity of medical services consumed from Q_0 to Q_1 (based upon a normative judgment that it is desirable to do so), either the demand for medical care can be increased from D_1 to D_2, or the supply can be increased from S_1 to S_2. Either of these policies will achieve the objective of increasing the use of medical care from Q_0 to Q_1. However, these alternative redistributive policies will differ in their costs and their effects on other population groups.

Demand and supply subsidies can be general, as when everyone in the population has access to that subsidy, or they can be targeted, such as providing the demand subsidy to only those with low incomes or subsidizing providers in low income areas. The cost of general versus targeted subsidies will differ as would the number of low-income persons receiving those subsidies under each approach.

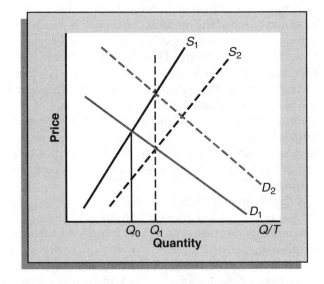

Figure 3-4. Alternative demand and supply policies to achieve a redistribution of medical care.

SUMMARY

The model of the medical care sector described previously also serves to enumerate the different subject areas of this book. To understand the medical care sector, it is necessary to learn about the theory of demand for medical care and the consequent derived demands within each of the other markets. In the demand section as in all other sections, the theoretical discussion of demand will be followed by a review of studies that have attempted to estimate the theoretical variables discussed. The review will be followed by a summary of empirical estimates of the factors that affect demand.

After analyzing the demand side of the medical care sector, the supply side of the different markets is examined. In this way it becomes possible to judge the efficiency of each of the different medical care markets: health insurance, hospital services, physician services, the market for physicians, the market for registered nurses, and the market for medical education. In addition to judging the efficiency of each of these markets, the relevant government policies that have an impact on these separate markets (such as health manpower legislation in the manpower markets) will be evaluated. Finally, public policy recommendations will be proposed for improving efficiency within each of these markets based upon an analysis of their market performance.

The overview presented here illustrates why medical care is said to be the output of the medical care sector. The efficiency of the separate markets and their interrelationship affects the efficiency with which medical care is produced, the cost at which it is produced, and the growth of expenditures in this sector. The evaluation of the efficiency of each of these markets is, therefore, of prime concern for public policy.

The foregoing model of medical care also illustrates the alternative approaches that may be used to redistribute medical services and the means for evaluating them. These two concepts, efficiency and redistribution (equity), will be the basis upon which both the separate markets and government policies will be analyzed throughout this book.

REVIEW QUESTIONS

1. With an increase in demand for medical care, how will different supply elasticities affect total medical expenditures?
2. Assume that the price of a specific input (e.g., registered nurses) was subsidized. Trace through the effect of such a policy in all the medical markets, and evaluate this policy in terms of its effect on the goal of increasing the level of the population's health. Second, evaluate this policy in terms of economic efficiency. Finally, evaluate this policy in terms of who benefits and who bears the cost.
3. Trace through each of the medical care markets the use of pre-authorization review of hospital admissions by managed care organizations.
4. Based on demographic projections, it is estimated that fewer female high school graduates will be available to pursue a nursing career. Trace through this demographic effect in each of the medical care markets.
5. Show how an increase in the quantity of medical care consumed can be achieved through either a demand or supply subsidy. What are the advantages and disadvantages of general versus targeted demand and supply subsidies?

REFERENCES

1. The description of the medical care sector in this section is based upon an article by Paul J. Feldstein and Sander Kelman, "An Econometric Model of the Medical Care Sector," in H. Klarman, ed., *Empirical Studies in Health Economics,* (Baltimore: Johns Hopkins University Press, 1970).

C H A P T E R

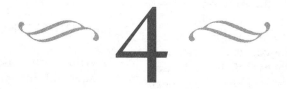

4

Measuring Changes in the Price of Medical Care

KEY TERMS AND CONCEPTS

- Consumer Price Index
- Medical Care Price Index
- Laspeyres and Paasche price indices
- Consumer expenditure survey
- Linking
- Actual versus list prices
- Quality change
- Cost of treatment price index

Learning Objectives

Upon completing this chapter, the reader should be able to:

- Appreciate the need for an accurate medical care price index (MCPI).
- Understand how the MCPI is constructed.
- Be aware of the weaknesses of the MCPI.
- Discuss how a treatment-based medical care price index differs from the current MCPI.
- Explain how an MCPI based on quality-adjusted treatment prices differs from an input-based MCPI.

THE USES OF A DEFINITION OF THE PRODUCT OF THE MEDICAL CARE INDUSTRY

How much has the price of medical care been increasing? Do rising Medicare expenditures indicate increased use of services, or are they the result of rising prices? Have physician fees fallen as a result of the increased supply of physicians? Has competition in medical care reduced the rate of increase in medical prices? The efficiency with which medical services are produced, the measurement of productivity change over time, the degree of price inflation, public policies to increase access to care, and the impact of market reforms are issues that are important for health policy. To be able to understand these issues, it is necessary to have accurate information on medical prices.

Accurate price information consists of two parts: a definition of the output being measured, and the actual price paid for that output. For example, how should the price of a hospital admission be measured? Should the hospital's list price be used? Large insurers and HMOs do not pay list prices, nor do Medicare and Medicaid. In fact, at any time, a hospital may have negotiated over 100 different prices for the same services with different organizations.

As difficult as it is to measure actual prices and their changes over time, measuring the output of the medical sector is even more difficult. A hospital admission today is not the same as one in 1985, and certainly not the same as one in 1965. The diagnoses treated in the hospital have changed, as have the services and medical technology available to treat those diseases. Patients do not demand a hospital admission or a physician visit, they demand a treatment for a particular disease. Hospital care, physician services, and home health care are actually inputs into a treatment.

From the patient's point of view, the demand for medical care is the demand for a treatment for some actual or perceived, current or potential, physical or mental disorder. After the patient consults a physician, a treatment is prescribed that often uses a combination of various inputs. Ideally, the costs and prices of medical care should be measured in terms of outputs, not just according to the inputs used in the treatment process. Using outputs rather than inputs would enable increases in input productivity and technological advances to be reflected both in the costs of providing a treatment and in its outcome.

To determine whether medical prices are increasing, it is necessary to analyze how medical treatment prices have changed over time. In the case of heart disease, the treatment uses a combination of drugs, hospital care, physician services, etc., and the combination of those services or inputs has changed over time. Further, new drugs are used in the treatment of heart disease, and the price of those drugs is more expensive than drugs previously used. However, the new drugs have reduced the use of the hospital, which has also increased in price. Thus not only has the combination of inputs used in treatment changed, but the inputs, such as drugs, are different and more expensive.

Crucial to measuring changes in the price of treating heart disease is determining how the outcome of that treatment has similarly changed. An accurate measure of output would have to be adjusted for quality improvements. Survival and quality of life, (outcomes of medical treatments) have improved over time. Unless the price of a treatment is adjusted for survival and quality of life, the data will indicate that input costs (hospital care, etc.) and overall treatment costs have increased. But this measure provides an inaccurate indication of rising treatment prices; patients treated for heart disease are clearly better off today than 30 years ago. Unless medical prices are adjusted for outcomes, medical prices increases overstate the amount of price inflation that has occurred.

Essential to any treatment measure of output is the necessity to adjust treatment costs for changes in treatment outcomes.

The beginning of the chapter focuses on the measurement of prices, starting with a description of the functions and limitations of the Consumer Price Index (CPI). This is followed by a detailed discussion of the medical care component of the CPI, which is still the most widely used index of medical care prices. The final section describes and evaluates several other approaches to measuring the price of medical care—those that are based on the use of medical treatments for specific conditions as the appropriate measure of medical care output.

THE CONSUMER PRICE INDEX

What Should the CPI Measure?

In the broadest terms, the Consumer Price Index (CPI) acts as a measure of inflation; that is, it records the change in the prices of goods that consumers purchase. The percentage change in the CPI from one year to the next is taken as a measure of the rate of inflation. In other words, it acts as the rate at which a family's income would have had to increase to keep up with rising prices to maintain a certain level of material welfare. Since the CPI acts as the major indicator of consumer purchasing power, many social welfare initiatives have been tied to the index. For example, social security benefit levels and Federal employee retirement pensions are adjusted using CPI data. Similarly, many union contracts contain provisions for automatically increasing wages in line with increases in the CPI. In all, the incomes of about half of the U.S. population are directly affected by changes in the CPI.

As an indicator of the nation's inflation rate, the CPI is used in economic formulas and calculations to correct for the effects of inflation. The CPI is used to deflate personal consumption expenditure data that is then used to construct national income accounts. Further, the CPI is used to more accurately estimate real growth in the economy and productivity of the labor force. In essence, policy makers use the CPI to reach an accurate assessment of economic data, which helps to determine monetary and fiscal policy.

The CPI is frequently referred to as a cost-of-living index. While the CPI does reflect the cost of goods and services that the average consumer purchases, it does not incorporate all of the contributors to personal utility that a cost-of-living index would require. If the CPI were a true cost-of-living index, then it should measure the cost of maintaining a given level of welfare or utility (or in terms of economic theory, of remaining on the same indifference curve). Accordingly, the cost of living is influenced by much more than the prices of goods and services that consumers buy. Tax rates influence the amount of gross income needed to maintain a certain level of welfare. Taxes that directly influence the prices of products, such as sales taxes, are reflected in the CPI, yet income taxes are not. On the other hand, governmental provision of free-of-charge services, such as highway improvements or fire protection, may increase the standard of living achievable at any level of income, but is not reflected in the CPI. One might argue that standards of living are also affected by changes in crime rates, environmental pollution, and other such factors essentially beyond the individual's control. Time costs, such as increased waiting time for treatments and procedures, also influence individual welfare. Unless the above factors are considered in a cost-of-living index, it is not necessarily true that a household is better off when its gross income increases faster than the prices of the goods and services it buys (1).

Aware of the difficulty of measuring the cost of maintaining a level of welfare, the Bureau of Labor Statistics (BLS) has attempted a more modest task and designed the CPI to measure the change in the cost of purchasing a fixed market basket of goods and services representing average consumption patterns during some base period. A price index of this type, in which individual prices are weighted by base-year quantities, is called a Laspeyres index.[1] Thus the CPI aims to measure how much the average household in its surveyed population will have to spend to buy the same market basket in the current year that it had bought in the base year.

---

1. It can be expressed by the following formula:

$$I_t = \frac{\Sigma_i Q_{bi} P_{ti}}{\Sigma_i Q_{bi} P_{bi}}$$

where I_t = value of the index in year t
   Q_{bi} = quantity of good i purchased in the base year
   P_{bi} = price of good i in the base year
   P_{ti} = price of good i in the year t

Such an index is often multiplied by some scaling factor so that it equals 100 in some particular year. Of course, if the index is multiplied by the same scaling factor in each year, percentage changes from year to year are not affected.

Even this limited view of the CPI, however, is not a simple task. The market basket purchased by the average household in the surveyed population is constantly changing, not only in response to price changes, but also in response to changes in incomes, tastes, and availability of new products and services not previously available to consumers. It is inaccurate to continue pricing the same goods and services without making an allowance for these changes. For example, if the healthcare portion of the CPI only measured penicillin among prescription antibiotics, the index would ignore the newer classes of antibiotics that have become the foundation of antimicrobial treatment. In the succeeding section, how the BLS resolves some of the major issues involved in constructing the CPI are discussed, together with the likely effects on the accuracy of the CPI.

ISSUES AND PROBLEMS IN CONSTRUCTING THE CPI

Population Coverage

The CPI was initially designed to measure price changes for urban wage earners and clerical workers. However, the definition of the covered population has changed over time (2). Until 1964, only families were included. At that time, single persons were added, and the stipulation that household income should be less than $10,000 was dropped. After the 1964 revision of the CPI, its coverage included about 45 percent of the total U.S. population. In the 1987 revision of the CPI, a CPI was constructed for two population groups, All Urban Consumers (CPI-U) and Wage Earners and Clerical Workers (CPI-W) (3). The CPI-U is based on expenditures of all urban consumer units without regard to income or employment status. Excluded from the CPI-U are all rural and farm residents, the military, and those in institutions. As of June 2003, approximately 87 percent of the total American population is included in the CPI-U (4).

The CPI-W is a more restricted sample that includes urban consumer units that receive more than one-half of their income from clerical or wage occupations, and one or more of the household members had to be employed for at least 37 weeks in an eligible occupation during the past 12 months. The CPI-W covers 32 percent of the total U.S. population. Organized labor has supported the continued use of the traditional index, which was the CPI-W, in contract escalation provisions because it believes that the more comprehensive index (CPI-U) will rise more slowly than the CPI-W.

Sampling Problems

The Bureau of Labor Statistics (BLS) updates the CPI market basket of goods and services about every 10 years. The CPI, as of June 2003, is based on a survey conducted in 1993 to 1995. The survey consists of two components: an interview survey to determine expenditures on the type and quantity of items that people purchase. Second, a diary, or record-keeping survey, in which individuals are asked to keep a two-week diary of small, frequently purchased items. The BLS assigns weights to different items in the CPI based on data from these consumer expenditure surveys.[2]

Several aspects of the BLS sampling methodology may bias the CPI. The major criticism has traditionally been that the 10-year intervals between surveys were not frequent enough to capture changes in consumption patterns. The BLS's weighting system was, until 1978, based on 1960 to 1961 information. Until the 1987 revision, spending patterns were based on 1972 to 1973 survey data. And until 1998, the CPI was based on buying patterns from a 15-year-old (1982 to 1984) Consumer Expenditure Survey. Currently, the CPI is based on 1993 to 1995 data. During any given 10 to 15 year period, consumption patterns change and new products are introduced. These changes, however, are not picked up in the CPI until a new revision appears.

---

2. The national CPI is built up from indexes calculated for a sample of cities. Separate city indexes are published. Differences between city indexes, however, do not measure price differences between cities, but only indicate price changes for each city since the base period.

Table 4-1 indicates changes in the relative weights of major groups of items over the years. The years 1935 to 1939, 1952, 1963, 1981, and 1996 were chosen because they correspond to major revisions in the CPI growing out of new consumer expenditure surveys. The 1981 weights are based on the 1972 to 1973 survey and were first incorporated in the CPI in January 1978. The 1996 weights are based on the 1982 to 1984 survey and were first incorporated in the CPI in January 1987. December 2003 was chosen because it was the most recent data available. The 2003 weights are based on the 1993 to 1995 survey and were first incorporated in the CPI in January 1998.

The most striking trends in Table 4-1 are the declines in the importance of food and the increase in transportation in consumer budgets. The weight assigned to food has fallen considerably despite the fact that, as Table 4-2 shows, its price has risen as fast as the all-items index. The decline in the importance of food in consumer budgets probably reflects low income elasticity. As per capita incomes have increased, a smaller fraction has been used to buy food. Food and housing remain, however, the most important elements in consumer budgets, together accounting, on average, for well over half of expenditures. As a percent of consumer spending, medical care has varied from 4.1 percent in 1935 to 1939 to a high of 7.4 percent in 1996, as measured by the CPI.

The CPI was previously based on seven major product groups of items (including food and beverages, housing, apparel, transportation, entertainment, and medical care, and other goods and services) but was revised into eight major categories in 1998, including the newly formed education and communications group. Table 4-2 presents values for the CPI and its major component groups from 1935 to 2003. Since all the component indexes are scaled to equal 100 in 1982 to 1984, those with the smallest values in 1935 increased the fastest in the period 1935 to 1982 to 1984. The major component groups with the highest values in 2002 have increased the fastest since 1982 to 1984. A one-point increase in an index is, of course, a smaller percentage increase today than it was in 1935. Table 4-2 shows that the indexes for the different major groups have had quite different patterns of increase over the years. Over the period as a whole, medical care has risen the most rapidly.

Table 4-1. Relative Importance of Major Components of the CPI, Selected Years (Percent)

Group	1935–1939	December 1952	December 1963	December 1981(a)	December 1996(a)	December 2003(a)
All Items	100.0	100.0	100.0	100.0	100.0	100.0
Food and beverages	35.4	32.2	25.2	17.5	17.5	15.4
Housing	33.7	33.5	34.0	46.0	41.2(b)	42.1(b)
Apparel and upkeep	11.0	9.4	10.6	4.6	5.3	4.0
Transportation	8.1	11.3	14.0	19.3	17.1	16.9
Medical care	4.1	4.8	5.7	4.9	7.4	6.1
Recreation(c)	2.8	4.0	3.9	3.6	4.4	5.9
Other goods and services(d)	4.9	4.8	5.7	4.0	7.2	9.6(e)

Source: U.S. Department of Labor, Bureau of Labor Statistics, *Handbook of Labor Statistics, 1989,* p. 485; data for December 1996 and 2003 come from Internet site http://stats.bls.gov/cpi/(accessed on February 12, 2004).

(a) CPI for All Urban Consumers.

(b) The rental equivalence approach to homeowner's costs: effective January 1985.

(c) Called "reading and recreation" before 1977, called "entertainment" between 1977 and 1996, and called "recreation" from 1997 to present.

(d) "Other goods and services" now includes tobacco and smoking products and personal care expenses. In pre-1997 index it included educational and personal care expenses, and tobacco products which were previously found under other categories.

(e) 2003 data include "Other goods and services" and "Education and communication."

Table 4-2. CPI and Major Groups, 1935–2003 (1982–84 = 100 unless noted)

Year	All items	Food	Housing	Apparel and Upkeep	Transpor- tation	Medical Care	Recreation(a)	Other(b)
1935	13.7	12.5	15.2	20.8	14.2	10.2	17.0	15.7
1945	18.0	17.3	18.2	31.4	15.9	11.9	25.4	20.0
1955	26.8	27.9	25.3	42.9	25.8	18.2	31.2	28.0
1965	31.5	32.2	29.2	47.8	31.9	25.2	39.1	33.0
1970	38.8	40.1	36.4	59.2	37.5	34.0	47.5	40.9
1975	53.8	60.2	50.7	72.5	50.1	47.5	62.0	53.9
1980(c)	82.4	86.7	81.1	90.9	83.1	74.9	83.6	75.2
1985(c)	107.6	105.6	107.7	105.0	106.4	113.5	107.9	114.5
1990(c)	130.7	132.4	128.5	124.1	120.5	162.8	132.4	159.0
1995(c)	152.4	148.4	148.5	132.0	139.1	220.5	153.9	206.9
2000(c)	172.2	167.8	169.6	129.6	153.3	260.8	103.3	271.1
2003(c)	184.0	180.0	184.8	120.4	157.6	297.1	107.5(d)	298.7

Sources: U.S. Department of Labor, Bureau of Labor Statistics, *Handbook of Labor Statistics, 1989*; data for 1990–2003 come from Internet site http://www.bls.gov/cpi/ (accessed on February 3, 2004).

Note: The 1978 and 1997 revisions brought about several definitional changes that have made it impossible to directly link pre- and post-1978 and 1997 indexes for "entertainment" and "other."

(a) It now includes video and audio. In pre-1997 index called 'Entertainment.' It included most of what was called "reading and recreation" in pre-1978 index; Entertainment excluded certain subcomponents found in "reading and recreation" such as TV and sound equipment, TV repair, and educational expenses.

(b) It now includes tobacco and smoking products and personal care expenses. In pre-1997 index, 'other' included educational and personal care expenses expenses, which in pre-1978 indexes were found under other categories. It also included tobacco products; it no longer included alcoholic beverages.

(c) CPI for All Urban Consumers.

(d) December 1997 = 100.

The major CPI product groups are divided into seventy expenditure classes, which in turn are subdivided into 211 item strata. The strata are the level at which the CPI is calculated. The weights of the item strata, as well as the higher levels of aggregation such as major product groups, are fixed until there is another major revision of the market basket. (Fixed quantity weights assume that there is no substitution between these strata.) The strata subdivide into a total of 305 entry-level items; some strata may contain only one entry-level item, while others may contain several. The BLS now samples these entry-level items in eighty-seven geographical areas based on the 1990 census.

The CPI is based on the principle of probability sampling. This method was introduced in the 1972 to 1973 CPI revision and has been used to determine how the price of an item changes over time. The underlying assumption is that the other items in that expenditure class are changing in price, on average, at the same rate as the item or items actually priced.

Within each geographic area sampled, a Point of Purchase survey is conducted in which consumers are asked how much they spend on each category of consumption and also where they make their purchases. Based on this survey, BLS selects a sample of outlets (or, in the case of the MCPI, medical providers). Within each selected outlet, one or more specific varieties of items are selected; the probability of the item selected is proportional to its sales based on the Point of Purchase survey.

Given this extensive sampling, there is still the problem mentioned above of outdated weights. Prior to 1998, the weights for the CPI were based on the 15-year-old, 1982 to 1984 Consumer Expenditure Survey. To help correct for the bias created by the outdated weights, the BLS instituted re-weighting of the CPI every five years (5). However, even the latest weights are not current at their time of introduction. The time involved in analyzing the survey data results in a 5-year lag time. These outdated weights may lead to an upward bias. For example, the fixed basket of goods may include branded drug X. While the price of branded drug X may remain stable over the course of 4 or 5 years, the emergence of substitute and generic medications may be more attractive and cheaper alternatives for consumers. A weighing system that is adjusted every 10 years may miss such changes. Studies within the health-care field have examined the issue of re-weighing. A study on heart attack treatment costs using a fixed-weight system similar to that of the CPI for the period of 1983 to 1994 based on the 1983 market basket found an upward bias in the rate of annual price increase at 1.7 percentage points per year compared to a system that re-weights items yearly. While this study was limited to a specific disease entity involving limited medical services, it does demonstrate the effect of the substitution bias within the framework of outdated weights (6).

Substitution Bias

Because the CPI calculates price changes based on the Laspeyres index (price data are based on the goods and services purchased in the base year), there is a substitution bias that overstates inflation. The substitution bias occurs because as prices of the base year goods and services increase, the consumer will choose a different set of goods and services that are less expensive. The BLS continues to price the base year goods and services and assumes that the consumer will purchase the same quantity of the item even though its price has risen. In fact, consumers will substitute away from those items for which price is rising more rapidly and this will lessen, to some extent, the impact of the general price increase. For example, as the price of movie theater tickets (included in the base year) increase, and video cassette recorder tapes (VCR tapes) do not (or increase less), VCR tapes become relatively cheaper; consumers may substitute some home viewing for theater viewing with no loss of overall well being. The additional income required to purchase the base-year market basket in a later year will generally exceed the increase necessary to buy a

market basket that is *equivalent in the eyes of the consumer* to that purchased in the base year.[3]

Studies have shown that the substitution bias has increased the CPI by 0.4 percentage points per year (5). To correct for substitution bias, in 1999 the BLS began to use a geometric mean estimator in its price calculations to permit limited substitution among products within item strata.[4] This correction has reduced the rate of growth by 0.25 percentage points in the aggregate CPI setting and has formed the basis for the C-CPI-U (8).

Quality Changes and New Products

As a price index for measuring inflation, price increases that result from improvements in product quality should be omitted from the index. For example, if a color television set is substituted for a black-and-white set, the index should not reflect the full price difference between the two since most of it will be due to product quality differences. If the CPI did not adjust for quality improvements in new cars, then

---

3. An index that used current-year quantities as weights would understate cost-of-living increases because it would put too much weight on items whose prices had increased relatively slowly. Such an index is called a Paasche index. Clearly, some sort of average of a Laspeyres and Paasche index will yield a better measure of cost-of-living changes than either one individually. The Laspeyres formula is used primarily because of the high cost of continually collecting information on weights.

4. The geometric mean estimator uses a set of fixed expenditure proportions as weights in averaging the prices of individual items within a CPI index. The Laspeyres or 'arithmetic mean' formula, uses fixed quantity weights. Using the arithmetic mean formula for all indexes did not allow for consumers switching from goods whose prices increased to lower-priced substitutes; thus the CPI was overstated. The geometric mean estimator is used for calculating the medical care commodities indexes while indexes for medical care services continue to use the 'arithmetic mean' formula, which is appropriate when there are low price elasticities for medical services (e.g., hospital and professional services) and when insured consumers pay only a portion of the price so substitution is less likely.

Source: Bureau of Labor Statistics,
http://www.bls.gov/cpi/cpigm02.htm

between 1967 and 1994 the price of new cars would have been 80 percent greater. For some products, such as with personal computers, consumer durables, apparel, and prescription drugs, quality change has been significant (9). Inadequate adjustment for quality change has led to an overstatement of inflation.

If the BLS considers the change in quality to be small, no adjustment for quality improvement occurs; this lack of quality adjustment, however, causes an upward bias in the CPI. When BLS adjusts for quality change, such as when new goods are substituted for older items, it is normally accomplished by linking. When the substitution is made, both the old and the new market baskets are priced. Percentage changes in the index prior to the link reflect percentage changes in the price of the old market basket; percentage changes after the link reflect percentage changes in the price of the new market basket. Thus, the price difference between the two market baskets at the time of the link is not reflected at all in the index.[5]

In many cases, linking appears to be a good method of changing the CPI market basket. If the link is made at a time when one product is beginning to replace another in the market but both are available and are purchased by some consumers, then the higher-priced one is worth the difference in price. However, when price changes are relatively small and quality improvements are large, linking understates the degree of quality improvement. For this reason, the BLS has explored other methods of making direct quality adjustments.[6]

Another important area where the BLS has been criticized is that new items are introduced too slowly into the CPI. Initially, a new item tends to have a relatively high price and then it declines as competitors enter the market and production expands. If consumers accept a new item while its price is relatively high and if the item is absent from the index until after its price has fallen, the index will fail to register that fall in price of an item already important in consumer budgets. This problem occurs, for example, with the introduction of new drugs. The CPI overstates inflation because it misses the price declines of new goods.

In addition to the timeliness issue, the CPI is biased because of inadequate price adjustment when new goods are substituted for goods they replace (the substitution effect). As the price of an item in the CPI increases, consumers will substitute toward less costly items that are not in the CPI. The new good, however, may also be different from the previous good in that it has certain quality improvements. Some new goods

---

5. The following is a simple hypothetical example of linking. Suppose that an EC has been represented by one item, black-and-white TV sets, and a decision has been made to price color sets instead. Let us say that the index for this EC was equal to 100 in year 1. The price of black-and-white sets rises from $150 to $165 from year 1 to year 2, which is an increase of 10 percent. The index, still based on black-and-white sets, rises to 110. At that point the link is made. Color sets go from $400 to $420 from year 2 to year 3, a 5 percent increase. The index, now based on the price of color sets, increases 5 percent to 115.5 in year 3. The $235 difference between the prices of color and black-and-white sets in year 2 never shows up in the index at all.

An Example of Linking

Year	B&W TV Sets	Index	Color TV Sets
1	$150	100	—
2	$165	110	$400
3	—	115.5	$420

6. The issue of adjusting for quality changes in a price index has received a great deal of attention from economists and statisticians. One proposed method for making such adjustments is the so-called hedonic technique. It can be applied to products for which many types are available at any one time; automobiles are perhaps the best example. Data is collected on the prices and characteristics of a number of different models at a point in time. Regression analysis is then used to estimate the contribution of different characteristics (in the case of the automobile, horsepower, fuel economy, interior room) to price. We can use this information to estimate what current models would have cost in the base year based on their characteristics. The difference between these prices and the current-year prices would be estimates of the pure price change. To date, BLS has not used this approach. For a more complete discussion of this subject, see John Muelbauer, "Household Production Theory, Quality, and the Hedonic Technique," *American Economic Review*, 64, December 1974: 977–994, and Zvi Griliches, "Hedonic Price Indexes for Automobiles: An Econometric Analysis of Quality Change," in *The Price Statistics of the Federal Government*, (Cambridge, Mass.: National Bureau of Economic Research, 1961), 173–196.

provide the same services as the previous good but with a greater variety of services; some are of higher quality and/or lower price, and others provide entirely new services previously unavailable, e.g., cellular telephones. It is difficult to estimate the extent of the CPI bias when a new good is substituted for another good because of price increases in the other good (substitution bias) and when a new good has quality improvements (quality bias).

It has been estimated that the overstatement of the CPI due to all of the various biases mentioned above is between 0.4 to 1.5 percent per year. This size of bias is significant given that the CPI is used to adjust federal revenues, such as Social Security payments and income tax brackets. A study conducted in 1996 for the U.S. Senate Finance Committee found that a 1.1 percentage point bias in the CPI would add $1 trillion to the federal deficit due to adjusted pension benefits and reduced tax collections over a twelve-year period (7). Further, that the current input approach toward measuring the MCPI results in an upward bias of 3.0 percent annually. Given these magnitudes, BLS is undertaking additional research to improve the accuracy of the CPI.

THE MEDICAL CARE COMPONENT OF THE CPI (MCPI)

Background of the MCPI

Rapidly rising medical prices have been the stimulus for proposals and legislation to reduce rapidly increasing hospital prices, physician fees, and prices of prescription drugs. Medical prices, which are a component of the CPI and have increased much more rapidly than the CPI, have caused the CPI to increase more rapidly than it would have otherwise. In December 2003 (relative weights are published once a year, thus December 2003 is the latest), medical care had a weight of 6.1 percent in the CPI-U, up from 4.9 percent in 1981 (but down from 7.4 percent in 1996), as shown in Table 4-1. An increase of about 13.5 percent in the MCPI would, in and of itself, increase the CPI by 1 percent. Through its effect on the overall CPI,

the MCPI influences the CPI and has far ranging effects on federal and private revenues and outlays as well as monetary policy to fight inflation. Determining the accuracy of the Medical Care Price Index (MCPI), therefore, is important for national policy as well as for evaluating the performance of the medical care sector.

The MCPI has two major components, medical care commodities and services. Commodities are further subdivided into prescription drugs and medical supplies and nonprescription drugs and medical supplies. The major component of the MCPI is medical care services, which consists of three expenditure categories: professional services, hospital and related services, and health insurance. (Health insurance premiums are not published, and the insurance category consists of only prices for administrative services and profits). Each of the above categories is subdivided into various item strata. Table 4-3 describes the rela-

Table 4-3. Relative Weights of Items in the MCPI (December 2003)

	U (%)	W (%)
Medical care	100.0	100.0
Medical care commodities	24.7	23.0
Prescription drugs	18.0	15.9
Nonprescription drugs and medical supplies	6.8	7.1
Medical care services	75.3	77.0
Professional services	45.3	45.4
Physicians' services	25.4	26.8
Dental services	11.7	11.5
Eye care	3.9	4.0
Services by other medical professionals	4.2	3.1
Hospital and related services	24.5	25.2
Hospital services	23.5	24.9
Nursing homes	1.0	0.3
Health insurance	5.6	6.4

Source: U.S. Department of Labor, Bureau of Labor Statistics, [Online information, 2004]. http://www.bls.gov/cpi/cpiri2003.pdf (accessed on February 12, 2004)

Note: Only health insurance premiums paid by the consumer are included in the CPI. The health insurance relative importance includes only that portion of the premium that is retained by the insurance carrier for adminsitrative cost and profit.

tive weights of the items included in the MCPI as of December 2003. These weights are based on the 1982 to 1984 Consumer Expenditure Survey data on quantities of medical goods and services consumed updated to 1996 prices. Note that the weights for the CPI-U and the CPI-W are very similar.

Table 4-4 presents an overview of movements in the MCPI and its component items since 1965. A glance at the table reveals that the "Medical Services" category has increased more rapidly than the "Medical Care Commodities" category. The fastest-rising component of the MCPI has been the "Hospital Room Rate," a close second is prescription drugs.

The BLS views the MCPI, like the CPI, as an index of the price of a fixed bundle of goods and services. Four important issues are raised by this approach. First, is the weighting of the MCPI (and its individual components) an accurate reflection of its importance to the CPI? Second, are the prices recorded by BLS accurate? Third, have the goods and services remained constant over time or have new services been introduced and quality increased? And fourth, how well do the goods and services priced by BLS represent what consumers are purchasing? These four issues are discussed next.

Table 4-4. Trends in the MCPI, Selected Years, 1965–2003 (1982–84 = 100 unless noted)

Item	1965	1970	1975	1980	1985	1990	1995	2000	2003
Medical care	25.2	34.0	47.5	74.9	113.5	162.8	220.5	260.8	297.1
Medical care commodities	45.0	46.5	53.3	75.4	115.2	163.4	204.5	238.1	262.8
Prescription drugs	47.8	47.4	51.2	72.5	120.1	181.7	235.0	285.4	326.3
Nonprescription drugs and medical supplies(a) (1986 = 100)						120.6	140.5	149.5	152.0
Medical care services	22.7	32.3	46.6	74.8	113.2	162.7	224.2	266.0	306.0
Professional services		37.0	50.8	77.9	113.5	156.1	201.0	237.7	261.2
Physicians' services	25.1	34.5	48.1	76.5	113.3	160.8	208.8	244.7	267.7
Dental services	30.3	39.2	53.2	78.9	114.2	155.8	206.8	258.5	292.5
Services by other medical professionals(b) (1986 = 100)						120.2	143.9	161.9	177.1
Hospital and related services				69.2	116.1	178.0	257.8	317.3	394.8
Hospital room	12.3	23.6	38.3	68.0	115.4	175.4	251.2		
Other inpatient hospital services(c) (1986 = 100)						142.7	206.8		
Other services(d) (1986 = 100)						138.7	204.6		
Hospital services (1996 = 100)								115.9	144.7
Nursing homes and adult daycare (1996 = 100)								117.0	135.2

Sources: U.S. Department of Labor, Bureau of Labor Statistics, Consumer Price Indexes, http://www.bls.gov/cpi/ (accessed on February 3, 2004).

Note: The only indexes available prior to 1978 are for urban wage earners and clerical workers. However, the table uses the more comprehensive All Urban Consumer indexes, which were introduced in 1978, for the year 1980. After the 1987 revision, all of the services include benefits paid by consumer-purchased insurance as well as consumer out-of-pocket expenditures.

(a) Excludes eyeglasses.

(b) Includes all consumer out-of-pocket expenses for eye care commodities.

(c) Consists of other hospital and inpatient services including nursing and convalescent home service.

(d) Consists of emergency room services, laboratory fees, and x-rays.

The Weight of the MCPI in the CPI

The population covered by the MCPI and the overall CPI is, of course, the same. Since 1978 when the population coverage was extended to include the elderly, the population included in the MCPI has become more representative of the general population.

Although the population has become more representative, an important factor affecting the weight of the MCPI is the *exclusion of services that are paid for by the government (Medicare and Medicaid) and by employer contributions to health insurance policies for their employees.* The CPI attempts to measure goods and services purchased out of pocket by consumers. However, in expanding the population coverage of the CPI, the BLS added groups for whom the government, through Medicare and Medicaid, pays a large portion of their medical care services. Previously when the aged, who are large consumers of medical services, were excluded, the weight assigned to medical care in the traditional CPI understated its importance in total consumption for the entire population. The relative weights of particular services within the MCPI were also different from the relative weights of those items in total U.S. medical care consumption. Hospital services, for example, are relatively more important for the elderly and unemployed than for urban wage earners and clerical workers. Dentists' fees are relatively less important.

The value of services not considered by the BLS because only consumer out-of-pocket payments are considered is substantial; in 1994, 37 percent of all medical care was purchased by governmental agencies, while 26 percent of all medical care was paid for by employers (5). In keeping with its general policy, the BLS does not attempt to reflect these governmental expenditures in the CPI weights. The MCPI is not designed as an index of the price of the bundle of medical care services *consumed* by its target population, but of those services *purchased* by it.

Table 4-5 shows how the weight of medical care within the CPI index would be different if the index covered the entire population and total medical expenditures rather than just consumer out-of-pocket payments. For 1975, 1985, 1995, and 2002, the CPI weight of medical care is compared with the weight of *consumer* expenditures on health services and supplies in personal consumption and with the weight of *total* expenditures on personal health care *plus* government purchases.

In the comparison years, both of the former weights are smaller than the weight of medical care in personal consumption plus government expenditures; this reflects the large role by government and employers in financing medical services. It appears that the CPI weight of medical care will continue to understate the importance of medical care in total consumption, particularly if the role of government in this sector continues to expand and the CPI fails to include such expenditures in determining its weights.

Table 4-6 describes how the weights of specific medical care components differ according to which expen-

Table 4-5. Weights of Medical Care in CPI, in Personal Consumption, and in Personal Consumption Plus Government Purchases, Calendar Years 1975, 1985, 1995, and 2002

	1975	1985	1995	2002
Weight of medical care in CPI	6.4	6.5	6.3	6.0
Weight of consumer expenditure on health services and supplies in personal consumption	4.8*(a)*	4.7	5.4	5.8
Weight of total expenditures on health services and supplies in personal consumption plus government purchases*(b)*	9.2	11.8	15.6	16.6

Sources: U.S. Department of Labor, Bureau of Labor Statistics, http://data.bls.gov/cgi-bin/dsrv (accessed on January 12, 2004); Centers for Medicare & Medicaid Services, Office of the Actuary: National Health Statistics Group, http://www.cms.gov/statistics/nhe (accessed on January 8, 2004); U.S. Department of Commerce, Bureau of Economic Analysis, http://www.bea.doc.gov/bea/dn/nipaweb/SelectTable.asp?Selected=N (accessed on January 12, 2004).

(a) 1972–1973 figure

(b) Total expenditures on health services and supplies (total National Health Expenditures) as a percentage of consumer expenditures plus government purchases. The difference between consumer expenditures plus government purchases and GNP is that GNP includes private investments and net exports. Neither private investments nor net exports are relevant in determining the weight of health care expenditures on consumer and government budgets.

Table 4-6. Relative Weights of Items in MCPI, in Consumer Expenditures on Health Services and Supplies, and in Total National Expenditures on Health Services and Supplies, Calendar Years 1975, 1985, 1995, 2002

	1975			1985			1995			2002		
	MCPI(a) (Dec. 1975)	Consumer(b) Expenditures (1972–73)	Total Expenditures	MCPI(a) (Dec. 1985)	Consumer Expenditures(b)	Total Expenditures	MCPI(a) (Dec. 1995)	Consumer Expenditures(b)	Total Expenditures	MCPI(a) (Dec. 2002)	Consumer Expenditures(b)	Total Expenditures
Medical services		80.1										
Hospital services	28.5	—(c)	40.2	26.4	26.6	39.3	30.7	31.2	35.4	22.9	31.5	31.3
Physicians' services	26.0	—(c)	18.3	27.0	27.2	19.5	25.7	24.8	20.4	25.4	22.8	21.9
Dental services	14.4	—(c)	6.1	15.1	15.7	5.1	14.5	14.1	4.6	12.8	13.1	4.5
Nursing home	—(c)	—(c)	6.6	—(c)	1.4	7.2	—(c)	1.4	7.9	1.4	1.5	6.6
All others(d)	15.5	0.0	13.1	8.8	8.7	13.2	6.9	7.0	17.0	8.9	6.1	15.2
Medical care commodities	12.0	16.5	11.9	18.9	16.9	10.2	17.4	16.4	9.8	23.3	19.9	13.7
Health insurance(e)	3.6	3.4	3.8	3.8	3.5	5.6	4.9	5.1	4.8	5.3	5.1	6.8
Total	100.0	100.0	100.0	100.0	100.0	100.0	100.1	100.0	99.9	100.0	100.0	100.0

Sources: U.S. Department of Labor, Bureau of Labor Statistics, *Relative Importance of Components of the Consumer Price Index, various issues;* U.S. Department of Labor, Bureau of Labor Statistics, *Consumer Expenditure Survey: Integrated Survey Data,* various issues, and personal correspondence, January 12, 2004; U.S. Department of Health and Human Services, Centers for Medicare & Medicaid Services, http://www.cms.gov/statistics/nhe (accessed on January 8, 2004).

(a) The index for all Urban Consumers is used.

(b) The amount of charges paid by consumer-paid health insurance has been allocated to specific services using the 1987 allocation rate provided to us by BLS.

(c) Data are not available. Prior to 1980, there is no breakdown of "Medical services" in the Consumer Expenditure Survey. Also, there is no breakdown of "Nursing home" from "Other Outpatient Services" in MCPI; they are included in "Hospital Services."

(d) "All others" in MCPI includes "Eye Care" and "Services by other medical professionals"; in Consumer Expenditures, it includes "Eye care services," "Services by other than physicians," "Lab test, x-rays," "Repair of medical equipment," and "Other medical care services"; in National Health Accounts (NHA), it includes "Other professional services," "Home health care," "Other personal health care," "Public health activities," "Research," and "Construction."

(e) Health Insurance has been allocated to different services according to the allocation rate used by CPI in 1987. Health insurance includes only that portion of the premium that is retained by the insurance carrier for administrative cost and profit.

Note: Totals may not add up to 100.0 due to rounding.

diture total is used (as described previously). Several components of medical care, such as hospitals and nursing homes, are constantly understated given the large role of government in paying for these services.

Accuracy of Measured Prices in the MCPI

For the MCPI, as with the CPI, BLS attempts to price items for which consumers have an out-of-pocket expenditure. For every such item, BLS attempts to measure a transaction price. A transaction price is the price a consumer actually pays for an item in the CPI market basket of goods and services.

The difference between hospital list prices (typically the charge to a full-paying patient) and the prices hospitals actually receive has been a major source of bias for the MCPI and, consequently, the CPI. Over time, there have been important changes in the percentage of patients who pay for hospital services completely out of pocket and the percentage of hospital list prices paid by private insurers and government.

Hospitals are paid different prices by different payers. Medicare changed from a cost-based per-day payment to a fixed price per admission, unrelated to list prices, starting in 1983. Medicare's price per admission also varies according to the patient's diagnosis. Medicaid typically pays hospitals a lower price than does Medicare. In addition to government payers, hospitals also charge self-payers (those without insurance) a separate price, while those who are uninsured and unable to pay may not be charged anything. Lastly, private insurers, HMOs, and Preferred Provider Organizations (PPOs) each negotiate separate prices with hospitals for their enrollees. Thus, a hospital may have upwards of 100 different prices. List prices are not indicative of actual prices received.

Over time, as competition among hospitals has increased, HMOs, PPOs, and private insurers have been able to negotiate larger discounts from hospitals' list prices. Thus the difference between list and transactions prices has increased. Previously, list prices increased faster than actual prices (this may have changed in the last several years as hospital competition has declined). Therefore, for many years the MCPI has been overstating the rise in hospital inflation, resulting in an upward bias in the MCPI.

Dranove, et al., studied the magnitude of the upward bias in hospital prices when list prices rather than transactions prices are used (10). Using data from California hospitals for the period 1983 to 1988, it was found that inflation in list prices exceeded the rise in actual prices by a factor of two.

Thus, although hospital services are underweighted in the MCPI because third party payers pay a large percentage of hospital care, the price of hospital services has risen very rapidly (faster than any other category in the MCPI) because hospital list prices were measured rather than transaction prices. Thus the bias in hospital prices has had a large impact on both the rise in the MCPI as well as on the CPI.

From a policy perspective, the upward bias in the hospital services index has hidden the impact that hospital price competition has had during the late 1980s and 1990s. (A similar problem has occurred with the price of physician services.)

Recognizing the problem between hospital list and actual prices, BLS is attempting to collect data on actual prices paid. In 1993, BLS developed a Producer Price Index (PPI) for both hospital and physician services based on the provider's transaction prices. (See the Appendix for an explanation of the PPI.) The PPI was used as a supplement to the CPI. Beginning in January 1997, the CPI pricing methodology for hospitals is similar to the PPI so as to more accurately reflect actual hospital prices.

In collecting transaction prices for the MCPI, however, BLS has relied on voluntary reporting by medical care providers, especially hospitals and physicians. Given the high degree of price competition within the healthcare environment, providers have been reluctant to give the BLS their actual price information. A General Accounting Office report in 1996 found that only 15 percent of hospital price quotes for the MCPI included the discounts from list price (11).

The difference between list and actual prices was also a problem for each of the other components of the MCPI. For example, with regard to physician services, BLS previously gathered data from physicians on their usual or customary charges for particular services instead of the more relevant average fee received by the physician. Customary charges differed from average prices *received* because customary charges were not actual prices, and not all charges were collected. For example, physicians participating in Preferred Provider Organizations discount their fees to a subset of patients. Further, customary charges changed at a different rate than the fees actually received by the physician. BLS moved to correct this problem in the 1987 revision of the CPI by collecting actual physician fee data by payer type.

The measurement of prescription drug prices is a major source of bias in the MCPI. The rise in drug prices has been a source of concern for many, particularly the aged, since Medicare does not cover prescription drugs, and a large part of the price is paid for out of pocket. The rise in BLS' prescription drug price index has been used by critics of the drug industry and by legislators to propose limits on rising drug prices. Researchers believe that BLS' approach to measuring drug price increases results in a serious overstatement of the rise in drug prices.

When a drug's patent protection expires and generic versions of the drug enter the market, consumers who act as though the branded and generic versions of the drug are equivalent benefit by paying less for the generic drug. Prior to 1995, however, the BLS defined products too narrowly, and close substitutes were treated as though they were new goods. Consequently, BLS did not measure price declines for those consumers who switched to the generic version. When a close substitute entered the market, such as with a generic drug, BLS "linked in" the generic drug to the index. Not all consumers of the branded drug, however, switch to the generic version. Consequently, the linking process is appropriate for those consumers since the generic version is not a good substitute. (When a generic version enters the market at a lower price than the branded drug, the branded drug often increases in price since those that continue to purchase the branded drug have a less price elastic demand.)

There are three problems with the BLS approach of linking, which assumes the generic version is a completely separate good. First, BLS does not include the generic version of the drug when it immediately comes on the market. Instead, there is a lag period. Drugs, similar to other products, have a life cycle. When they are first introduced their prices are relatively high, and later in the cycle their prices decline. By linking the

generic version after a lag time, BLS misses the decline in price of that drug.

The same lag problem occurs with new branded drugs. New drug prices frequently decline after their introduction as production expands and competition occurs among drugs in the same therapeutic class. Because the price of the new branded drug is higher than existing, competitive, drugs, the higher price purchasers are willing to pay reflects a difference in actual or perceived quality. It is thus appropriate for BLS to link these new drugs into its index and treat them as a new good. However, by the time BLS links these new drugs into the drug price index, their price may have already declined as "me-too" drugs are developed for the same disease, resulting in an overstatement of the index.

Second, the weight given to the generic drug by BLS in its index is too small. Even though BLS picks up the generic drug late, its market share continues to grow, and thus its weight in the index should continue to increase.

Third, because the generic drug is treated as a separate good and linked in, the price decline experienced by those consumers who switch to the generic drug is not reflected in the BLS drug price index.

Studying only a limited number of drugs to illustrate the problem of the prescription drug price index, researchers contrasted the BLS approach with alternative methods (12). The BLS approach assumes that the entry of generic drugs, once the patent protection of a branded good expired, was equivalent to a completely new product and not to be compared to the branded product. The BLS approach resulted in a 14 percent price increase over a 45-month period. An alternative approach that assumes the generic and brand name drugs are perfect substitutes results in a 53 percent decline in price. (An adjusted Paasche index, preferred by the researchers, declined by 48 percent.) Additionally, prior to 1996, emphasis on older drugs exacerbated the bias. A study estimated the bias caused by over-sampling older drugs to be near 3 percent. To correct for this, the BLS now adds to the drugs sampled in the market basket with additional supplementary drugs for more accurate pricing (5).

Given this disparity between new and old drugs, BLS instituted changes in how prescription drugs were measured to correct for the dual problem of frequent introductions and substitutability. A revision in 1995 treated branded and generic drugs as equivalent 6 months after patent expiration with the probability of being chosen and included in the index between the two versions being proportional to their respective sales (8). Thus BLS' drug price index has had a significant upward bias.

Quality Changes and New Products

A third major problem with the MCPI is in regard to changes in quality. The BLS measures inflation by calculating price changes in a constant quality basket of goods and services. It is particularly difficult, however, to control for quality when measuring changes in prices of medical services. For example, the outcome of open heart surgery has improved over time, less invasive surgical techniques are being used, and innovative drugs have lessened the need for surgical intervention and prolonged life expectancy. Similarly, with regard to physician services, medical knowledge has improved, physicians are better trained than in the past, and together with improved technology, their diagnoses and treatment of illnesses have been improved. A physician visit is not the same product or of similar quality as a visit 10 or 20 years ago.

The intensity (inputs) of medical services has increased over time, and medical outcomes have improved. The approach taken by BLS, however, has generally been to ignore quality change and assume that any price increase is solely due to inflation.[7]

Recently the BLS made minor adjustments in its methodology to account for the changing nature of medical care. Driven by cost-cutting pressures, procedures that were performed in an inpatient setting have been shifted to an outpatient facility. As less intensive procedures that once required inpatient care, such as colonoscopies, have been shifted to an outpatient setting, inpatient procedures and treatments have become more intensive and expensive. As more formerly inpatient surgeries have been shifted to an outpatient setting, the average outpatient encounter has also become more expensive. Prior to 1997, the CPI measured inpatient and outpatient hospital services as separate cost entities. As the average price of each setting increased, the hospital services portion of the CPI overestimated price growth. In recognition of this problem, the BLS began treating inpatient and outpatient care as one category to capture the effect of the shift to outpatient care.

The problem of quality adjustment is particularly troublesome for hospital services, since it is the fastest increasing component of the MCPI (13). Prior to 1972, hospital services were represented in the MCPI by daily room charges only. The index of semiprivate room charges was frequently cited as an index of the price of hospital care. This use of the semiprivate room charge not only ignored problems of quality change, but also presumed that the prices of other inpatient services not included in the basic room charge were changing at the same rate.[8] In 1972, an expanded hospital service charge index was introduced. It included the semiprivate room charge, the operating room charge, and the charges for eight specific ancillary services. The 1978 revision specified a much larger number of services for pricing.

Prior to 1997, the items that were priced in the Hospital and Related Services Index were individual components of a hospital admission. Further, the most important component in the hospital service

---

7. Except, apparently, when an obvious method of adjustment is available. For example, in 1961 obstetricians' fees for obstetrical cases were substituted for general practitioners' fees for the same service. The obstetricians' fees were linked in—that is, the difference between their fees and those of general practitioners was attributed entirely to a quality difference. Similarly, if a service (e.g., a throat culture) were routinely given to all patients as part of a limited office visit, then that new service would be linked in to the price of that type of visit.

8. The room charge index is also sensitive to changes in hospital pricing policies that may not affect the overall level of hospital charges. The extremely rapid increase in the semi-private room charge index immediately after the introduction of Medicare was probably in part due to a movement away from the traditional policy of keeping room rates below average costs (since patients could compare different hospitals' room charges before entering the hospital) and having very high price mark-ups over cost on ancillary services (once in the hospital patients no longer had a choice of sellers of such services).

charge index was the basic room charge, which was not a constant-quality item. Although BLS recognizes that service quality might include patient satisfaction, mortality rate from surgical procedures, frequency of postoperative infections, patient functional health status, and even intensity of resource utilization, BLS believed that no single measure could, by itself, offer a measure of the quality of a hospital service. Since increased hospital prices are minimally adjusted for quality improvements, BLS seriously overstated the rise in hospital and medical prices.

As previously noted, prior to 1997 the CPI measured hospital use by the day. As the average length of a hospital stay began to decrease in the early 1980s, the reduced stay led to an overall lower price per hospital admission compared to the assumption of a constant stay. However, the greater intensity of care during the shortened stay led to higher prices per day. The BLS approach of pricing by hospital *day* indicated a higher hospital inflation rate and failed to capture the overall savings derived from an abbreviated hospital admission.

To adjust for the shortened length of stay and higher price per day, the BLS instituted reporting per hospital *stay* in 1997. (The reduced length of hospital stay was thus used as a proxy for improved quality.) This change in pricing involved surveying the types of hospital admissions based on the primary diagnosis for treatment. The BLS then samples individual patient bills from hospital medical records. Using this treatment data from the initial period, the CPI then compares out-of-pocket prices for similar hospital treatment episodes over different time periods.

A TREATMENT APPROACH TO MEASURING THE RISE IN MEDICAL PRICES

The BLS constructs its MCPI by measuring how a fixed set of inputs (a hospital stay, a physician office visit, drug prices, etc.) have increased over time. However, when people become ill, they are not interested in purchasing a specific set of inputs, but rather a treatment for their illness. The specific goods and services that function as inputs—physician visits, hospital bed days, prescription drugs, and so forth—

function as inputs that are combined to produce medical treatments. It is therefore reasonable to measure the cost of medical care by looking at specific illnesses and determining how the average cost per treatment episode has changed over time. Economists have found this cost-of-treatment approach to measuring medical care costs conceptually appealing.

A treatment approach for measuring changes in medical prices could incorporate the effects on prices of improvements in quality, new medical technology, new drugs, as well as input substitution for providing a medical treatment. Treatment for a medical condition can be provided entirely in the hospital, or it can be provided in part with hospital care, outpatient services, and home health care. With improvements in medical technology and the movement toward managed care, many surgical procedures previously performed in the hospital are now performed in outpatient surgery centers, thereby reducing the price of that treatment. The costs-of-treatment index would increase less and perhaps even decline, depending on the net effect of input substitution and improved quality.

Further, a treatment approach to measuring medical prices would facilitate adjustments for changes in treatment outcomes. The probability of recovery might be increased, there may be a reduction in the amount of pain, and improvements may occur in the patient's wellbeing and lifestyle.

In 1962, Anne Scitovsky detailed a proposal for a treatment index based on the treatment costs for specific illnesses aggregated into a composite index, weighting each component by the percentage of total medical expenditures spent on that illness in a base year (14). This procedure is analogous to the method by which the various component indexes are aggregated into the all-items CPI.

Recognizing that her proposed index would not automatically adjust for such changes in the quality of treatments, Scitovsky suggested that for each illness included in the calculation of the index, a single objective indicator of quality be chosen. For example, the number of live births per 100 pregnancies might be the quality measure for maternity cases. Using quality indicators to adjust the individual costs-of-treatment indexes would have "the great merit of making possible more complete and systematic correction for quality changes," Scitovsky argued. (The issue of how to deal with changes in the quality of treatments is a major point of contention in the debate over the merits of this approach to measuring the cost of medical care.)

A modification of the original Scitovsky idea arose out of a comment by Yoram Barzel. Using the example of polio, he argued that although the costs of treating individual cases of polio may have remained constant or possibly increased, the introduction of the polio vaccine has led to a drop in the total cost of polio because its incidence has been curtailed. Barzel contended that it is more appropriate to look at the *expected* treatment costs of an illness rather than at the treatment costs of cases that actually occur (15).

The prevention of an illness clearly represents an output that is superior to the successful treatment of the illness. Measuring the price of a specific treatment over time ignores the influence of preventive medical care. An index that measures the costs of medical treatments should reflect the role of preventive care, otherwise it gives a misleading view of changes in the price of care and the productivity of the industry.

Not all prevention, however, is the result of the medical sector. Prevention may occur because of changes in personal health habits, environmental improvements, information gathered from different sources, and so on. Thus using an expected cost of treatment approach would attribute a lower expected cost of treatment solely to the medical care industry, which would overstate productivity improvements in medical care and thereby result in a downward bias in the index.

Recent Cost-of-Treatment Studies

Several studies have recently been completed using the cost-of-treatment approach to indicate the extent of bias in the MCPI. The researchers constructed two new indexes of medical care prices, which they then applied to a particular disease: heart attack (acute myocardial infarction, or AMI). The two indexes were a Service Price Index and a Cost of Living Index (6). Conceptually, this approach results in a price index of particular medical treatments over time.

The Service Price Index focuses on the services (inputs) actually used in treatment and is somewhat similar to the current MCPI which also measures how the price of a given set of services (inputs) have changed over time. Neither the Service Price Index nor the MCPI adjust rising prices for quality improvements or for changes in inputs.

The Cost of Living Index is an attempt to incorporate quality changes. While the Service Price Index measures how the price of a treatment has changed, using a constant set of services, the Cost of Living Index adjusts the increase in treatment price by subtracting the additional value gained from the treatment. In effect, this index adjusts for quality by considering how much more consumers would be willing to pay for better quality treatments, that is, to have the current medical treatment at current prices compared to the previous (base period) treatment at previous prices.

Heart attacks were chosen as the treatment to be studied because heart disease (which is more inclusive than heart attacks) accounts for almost one-seventh of medical spending, and treatment costs for heart attacks have risen rapidly in recent years. Heart attacks are also a readily definable episode with a beginning and a measurable outcome, survival. Given the outcome measure, it becomes easier to establish a value for such a treatment than for other types of treatment with different types of outcomes.

Two sources of data were used for the study: detailed data on services, prices, the discharge abstract, and demographic information for all heart attack patients admitted to a single major teaching hospital for the period 1983 and 1994 and, second, data on Medicare patients who had a heart attack between the period 1984 and 1994.

Neither the Service Price Index nor the Cost of Living Index were adjusted for factors affecting the incidence of illness, such as changes in lifestyle which would affect the expected cost of heart disease. Further, the authors recognize that if their study were to be extended to examine the price of all medical services, then multiple treatment indexes would have to be calculated and adjustments made for their changing weights over time.

The authors found that the rise in the Service Price Index rose less rapidly than a method based on the

MCPI. The study results are summarized in Table 4-7. All of the annual percent increases are adjusted for inflation. Over the time period studied, 1983 to 1994, the MCPI rose 3.4 percent per year. The Hospital Services component of the MCPI rose even more rapidly, 6.2 percent annually.

As discussed above, for many years the BLS used list prices for a constant set of services over time. As a comparison with their treatment approach, the authors constructed a "synthetic" MCPI that was based on list prices for hospital services used in treatment of a heart attack. (The synthetic MCPI allowed for changes in the use of the hospital.) The synthetic MCPI increased by 3.3 percent annually, more slowly than the BLS' Hospital Services Index of 6.2 percent.

The authors constructed a second synthetic treatment MCPI that used actual prices (based on the hospital's accounting costs) rather than list prices. This index rose even more slowly, by 2.4 percent annually.

By measuring changes in prices of a fixed set of inputs, the BLS' MCPI cannot adjust for changes in the mix of treatments provided to patients with a heart

attack, which have changed over time. In 1984, 65 percent of heart attack patients at the hospital studied received medical management, but by 1994 only 23 percent of patients were treated with this approach. Similarly, the comparable percentages for the earlier and the more current period were: catherization only, 20 percent and 21 percent; angioplasty, 3 percent and 30 percent; and bypass surgery, 11 percent and 27 percent. There has been a dramatic shift over time to more expensive treatment methods.

Even within each of these treatment methods there have been shifts in the inputs used for treatment. For example, the use of operating room time increased by 38 percent for bypass surgery patients, while their length of stay declined by 22 percent.

To account for this shift to more expensive treatment methods and shifts in the use of inputs within each treatment type, the authors developed a set of additional Patient Weighted Price Indexes (PWPI) that could be re-weighted (or "chain weighted") at different time intervals. One chain weighted PWPI re-weights the mix of treatments every 5 years; the other recalculates the weights every year. These chain weighted indexes are compared to a price index, similar to the MCPI (referred to as the Laspeyres PWPI) that does not re-weight the change in mix of treatments for heart attack patients. Over the time period studied, the Laspeyres Index increased by 2.8 percent per year. The 5-year chain weighted index rose 2.1 percent per year, and the chain weighted index that was re-weighted annually increased by only 0.7 percent per year.

The main reason for the lower rate of increase in the latter index is the weight placed on room charges. The length of stay in the hospital decreased sharply over that time period (36 percent), while the hospital room charge increased by 60 percent. Unless these changes in input use are recognized by more frequent re-weighting which would have captured the decrease in length of stay, the MCPI is likely to have a serious upward bias. The BLS has responded with more frequent re-weighting schemes, but this study illustrates the difficulty inherent in measuring a treatment that can be performed in many different ways.

The above treatment indexes did not attempt to adjust prices for changes in the treatment outcome. To

Table 4-7. Annual Rates of Change in Various Medical Price Indices, Adjusted for Inflation, 1983–1994

Index	Real Annual Change
Service Price Indices	
Basic Components Price Indices	
MCPI	3.4%
Hospital Component	6.2
Room	6.0
Other Inpatient Services	5.7
Synthetic MCPI for MTH—Charges	3.3
Synthetic MCPI for MTH—Costs	2.4
Patient Weighted Price Index—Laspeyres	2.8
Patient Weighted Price Index—5-Year Chain Index	2.1
Patient Weighted Price Index—Annual Chain Index	0.7
Cost of Living Index (1984–1994)	–1.1%

Source: This table is based on David M. Cutler et al., "Are Medical Prices Declining? Evidence From Heart Attack Treatments," *The Quarterly Journal of Economics,* 113(4), November 1998: 991–1024.

remedy this, the authors constructed a Cost of Living Index to adjust treatment costs for changes in life expectancy. To calculate this, it was necessary to estimate the value of an additional year of life less the costs of producing that additional year. (To place a value on the additional years remaining after a heart attack, several different values of an additional life year were used.)

When the BLS approach was contrasted with the Cost of Living Index, the authors found that the latter index actually *decreased (adjusted for inflation) by about 1 percent per year; a difference of 4 percent per year between the two indexes.*

The authors conclude that by adjusting for both differences between list and actual prices paid and by including changes in the mix of treatments actually used (annual chain weighted PWPI), the result is a much slower rate of increase in medical prices, about 0.7 percent per year as compared to 3.3 percent per year (synthetic MCPI-charges) adjusted for inflation. Further, *if the MCPI were actually a Cost of Living Index, then medical prices would be falling rather than increasing.*

Thus the MCPI approach substantially overstates the amount of price inflation. Further, rather than the rapid price increases that have been indicated by the MCPI, the inflation-adjusted price of medical care may actually have been falling over this time period. (The authors caution that the estimate of the Cost of Living Index is dependent upon the assumed value of life.)

Assuming that the results of the above study can be generalized to other medical services, the MCPI seriously overstates the rise in medical price inflation.

While this study provides some indication as to how much the MCPI is upward biased, it should be kept in mind that the study is based on data from one teaching hospital, using one disease type (heart attack patients) where the services are provided within the hospital, and uses one outcome measure, additional life years. Constructing a new MCPI price index based on this approach would be highly useful, but also quite difficult.

A similar disease-based approach was used to study acute depression (16). In this case, the outcome measure was treatment of depressive symptoms rather than mortality. Further, to correct for quality variations among the different treatments available to clinicians, the researchers utilized standard of care guidelines based on both the federal government's Agency for Health Care Policy Research and the American Psychiatric Association recommendations. The standards included various treatment options, including psychotherapy, pharmacological therapy (using different classes of anti-depressant medications), and combination treatments. Price indexes were constructed based on these standards, weighted by expenditure amounts on differing types of treatment methods. Nine treatment bundles were identified from clinical research that resulted in similar outcomes, later aggregated into five standards by the researchers. The implicit assumption is that similar outcomes from alternative treatments approximate similar utility levels among consumers. From these data, various indexes were constructed, including a Producer Price Index, an index based on out-of-pocket costs paid for by the consumer (equivalent to the MCPI), and other indexes based upon assumptions of substitutability of treatments.

The pricing data set was derived from insurance claims processed during the years 1991 through 1995 from four large self-insured employers comprising 428,168 enrollees. The data were retrospectively sorted to define those patients diagnosed as having major depression based on the ICD-9 diagnostic codes, and treated as outpatients. Over 10,000 cases were identified. However, only 20 to 25 percent of those cases received treatment consistent with the standards of care.

The authors priced the treatment bundles for the periods of 1991 and 1995 using producer prices (PPI) and consumer out-of-pocket prices (CPI). (The PPI prices of the treatment include the total of all the payments to providers from all payers including insurers and patients, who typically pay co-payments and deductibles). Patient out-of-pocket payments (CPI) changed during the study period because of changes in insurance benefit design, such as increased cost sharing and greater use of out-of-network providers by patients as managed care plans used more restrictive provider networks. Table 4-8 presents the results of the study based on the PPI approach, while Table 4-9 summarizes the results using the CPI approach.

For both the PPI and CPI analyses, Laspeyres (base period quantity fixed weights) and Paasche (final period quantity weights) indexes were used. Both the Laspeyres and Paasche indexes were calculated with fixed (constant) weights and chain (updated) weighted.

The general conclusion using the PPI treatment approach presented in Table 4-8 is that over the time period studied, the price of treating acute major depression either remained the same or decreased slightly. In contrast, the BLS' PPI approach, using inputs rather than a treatment, over this same time period increased by 5 percent and for antidepressants increased 20 percent.

Table 4-9 compares the treatment approach to BLS' input approach based on consumer out-of-pocket payments. Over the time period studied, the price of treating acute major depression rose between 27 and 33 percent, depending upon whether the Laspeyres or Paasche index is used and whether it is fixed or chained weighted. In contrast the BLS' CPI indexes for Medical Care and for Prescription Drugs rose by 27 and 18 percent, respectively. (As discussed above, consumer out-of-pocket payments using the treatment approach increased because of increases in their cost sharing rather than price increases.)

Table 4-8.   Producer Price Index (PPI) Treatment Price Indexes for Acute Major Depression

Price Index	1991	1995
Fixed Weights		
Laspeyres	1.00	.98
Passche	1.00	1.00
Chained Weights		
Laspeyres	1.00	.97
Passche	1.00	.98
BLS PPIs*		
Aggregate PPI	1.00	1.05
Antidepressants	1.00	1.20

Source: Adapted from Ernst Berndt, Susan Bresch, and Richard Frank, "Treatment Price Indexes for Acute Phase Major Depression" in David M. Cutler and Ernst Berndt, eds., *Medical Care Output and Productivity* (University of Chicago Press, Chicago), 2001, p. 491.

*BLS indexes are normalized to appropriate base year.

Table 4-9.   Consumer Price Indexes (CPI) Treatment Price Indexes for Acute Major Depression

Price Index	1991	1995
Fixed Weights		
Laspeyres	1.00	1.27
Passche	1.00	1.33
Chained Weights		
Laspeyres	1.00	1.28
Passche	1.00	1.32
BLS CPIs*		
All Items	1.00	1.12
Medical Care	1.00	1.27
Prescription Drugs	1.00	1.18

Source: Adapted from Ernst Berndt, Susan Bresch, and Richard Frank, "Treatment Price Indexes for Acute Phase Major Depression" in David M. Cutler and Ernst Berndt, eds., *Medical Care Output and Productivity* (University of Chicago Press, Chicago), 2001, p. 491.

*BLS indexes are normalized to appropriate base year.

This study finds that price indexes using the PPI treatment approach generate lower price inflation than the less accurate treatment approach based on consumer out-of-pocket payments and also lower than the price inflation indicated by BLS' PPI and CPI, which uses an input approach (as shown at the bottom of Table 4-8 and Table 4-9).

Evaluating the Cost-of-Treatment Approach

The results of the above studies clearly show that in the absence of adjustments for changes in actual prices paid, changes in the mix of treatments, and improvements in treatment outcomes, the MCPI has a serious upward bias. In evaluating the merits of the costs-of-treatment approach to measuring the costs of medical care, it is important to consider whether a practical method exists for making adjustments for changes in treatment quality.

Three serious problems hinder the implementation of a cost-of-treatment approach. The first is that the quality of a medical treatment is truly multidimensional; a single quality indicator for each illness might be too simplistic. The probability of recovery, the expected number of disability days, the probable extent of physical impairments once recovery is completed, the painfulness of the treatment, and the amenities provided along with it are only some of the relevant aspects of the quality of a treatment. Determining how different treatment methods affect these different aspects of quality might be very costly, although such information would obviously be useful for other purposes besides the construction of a medical care price index.

The second problem, which would still be troublesome even if complete information existed on the technical aspects of the outcomes of different treatment methods, arises when placing values on differences in treatment quality. What value, for example, should be placed on a slightly lower probability of death from a particular disease, or on a little less pain? The problem of determining such values is as much conceptual as technical; its solution is not clear. A reduction in the frequency of miscarriages certainly represents an improvement in the quality of maternity care, however, is it appropriate to assume that an obstetrician who is 99.9 percent successful in delivering babies is exactly twice as good as one who delivers only one live birth for every two cases handled? A doubling of the success rate in delivering babies or in treating an illness might imply more than a two-fold increase in quality. But exactly how much more? This is the kind of question that must be answered if a cost-of-treatment index is to be adjusted correctly for changes in quality of treatments.

Third, should the *expected* treatment cost of an illness be used rather than the average costs of cases actually treated? Since expected treatment cost is the probability of contracting an illness multiplied by the average cost of treatment, it can be influenced by preventive medical care. Capitation payment provides HMOs and their providers with a financial incentive to substitute preventive services for more costly acute care. In principle, an expected-costs-of-treatment index could be calculated in the manner described earlier. For each illness, the total costs of treatment would be averaged over the number of cases treated plus the number of cases prevented. However, it is not simple to distinguish the number of cases eliminated by preventive medical care alone.

Incidence rates of illnesses are influenced by many factors, including nutrition, personal health habits, lifestyle, and environmental factors such as pollution levels. Simply comparing the incidence of an illness in a base year with that in a later year and taking the difference as a measure of the effects of preventive care is unsatisfactory. Other factors may be responsible for the difference. If birthrates go down and less is spent on maternity care, for example, does this mean that the medical care industry is more productive? Is it more productive if the nation decreases its consumption of cigarettes and the incidence of lung cancer goes down? Surely the answer is no in both cases. Ideally, then, the effects of preventive care on incidence rates should be computed separately from those of other factors when preparing an index of expected treatment costs. Multivariate statistical techniques might be used for this task, but it is questionable whether precise estimates could be obtained.

Despite its limitations, the costs-of-treatment approach retains a theoretical appeal; it would enable more meaningful comparisons to be made of the cost of medical care, both cross-sectionally and over time.

SUMMARY

The current Medical Care Price Index has a number of serious limitations that result in an upward bias in both the MCPI as well as in the CPI, of which it is a component. Although the MCPI has become more representative of the U.S. population, the index only measures consumers' out-of-pocket expenditures rather than what consumers consume, including what third-party payers spend on their behalf, leading to a smaller weight of the MCPI in the overall CPI.

The MCPI infrequently re-weighs the basket of goods and services purchased by consumers thereby neglecting to account for substitution bias (consumers switching to less expensive services as base-period services increase in price) and incorporating new goods and services too late in the MCPI. In the most recent CPI revision, the price data collected from medical providers is becoming more representative of what patients, insurance companies, and other organizations actually pay the provider. However, in many cases the MCPI still relies on list prices rather than actual or transactions prices. Given the extensive discounting that occurs among hospitals and physicians, there is a large divergence between list and actual prices. All of the problems result in an upward bias in the MCPI.

An important conceptual problem with the MCPI is its emphasis on pricing inputs (such as a hospital stay and a physician visit) rather than an output approach, namely the treatment for an illness. The fixed-bundle-of-goods-and-services method of pricing medical care used by the BLS yields results that are difficult to interpret. Pricing the treatment of an illness seems a more appropriate concept of medical care output than pricing the inputs used in all treatments. Using a cost-of-treatment approach allows for substitution of inputs and the introduction of new inputs. Frequent re-weighting of the inputs used in treatment would further improve the cost of treatment approach. Aggregating the distribution of treatments by their cost would be an alternative measure of the price of medical care.

Finally, an accurate measure of how medical prices are changing over time should adjust for changes in treatment outcomes and quality of care. Studies that have attempted to account for treatment outcomes using the cost-of-treatment approach find that the MCPI greatly overstates the amount of medical price inflation.

The difficulty in accounting for quality change, the introduction of new products, substitution bias, transaction prices, more frequent re-weighting, and so on, raises questions about what the MCPI does and what it ought to measure. There is serious concern that the MCPI greatly overstates the amount of medical price inflation.

Still, enormous practical difficulties and perhaps considerable cost would be involved in actually constructing a costs-of-treatment index as a substitute for the MCPI. In addition, some conceptual problems involved in this approach have not been solved adequately, most notably the issues of how to deal with changes in the quality of medical treatments and how to take account of the preventive aspects of medical care.

As medical care as a percent of GDP and government expenditures continues to increase rapidly, it becomes increasingly important for public policy to measure whether these increased expenditures represent greater value for which consumers are willing to pay.

APPENDIX 1: THE PRODUCER PRICE INDEX

The Producer Price Index (PPI) measures the average change in prices received by producers for their products. These data are collected from domestic producers based on the transaction prices of their goods and services. Unlike the CPI which collects data based on consumer out-of-pocket payments, the PPI includes price information from all sources, both public (e.g., Medicare) and private sources (e.g., third-party insurance payments). This producer price information is reported by industry and is a price index of the output of that industry. However, the PPI has not constructed an aggregate price index for the medical care sector. Instead, it collects price information from separate industries within medical care; hospitals, physician's offices, and nursing homes are each considered separate industries. While no aggregated medical care PPI has existed, plans are in place to begin calculating aggregate PPI data beginning in January of 2002.

The PPI has some of the same problems as the CPI. The PPI uses a Laspeyres weighting procedure, which relies on fixed weights thereby not allowing for substitution until the revision period. Also, the PPI does not adjust for quality.

Similar to the CPI, the PPI for hospitals prices the entire bundle of services provided during the hospital stay. However, unlike the CPI, the PPI collects hospital price data for all the types of payers, government, private insurance, etc. All hospital episodes are categorized by diagnostic and DRG (diagnostic related group, used by Medicare) codes, which allows for comparison of treatment costs specified to the disease entity over time. When BLS reprices the hospital admission, it also inquires whether the length of stay has changed for that diagnostic admission; if it has, then it is treated as a change in quality, not as a price change. A change in the average length of stay is the only quality adjustment made in the PPI for hospitals.

The PPI for hospital services has been published since December 1992.

Like the hospital PPI, the BLS collects data from all physician practices based on a stratified (by size and specialty) random sample. From the sample of physician offices, patient bills are randomly selected and categorized by diagnostic codes and services provided. The items on the patient's bill are kept constant (until the next major revision) and are re-priced monthly to gauge changes in prices using the Laspeyres price index formula. However, similar to the CPI, the use of a constant bundle of items precludes quality and treatment adjustments; in effect, it ignores substitution.

In addition to a lack of substitution within the physician and hospital services categories, there is the artificial separation between the hospital PPI and the physician services PPI, which ignores the possibility of substitution *between* the two services. Thus the PPI precludes any calculation of the benefits to consumers of shifts in care settings between hospital outpatient clinics and physician offices when similar services are provided in both settings.

BLS has published their PPI for physician services since December 1993.

Although the PPI is supposed to be based on transaction prices received by producers, the problem of differential pricing for different customers that creates upward biases in the CPI is also prevalent in the PPI. A study by Catron and Murphy (1996) (17) found that in 1995, 43.4 percent of inpatient price quotes and 64.6 percent of outpatient price quotes were based on list prices. Given the frequency of discounts within the hospital and physician payment system, reporting list prices provides an upward bias to the PPI price estimates.

The weights used in the PPI are recalculated more frequently than the CPI, every 5 years instead of every 10 for the CPI. In addition, it only takes 1 to 2 years to introduce those new weights in the PPI, whereas it takes about 3 to 4 years before the new weights are introduced in the CPI.

The PPI has a different purpose from that of the CPI. The CPI is a price index of the goods and services that consumers spend out of pocket and measures how much consumers would have to spend to buy the same basket of goods and services over time. The PPI measures the price of an industry's output, including the prices paid by all payers for that output. Thus, since the PPI includes governmental and third-party payments, industry-wide patterns can be evaluated, as for example, the impact of new technology or the effects of public policy changes on the price of an industry's output (8) (Berndt et al., 2000, 164). Further, the PPI can be used for comparing how the price of that industry's output has changed relative to the costs of that industry's inputs over time; an input price index by industry, however, is lacking.

APPENDIX 2: HEALTH INSURANCE PREMIUMS AS A MEASURE OF THE PRICE OF MEDICAL CARE

Prior to 1964, BLS directly priced health insurance premiums in the MCPI by pricing the most widely held Blue Cross-Blue Shield family plan in each sample area (the premiums of health insurance plans not priced were assumed to change at the same rate as those that were priced). Health insurance premiums may change in response to any of four types of changes: (1) changes in the price of medical services covered by the policy, (2) changes in administrative costs and profits, (3) changes in insurance benefits, and (4) changes in average utilization by enrollees. When measuring changes in premiums directly, BLS was unable to control for changes in benefit coverage or changes in use of services by enrollees which BLS considered to be quality changes. For that reason, BLS switched to indirect pricing of health insurance premiums.

Currently and since the 1964 CPI revision, BLS no longer directly prices health insurance policies. Instead, it does so indirectly by pricing a bundle of services representing those covered by health insurance. Insurance expenditures are placed into three categories: changes in the prices of medical care items covered by health insurance policies, changes in the cost of administering policies, and changes in the cost of maintaining reserves and profits. Most of the weight for health insurance is assigned to the first category; within this category, expenditure weights for each benefit area are allocated to each specific medical input index. Health insurance in the MCPI currently only includes those two expenditure categories not spent on medical services, namely administrative cost and profit. The insurance component is the result of a weighted average of the overhead of commercial insurers, Blue Cross Blue Shield, HMOs, and supplementary policies for Medicare Part B. The health insurance component still represents premium payments made by consumers only.

Given the criticisms of the current MCPI and the policy implications of its significant annual upward bias, BLS has, since 1999, begun testing an alternative MCPI by again directly pricing health insurance premiums (18). This new experimental health insurance index contains two item strata: Health Insurance Other than Medicare and, second, Medicare and Consumer Paid Medicare. The first is defined as the total out-of-pocket expense paid by consumers for health insurance. The second item strata only includes consumer payments for the Medicare Part B premium. (If BLS adopts direct pricing of premiums, then the insurance weights would have to be removed from the medical care input indexes.)

The experimental, new, health insurance index still faces some formidable challenges. A health insurance policy is not a constant-quality good over time. To be able to measure pure price changes in insurance premiums, BLS must be able to factor out from premium changes any changes that have occurred in benefits, quality of care (including technological improvements), and utilization by its enrollees. Each of these will affect changes in the insurance premium. Changes in medical care prices, such as increased hospital and physician fees, as well as increased insurer administrative costs, would be considered price effects. Premium changes due to benefit and utilization changes would generally be considered quality changes and, as such, should be used to adjust the premium.

Benefit levels in insurance policies may be increased or decreased. New services may be added or dropped, cost containment programs that restrict use of services may be added, and deductibles and co-payments may be increased or decreased. Any of these changes represent changes in quality; therefore the premium should be adjusted accordingly since premium changes due to benefit changes are not pure price changes. For example, if preventive care is added, the dollar value of this change should be subtracted from the premium because the consumer is receiving a different level of coverage than under the previous benefit level.

Technological changes that reduce the cost of treatment (a new prescription drug that eliminates the need for surgery) or increases the chance of recovery would lower the cost of treatment for a given outcome. The insurance premium should be adjusted down for a quality change.

Changes in average utilization by the policyholder will affect the premium, but in certain cases it is not clear whether the premium should be adjusted for some types of utilization changes. Demographic changes, such as an older insured population, will increase the demand for care; as the insured group has a higher risk level, the premium will increase. Clearly this is considered a quality change, and the premium should be adjusted down for increased risk levels of the insured group. Similarly, if the insurance benefit includes prescription drug coverage and the demand for drugs increase because of new drugs being developed or because of drug company advertising, then the consumer is realizing more coverage for the same premium, and the premium should also be adjusted downward.

However, if a new disease develops (such as AIDS), the premium will increase because of increased insurance expenditures on treatment. The insurer would likely view this increased use as a quality increase (hence the premium should be adjusted down) because the insurer is incurring greater risk and potential expenses. However, if an inexpensive cure is developed lowering the risk of the disease and its treatment cost, this would be considered a (quality) price (premium) decrease; but to do so, the disease and its treatment cost would have had to have been treated as an increase in price so that both effects would eventually be balanced out—the consumer is at the same level of health as before. If the new disease were initially treated as a quality change and the cure also as a (quality) price decrease, then the premium would be lower for the same level of health, which would not be correct. Therefore, it is not clear whether certain utilization effects should be treated as quality or price effects.

In addition to theoretical and practical difficulties of adjusting for the above factors affecting premiums, implementing direct pricing of insurance premiums involves a number of technical problems, such as more frequent sampling. Unless BLS incorporates new insurance policies (such as defined contribution plans) in a timely manner when they enter the market, BLS will not be able to accurately weigh the mix of policies and their effect on premium changes.

Direct pricing of insurance is subject to many basic problems that plague the other methods of pricing medical care that were examined: How can the component of price change that represents the value consumers place on increased quality (or loss they attach to lower quality) be quantified? Adjusting insurance premiums for quality change would be at least as conceptually and practically difficult as adjusting a costs-of-treatment index.

REVIEW QUESTIONS

1. Evaluate the present Medical Care Price Index. What should the MCPI conceptually measure? What are its limitations?
2. What is the difference between the Laspeyres price index and Paasche price index?
3. Contrast the treatment and MCPI approaches for measuring changes in the price of medical care.
4. What are the difficulties in constructing a treatment price index?
5. How does the Producer Price Index (PPI) differ from the CPI?
6. What are some of the difficulties in constructing an insurance price index?

REFERENCES

1. For a further discussion of the appropriateness of the CPI as a cost-of-living index, see Janet L. Norwood, "Indexing Federal Programs: The CPI and Other Indexes," *Monthly Labor Review,* 104(3), March 1981: 60–65.
2. See U.S. Department of Labor, *The Consumer Price Index: History and Techniques,* Bulletin 1517, 1966, especially p. 84. Also see Ina K. Ford and Philip Sturm, "CPI Revision Provides More Accuracy in the Medical Care Services Component," *Monthly Labor Review,* 111(4), April 1988: 17–26.
3. For a general discussion of the 1987 revision of the CPI, see Ford and Sturm, Ibid., and Charles Mason and Clifford Butler, "New Basket of Goods and Services Being Priced in Revised CPI," *Monthly Labor Review,* 110(1), January 1987: 3–22.
4. Bureau of Labor Statistics, "Consumer Price Index: September 2002," *News,* United States Department of Labor, Bureau of Labor Statistics, ftp://ftp.bls.gov/pub/news.release/History/cpi.07162003.news, June 2003.
5. Joseph P. Newhouse, "Medical Care Price Indices: Problems and Opportunities, the Chung-Hua Lectures," Working Paper Series, National Bureau of Economic Research, 8168, 2001, 1–53.
6. David M. Cutler, Mark McClellan, and Joseph P. Newhouse, "The Costs and Benefits of Intensive Treatment for Cardiovascular Disease," in Jack Triplett, ed., *Measuring the Prices of Medical Treatments,* Brookings Institution Press, Washington, D.C., 1999, 34–71.
7. Michael J. Boskin, Ellen R. Dulberger, Zvi Griliches, et al., *Toward a More Accurate Measure of the Cost of Living: Final Report for the Advisory Commission to Study the CPI,* Washington, D.C., U.S. Senate Finance Committee, December 4, 1996. Also see Michael J. Boskin & Dale Jorgenson, "Implication of Overstating Inflation for Indexing Government Programs and Understanding Economics Progress," *American Economic Review,* 87(2), May 1997, 89–93.
8. Ernst R. Berndt, et al., "Medical Care Prices and Output," in *Handbook of Health Economics,* vol. 1A, eds. A. J. Culyer and J. P. Newhouse, (New York: North-Holland Press, 2000), 119–180.
9. Brent R. Moulton, "Bias in the Consumer Price Index: What Is the Evidence?," *Journal of Economic Perspectives,* 10(4), Fall 1996, 159–177.
10. David Dranove, Mark Shanley, and William D. White, "How Fast Are Hospital Prices Really Rising?," *Medical Care,* 29(8), August 1991, 690–696.

11. U.S. Government Accounting Office, "Consumer Price Index: Cost-of-Living Concepts and the Housing and Medical Care Components," Report to the Ranking Minority Member, Committee on Banking and Financial Services, House of Representatives, Washington, D.C., August 1996, GAOO/GGD-96-166.

12. Zvi Griliches and Ian Cockburn, "Generics and New Goods in Pharmaceutical Price Indexes," *American Economic Review*, 84(5), December 1994, 1213–1232.

13. Elaine Cardenas, "The CPI for Hospital Services: Concepts and Procedures," *Monthly Labor Review*, 119(7) July 1996, 32–42.

14. Anne Scitovsky, "An Index of the Cost of Medical Care—A Proposed New Approach," in Solomon J. Axelrod, ed., *The Economics of Health and Medical Care* (Ann Arbor, Mich.: Bureau of Public Health Economics, University of Michigan, 1964): 128–147. Also see Anne Scitovsky, "Changes in the Costs of Treatment of Selected Illnesses, 1951–65," *American Economic Review*, 57(5), December 1967: 1182–1195; Anne Scitovsky, "Changes in the Costs of Treatment of Selected Illness, 1971–1981," *Medical Care*, 23(12), December 1985: 1345–1357.

15. Yoram Barzel, "Cost of Medical Treatment: Comment," *American Economic Review*, 58(4), September 1968: 937–938.

16. Ernst R. Berndt, Susan H. Busch, and Richard G Frank, "Treatment Price Indexes for Acute Major Depression," in David M. Cutler and Ernst R. Berndt, eds., *Medical Care Output and Productivity*, (The University of Chicago Press: Chicago), 2001, 463–505.

17. Brian Catron and Bonnie Murphy, "Hospital Price Inflation: What Does the New PPI Tell Us?" *Monthly Labor Review*, 119(7) July 1996, 24–31.

18. Elaine Cardenas, et al., "Premium Pricing: Is It Time for a Directly Priced Health Insurance Index in the U.S. CPI," Working Paper, June 2003. Also see "Appendix: Test of Direct Pricing of Health Insurance Premiums," in Ina K. Ford and Philip Sturm, "CPI Revision Provides More Accuracy in the Medical Care Services Component," *Monthly Labor Review*, 111(4), April 1988, 17–26.

CHAPTER

5

The Demand for Medical Care

KEY TERMS AND CONCEPTS

- Demand versus need
- Efficiency in consumption
- Consumer sovereignty
- Determinants of demand
- Price and income elasticities
- Time costs
- Cross-price elasticities
- Physician as the patient's agent

Learning Objectives

Upon completing this chapter, the reader should be able to:

- Understand the difference between need and demand.
- Discuss how a demand analysis is used for forecasting demands for medical care.
- Explain the important role of the physician as the patient's agent.
- Appreciate the importance of prices, incomes, and time costs as factors affecting demands for medical services.
- Apply demand analysis for explaining changes in medical expenditures.

THE PURPOSE OF DEMAND ANALYSIS

One of the purposes of an analysis of the demand for medical care is to determine those factors which, on the average, most affect a person's utilization of medical services. At any point in time many factors influence the consumer's choice to seek medical treatment of a given intensity. It would be virtually impossible to explain completely every individual's utilization of medical services, but certain factors are important for most persons. Demand analysis seeks to identify which factors are most influential in determining how much care people are willing to purchase. The better our understanding of those factors, the better we will be able to explain variations in utilization among population groups and between areas.

Such an understanding will also enable us to forecast future utilization more accurately. To do so, each of the factors affecting demand is forecasted separately. If, for reasons of social policy, it were desirable to increase a certain population group's use of medical care, then by our understanding of which factors affect demand, such a change could be achieved. Thus an understanding of which factors affect demand and to what extent each affects demand will enable us to explain variations in use of medical services. That knowledge can be used to forecast demand more accurately and to bring about changes in utilization if so desired.

DEMAND VERSUS NEED AS A BASIS FOR POLICY AND PLANNING

At various times it has been proposed that the planning of health facilities and health manpower be based solely upon estimates of need for medical care in the population. Need has generally been defined as the amount of medical care that medical experts believe a person should have to remain or become as healthy as possible, based on current medical knowledge.[1] The Lee and Jones research of the 1930s was one of the classic studies using medical need as the basis for determining physician requirements in the country (1). The Hill-Burton formula for planning hospital facilities (initiated late 1940s) also used need as the criterion for the number of beds required in an area. Four and one-half beds per thousand population was the standard for determining whether additional beds should be built. (If population density was fewer than six persons per square mile, then the standard became 5.5 beds per thousand).

The assumption underlying the use of need as a basis for public policy in medical care is that need itself is (or should be) the main determinant of hospital and physician use. Need, however, is only one factor affecting demand for care; basing resource allocation decisions solely on medical need will result in a misallocation. If the estimated quantity of services required to meet medical need exceeds the quantity that people will actually use, then there will be an underutilization of hospitals and physicians, resources that could have been used elsewhere or in another manner. If, on the other hand, people demand more medical care than would be provided based solely on a need criterion, then there will be excess demand and increased waiting times. Shortages of facilities and manpower are costly because they waste a patient's time—time that could have been spent in a more productive manner.

Thus planning based solely on medical need is likely to result in the use of either too few or too many resources. These consequences are shown in Figure 5-1. Planning according to medical need is shown by a vertical line since need is independent of price. (Need is also independent of the prices of other services, of the patient's income, and whether the patient has insurance coverage. Changes in these economic factors affecting demand would not change need, as medically defined.) The number of medical facilities determined by need is shown along the horizontal

---

1. J. Jeffers et al., state: "An accurate specification of a population's 'needs' for medical services requires perfect knowledge of the state of its members' health, the existence of a well-defined standard of what constitutes 'good health,' and perfect knowledge of what modern medicine can do to improve ill (or below standard) health. It must be acknowledged that existing diagnostic procedures are not capable of providing perfect knowledge of the state of any population's, or even an individual's, health. It also must be acknowledged that a clear-cut consensus as to what constitutes 'good health' does not exist among health professionals." James R. Jeffers, Mario F. Bognanno, and John C. Bartlett, "On the Demand Versus Need for Medical Services and the Concept of 'Shortage,'" *American Journal of Public Health,* 61(1), January 1971: p. 47.

axis (e.g., Q_0 equals four beds per 1,000 population). If utilization is less than need (Q_1) or greater than need (Q_2) at a given price (P_0), then either too many ($Q_0–Q_1$) or too few ($Q_2–Q_0$) resources will be allocated to medical facilities.

When need is viewed as only one factor affecting demand, then greater or lesser needs for care would be represented by different demand curves; for example, D_2 may include a greater amount of need than D_1. Changes in medical need cause a *shift* in the demand for care. If preventive care reduces the future need for acute medical services, this reduction in illness would be shown by a *shift to the left* in the demand for acute care (e.g., from D_2 to D_1).

Planning according to demand would reduce the waste of unused resources and/or the opportunity cost of patients' time. If utilization is less than medical need (e.g., utilization equals Q_1), then by understanding the factors that affect demand and the extent to which demand can be changed when each of these factors is changed, demand can be increased so that quantity demanded at the market price equals med-

ical need. (For example, if the price elasticity of demand for preventive care is –0.3, reducing that price by 10 percent will result in a 3 percent increase in the quantity demanded of preventive care.) Conversely, if a decrease in utilization were desired because patients are staying too long in the hospital when they could be less expensively cared for at home (e.g., utilization equals Q_2), then the price of home health care to the patient (a substitute to inpatient care) could be reduced (by including home health coverage in the patient's insurance), thereby shifting the demand for hospital care to the left.

Using demand analysis does not mean that medical need is disregarded. Instead, additional demand factors as well as need are used to estimate utilization. The emphasis, then, is on accurately forecasting demand (by type of facilities, health manpower, etc.). Once demand has been forecast, it can then be decided, based on value judgments, whether demand should be increased or decreased.

Planning according to medical need alone is based on the assumption that medical need should be the *only* criterion for determining utilization, which is a value judgment that not everyone shares. Everyone may not place the same value on fulfilling all or even a certain percentage of their medical needs. Some may not be willing to pay the necessary price or to spend the necessary time to receive all the medical care that medical experts believe they should receive. Disregarding demand factors is likely to result in a waste of resources as well as a failure to ensure that those persons with the greatest need receive care; low income persons will not be able to afford the care in facilities built based on community need.

Underlying demand analysis is the assumption that people allocate their scarce resources among different goods and services in a way that maximizes their utility. Some persons might say, however, that medical care does not provide any utility, since the patient does not desire to purchase it. Many goods fall into this category: auto repair services, legal services, and home repairs. The desirability of the service is not relevant to the applicability of demand analysis. "Undesirable" services could simply be redefined (as

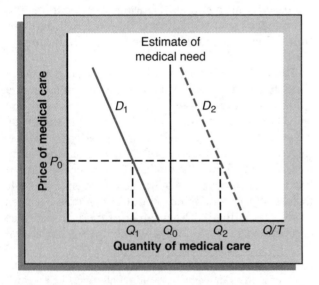

Figure 5-1. Need versus demand as the basis for planning in medical care.

in the case of medical care) to mean those services that provide benefits by alleviating or eliminating illness.

As the price of medical services is reduced, there will be, on average, an increase in the quantity demanded. At some point, the marginal benefits derived from additional units of medical care declines. For example, diagnostic uncertainty decreases as more specialists' services and tests are used. In addition, the probability of recovery from particular illnesses varies depending upon the quantity of medical care used. Some medical services provide reassurance to patients; others provide amenities. Some medical services are a substitute for services performed by the family in the home. Patients and their families differ in their perception of the value of these different aspects of medical care, which reflects differences in the amounts they are willing to pay for these perceived benefits.

There is great variability in the use of medical care due to the unpredictability of the individual incidence of illness. Variability in medical care use and in incidence of illness, however, averages out over large groups of individuals. It is therefore possible to forecast the average demand for care, as opposed to the demand by any particular individual. The estimated demand curve represents the average of many individuals' perceived benefits from additional units of medical care in relation to the price they are willing to pay for those additional benefits.

Since patients differ in both their perception of medical benefits and in their willingness to pay for additional medical services, who is to judge how much medical care should be used? If the patient makes this determination, then, as is the case in a market-oriented system, he or she would use medical services to the point where the marginal benefit of the last unit equals the price paid (the patient's marginal cost) for that unit. If, however, medical need were the criterion for rationing medical care, then regardless of the patient's willingness to pay, he or she would not be allowed to receive more medical care than others believe they need (the marginal benefit to the patient of additional visits exceeds their marginal cost).

In most markets in the United States, output quantity and quality are based upon the concept of consumer sovereignty. Consumers are assumed to be the best judge of how to use their resources to increase their own utility; how they choose to spend their money, together with the cost of producing those goods, determines the variety and quality of the goods and services being produced.[2] The concept of consumer sovereignty in medical care is not uniformly accepted by health professionals, whose task it then becomes to develop an alternative set of criteria sufficiently specific to determine not only the quantity of resources to be spent on medical care, but also the method by which these limited resources are to be allocated among different patients and institutional settings. These alternative criteria must substitute for all those allocative functions that would, in a system of consumer sovereignty, be performed by prices and differing consumer demands. In addition, an alternative system should make explicit the values underlying its distribution of medical care.

The determination of optimal output in a market, whether it is made with respect to medical care demand, the manpower markets, or the health education markets, is based upon the concept of marginal benefits and marginal costs. When the marginal benefits of a service are equal to the marginal costs of producing that service, the output of that service is considered to be optimal. If the marginal benefits are either greater or less than the marginal costs of producing a service, consumption in that market is considered to be economically inefficient (i.e., resources are misallocated in that they are not placed in their highest-valued uses). Efficiency in consumption, therefore, is one criterion by which the output of different medical care markets will be evaluated. The other criterion is efficiency in production: whether the output is produced at minimum cost. Economic efficiency in consumption and in production are criteria that economists use to evaluate the performance of different markets. In medical care, the criterion of

---

2. Deciding whether incomes should be redistributed is independent of deciding who should determine the goods and services to be produced in society. If society determines that certain population groups do not have sufficient incomes, their incomes can be supplemented.

efficiency in production is more widely accepted than is the criterion of efficiency in consumption, for which some persons would prefer to substitute a need criterion or a government system, such as in Canada. Applying the criterion of efficiency in consumption to each medical care market, however, should sharpen the debate on the underlying values and criteria for defining optimal output in each market; should consumers' or health professionals' (or government administrators') perception of marginal benefits prevail?

Whether or not people accept the criterion of efficiency in consumption, demand for medical services must still be analyzed if we are to be able to more accurately forecast use of services.

A MODEL OF THE DEMAND FOR MEDICAL CARE

The Demand for Medical Care Derived from the Demand for Health

The traditional theory of consumer demand assumes that consumers purchase goods and services for the utility provided by those specific purchases. A reformulation of consumer demand, however, draws a distinction between goods and services purchased in the market and more fundamental objects of choice, referred to as commodities (2). If the commodity demanded by consumers is good health, then health can be as the output of a production function whose inputs are goods and services purchased in the market, as well as by the time devoted to preventive measures. Within this framework, the demand for medical care (an input in the health production function) is derived from the more basic demand for health.

According to Michael Grossman (3), consumers have a demand for health for two reasons: (1) it is a consumption commodity—fewer sick days makes the consumer feel better, and (2) it is an investment commodity—a state of health will determine the amount of time available to the consumer for both market and non-market activities. A decrease in the number of sick days will increase the time available for work and leisure activities; the return to an investment in health is the monetary value of the decrease in sick days.

A view of medical care demand as being derived from the demand for health implies the following. First, increases in age result in an increase in the rate at which a person's stock of health depreciates. Over the life cycle, people will attempt to offset part of the increased rate of depreciation in their stock of health by increasing their expenditures on and use of medical care. Second, the demand for medical care will increase with increases in a person's wage. The higher their wage, the greater the value of an increase in the number of healthy days. A consumer who is paid a high wage will also substitute purchases of medical care services for his or her own time when producing the commodity health. We would thus expect to observe a positive relationship between increased wages and greater expenditures on the demand for medical care. Third, it is hypothesized that education has a negative effect on the demand for medical care. More highly educated people are presumed to be more efficient in producing health. They are, therefore, likely to purchase fewer acute medical care services.

This view of medical care demand provides a rationale for including in the demand model certain factors believed to affect demand, traditionally known as taste variables, because they influence the individual's demand for health. The importance of the patient's time in relation to the demand for medical care will also be included in the demand model. Analyzing the demand for medical care as being derived from the individual's demand for health provides a better basis for determining which factors should be included in a model of demand for medical care, and for hypothesizing their effects.

Determinants of the Demand for Medical Care

A discussion of the demand for medical care requires an economic framework not only for surveying the literature on factors affecting demand, but also for evaluating empirical research on demand. If a demand study excludes relevant factors affecting demand, perhaps because they are not easily measured or because the investigator is unaware of their importance, then its results are likely to be inaccurate.

Variations in the demand for medical care are determined by a set of patient and physician factors. The patient's demand for medical care is essentially the demand for a treatment, and variations in demand are a result of variations in the number, type, or quality of treatments demanded. The patient typically initiates this demand. The physician then combines various inputs to provide a treatment of a given quality. The patient's determinants of demand are his or her incidence of illness or need for care, a set of cultural-demographic factors, and economic factors. The roles of the physician as advisor to the patient and as a supplier of a service are discussed separately below.

Empirical studies on the demand for medical care should thus describe, first, how different factors affect the patient's demand for medical care, and second, what determines how the physician will provide care for a given treatment. For purposes of clarity, the patient and physician phases will be described sequentially, although they occur simultaneously. The aim of empirical research, then, is to derive an estimate of the relationship between patient and physician factors and use of medical care.

The assumption of choice is implicit in studies of demand. Choices are made with respect to the amounts of medical care purchased and of the combinations of components of care that produce a treatment. If choice in these areas were not possible, much less variation in medical care use would be observed when non-medical factors, such as the patient's education and income, are analyzed. Less variation would also exist in the manner in which a treatment is provided. The degree of choice by both the patient and physician depends on two factors: knowledge and the availability of substitutes. Non-economists have often assumed that there are no close substitutes in treatment methods or (facilities) for specific illnesses. Even if this were true, which it is not, families might still differ in their demand for medical services because they attach different values to the expected benefits of increased use or because their knowledge of these benefits varies. The substitutability of components in providing a medical treatment has been increasing over time. Not only are ambulatory services and home health care partial substitutes for hospitalization, but also the increased use of outpatient surgery provides an additional substitute for hospital care. These, then, are the reasons underlying the assumption that the patient exercises choice in his or her demand for medical care, and the physician exercises it in the treatment provided.

Factors Affecting the Patient's Demand for Medical Care

As we have noted, the factors affecting a patient's demand for medical care are incidence of illness, cultural-demographic characteristics, and economic factors. The first two, stemming from the family's perception of a medical problem and their belief in the efficacy of medical treatment, shape the consumer's desire (perceived marginal benefits) for medical care. When translating this desire into an expenditure, the family is constrained by its available resources. Determining the amount to spend on medical care becomes a part of the family's problem of allocating scarce resources among alternative goods and services. Each of these general factors affecting a patient's demand for care is discussed below.

Actual or perceived illness or desire for preventive medicine determines whether or not an individual is in the market for medical care at any point in time. The onset of illness and the use of a hospital is for many people an unexpected occurrence. Thus, for individuals, illness may be considered a random event, but with respect to the age and sex of the population as a whole, illness has a fair degree of predictability. As individuals age, the incidence of illness increases, and morbidity patterns change; chronic diseases become a more important determinant of the need for medical care. As shown in Figure 5-2, medical expenditures begin to increase at ages 45 to 64 years of age; after age 65, medical expenditures rise very sharply.

Women have higher medical expenses than men until age 45; after age 45, medical expenditures for men exceed those of women.

Although these demographic characteristics may not affect each of the components of medical care in the same manner, they are important in explaining variations in the use of these services.

Marital status and number of persons in the family also affect the demand for medical care. Single persons generally use more hospital care than do married persons. The availability of people at home to

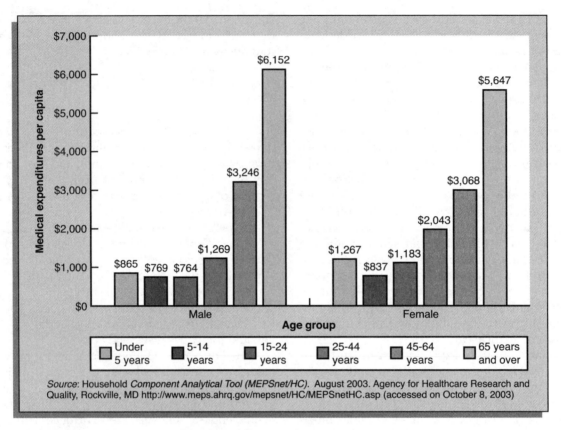

Figure 5-2. Medical expenditures per capita, by age and sex, United States, 2000.

care for an individual may substitute for additional days in the hospital. Family size also affects demand; a larger family has less income per capita (although not necessarily proportionately less) than does a small family with the same income.

Higher levels of education may lead to increased efficiency in a family's purchase and use of medical services. More years of education within the household may enable a family to recognize the early symptoms of illness, resulting in a greater willingness to seek early treatment and/or change their lifestyles. Such families are likely to spend more for preventive services and less for more acute illnesses later. Years of education in a household may be a proxy measure for a greater awareness of the need for medical care, for different attitudes toward seeking care, and for

greater efficiency in its purchase and production. As shown in Figure 5-3, controlling for age by examining those aged 45 to 64, persons with higher educational levels have lower *overall* medical expenditures; although they have higher expenditures for office visits, these are offset by their much lower hospital expenditures.

Although it is important to determine the effect that cultural-demographic factors have on the demand for medical services, such factors are not subject to sudden changes, nor are they generally the instrument of public policy. The age structure changes gradually, as do attitudes and educational level. The effect that economic factors have on the demand for medical services is of more immediate value for purposes of forecasting and policy.

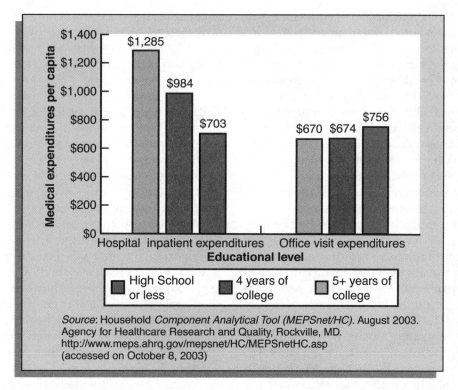

Figure 5-3. Medical expenditures per capita for people 45 to 64 years of age, by educational level and by use of different services, 2000.

The economic factors contributing to the demand for medical services are income, prices, and the value of the patient's time. They affect not only whether a patient will seek medical care, but also the extent of the care once treatment is undertaken. Economic factors may not have much of an effect on whether a maternity patient goes to a hospital (although they may influence the choice of hospital), but once she has been admitted, they have affected her length of stay. Each of these economic factors is briefly discussed.

Estimates of income elasticity derived from survey data using the individual as the unit of observation have typically been close to zero, while estimates based on more aggregate levels of observation, such as time series analyses of national income and national health expenditures data have been greater

than +1 (4). There are several reasons why analyses based on survey data are misleading.

The manner in which family income is measured must be understood if the effect of income, as it is derived from medical care surveys, is to be interpreted correctly. A family's income in any given year may be abnormally low or high because of the temporary loss of employment, ill health, windfall gains, or other unexpected events. Empirical evidence suggests that total consumption is not raised or lowered to correspond with temporary changes in income. Rather, a family's level of consumption is determined primarily by its expected normal or permanent income (5). If transitory income has little or no effect on total expenditures and families that are sick are likely to be below their normal incomes, then survey data that merely shows the relationship between income and expenditures includes both permanent and transitory income. Since transitory income is included in the income reported by the survey (although it presumably has little effect on expenditures), the reported survey relationship between income and expenditure is likely to be understated. If the effects of transitory income can be removed, the income elasticity of medical expenditures will be increased. Thus the difficulty of determining the relationship between permanent incomes and medical expenditures based on survey data is an important reason why the effect of income on medical care expenditures is low.

Another reason why estimates of income elasticity derived from survey data are biased downward is that employer contributions to health insurance premiums are not normally included in survey data as either income or expenditures. Such employer contributions do not constitute taxable income for employee recipients. The higher the income tax bracket, the larger the potential tax saving to the employee and the greater is the incentive to have the employer pay for health insurance. Further, if persons with higher incomes have a greater proportion of their medical expenditures paid by third-party payers, then survey data based on an individual's out-of-pocket expenditures will not include expenditures paid by insurers. Therefore, employer-paid health insurance understates the true income elasticity.

When observations representing higher levels of aggregation (such as national income and national health expenditures) are used for analyzing income elasticity, transitory income effects and variations in health status are averaged out, and employer-paid health insurance is included in both incomes and expenditures. Once the data is corrected for these effects, estimates of income elasticity of medical care expenditures are generally greater than +1; that is, a 10 percent increase in income will lead to a 10 percent increase in expenditures on medical care. Different components of medical care, however, have different income elasticities of demand; for example, dental care being much greater than +1 and hospital care being less than 1.

The price of a service and the use of that service are, according to economic theory, inversely related:

as the price is reduced, purchase or use of the service will increase. Knowledge of price elasticity of demand for medical services is therefore of great importance for public policy. Many persons have generally assumed, however, that prices have very little effect on use of medical services. If national health insurance is to result in greater use of medical services, its proponents must assume that the use of medical services is responsive to changes in price; if not, national health insurance will not result in any changes in use but merely in a redistribution of income.

It is useful to clarify why market demand curves are negatively sloped. People often think of medical services as being emergent, such as an auto accident or the need for heart surgery, in which case price is unimportant. In such life-or-death situations, people will not buy more or less medical care if the price is changed. Medical services, however, consist of more than emergency cases. There are many situations where a person might delay having a surgical procedure or which surgeon will perform that procedure depending upon the price they may have to pay, or whether to see a physician and/or a specialist for a health concern. Many medical services are postponable, can be performed in different institutional settings, or simply provide the patient with reassurance. The use of these services is more responsive to prices.

The market demand for medical services or for any of its components (such as the demand for physician services) is the horizontal summation of thousands (within a community) or millions (large urban areas) of individual demands for that service. *Even though many individuals may not change their use of medical services when the price of that service changes, some persons might do so.* Those who go to the hospital or physician for emergency reasons are added together with those who use services for other reasons. Further, even though many persons may not be aware of the price that is being charged, others are. Thus when the demands for medical services are added up, namely how much each person will demand at different prices, the slope of the demand curve is based on those individuals that are responsive to price as well as those who enter the market at a lower price.

Obviously the market demand for specific services whose use is more emergent will have price inelastic demands compared to those services that are less emergent. And when the market demands for all of these services are added together, the slope of the demand curve will reflect the use of the less emergent services.

Thus as in any market *it is not the average person but the marginal purchaser—those who are responsive to price—that provides the demand curve with its negative slope.*

Figure 5-4 illustrates how individual demands are summed to obtain the market demand. Individual demand curves are represented by d_A, d_B, d_C, and d_D. The first two demand curves are completely price inelastic; those individuals will purchase the same quantity regardless of the price. Individuals d_C and d_D, however, will change their quantity demanded based on price. To derive the market demand curve, the quantities each person will buy at each price are summed up. When these four demand curves are horizontally summed to derive the market demand curve, the market demand curve's negative slope is based on individuals represented by d_C and d_D.

Before discussing estimates of price elasticity of demand for medical services, it would be useful to

discuss what is the relevant price variable. Patients do not usually pay the medical provider's stated price or charges. The total (as in the case of Medicaid patients) or part of the price is paid by an insurer or by the government on the patient's behalf. Any estimate of price elasticity of demand should be based upon the net or the out-of-pocket price paid by the patient. Health insurance is one of the most important factors reducing the patient's price. Insurance coverage represents a movement down the individual patient's demand curve, which increases the quantity of services demanded. For all individuals, the existence of insurance coverage represents a *shift* in the overall demand for medical care.

The effect of insurance on the individual's demand for care and on the aggregate demand for care is explained graphically and more completely in the Appendix to this chapter. Although, as will be discussed, estimates of price and insurance elasticities have generally been found to be inelastic with respect to demand for medical services, these estimates vary by type of medical service and by seriousness of illness.

Certain institutional settings can substitute for others in treatment of an illness. An analysis of the

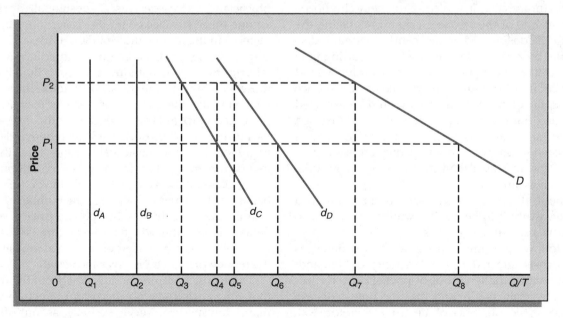

Figure 5-4.   Summing individual demands to obtain market demand.

demand for any one component may be inaccurate if it omits the substitutability and demand for other components. Because a patient can be treated for an illness with different combinations of hospital care, outpatient services, and home health care, different lengths of stay in the hospital may reflect differences in the use of other institutional settings. Therefore, a demand analysis of any one component of care should include net prices to the patient of substitutes and complements. Again, the relevant price to the patient of these substitutes and complements is the out-of-pocket, not the stated, price.

One important reason why estimated price elasticities of demand for medical care is expected to be low is that time costs may represent a relatively large portion of the total price of ambulatory medical care. In addition to prices and income, the consumer's time is a constraint that affects the type of goods and services purchased. Consumer time may be considered an input into the production of a good or service. Cooking a meal and consuming it at home, for example, requires more consumer time than does eating in a restaurant.

When time costs are high, people will substitute purchased services for their own time. Since time has an opportunity cost, it is also scarce and should be viewed as one of the resource constraints facing the consumer. Consumer demand can be better understood and more accurately forecast by including time costs as well as the money costs of consuming a good or service. If either time or money costs of a service decrease, the quantity demanded would be expected to increase. For example, people with higher earned incomes, such as businessmen, typically have a higher cost of time; consequently, they have a higher demand for air travel than do those with low time costs, such as students.

In medical care, time is used in traveling to a provider, waiting to be treated, and, with regard to preventive care, time to exercise.

The following example illustrates how differences in time costs affect the price elasticity of demand. Assume that the patient's out-of-pocket price for visiting a physician is $20, and that the time costs are equal to $30; the total price of the visit is therefore $50. Assuming the elasticity of the medical service with respect to the total price were –1.0 (meaning that a 10

percent change in the total price results in a 10 percent change in use), and assuming the out-of-pocket price dropped 50 percent (from $20 to $10), the result would be only a 20 percent decrease in the total price of care (from $50 to $40). This 20 percent change in the total price would lead to a 20 percent change in use because the price elasticity is –1.0. Thus, when an out-of-pocket price is reduced by 50 percent and use increases only 20 percent, the calculated price elasticity is –0.4. The demand for that service is thereby estimated to be price inelastic. Thus, as time costs contribute a larger proportion of the total price, the calculated price elasticity of demand becomes smaller, while the time price elasticity increases (6).

As private insurance, Medicare, and Medicaid covered a greater portion of the bill, time costs began to represent a greater portion of the patient's total cost. Subsequent increases in co-payments by private insurers to reduce the rise in insurance premiums have important implications for the consumption of medical services for persons with different time costs. One study examining the effect of an increase in patient co-payment (from no out-of-pocket price to the introduction of a 25 percent co-pay), found that the demand for physician services decreased substantially, primarily among those enrollees with the *lowest* time costs. The increase in the money price of the service, a 25 percent co-payment, represented a much larger increase in total price to persons with low time costs than it did for those with higher time costs. For example, home visits, which involve the lowest time costs for the patient, experienced twice as large a decline as other types of visits. Further, enrollees decreased "their demand for care of minor illnesses considerably more than their demand for medical care of other conditions" (7). Nonprofessionals (i.e., those with lower time costs) had a much greater reduction in the number of annual examinations as their out-of-pocket price increased. Female dependents who have lower time costs than female subscribers had a larger reduction in visits when the money price of a visit was increased.

Three policy implications follow from the findings that time costs have an important effect on the demand for medical services. First, as out-of-pocket prices to patients decrease, demand for medical care becomes more responsive to the cost of time. If the quantity supplied of medical care does not increase sufficiently to meet increased demands (as occurs under the Canadian health care system), then those who can afford to wait are more likely to receive care. Time, not price, is the rationing method used. Those with a low time cost are more likely to receive care than are those with a high opportunity cost of time.

Second, society has determined that certain population groups should receive an increase in their use of medical services, such as providing prenatal care to low income pregnant women. Although the money prices to these groups have been reduced, it may be desirable to reduce their time costs to further increase their use of services. Locating clinics closer to these population groups and/or decreasing their waiting times will lower their time costs and increase utilization.

Third, when the number and size of hospitals and medical groups is planned, patient time costs should be considered together with institutional costs as the relevant costs to be minimized. Consumers are willing to pay higher money prices to decrease their travel (time) costs. Neglecting time costs will result in fewer but larger facilities, thereby increasing patients' travel costs. In competitive markets, the size distribution and location of hospitals and medical groups typically minimize both travel time and facility costs.

The Role of the Physician in the Demand for Medical Care

In non-medical markets, the consumer, with varying degrees of knowledge, selects the goods and services that he or she desires. In medical care, however, the patient does not decide, for example, what hospital to enter or the form of treatment he or she is to receive; instead, the patient selects a physician who then makes these choices. When acting on the patient's behalf, the physician, as the patient's agent, uses their awareness of the patient's financial resources and medical needs to act as the patient would if he or she had the knowledge and medical authority to make the decision (8). When choosing the components of care to be used in treatment, the physician is guided not only by their efficacy, but also by their relative prices to the patient. For example, before the 1980s Blue Cross only covered

inpatient hospitalizations. If a patient had Blue Cross insurance and could be treated either as an outpatient or as an inpatient, it was less costly *to the patient* to be hospitalized. This choice of treatment settings by the physician on the patient's behalf, however, resulted in higher total health care costs.

Evidence that physicians made such choices on the patient's behalf is documented in many studies relating hospital utilization to the patient's insurance coverage. Although physician behavior is also affected by other factors discussed below, the fact that they often act in the patient's financial and medical interest can be used to predict medical and hospital use according to the patient's financial, socio-demographic, and medical characteristics. The more likely a physician is aware of and acts in accordance with the patient's needs, desires, and financial interests, the stronger is the empirical relationship between such patient characteristics and use of medical services.

After the 1960s, as health insurance became more comprehensive (lower patient out-of-pocket payments) and physicians were paid fee for service, financial constraints became less important to both patients and their physicians, and physicians prescribed the highest quality of medical care for their patients. This was rational behavior on the part of both physician and patient since the marginal benefit of additional tests and other services, no matter how small, was probably greater than the out-of-pocket price the patient had to pay. The physician was able to practice what Victor Fuchs referred to as the "technologic imperative" (9). In other words, medicine was able to prescribe the best care that was technically possible. No consideration was given as to whether the marginal benefits of that additional care exceeded the marginal costs of producing it.

With the development of managed care in the 1980s, utilization review programs prevented the physician from acting solely in the patient's interest. Physicians found it difficult to prescribe hospital care and/or a length of stay that satisfied the patient's preferences when it conflicted with guidelines on appropriateness of hospital admissions and length of stay. Managed care has weakened the relationship between utilization and patient characteristics (both economic and non-economic).

There is a more important reason why the physician may not act solely in the patient's interest. As one of the inputs into the patient's medical treatment, the physician has an economic interest in the manner in which a treatment is provided. The physician has a dual role. A physician is both the patient's advisor and a supplier of medical services. As a supplier of a service, the physician has a financial stake in the services used in treatment. In prescribing care to a patient, the physician is acting not only as the patient's agent, but also in his or her own interest as a supplier of services. One of the more obvious examples of the effect of this dual role is when physicians prescribe additional tests for the purpose of protecting themselves against a possible malpractice suit. The physician is able to shift certain costs from themselves to the patient and the patient's third-party payer.

According to traditional economic theory, an increase in the supply of physicians would lead to a movement down the market demand curve for physician services with a consequent decrease in price and an increase in quantity demanded of physician services. With a price inelastic demand for physician services, a decrease in price would decrease physician incomes.

Contrary to traditional economic predictions, when the supply of physicians (the physician-to-population ratio) increased, researchers did not observe a decrease in physician incomes, but instead found that physician fees and utilization increased. The empirical findings of higher physician-to-population ratios leading to higher physician prices and utilization gave rise to the belief that physicians could create their own demand.

According to the demand creation hypothesis, when the physician supply increases and the demand facing each physician decreases, physicians will prescribe additional treatments in order to maintain their incomes. When faced with a relatively high demand, a physician will have little incentive to prescribe additional treatments that may or may not be needed. When demand falls however, physicians are hypothesized to increase both their output and price to maintain their incomes. Given the lack of patient information regarding treatment needs and extensive insurance coverage, the physician is able to take advantage of their advisory role and recommend additional services.

(Many similar advisor-supplier relationships exist with purveyors of other goods and services that consumers purchase—for example, legal services, real estate agents, and auto mechanics.)

Prior to managed care, tissue review committees within a hospital were relied upon to reduce unnecessary surgery. The problem with such institutional arrangements (which were not very successful) was that other physicians in the hospital were financially unaffected by the medical practice of their colleagues; thus they had little incentive to become concerned with their colleagues' behavior.

Managed care relied upon two general approaches to limit physician-induced demand. First, by increasing patient and/or insurer knowledge, the physician's ability to create demand is reduced. The patient (or the insurer acting on the patient's behalf) can obtain additional information by having the insurer require prior approval for certain types of surgery and also paying for a second opinion from another physician whenever surgery is recommended. A second approach used by some insurers was to provide their participating physicians with a financial incentive to reduce unnecessary services. Some insurers capitated their physicians; the physician or medical group received a monthly payment per enrollee regardless of the quantity of medical services provided to the patient.

In summary, there is a potential conflict in the physician's role as both an advisor to the patient and as a supplier of a medical service. To the extent that the physician acts as the patient's agent, considering the patient's needs and financial resources, a strong relationship between patient characteristics and their demands for medical care would be expected. On the other hand, to the extent that the physician is also concerned with maintaining their income, there is a concern that the physician will induce demand for their services and the relationship between patient factors and their demands for care will be less obvious. Demand inducement is more likely to occur when physicians are paid fee for service, the patient has extensive insurance coverage, the patient has limited information, and the insurer has limited incentive to be concerned with physician behavior. Under pressure from large employers, the health insurance market has become price competitive; insurers have therefore become more concerned with monitoring their physicians' behavior. As a consequence, demand inducement has declined. (The role of the physician as the patient's agent is discussed more extensively, together with appropriate diagrams, in Chapter 10 on "The Physician Services Market.")

A Review of Selected Empirical Demand Studies

A number of studies have attempted to estimate price and income elasticities of demand for medical services. These studies have been based on the fee-for-service system and have differed with regard to the theoretical variables included in the demand model, the measurement of the theoretical variables, data, statistical techniques, and methods used for analysis. Most of the demand studies have attempted to estimate the relationship between economic factors and total medical care expenditures, as well as separately for expenditures on hospital and physician services while holding constant the effect of other non-economic factors. Very few studies have been able to measure the effect of economic factors by type of medical diagnosis or by seriousness of illness. Ideally, it would be desirable to know price elasticities at different deductible, coinsurance levels, and incomes, holding constant such factors as health status, time prices, and non-economic factors. It would then be possible to forecast more accurately changes in utilization if prices were increased or decreased, as under proposed national health insurance plans.

When expenditures rather than visits or hospital utilization are used as the dependent variable, estimated price and income elasticities are generally higher, presumably because expenditures include some measures of quality. Physician visits, hospital admissions, and patient days do not enable the investigator to differentiate between visits that include a greater intensity of services, use of specialists, or changes in the length of the visit. Expenditure data reflect quality as well as quantity of services; therefore, price and income elasticity estimates based on expenditure data partly measures the demand for

quality in addition to quantity. When expenditure data is used, however, it is particularly important that prices be accurately measured. If, for example, a physician charged a higher price to higher-income persons, part of the difference in expenditures between high- and low-income persons was a result of price differences and not of differences in quantity or quality.

The importance of time costs on demand has often not been included in statistical demand studies. Only a few studies have estimated time-price elasticities. Failure to include time explicitly as a factor affecting demand for services may result in incorrectly attributing its effect to other factors.

Demand studies have also differed with respect to the inclusion of substitutes and complements in the demand model. The demand for hospital care depends, in part, on the price of home health care. The availability of data on substitutes and complements has generally been limited. Excluding such factors from the statistical estimation of demand may affect the price elasticities of demand for hospital services or other services whose demand is being analyzed.

The measurement of income has also distorted the results of demand studies. Ideally, it is desirable to measure the effect of usual or permanent income, but when surveys collect income data, the incomes of those surveyed may be temporarily high or low. If, for example, a person is sick and his or her income is temporarily low but their expenditures are related to their usual income, the person will show up in the survey as having a low income but a high expenditure. Thus, if demands for medical services are related to usual and not temporary income, the estimate of income elasticity will be too low when it is measured using temporary incomes.

Data used in demand studies has also differed by level of aggregation. Some studies have been based on state averages; others have used individuals as the unit of observation. In those studies where the level of aggregation encompasses a state, certain factors known to affect demand (such as age) may turn out to be statistically insignificant because there is insufficient variation between states according to age. Use of individual data, however, has generally resulted in lower elasticity estimates. When individual data is used, it is often difficult to separate the effect of economic factors from all other variables.

The databases from which elasticity estimates were derived have changed over time. Initially, researchers used state data, which included only gross measures of prices and the proportion of the population with insurance coverage. Subsequently, there were a number of studies that used claims and premium data from specific insurance companies. Comparisons have also been made between individuals having different insurance policies. Occasionally natural experiments were available, as when an employer introduced a co-payment in their employees' insurance plan. The RAND Health Insurance Study was designed as an experiment, and many studies have been published using the RAND data on the effect of prices on use of services. As the data has improved, it has become possible to develop better measures of prices, as well as to show the effect of income-related co-payments and health status.

The foregoing discussion of empirical demand studies provides some indication of the great variety of variables used, how economic factors are measured, and data sources. Such studies have also used different methods of statistical estimation. Most studies have used a single-equation approach, although some have used simultaneous equations. Differences in statistical estimation methods could also result in different elasticity estimates. Given these differences in approach, data, and methods, it is not surprising that large variations exist in the statistical estimates of price and income elasticities.

The following is a brief summary of the results of statistical demand studies. Estimates of the price elasticity of (market) demand for hospital, physician, and other providers' services are shown in Table 5-1. (Price elasticity estimates for individual health insurers, physicians, and hospitals are shown in their respective chapters.)

The market demand curves for hospital and physician services are price inelastic. The price elasticity for hospital admissions and physician visits are roughly −0.2. Market demand curves are less price elastic than demand curves facing individual providers since there are fewer good substitutes to all hospitals or all physicians than for individual providers.

Table 5-1. Selected Results on Price Elasticities of Demand for Medical Care

Study	Dependent Variable	Elasticity
W. G. Manning et al. (1987)	hospital admissions	−0.14 to −0.17 (depending on co-ins)
M. S. Feldstein (1977)		−0.20
J. Newhouse and C. Phelps (1976)		−0.17
G. J. Wedig (1988)	physician visits	−0.11 to −0.35
W. G. Manning et al. (1987)		−0.17 to −0.31 (depending on co-ins)
Newhouse, Phelps, and Marquis (1980)		−0.09 to −0.13
F. Goldman and M. Grossman (1978)		−0.03 to −0.06 (pediatric visits)
J. Newhouse and C. Phelps (1976)		−0.16
Lamberton, Ellingson and Spear (1986)	nursing home services	−0.76
B. R. Chiswick (1976)		−0.73 to −2.40 (different proxies for price)

Sources: B. Chiswick, "The Demand for Nursing Home Care: An Analysis of the Substitution Between Institutional and Noninstitutional Care," *Journal of Human Resources,* Summer 1976, 11(3), pp. 295–316; M. Feldstein, "Quality Change and the Demand for Hospital Care," *Econometrica,* October 1977, 45(7), pp. 1681–1702; F. Goldman and M. Grossman, "The Demand for Pediatric Care: An Hedonic Approach," *Journal of Political Economy,* April 1978, 86(2), pp. 259–280; C. E. Lamberton, W. D. Ellingson, and K. R. Spear, "Factors Determining the Demand for Nursing Home Services," *Quarterly Review of Economics and Business,* Winter 1986, 26(4), pp. 74–90; W. G. Manning et al., "Health Insurance and the Demand for Medical Care: Evidence from a Randomized Experiment," *The American Economic Review,* June 1987, 77(3), pp. 251–277; J. Newhouse and C. Phelps, "New Estimates of Price and Income Elasticities for Medical Services," in R. Rosett, Ed., *The Role of Health Insurance in the Health Services Sector* (New York: National Bureau of Economic Research, 1976); J. P. Newhouse, C. E. Phelps, and S. Marquis, "On Having Your Cake and Eating It Too: Econometric Problems in Estimating Demand for Health Services," *Journal of Econometrics,* August 1980, 13(3), pp. 365–390; G. J. Wedig, "Health Status and the Demand for Health: Results on Price Elasticities," *Journal of Health Economics,* June 1988, 7(2), pp. 151–163.

Insurance coverage for hospital services (and physician in-hospital services) is currently quite high; approximately 90 percent of the hospital bill is paid for by private or public insurance. It is therefore unlikely that hospital use will increase rapidly if the remaining out-of-pocket prices were to be paid for under any form of national health insurance. Also, utilization review methods would serve to limit increases in hospital use if the remaining financial barriers were removed. Physician office visits, however, have less-complete insurance coverage. Thus any policy that lowers the price of physician office visits could result in an increase in demand for physician services.

The demand for nursing home care among private pay patients appears to be price elastic, on average between –0.7 and –2. Thus policies to include nursing home care under Medicare or a new long-term care program would result in large increases in use and expenditures.

The estimates of elasticity of demand with respect to time, shown in Table 5-2, are surprisingly high: –1 on the number of sick child visits (using the parent's wage as the opportunity cost of time); –0.6 to –1 with respect to travel time to a public outpatient department and –0.2 to –0.3 to a private physician's office. Waiting time elasticities of demand are lower, between –.05 and –.12.

When income elasticities of demand for medical expenditures are estimated based on aggregations of individuals or through national data over time, medical services are found to be income elastic; between +1.0 and +1.3; that is, as income increases by 10 percent, expenditures on medical care will increase by as much as 13 percent. These results are shown in Table 5-3.

There is a difference in estimated income elasticities when aggregated data as compared to individual data is used. As discussed earlier, persons with higher income are more likely to have employer-paid health insurance; the growth in insurance coverage, both as a percentage of the bill paid and in terms of the type of medical services covered, is income related. Thus at any point in time, the relationship between out-of-pocket expenditures and income is positive but not income elastic. Over time, however, the income effect (which includes the amount paid by insurance) is more pronounced. Thus using national data on total medical expenditures and income over time includes all medical expenditures whether they are paid directly by the consumer or through government, and variations in temporary income and health status are diminished.

The finding that medical expenditures are income-elastic suggests that as the economy grows, expenditures on health care will increase by a greater percentage. Medical care is, therefore, likely to continue to absorb an increasing share of our country's resources.

The income elasticity of demand for physician services, except for pediatric visits, appears to be inelastic.

Table 5-2.   Time-Price Elasticities for Physician Services

Study	Dependent Variable	Elasticity
J. P. Vistnes and V. Hamilton (1995)	physician visits	–1.05
R. M. Coffey (1983)		–0.09
F. Goldman and M. Grossman (1978)	physician visits	–0.06 to –0.07
J. Acton (1976)	(travel time)	–0.06 to –1.00 (to public outpatient dept.)
		–0.25 to –0.37 (to private physician's office)
J. Acton (1976)	physician visits	–0.12 (to public outpatient dept.)
	(waiting time)	–0.05 (to private physician's office)

Sources: J. Acton, "Demand for Health Care Among the Urban Poor with Special Emphasis on the Role of Time," in R. Rosett, Ed., *The Role of Health Insurance in the Health Services Sector* (New York: National Bureau of Economic Research, 1976); R. M. Coffey, "The Effect of Time Price on the Demand for Medical-Care Services," *The Journal of Human Resources,* Summer 1983, 18(3), pp. 407–424; F. Goldman and M. Grossman, "The Demand for Pediatric Care: An Hedonic Approach," *Journal of Political Economy,* April 1978, 86(2), pp. 259–280; J. P. Vistnes and V. Hamilton, "The Time and Monetary Costs of Outpatient

Table 5-3. Estimated Income Elasticities of Demand for Medical Services

Study	Dependent Variable	Elasticity
U-G Gerdtham et al. (1992)	medical services	1.33
T. Getzen and J. P. Poullier (1992)		1.39
R. E. Leu (1986)		1.18 to 1.36
J. P. Newhouse (1977)		1.31
E. Kleiman (1974)		1.22
P. Feldstein and J. Carr (1964)		1.00
F. Goldman and M. Grossman (1978)	physician services	1.32 (pediatric visits)
V. Fuchs and M. Kramer (1973)		0.57
R. Andersen and L. Benham (1970)		0.41
M. Silver (1970)		0.85
C. E. Lamberton, W. D. Ellingson and K. R. Spear (1986)	nursing home care	1.07
W. J. Scanlon (1980)		2.27
B. R. Chiswick (1976)		0.55 to 0.89
P. Feldstein (1973)	dental services	1.22
R. Andersen and L. Benham (1970)		1.24
M. Silver (1970)		2.39 to 3.22

Sources: R. Andersen and L. Benham, "Factors Affecting the Relationship Between Family Income and Medical Care Consumption," in H. Klarman, Ed., *Empirical Studies in Health Economics* (Baltimore: Johns Hopkins University Press, 1970); B. Chiswick, "The Demand for Nursing Home Care: An Analysis of the Substitution Between Institutional and Noninstitutional Care," *Journal of Human Resources,* Summer 1976, 11(3), pp. 295–316; P. Feldstein and J. Carr, "The Effects of Income on Medical Care Spending," *Proceeding of the Social Statistics Section of the American Statistical Association* (1964); T. Getzen and J. P. Poullier, "International health spending forecast: concepts and evaluation," *Social Science and Medicine,* 34(9), pp. 1057–1068; V. Fuchs and M. Kramer, *Determinants of Expenditures for Physicians Services in the United States, 1948–1968* (New York: National Bureau of Economics Research, Occasional Paper 117, 1973); Ulf-G. Gerdtham et al., "An Econometric Analysis of Health Care Expenditure: A Cross-Section Study of the OECD Countries," *Journal of Health Economics,* May 1992, 11(1), pp. 63–84; P. J. Feldstein, *Financing Dental Care: An Economic Analysis* (Lexington, MA: DC Health 1973); F. Goldman and M. Grossman, "The Demand for Pediatric Care: An Hedonic Approach," *Journal of Political Economy,* April 1978, 86(3), pp. 259–280; E. Kleiman, "The Determinants of National Outlay on Health," in M. Perlman, Ed., *The Economics of Health and Medical Care* (London: Macmillan, 1974); C. E. Lamberton, W. D. Ellingson, and K. R. Spear, "Factors Determining the Demand for Nursing Home Services, *Quarterly Review of Economics and Business,* Winter 1986, 26(4), pp. 74–90; R. E. Leu, "The Public-Private Mix and International Health Care Costs," in Culyer, A. J. and B. Jonsson, Eds. *Public and Private Health Services* (Oxford: Basil Blackwell, 1986): pp. 41–63; J. P. Newhouse, "Medical-Care Expenditures: A Cross-National Survey," *Journal of Human Resources,* Winter 1977, 12(1), pp. 115–125; W. J. Scanlon, "A Theory of the Nursing Home Market," *Inquiry,* Spring 1980, 17(1), pp. 25–41; M. Silver, "An Economic Analysis of Variations in Medical Expenses and Work Loss Rates," in H. Klarman, Ed., *Empirical Studies in Health Economics* (Baltimore: Johns Hopkins University Press, 1970).

More recent studies find that the income elasticity of demand for nursing home care by private-pay patients was estimated to be highly income elastic, between +1 and +2.2. Dental care is also highly income elastic; estimates range from +1.2 to +3.2.

The RAND Health Insurance Experiment (RAND) was a controlled experiment to determine the effect of different insurance co-payments on use of medical services; as such, it has greatly increased our knowledge of the effect of deductibles and income-related cost sharing on the demand for medical services (10). Under the experiment, participants were randomly assigned to one of fourteen insurance plans for three to five years. One of the insurance plans provided free care (no deductibles or cost sharing), while the others involved different cost-sharing percentages. The cost-sharing plans differed according to the family's coinsurance rate, which was 25, 50, or 95 percent. The 95 percent plan was the same as an income-related catastrophic plan. The maximum annual dollar expenditure of the family under these plans was income related; it was 5, 10, or 15 percent of income, up to a maximum of $1,000.

The RAND study concluded, consistent with traditional economic theory, that as the coinsurance rate rose, overall use and expenditure fell for adults and

Table 5-4. Differences Between Plans in Predicted Total Expenditures per Person and in the Probability of One or More Physician Visits or Hospital Admissions (All Participants)

	Expenditures	Physician Visits (Probability as a Percent of Free Plan)	Hospital Admissions (Probability as a Percent of Free Plan)
Free care	$430	100	100
25 percent coinsurance	81%	93	79
50 percent coinsurance	67%	89	71
95 percent coinsurance	69%	82	75
Individual deductible plan, 95 percent coinsurance	77%	87	88

Source: Adapted from Joseph P. Newhouse et al., *Some Interim Results from a Controlled Trial of Cost Sharing in Health Insurance,* (Santa Monica: R-2847-HHS, RAND Corporation, January 1982).

children combined. These results are presented in Table 5-4. Compared to the free care plan, a coinsurance rate of 25 percent resulted in a 19 percent decline in expenditures; higher coinsurance rates, 50 and 95 percent (subject to a with a maximum out-of-pocket amount), resulted in over 30 percent declines in expenditures. In other words, per-person expenditures in the free care plan was 23 percent higher than in the 25 percent plan, and 50 percent higher than in the 50 percent coinsurance plan. The probability of a physician visit in a year was 7 to 18 percent lower in the cost-sharing plans than in the free care plan, while hospital admissions were 21 to 29 percent lower. For the Individual Deductible Plan, which had coinsurance for ambulatory services (95 percent) and free inpatient services, the respective probabilities were 13 and 11 percent lower than the free plan.

Price elasticities for the 0 to 25 and 25 to 95 percent ranges of coinsurance were calculated according to the type of care received by the patient (e.g., outpatient, hospital, and all care). As shown in Table 5-5, for the 0 to 25 percent plan, the price elasticity was –0.17 for each of the above types of care. Under the 25 to 95 percent plan, the elasticity estimates were –0.31, –0.14, and –0.22 for outpatient, hospital, and all care, respectively. For outpatient care under the 25 to 95 percent plan, these estimates varied according to whether the treatment was for well care (–0.43) or for chronic care (–0.23).

A concern with increased cost sharing is that it delays seeking needed medical care. Further, that lower use rates associated with increased cost sharing may have adverse health effects on individuals. To examine these effects on health, the RAND study included

Table 5-5. Price Elasticities for Various Types of Care

Range of Nominal Coinsurance Variation	Type of Care					
	Outpatient				Hospital	All Care
	Acute	Chronic	Well	All		
0–25 Percent	.16	.20	.14	.17	.17	.17
25–95 Percent	.32	.23	.43	.31	.14	.22

Source: W. G. Manning et al., "Health Insurance and the Demand for Medical Care: Evidence from a Randomized Experiment," *The American Economic Review,* June 1987, 77(3), pp. 251–277.

measures on self-reported health status indicators, measures of physiologic health, and health practices, such as smoking, weight, and use of preventive services (11). Since participants were randomly assigned to health insurance plans, differences in use rates were due to cost-sharing provisions of the plan and not to the health of the participants. Individuals with the free care plan improved on three of the eleven health status indicators, vision, blood pressure, and dental health. Free care members scored better on three of the twenty-three physiologic measures (two vision measures and blood pressure). The effect of the free care had small effects on health practices; blood pressure control and early detection of cancer improved, although they were offset by decreases in other health practices. The authors state that ". . . the average appraised mortality risk for people on the free plan was very close to the risk for those with cost sharing." Even when those at elevated risk were compared, the effect ". . . rarely differed between insurance plans."

The authors concluded by saying that "Despite the limited gains in health, free care leads to large differences in utilization for the healthy. Because most people are healthy, it is expensive and inefficient to use free care for all as the method to assure the health needs of the few."

The impact of cost sharing, however, was found to have a larger effect on lower-income persons, particularly children (12). A panel of experts divided episodes of care into those in which medical care produces usually effective treatments and usually less-effective treatments. It was determined that for those conditions in which medical care is highly effective, the probability of poor children in the cost-sharing plan having an episode of treatment was 44 percent less than children in the free plan; for non-poor children, the probability was only 15 percent less. Poor adults in the cost-sharing plan had a 41 percent lower probability of seeking treatment than adults in the free plan, while for non-poor adults it was 29 percent lower.

The poor are at greater risk of not receiving treatment when such treatment would be effective than are the non-poor, particularly poor children. This finding should be kept in mind with regard to any government proposals for national health insurance in which cost sharing is not income related.

AN APPLICATION OF DEMAND ANALYSIS: EXPLAINING ANNUAL CHANGES IN PERSONAL MEDICAL EXPENDITURES

Personal health care expenditures have increased from $23.7 billion in 1960 to $1.34 trillion by 2002. The average annual rates of increase have, however, varied over time. Before the introduction of Medicare and Medicaid in 1966, personal health care expenditures increased at an annual rate of 8.3 percent. Afterward, the annual percentage increases became more rapid. Between 1965 and 1975 and between 1975 and 1985, it was 12.5 and 12.7 percent per year, respectively. Between 1985 and 1995, the annual rate of increase slowed to 8.8 percent per year and further slowed to 6.5 percent over the period 1996 to 2002.

These rapid increases in medical expenditures in the post-Medicare period have been the result of increased demands for medical care, the increasingly large involvement of government in the financing of medical care, and increases in the costs of providing such services, including new technology. Together, these changes in demand and supply have resulted in increased prices and quantities for medical services, each of which constitute a part of the increase in medical expenditures.

A detailed analysis of changes in medical care expenditures would examine a number of demand and supply factors, several of which change gradually from one year to the next. This illustration examines just several of the more important factors to be included in a demand analysis. Included are the price of medical services, which has increased sharply, population growth and the aging of the population, and the increase in personal income. The changes in prices, incomes, population and its changing composition can be used to provide a rough approximation of the importance of these demand factors in contributing to increases in medical care expenditures during different time periods (13).

As shown in Table 5-6, the rise in the price of medical care as measured by the Medical Care Price Index contributed substantially to each period's increase in medical care expenditures. Before 1965, medical prices contributed less than 30 percent of the annual percentage increase in expenditures. However, after the introduction of Medicare and Medicaid in 1966, the increase in medical prices contributed between 50 and 75 percent of the annual percentage increase in medical expenditures. When the rate of increase in medical prices is subtracted from the rate of increase in medical expenditures, the result is the average annual percentage increase in the *real* quantity of medical care purchased. (The accuracy of the Medical

Care Price Index as a measure of medical care inflation is discussed in Chapter 4, "Measuring Changes in the Price of Medical Care.")

To explain changes in the quantity of medical care purchased during this period, it is necessary to first adjust for changes in the population, which then results in the annual percentage increase in the quantity of medical care per person. Subtracting the rate of increase in population from the rate of increase in real medical output yields the annual percentage increase in quantity of medical care per person during this period. As shown in Table 5-6, population changes

Table 5-6.   Factors Affecting Changes in Personal Health Care Expenditures

Factor	Average Annual Rate of Change %				
	1960–1965	1966–1975	1976–1985	1986–1995	1996–2002
Personal health care expenditures	**8.3**	**12.5**	**12.7**	**8.8**	**6.3**
Accounted for by:					
Rise in price of medical care (CPI Medical Care)	2.5	6.6	9.1	6.9	3.8
Population increase (resident population)	1.5	1.1	1.0	1.0	0.9
Rise in real personal income per capita, increasing medical expenditures by an equal percentage (income elasticity = 1.0)	3.4	2.4	1.8	1.1	1.7
Decline in quantity demanded because of rise in relative price of medical care (price elasticity = −0.2)	−0.3	−0.2	−0.4	−0.7	−0.3
Changes in population distribution (aging population)	0.0	0.3	0.3	0.3	0.3
Total accounted for	**7.1**	**10.2**	**11.8**	**8.6**	**6.4**
Unexplained residual	**1.2**	**2.3**	**0.9**	**0.2**	**−0.1**

Sources: Data on 'personal health care expenditures' from Centers for Medicare & Medicaid Services, Office of the Actuary, National Health Statistics Group, http://www.cms.gov/statistics/nhe (accessed on January 8, 2004).

Data on 'resident population' from U.S. Census Bureau, *Statistical Abstract of the United States, 2002,* http://www.census.gov/prod/2003pubs/02statab/pop.pdf (accessed on January 13, 2004).

Data on 'personal income per capita' from U.S. Department of Commerce, Bureau of Economic Analysis, http://www.bea.doc.gov/bea/regional/spi/drill.cfm (accessed on January 13, 2004).

Data on 'consumer price index' from U.S. Department of Labor, Bureau of Labor Statistics, http://www.bls.gov/cpi (accessed on January 13, 2004).

Household Component Analytical Tool (MEPSnet/HC). August 2003. Agency for Healthcare Research and Quality, Rockville, MD. http://www.meps.ahrq.gov/mepsnet/HC/MEPSnetHC.asp (accessed on January 13, 2004).

explain only a small part of the overall rate of increase in medical expenditures, particularly in the post-1965 period. During the latter period, population was increasing at approximately 1 percent per year, while medical expenditures were increasing more rapidly than previously.

Per capita incomes (real, adjusted for inflation) were rising (although at different annual rates of increase) during the different periods examined. If an income elasticity of +1.0 is assumed—that is, demand for medical care will increase at the same rate as the increase in income—then part of the annual percentage increase in medical care can be accounted for by increased per capita incomes.

Medical care prices have been increasing at a faster rate than prices in the rest of the economy. Thus, the rate of increase in medical prices relative to the prices of other consumer goods and services can be used to represent an increase in the price of real medical care services. An increase in the price of a service would be expected to decrease the quantity demanded of that service. The magnitude of the decrease in quantity demanded depends upon its price elasticity of demand. Assuming that the price elasticity of demand for medical services is –0.2 (which means that the demand for medical care is relatively price inelastic), a 1 percent increase in price would lead to a 0.2 percent decrease in quantity demanded. With reference to Table 5-6, the quantity demanded of medical care will decline by 0.2 multiplied by the *relative* rate of increase in the price of medical care.

Over time the composition of the population has changed. In 1965, 9.2 percent were over 65 years of age. By 2000, 12.4 percent were 65 and over. Since those over 65 have greater demands for care than the rest of the population, an adjustment was made for the aging of the population.

When the above factors affecting demand are summed up for the different time periods, most of the annual percentage increase in medical expenditures can be accounted for. The amount of the unexplained residual was greatest (2.3 percent per year) in the period right after the introduction of Medicare and Medicaid, 1965 to 1975, than in the subsequent ten-year periods (0.9 percent, 0.2 percent, and –0.1 percent annually).

The large unexplained residual in the post-Medicare period, which is the percentage increase in real medical care output that cannot be explained by the demand factors described, most likely represents changes in the medical care product. A hospital admission in 1965 is not the same service as a hospital admission today; the treatment for heart disease and cancer is also very different today than previously. When medical prices were used to adjust expenditures to determine real output increases, it was assumed that the price increases were pure price increases, and that the output produced was similar over time. Innovations in medical technology have, however, changed the medical product over time. Further, after Medicare was introduced, hospitals increased their service quality by adding more facilities and services and increasing ratios of personnel per patient, both of which would contribute to an increase in real expenditures per person in the post-Medicare period. Similarly, there has been greater use of (more expensive) specialist services over time, which would also represent a higher quality service and not just a price increase. If the foregoing analysis had been able to include these additional factors, price increases would have been smaller (since it also reflects changes in product and quality over time), and that the size of the unexplained residual would have been lower.

The unexplained residual has become smaller in subsequent time periods, becoming negative in the most recent time period. This negative residual most likely reflects the more competitive structure of the medical care industry with the introduction of managed care and lower rates of increase in utilization and provider prices and, consequently, expenditures due to managed care.

SUMMARY

An understanding of the factors affecting demand for medical services is essential if one is able to explain differences in demand among different population groups. In addition to need, there are economic factors, such as out-of-pocket price, time costs, and income, as well as cultural and demographic factors. Although all these factors are important in a demand analysis, economists are particularly concerned with the economic factors since they change more quickly. It is also through changes in the economic factors, such as out-of-pocket prices and time costs, that public policy is able to change demands for care.

Estimates of price and income elasticities (the percent change in quantity of medical services resulting from a 1 percent change in price or income) are important for quantifying differences in demand and for forecasting demand for medical services.

The role of the physician as the patient's agent has been subject to a great deal of discussion and research. A physician can be hypothesized to act as either a perfect or imperfect agent on behalf of the patient. When the physician is a perfect agent, the physician is expected to act solely in the patient's interest, prescribing treatment according to both the patient's medical needs and economic resources. As an imperfect agent, the physicians manipulate information to benefit themselves as well as the patient. In a fee-for-service setting, imperfect physician agents induce additional demand for their services in order to maintain or increase their income.

To counteract fee-for-service physicians who act as imperfect agents, insurance companies have introduced cost containment approaches (such as utilization management) which attempt to correct the imbalance of information between the physician and the patient. When physicians are capitated, it becomes necessary to monitor physician behavior to prevent imperfect physician agents from decreasing patient access to care.

APPENDIX: THE EFFECT OF COINSURANCE ON THE DEMAND FOR MEDICAL CARE

A diagram may clarify the effect of coinsurance on the demand for medical care. Figure 5-5 shows the relationship between the price of medical care and the quantity demanded, with all of the other determinants of demand being held constant. When the price

is P_1, the quantity demanded will be Q_1. When insurance has a coinsurance feature, the person using medical services would have to pay the amount of the coinsurance, which is the difference between the proportion that the insurance pays and the price charged. The price paid by the patient would be P_2, which is, for example, 20 percent of P_1; the third-party payer would pay the remainder of the price, P_1–P_2. As a result of the 80 percent price reduction, the patient will now demand Q_2 of medical services. (The actual increase in quantity demanded as a result of the decrease in price due to coinsurance will depend upon the size of the coinsurance and the price elasticity of demand.) As long as there is some responsiveness of price to quantity demanded, coinsurance will increase demand by lowering the price the patient will pay for medical care.

Although insurance coverage represents a *movement* down an individual's demand curve, the aggregate effect of an increase in coverage is to cause a *shift* in the demand for medical care. For example, according to the demand curve represented by D_1 in Figure 5-6, an individual would demand Q_1 units of medical care if the out-of-pocket price were $10 per unit. If the

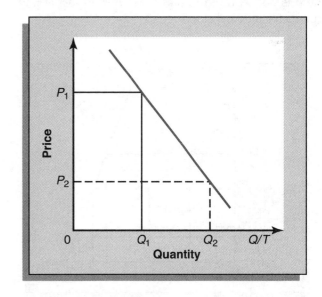

Figure 5-5. The effect of co-insurance on the demand for medical care.

individual were now provided with insurance requiring that only 20 percent of the total price be paid, then at a price of $10 per unit the individual need only pay $2. Therefore, the individual would move down their demand curve and consume Q_2 units at a price of $2 per unit. The actual price of Q_2 units, however, is not $2 per unit but $10 per unit; the third-party payer pays 80 percent, or $8 per unit. Thus, the actual demand curve for medical care has shifted to the right. Similarly, if the initial price were $15, the patient with demand curve D_1 would consume Q_3 units of medical care. With the introduction of a 20 percent coinsurance program, the patient would move down their demand curve and consume Q_4 units at a price of $3 per unit. The total price per unit at Q_4 is, however, $15 per unit. Each of the points on the original demand curve (D_1) now represents only 20 percent of the total price. The new demand curve (D_2) represents the relationship between the total price per unit (20 percent of which is paid for by the patient and 80 percent by the third-party payer) and the quantities demanded at these different prices. (As the patient's copayment becomes less, the demand curve will rotate to the right; it will become completely vertical when the patient is not required to make any out-of-pocket payments for medical care.)

Analyzing the effect of insurance becomes more complicated when there is a coinsurance provision *and* a rising supply curve for medical care. For example, according to Figure 5-7, the patient's original demand curve is D_1. The provision of health insurance with a coinsurance feature (for simplicity, it is assumed to be 50 percent with the remainder being paid by the government) will result in a shift in demand to D_2, which represents the amount that both the patient and the government will pay for medical care. Every point on demand curve D_2 represents a doubling of the price for a given quantity over D_1 since it is a 50 percent coinsurance program. So far, the analysis is similar to the previous example. However, since the new demand curve (D_2) intersects the supply curve at a higher price than previously, a new equilibrium price and quantity of medical care, P_2 and Q_2, will be established. Q_2 is thus the only quantity at which the public pays one-half the price of the medical care ($P_2/2$) that is also an equilibrium position. Therefore, the price the consumer will pay with a 50 percent coinsurance is greater than 50 percent of the original market price ($P_1/2$). The introduction of a percentage co-payment feature does not mean that the consumer's price will be a similar percentage of the original market price, nor does it mean that the amount of

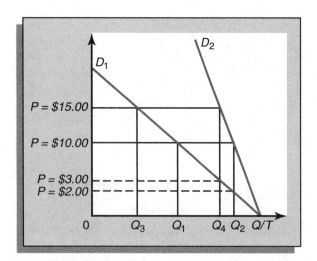

Figure 5-6. Insurance as a shift in the aggregate demand for medical care.

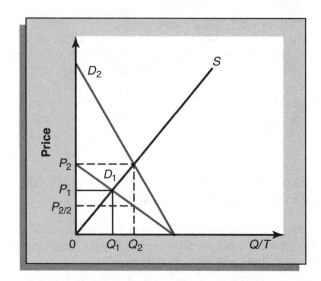

Figure 5-7. The effect of co-insurance on the aggregate demand for medical care with a rising supply curve.

care used will increase by that same proportion. The greater the co-insurance paid for by the government (or other third party), the greater will be the consumer's use of medical services, but the actual price the consumer must pay and the amount actually consumed will depend upon the elasticity of both demand and supply. The more elastic demand and supply are, the greater will be the increase in quantity and the less the rise in price.

REVIEW QUESTIONS

1. If the price of medical care were set to zero for everyone, would individual demands for medical care still differ? Under what conditions would you favor a "negative" price for medical care?
2. Why do economists tend to reject the concept of need as the sole determinant of use in favor of the concept of the demand for medical care?
3. What are the various consequences if hospital planning in the United States is done according to need (or the use of bed-to-population ratios) rather than demand?
4. What variables should be included in a comprehensive measure of the price a person pays to consume medical care?
5. Define cross-price elasticity of demand. What is the meaning (in words) of a cross-price elasticity of demand of +6.5? Would you expect the goods to be substitutes or complements?
6. Discuss the determinants of the demand for medical care.
7. Why are estimates of income elasticity of demand for medical care higher when national time series data is used compared to using estimates derived from survey data on individuals?
8. Evaluate the statement, "Medical care is never free, although the individual recipient may pay nothing."
9. How can a model of demand for hospital care be used to explain changes in hospital utilization over time?
10. How can a model of demand for medical care be used to explain the rise in medical expenditures over time?
11. How would you use the results of a demand analysis to suggest recommendations to increase the utilization of ambulatory medical care by those with low incomes?
12. What factors might cause physicians to experience an increase in the number of requests for annual physical examinations even though they do not change their fees for this service?
13. It has been said that extensive (both public and private) insurance coverage resulted in an "erosion of the medical marketplace." Explain this statement.

REFERENCES

1. Roger Lee and Lewis Jones, *The Fundamentals of Good Medical Care* (Chicago: University of Chicago Press, 1933).
2. Kevin J. Lancaster, "A New Approach to Consumer Theory," *Journal of Political Economy,* 74(2), April 1966, 132–157.
3. Michael Grossman, "The Human Capital Model," in *Handbook of Health Economics,* vol. 1A, eds. A. J. Culyer and J. P. Newhouse, (New York: North-Holland Press, 2000), 347–408.
4. An excellent review article examining income elasticities derived from data using observations of different levels of aggregation is Thomas E. Getzen, "Health Care Is An Individual Necessity and a National Luxury: Applying Multilevel Decision Models to the Analysis of Health Care Expenditures," *Journal of Health Economics,* 19(2) March 2000, 259–270.
5. The distinction between permanent and transitory components of income and their relationship to consumption are discussed by Friedman in terms of his permanent income theory of consumption in Milton Friedman, *A Theory of the Consumption Function* (Princeton, N.J.: Princeton University Press, 1957).
6. For a more complete discussion of the role of time in the demand for medical care, see Jan P. Acton, "Nonmonetary Factors in the Demand for Medical Services," *Journal of Political Economy,* 83(3), June 1975, 595–614. See also Charles E. Phelps and Joseph P. Newhouse, "Coinsurance, the Price of Time, and the Demand for Medical Services," *Review of Economics and Statistics,* 56(3), August 1974, 334–342.

7. Anne A. Scitovsky and Nelda M. Snyder, "Effect of Coinsurance on Use of Physician Services," *Social Security Bulletin,* 35(6), June 1972, 3–19.

8. For a discussion on agency theory, see Thomas G. McGuire, "Physician Agency" in *Handbook of Health Economics,* vol. 1A, eds. A. J. Culyer and J. P. Newhouse, (New York: North-Holland Press, 2000), 461–536.

9. Victor Fuchs, "The Growing Demand for Medical Care," *The New England Journal of Medicine,* 279(4), July 25, 1968, 190–195.

10. A shorter version of the study results without appendices is contained in Joseph Newhouse, et al., "Some Interim Results From a Controlled Trial of Cost Sharing in Health Insurance," *The New England Journal of Medicine,* 305(25), December 17, 1981, 1501–1507. See also Emmett B. Keeler and John E. Rolph, "How Cost Sharing Reduced Medical Spending of Participants in the Health Insurance Experiment," *Journal of the American Medical Association,* 249(16), April 29, 1983, 2220–2222.

11. Emmett B. Keeler, et al., "Effects of Cost Sharing on Physiological Health, Health Practices, and Worry," *Health Services Research,* 22(3), August 1987, 279–306.

12. Kathleen N. Lohr, et al., "Use of Medical Care in the RAND Health Insurance Experiment, Diagnosis and Service-Specific Analyses in a Randomized Controlled Trial," *Medical Care,* 24(9), Supplement, September 1986, S1–S87.

13. The discussion in this section is based on an earlier article by Victor Fuchs, "The Growing Demand for Medical Care," *The New England Journal of Medicine,* 279(4), July 25, 1968, 190–195.

CHAPTER

6

The Demand
for Health Insurance

KEY TERMS AND CONCEPTS

- Deductibles and co-insurance
- Indemnity versus service benefits
- Expected and actual utility
- Decreasing marginal utility of wealth
- Risk aversion
- Probability of loss occurring
- The size of the expected loss
- Pure premium
- Loading charge
- Tax-exempt employer paid health insurance
- Adverse selection
- Preferred risk selection
- Moral hazard
- Optimal amount of health insurance

Learning Objectives

Upon completing this chapter, the reader should be able to:

- Describe the concepts of deductibles, co-payments, stop loss coverage, and catastrophic insurance.
- Understand why utility theory is used to explain the demand for health insurance.
- Explain the theory underlying the demand for health insurance.
- Discuss why consumers would be worse off if they were required to purchase insurance covering all their medical expenses.
- Analyze the effect that tax-exempt employer-paid health insurance has had on the demand for health insurance.
- Appreciate why adverse selection occurs and its effects on insurance markets.
- Understand why preferred risk selection occurs and methods to eliminate it.
- Explain moral hazard and how it increases health insurance premiums.

APPROPRIATENESS OF HEALTH INSURANCE COVERAGE

Although the number of services covered and the percentage of the bill paid by health insurance have increased over time, insurance coverage still varies greatly by population group, by services covered, and by percentage of the medical bill covered. In pointing to the percentage of the medical bill covered by insurance as a measure of its "adequacy," anything less than 100 percent coverage (or at least a "high" percentage) is deemed by some to be "inadequate." The policy recommendations that follow from such a normative judgment are based either upon the assumption that inadequacy is a result of insufficient financial means on the part of consumers for purchasing the appropriate amount of insurance, or that the inadequacy is a result of the health insurance industry's failure to provide more appropriate coverage. The recommendations based upon this normative judgment of inadequate health insurance are that the government should either provide comprehensive coverage under its own auspices or subsidize the purchase of health insurance.

To determine the "appropriateness" (or optimal amount) of health insurance coverage in the United States, appropriateness in an economic sense must be defined. It is also important to determine whether there are market conditions that distort the consumer's ability to select the economically appropriate quantity of health insurance coverage. In this chapter, therefore, the determinants of the demand for health insurance are examined. In a subsequent chapter, the economic efficiency of the health insurance market is examined to determine whether there are (or have been) distortions on the demand or supply side of that market that result in either "too much" or "too little" (or insufficient varieties) of health insurance offered. The conclusions with respect to the supply side of that market should indicate the appropriate role of government, if any, as a regulator or provider of health insurance.

HEALTH INSURANCE TERMINOLOGY

As a preface to the analysis of the demand for health insurance, a brief discussion of a number of concepts used in health insurance is in order.

Deductibles

When consumers pay a flat dollar amount for medical services before their insurance picks up all or part of the remainder of the price of that service, this is referred to as a deductible. Deductibles may be set in a number of ways: they may apply to each unit of service, or they may be cumulative—for example, once $250 has been paid by the consumer for medical services within a year, the insurer will pay the full amount of additional services. Deductibles may apply on a family basis or for each individual. Deductibles may also be related to family income, with higher deductibles being required of persons with higher family incomes, as has been proposed under certain national health insurance schemes.

An important reason for using a deductible is that it lowers the administrative costs of claims processing when there are many small claims and the cost of handling these claims is high. These transaction costs are likely to exceed the amount people are willing to pay for insurance against small claims. Typically, people are more willing to pay the transaction costs of handling large unexpected claims. Thus, by eliminating the transaction costs for small claims, the consumer is more likely to be able to buy insurance (at a lower premium) for protection against large medical expenditures. A large percentage of families incur small medical expenditures within a year, while a small percentage of families incur very large expenditures. This phenomenon is illustrated in Figure 6-1A. The insurance costs of covering medical expenditures would obviously be lowered if a deductible were placed at the low end of the expenditure spectrum, as indicated by line A in Figure 6-1A. Further, the deductible provides the consumer with an incentive to shop around for the best price when the deductible is greater than the price of the service.

The case against deductibles is generally made on the grounds that the deductible, no matter how small, may be a deterrent to needed care. Further, a flat deductible, irrespective of family income, is a greater burden on low-income families than on high-income families.

The effect of the deductible on use of services is complex. If there is a deductible, once the deductible is exceeded and additional services are free, the deductible will have no effect on decreasing the use of

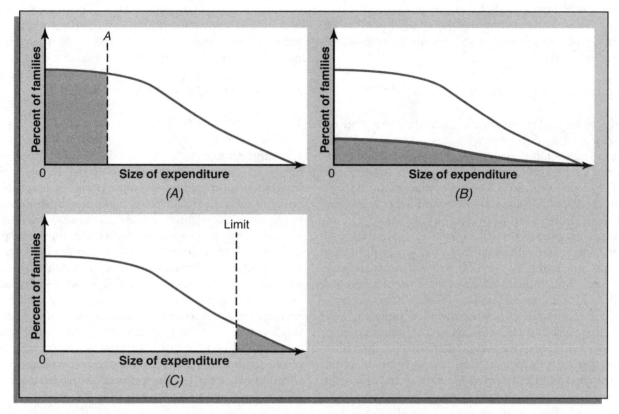

Figure 6-1.   The expected distribution of family medical expenses with different types of co-payments; (A) the imposition of a deductible; (B) a co-insurance provision; (C) a maximum or limit to coverage.

services. Once the deductible has been paid, the patient will use the services as though their price were "zero." If the deductible has not been exceeded, the price of the services will determine (other factors being held constant) how much they will be used. A deductible by itself, therefore, will either tend to result in greater use of services (similar to a zero price) when a low deductible is used, or if the deductible is high, it will tend to make insurance coverage irrelevant to many users of care. The effectiveness of a deductible depends upon the size of the deductible, the expected medical expenditures of the family (if on a family basis), and on family income.

Co-insurance

When the insurer reimburses the patient for a certain fraction of the price of the service, the arrangement is termed co-insurance. A co-insurance level of 80 percent in effect lowers the price to the patient of those covered services by 80 percent. The patient pays the remaining 20 percent themselves. If the price of the service rises, the insurance would pay 80 percent of the new, higher price. Co-insurance levels can also vary by service covered and by family income. The advantage of co-insurance is that it reduces the price of the service and still provides the patient with an incentive to seek out less costly providers. The effectiveness of a co-insurance feature depends upon how responsive the patient's use of services is to lower prices, which is the price elasticity of demand. If use is not responsive to price, co-insurance will merely be a way of reducing the cost of the insurance package to the consumer. Depending upon the level of co-insurance and the price elasticity of demand, co-insurance can change the distribution of medical expenditures, as shown in Figure 6-1B. Co-insurance would result in the consumer's paying for the shaded portion of Figure 6-1B, while the insurer pays for the remainder of the medical expenses.

Stop Loss Levels, Limits, and Maximums

Deductibles and co-insurance can add up to a large financial loss to a person who has a serious illness. Insurance, therefore, includes a "stop loss." Once the patient's out-of-pocket medical expenses (deductible and co-insurance) reach a certain dollar amount (typically $2,500), then the patient is no longer responsible for additional out-of-pocket payments.

While stop loss levels are meant to protect the patient from a large financial loss, "limits" and "maximums" are similarly used to protect the insurance company from large losses. Insurance companies often include $1 million or $2 million lifetime limits on how much they are willing to reimburse for a patient's medical expenses. Expenditures above that limit become the responsibility of the patient. Previously, when Blue Cross provided a benefit that just covered hospital care, it used a limit that provided for a maximum of 30 days in the hospital. Mental health benefits have typically had low maximums, typically $50,000. (Legislation enacted in 1996 requires mental health benefits to be the same as medical benefits.)

Medical expenditures excluded by limits and maximums generally comprise the tail of the distribution, as shown in Figure 6-1C. Large expenditures, incurred by a small percentage of families, are generally not responsive to prices; to exclude this part of the distribution from coverage appears to be particularly unwise since large, unexpected losses to a small percentage of the population meet the criteria defining insurance risks. If the objective of using limits were to enable the insurance company to lower its insurance premium to consumers, an alternative approach would be to use a small deductible for the many families that have small expenditures. This front-end deductible, when applied to many families, would be less of a financial hardship than would a catastrophic expense befalling a small percentage of the population.

Insurance coverage for the tail of the distribution (i.e., large expenditures incurred by a small percentage of the population) is referred to as major medical or catastrophic insurance. Major medical coverage was an innovation introduced by the commercial insurance companies in the late 1940s to compete with Blue Cross, which until that time was the dominant health insurer selling hospitalization insurance up to a maximum number of days.

Other Forms of Coverage

Insurance contracts may include any or all of the above in various combinations of deductibles, co-insurance, and limits. Other aspects of insurance coverage should also be briefly mentioned. Some coverage may specifically exclude (or impose a waiting period) certain diseases for which the potential insurance purchaser was treated in the previous year; this is referred to as a pre-existing condition. Allowing immediate coverage for pre-existing conditions would be like allowing a person whose house was on fire to buy insurance to cover his loss; a person would have no incentive to buy insurance while they were healthy. Other kinds of insurance coverage may include continuation of salary if a person becomes ill, or disability benefits if a person is unable to be fully rehabilitated once an illness has been incurred.

Indemnity versus Service Benefits

When Blue Cross was started in the 1930s, it provided a "service" benefit for hospital care, which meant that the price to the patient for the stay in the hospital (up to a maximum period) was reimbursed in full to the hospital. The patient was not responsible for any deductibles or cost-sharing. An indemnity benefit, offered by commercial insurers, differed from a service benefit in that it reimbursed the patient, not the hospital, a pre-determined amount for the patient's medical costs. The amount of reimbursement was often a fixed dollar amount per hospital day or admission or a percentage of the bill. The patient had an incentive to minimize the cost of the illness. Naturally, the hospitals that founded Blue Cross preferred the service-benefit approach since it meant that they would be reimbursed for all their services and the patient would have no incentive to shop around for the least expensive hospital or a less costly non-hospital provider. By providing coverage only for hospital care, Blue Cross made non-hospital services more costly to the patient; therefore, hospital use was encouraged when other, less costly settings could have been used to treat the patient. Further, hospitals would incur lower collection costs if they could bill Blue Cross for all their patients than having to collect from each patient. A more detailed discussion of the Blue Cross service benefit policy and a comparison between it and an indemnity policy is provided in Appendix 1 of this chapter.

THE THEORY OF DEMAND FOR HEALTH INSURANCE

People buy health insurance to protect themselves against the possibility of a large financial expense if they become ill. An illness, and consequently medical expenditures, is unpredictable for an individual. The person can save for the possibility of a serious illness, but for some illnesses the probability of it occurring is low and the amount to be saved would be very large. Insurance companies pool risks; that is, within a large population group with similar characteristics, the insurer is able to more accurately calculate the probability of an event occurring. By paying an insurance premium, people can protect themselves while not having to save a large amount for a possible catastrophic financial loss.

The consumer's demand for health insurance represents the amount of insurance coverage that he or she is willing to buy at different health insurance premiums, (actually, at different amounts of the loading charge, which is the amount above the pure or actuarially fair premium). Additional insurance coverage (either greater comprehensiveness, additional benefits, or less restricted access to providers) will be purchased if the insurance premium (loading charge) declines. The consumer's marginal benefit of increased comprehensiveness of insurance declines the more comprehensive the coverage. *When the marginal benefit of additional coverage equals the marginal cost (to the consumer) of buying that additional coverage, then the "appropriate" amount of insurance will have been purchased.*

According to this definition, 100 percent coverage of all medical expenses would be demanded by the consumer only when insurance is sold at its pure premium; that is, no administrative cost is added.[1] At positive administrative prices for insurance, the consumer would demand less than 100 percent coverage. This is because the marginal benefit of the last unit of insurance coverage would be purchased only if the price of that additional coverage to the consumer were very small. Adding an administrative price to the pure premium would cause the total price of those last units to be greater than their marginal benefits. The consumer would purchase additional coverage only to the point where the benefit of additional coverage equaled the total price of additional coverage.

Keeping in mind that the appropriateness of the amount of insurance coverage consumers will buy will be related to their perception of the value of additional coverage compared with the additional cost of that coverage, the demand for health insurance will be examined under two conditions. It is first assumed that there is no "moral hazard." The demand for medical care is assumed to be completely price inelastic; that is, patients cannot affect the size of their loss once they are ill (1). The second situation analyzes the demand for health insurance when moral hazard exists; when insurance lowers the price of medical services, patients will increase their use of those services.

To understand the factors that affect the demand for health insurance, it is necessary to be familiar with the economic theory underlying the purchase of insurance. This discussion should clarify why people buy insurance for some risks and not for others. The economic theory of insurance is then used to predict the type of insurance expected to be most prevalent in the health field.[2]

---

1. This statement assumes that the demand for medical services is completely price inelastic. As discussed later, the existence of price sensitivity with respect to medical services, that is, moral hazard, will result in consumers purchasing insurance policies that cover less than 100 percent of medical services.

2. Throughout this analysis, for the sake of simplicity, it is assumed that utility functions are independent, that is, the degree to which others have insurance to cover their medical loss does not affect an individual's desire to subsidize another person's purchase of insurance.

Underlying the demand for insurance is the assumption that an individual wishes to maximize his or her utility, which is the usual assumption made in demand analysis. Since a person does not know whether they will have an illness (consequently, a loss of wealth to pay for it), the individual who seeks to maximize his or her utility when subject to uncertain events seeks to maximize his or her *expected* utility. That is, the person can choose between two alternative courses of action:

1. He or she can purchase insurance and thereby incur a small loss in the form of the insurance premium, or

2. He or she can self-insure, which means facing the small possibility of a large loss in the event that the illness occurs, or the large possibility that the medical loss will not occur.

To determine whether consumers will purchase insurance for an unexpected medical event or self-insure and bear the risk themselves, it is necessary to compare course 1 and course 2 to determine which choice provides them with a higher level of utility.

The use of expected utility, as discussed by Friedman and Savage in their classic article (2), assumes that the consumer selects among alternative choices according to whether one choice is preferred to the others, and ranks these choices according to how much one choice is preferred over another (i.e., cardinal rankings). Although one can think of the utility function as having no unique origin or unit of measure, once some unit of measure and a point of origin are accepted, the utility function of an individual can be described for all levels of wealth. Further, for an individual to purchase insurance, he or she must believe that the marginal utility of wealth is decreasing; although the preference is for more wealth rather than less wealth, additional wealth has a lower marginal utility. The relationship between total utility and wealth is shown in Figure 6-2A; as will be shown, unless the utility function exhibits this relationship to wealth, the "rational" individual will not purchase insurance.

To illustrate an individual's choices when trying to decide whether or not to purchase health insurance, we will assume that if an illness occurs, it will cost $8,000. If the individual is currently at W_3 (meaning that his or her wealth is $10,000), then if the event occurs, $8,000 must be paid out, thereby moving the in-

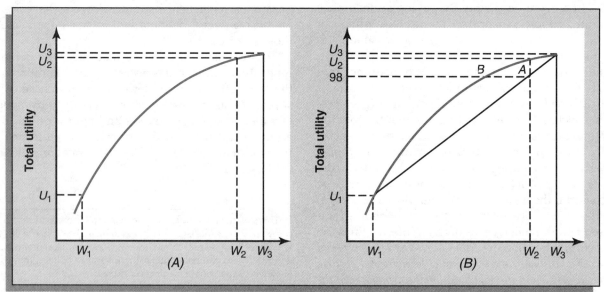

Figure 6-2. The relationship between total utility and wealth; (A) diminishing marginal utility with increased wealth; (B) expected utility.

dividual to wealth position W_1. (The corresponding utility levels at W_3 and W_1 are U_3 and U_1, respectively.) Let us assume that the probability of the individual's requiring medical services costing $8,000 is 0.025—that is, 2.5 percent. The "pure (or actuarially fair) premium" of the insurance that would cover the actuarial value of the expected loss would therefore be $0.025 \times \$8,000 = \$200$.

The pure premium is a function of *both* the size of the expected loss ($8,000) and the probability of it occurring (0.025) *for a large group of people* (the law of large numbers). If the person were to buy insurance priced at the actuarial value of the expected loss, he or she would pay $200, thereby reducing their wealth, with certainty, to point W_2 on Figure 6-2A, which represents $9,800. Let us further assume that as a result of purchasing insurance and decreasing one's wealth to $9,800, the individual is now at U_2, which is equivalent to being at a total utility level of 99, U_3 being 100 and U_1 being 20. The choices facing the individual therefore are:

a. To purchase insurance for $200 and move to a lower level of utility, 99, or

b. Not to purchase insurance and have a 2.5 percent chance that he or she will incur an $8,000 loss and thereby move to a utility level of 20 (U_1) which is associated with a wealth position of $2,000, or face a high probability of 97.5 (100 - 2.5 percent) that a loss will not be incurred and thereby remain at a wealth position of $10,000 with an associated utility level of 100.

To compare choices *a* and *b*, we must use expected utility. The expected utility of choice *b* is the weighted sum of the utilities of each outcome, with the weights being the probabilities of each outcome. Therefore, the expected utility of choice *b* is

$$P(U_1) + (1 - P)(U_3) = 0.025(20) + 0.975(100) = 98$$

To determine whether a person would buy health insurance, we compare the utility level of choice *a*, which represents purchasing insurance and thereby leaves the person at utility level $U = 99$, with the ex-

pected utility level of choice *b*, which represents not purchasing insurance and thereby results in an expected utility level $U = 98$. Since the utility level of choice *a* is greater than that of choice *b*, we predict that the person would purchase insurance. In this example it is assumed that the insurance is sold at the actuarially fair premium and that the utility function with respect to wealth is similar to the one described in Figure 6-2A—namely, diminishing marginal utility with respect to increased wealth.

The expected utility of choice *b*, $U = 98$, is shown in Figure 6-2B, by the straight line drawn on the utility curve extending from U_3, W_3, to U_1, W_1. The straight line represents expected utility for different probabilities that the illness will occur. The *lower* the probability that the event will occur, the closer the expected utility will be to the point farthest to the right on the utility curve. As the probability that the loss will occur increases, the expected utility value moves down to the left on the straight line, closer to the point represented by U_1 on the curve. In other words, if the loss is certain to occur, the individual will be at W_1 ($2,000) with a corresponding utility level of U_1 ($= 20$). Since the calculation of expected utility is based on the weighted sum of the probabilities of being at the different utility levels, as the probability of being at U_1 increases, the expected utility estimate declines in a linear fashion.

To show that expected utility declines linearly, the probability of the event occurring can be assumed to increase from 0.05, to 0.10, to 0.15, to 0.20. The expected utility of each of these events would then be as follows:

$$
\begin{aligned}
P(U_1) + (1 - P)(U_3) &= 0.05(20) + 0.95(100) = 96 \\
&= 0.10(20) + 0.90(100) = 92 \\
&= 0.15(20) + 0.85(100) = 88 \\
&= 0.20(20) + 0.80(100) = 84
\end{aligned}
$$

Because the individual's actual utility curve (decreasing marginal utility with respect to wealth) is always above the expected utility line (constant marginal utility with respect to wealth), the individual will always buy insurance if it is sold at its actuarially fair value (its pure premium). Thus, a risk-averse person will prefer to take a certain loss (the premium) rather than accept the uncertainty of a loss, even though the expected value of the loss is equal.[3]

Insurance, however, is never sold at its pure premium because there are administrative, claims processing, and marketing costs. These costs are referred to as the *loading charge* and are, in effect, the price of insurance. To determine whether or not an individual, as represented in Figure 6-2B, will buy insurance when there are these additional costs, the maximum amount above the pure premium he or she would be willing to pay for insurance must be calculated.

Referring back to Figure 6-2B, W_3-W_2 represents the dollar amount of the pure premium for an $8,000 loss that has a 2.5 percent probability of occurring. Since the utility level with insurance is greater than the expected utility level (99 versus 98), *the person purchasing insurance will be willing to pay an amount above the pure premium that makes the actual utility level after the additional payment equal to the expected utility level.* When the actual utility level is equal to the expected utility level (at U = 98), the person will be indifferent as to whether he or she purchases insurance or self-insures. If an additional payment (loading charge) places the individual's actual utility level below his or her expected utility level, the person would be better off by self-insuring; that is, the person would be willing to pay an amount above the pure premium as long as his expected utility is not greater than his actual utility.

---

3. In a thought provoking new book, John Nyman presents a controversial new theory of demand for health insurance. In his book, Nyman discusses the new theory of health insurance and contrasts its assumptions, predictions, and policy implications with the conventional theory. For example, the conventional theory holds that consumers purchase insurance because they prefer a certain loss (the insurance premium) to an uncertain loss of the same magnitude. Nyman finds the opposite to be correct, claiming that the decision to purchase insurance has little, if anything, to do with preferences regarding risk. Further, rather than being discretionary and inefficient as analyzed according to the conventional theory moral hazard, according to Nyman, makes the consumer better off and represents a central motivation for purchasing insurance. The opposing theories imply both different cost containment policies and justifications for government intervention in health insurance markets. John A. Nyman, *The Theory of Demand for Health Insurance*, (Stanford University Press: Stanford, California) 2003.

This discussion is illustrated in Figure 6-2B. Point A is the expected utility without insurance. If one draws a straight line from Point A to where it crosses the actual utility curve, then at Point B, a person's actual utility level and expected utility level are the same, U = 98. The distance from Point A to Point B on the wealth axis is the additional amount above the pure premium that a person would be willing to pay for that insurance. At every point along the expected utility line (which represents a different probability of the event occurring), there is an additional amount above the pure premium that a person would be willing to pay for insurance. At points close to W_1, which represent a high probability that a person will incur a large enough loss to leave him or her at wealth position W_1, a person would be willing to pay a smaller amount above the pure premium; the distance between the expected utility line and the actual utility curve, which would leave him or her at the same level of utility, is closer at that point.

As shown in Figure 6-3A, with an expected utility level at Point E, the pure premium would be W_3-W_4, which is a large amount since the probability of the loss occurring is quite high. A person would be willing to pay an additional amount above the pure premium equal to the distance EF, since at Point F expected utility is equal to actual utility. Any amount greater than EF would place the person at a lower point on his or her actual utility curve. Actual utility would then be less than the expected utility of not buying insurance. The amount above the pure premium, which is equal to the distance EF, is smaller than at another part of the graph, for example, CD. At Point C, a person is willing to pay an additional amount equal to CD, which would make the actual utility level indicated by D equal to the expected level indicated by C. CD is greater than EF because the probability of the loss's occurring is larger at Point E.

As the loss becomes almost certain to occur, the person can save for the event instead of paying the same amount (equal to the pure premium) to an insurance company *plus* an additional amount (loading charge) to cover other insurance company costs. In the case of near-certain events such as annual medical or dental checkups (probabilities approximately 1.0), it would be cheaper to self-insure. At large probabilities and at very small probabilities (very rare events), a person is willing to pay less over the pure premium than at other, more intermediate probabilities.

Another factor that influences how much above the pure premium the person is willing to pay for insurance is the magnitude of the expected loss. When the expected loss is relatively large, as shown in Figure 6-3B, a person can lose W_3–W_1 ($8,000) if the illness occurs and they do not have insurance. If, on the other hand, the loss is relatively small, as for a visit to the dentist for a filling, this loss will be represented by a smaller possible loss in wealth if it occurs, W_3–W_5. The expected utility line for the large loss is AC; for the small loss it is AB. The distances W_3–W_1 (expected utility line AC) and W_3–W_5 (expected utility line AB) represent different-sized losses with the same probabilities of occurrence. The area between the actual utility curve and the expected utility line is much greater for the large loss than for the small one. Given the same probability that either the large or the small loss will occur, a person is willing to pay a larger amount above the pure premium for the large loss than for the small one.

To determine the demand for health insurance, we must now combine the preceding discussion of risk aversion (the individual's total utility curve that increases but at a decreasing rate), the probability that a loss will occur, the magnitude of that loss if it should occur, and information on the price of insurance—that is, the amount charged above the pure premium. To illustrate the price-quantity relationship of the demand for health insurance, reference is made to Figure 6-4.

The price of insurance along the vertical axis in Figure 6-4 is the amount *above* the pure premium (the loading charge) that the person must pay for insurance; along the horizontal axis is the probability that the event will occur. The curved line starting at 0 probability of the event occurring and ending at a probability of 1.0 (certainty) is the amount above the pure premium that the person is willing to pay for insurance. This area is taken from the previous figures and is merely the distance between the actual utility curve and the expected utility line. Since insurance is never sold at a price just equaling the pure premium (included are costs for marketing, administration, and

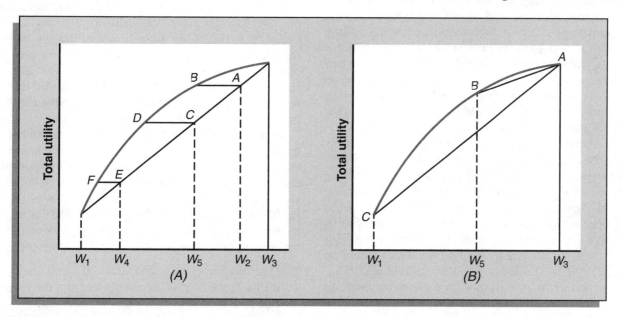

Figure 6-3.   The amount above the pure premium an individual is willing to pay for health insurance; (A) according to different probabilities of the event occurring; (B) according to different magnitudes of the expected loss.

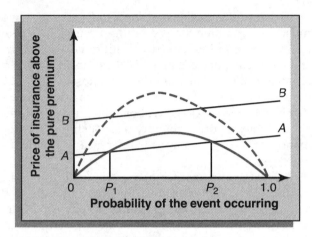

Figure 6-4. The relationship between price of insurance and quantity demanded.

claims processing), the price of insurance is represented by line AA in Figure 6-4. The reason it increases as the probability of the event's occurring increases is that there are greater administrative costs (such as recordkeeping and verification) when claims are more frequent (have a higher probability of occurring). Since line AA intersects the solid curved line representing the amount above the pure premium the person is willing to pay for insurance, the person will buy insurance for events that fall between P_1 and P_2. Between those two points the price the person has to pay for insurance is *less* than the amount he or she would be willing to pay, meaning that he or she would be better off (at a higher level of utility) if the insurance were purchased.

The price of insurance (the loading charge) is *greater* than the amount he or she is willing to pay for events that have either a very small probability of occurring (the area $0–P_1$) or a very high probability of occurring (to the right of P_2). Based upon Figure 6-4, we would predict that illnesses having both a very small probability of occurrence as well as those that have a high probability of occurrence (i.e., routine care) would be unlikely to be insured against by individuals. If required to purchase insurance for these two events, an individual would be worse off, since the marginal benefits to be derived from that coverage would be smaller than the marginal costs (price) of insurance!

If the price of insurance were to rise to line BB, we would expect the individual represented by the solid curved line to self-insure—that is, to demand *less* insurance coverage. With a higher price of insurance, the new price *exceeds* the additional amount above the pure premium the individual is willing to pay. Regardless of the probability of the event's occurrence, the individual would be worse off if more had to be paid for insurance than he or she was willing to pay. Only if the magnitude of the loss, as shown by the dashed curved line, were greater than price line BB would the individual purchase insurance for that probable loss. Thus, as the price of insurance rises, the individual will be less likely to insure for certain events. This inverse relationship between the price of insurance and the quantity of insurance demanded is the demand schedule for insurance.

A person is also more likely to insure against events that have a greater magnitude of loss than against events with smaller possible losses. This aspect of the demand for health insurance can be seen with reference to the price of insurance (BB) in Figure 6-4 and the two curved lines representing different possible losses. Referring back to Figure 6-3, we saw that the amount above the pure premium that a person was willing to pay was less for small losses than for large losses given the same probability of the event occurring. One interesting implication of this relationship between the price of insurance and the size of the loss is that as the cost of medical care has risen, so has the size of the probable loss, and this by itself has resulted in an increase (a shift to the right) in the demand for health insurance.

In summarizing the theory of the demand for health insurance, attention should be drawn to two areas: (a) the factors that affect the demand for health insurance, and (b) the welfare implications (is the person better or worse off?) of requiring an individual to purchase health insurance against all types of medical illness, the routine as well as low-cost services. The following factors would affect the demand for health insurance:

1. *How risk averse is the individual?* If he or she has a utility curve that is increasing but at a decreasing rate (i.e., diminishing marginal utility with respect to increased income), the individual is willing to pay an amount above the pure premium for insurance coverage. (Risk averse people have a greater demand for insurance.)

2. *The probability of the event occurring.* As shown in Figure 6-3, for those events that have a very low or a very high probability of occurring, a person is willing to pay less above the pure premium than for events that have a more intermediate probability of occurring. (The demand for health insurance is lower when the probabilities of the event occurring are either very high or very low.)

3. *The magnitude of the loss.* The larger the magnitude of the loss, as in Figure 6-3, the greater will be the amount above the pure premium that the individual is willing to pay for insurance. (The demand for insurance will be greater the greater the size of the loss.)

4. *The price of insurance* (also known as the loading charge). The higher the price of insurance (the amount above the pure premium), the individual will insure against fewer events. (The higher the price, the lower the quantity demanded of insurance.)

5. *The income of the individual.* The size of a person's income and wealth will affect the amount above the pure premium they are willing to pay for health insurance. At both low and high incomes, the marginal utility of income is either relatively high or low so that such persons might prefer to self insure (3); the distance between the expected and actual utility curve is less at both high and low incomes than for intermediate income levels.

Low-income persons, in addition to not willing to spend much above the pure premium for insurance, also have available a low-priced substitute if they become ill—Medicaid.[4] (There may also be an "income" effect even if sold at the pure premium; insurance may be too expensive for a person with low income.) However, those with high incomes have an incentive to purchase employer-paid health insurance because it is a fringe benefit and is not considered to be taxable income. The tax treatment of health insurance is discussed below.

The demand for health insurance is affected by the tax treatment of health insurance premiums. Employer-paid health insurance premiums are excluded from the taxable income of the employee (not just federal taxes, but state, Social Security, and Medicare payroll taxes as well). This tax subsidy for the purchase of health insurance lowers the price of insurance to those with a high income. As employee incomes increase and move into higher tax brackets, they have a greater incentive to have their employer buy fringe benefits with *before-tax* income than for them to buy the same service with their *after-tax* income.

The favorable tax treatment of employer-paid health insurance lowers the price of insurance and led to a much greater demand for insurance than would have otherwise occurred. (See Appendix 2 for a graphical illustration of this issue.) It has been estimated that in 2001, this tax incentive for the purchase of health insurance resulted in a loss in federal government revenues (excluding lost state income taxes) of approximately $120 billion a year (4). The tax treatment of health insurance coverage is, in effect, a subsidy for the purchase of health insurance, and the subsidy is greater for persons in higher income tax brackets.

For example, when an employer buys health insurance for an employee in a 30 percent marginal tax bracket, the employee purchases that insurance *at less than its pure premium. The price of health insurance to the employee is the loading charge minus the employee's tax rate multiplied by the total premium.* Assume that the pure premium is $5,000 per year and that the loading charge is 10 percent of the premium, or $500. The total premium is therefore $5,500 per employee. If the employer gave the employee a wage increase of $5,500 to buy insurance and the employee then paid taxes on the $5,500, the employee would only have $3,850 to buy that insurance (0.30 × $5,500 = $1,650;

---

4. Expansions of public insurance programs, such as Medicaid and the State Children's Health Insurance Program (SCHIP) enacted as part of the 1997 Balanced Budget Act (to increase insurance coverage of children whose family income exceeded Medicaid eligibility limits), have resulted in the substitution of public insurance for private insurance, termed "crowd-out." The substitution of public for private insurance is more likely to occur as eligibility levels expand to those with higher incomes who are more likely to have private insurance. Empirical estimates of the "crowd-out" effect vary greatly, up to 45 percent of Medicaid enrollment increases from expanded eligibility may be from crowding out private insurance. Richard Kronick and Todd Gilmer, "Insuring Low-Income Adults: Does Public Coverage Crowd Out Private?," *Health Affairs,* 21(1), January/February 2002, 225–239.

$5,500 – $1,650 = $3,850). The employee would either have to buy a less expensive health plan or use an additional $1,650 of his or her own money to buy the $5,500 health plan. When the employer buys the insurance for the employee with the $5,500 before it is taxed, then the employee can have the $5,500 health plan. The employee saves $1,650 when the insurance is purchased with before-taxed income. This is the same as the employee paying only $3,850 in after-tax dollars for a health plan that costs $5,500.

Tax-exempt employer-paid health insurance provides a tax subsidy to purchase health insurance. In the above example, the tax subsidy equals $1,650. The tax subsidy enables the employee to buy the insurance at less than its actuarially fair value! The *effective price of insurance* to an employee in a 30 percent tax bracket would be *minus* $1,150; it is $1,150 less than the loading charge ($500 –0.30 × $5,500 = $500 – $1,650 = –$1,150).

The tax subsidy is even greater than shown in the above example. An employee in a 30 percent federal tax bracket must also pay state taxes, Social Security taxes, and a Medicare payroll tax. Assuming state taxes are 5 percent, Social Security taxes 7.5 percent, and the Medicare tax is 1.45 percent, then the marginal tax rate for an employee earning $100,000 would be about 44 percent. Thus the advantage to that employee of having the employer purchase health insurance is a tax saving of $2,420 ($5,500 × 0.44 = $2,420) or an effective price of insurance that is $1,920 *below* the loading charge ($500 –0.44 × $5,500 = $500 –$2,420 = –$1,920).[5]

Tax-exempt employer-paid health insurance provides employees in higher tax brackets with an incentive to buy insurance with before-tax dollars; their tax subsidy exceeds the price (loading charge) of the insurance, thereby lowering the price of insurance. (The price elasticity of demand for health insurance has been estimated to be between –0.2 to –1.0) (5). Thus an important reason for the increasing comprehensiveness of health insurance coverage for small claims ("first-dollar coverage") is that the premium for such losses is *less* than the actuarial value of such losses as the individual moves into higher and higher tax brackets. Government tax policy has stimulated the demand for health insurance and has increased its comprehensiveness.

Marginal tax brackets have been declining over time. The highest tax bracket decreased from 87 percent in 1963 to 70 percent in 1980 to 39 percent currently. This decline in marginal tax brackets *increased* the effective price of health insurance and has likely led to a decline in its comprehensiveness.

Previously, cost-based reimbursement and the use of service benefit policies removed any incentives that may have existed either for the patient to shop around or for the provider to provide care more efficiently. These policies increased the magnitude of a medical loss and thereby increased the demand for health insurance. If the provider's costs are reimbursed in full, regardless of what other hospitals may charge, and if the patient is not required to pay any portion of the hospital's bill, as is the case under a service benefit policy, then any incentives for cost constraint on either the demander or the supplier have been removed. This method of provider reimbursement, preferred by hospitals and accepted by Blue Cross, increased hospital costs, increased the magnitude of the probable loss due to a hospital episode, and thereby resulted in a further *increase* in the demand for protection against such large losses.

An important factor affecting the price of insurance (loading charge) is whether the individual is part of a large employee group. Group policies are sold at substantially lower prices than individual policies. In part, the reduced price reflects economies of scale in administering the insurance contract; the group handles some administrative and claims processing costs itself and it is less expensive to market to a group than to the same number of separate individuals. (Another reason for lower prices to group members, discussed below, is that there is less likelihood of adverse selection. Individuals seeking to purchase health insur-

---

5. Economists believe that the employer's share of Social Security and Medicare payroll taxes are shifted to the employee in the form of reduced wages making those taxes double the above amounts, resulting in a marginal tax rate of almost 53 percent in the above example. For a graphical illustration of who bears the burden of payroll taxes, see the Chapter on National Health Insurance, Figure 19-4.

ance may be doing so because they expect to use such coverage in the near future. To guard against such self-selection and the possibly higher risks associated with it, the price of the policy will be higher to an individual than to a person who is a member of a group which they joined so as to have a job rather than because they were ill and wanted insurance.) The higher price of insurance (the loading charge) to persons who are not part of a group leads to a smaller quantity demanded for health insurance.

Whether or not a group is self-insured will affect the group's expected loss (hence the insurance premium), and consequently, the demand for insurance. In the last 20 years, state legislatures have enacted more than 1500 state mandates. Insurance companies are required to include in their insurance policies their respective state mandates. These mandates are generally of three types: coverage for specific medical conditions, such as substance abuse, in vitro fertilization, and hair transplants (Minnesota), the services of specific health providers, such as chiropractors and optometrists, and inclusion of certain population groups, such as newborns and the handicapped.

A self-insured employer is exempt from state regulation, including state mandates and state health insurance premium taxes, according to the 1974 federal Employee Retirement and Security Act (ERISA). These cost savings are significant and are an important reason why many large firms have become self-insured (6). It is believed that more small businesses would offer health benefits to their employees if state mandates were eliminated. The additional cost of state mandates exceeds the amount above the pure premium that individuals are willing to pay to be insured, leaving them with the only option of being self-insured.

One additional factor affecting the price and demand for health insurance is technology (7). The growth in medical technology over the last several decades has made it possible to treat certain diseases that were previously untreatable. These treatment costs, however, are quite large; for example, organ replacements and survival of low birthweight babies cost hundreds of thousands of dollars. Once a treatment for a previously untreatable condition becomes

available, there is an increased probability that an individual may require such a treatment. Further, the magnitude of the loss is increased. Both of these factors, the probability of a loss and its magnitude, will cause an increase in the demand for health insurance.

It has been said that there are three stages of technology development. The first is "nontechnology," in which hospital and medical care offers little hope of recovery or improvement from the disease, thus treatment costs are low. The second is "halfway technology," which treats the disease once it has been incurred, for example, organ transplants or surgery for cancer patients. Halfway technology is typically very expensive. The third stage is "high technology." This stage is characterized by an understanding of the disease process thereby making it possible to prevent the onset of the disease. An example of technology in this stage is immunizations. Technology is relatively inexpensive in this stage.

In the last three decades, the medical sector has been characterized by the development of halfway technologies for many diseases. These technological developments, by raising the probable loss of a medical event, have increased the demand for health insurance.

Health insurance provides for treatment of an illness with whatever technology is currently available as contrasted with providing only the state of technology available at the time the contract was written. The demand for health insurance is increased when the latest (non-experimental) technology is covered since the probable loss is increased if halfway technology becomes available to cover a previously untreatable illness. The insurance premium, however, is also increased since the new technology is costly. "In the long run, the price of private health insurance depends upon the state of technology" (8). As the premium increases, the quantity demanded decreases, leading to a larger number of uninsured.

In addition to which state of technology is covered, the method used by the insurer to pay for the new technologies has further increased the price of insurance. Previous retrospective cost-based payment to hospitals (and no out-of-pocket payment by patients) eliminated provider efficiency incentives while providing an incentive to the patient and physician to perform the service as long as there was some positive marginal benefit, even though the marginal benefit was less than the resource costs of providing the treatment. Thus the insurance system encouraged the development of halfway technologies while increasing the cost of insurance.

There is a circular process to the demand for health insurance and the development of technology. While technology has increased the demand for insurance, insurance has stimulated the growth of technology. The investment in technology depends upon its profitability, which is related to the potential size of its market, whether insurance (either private or government) will pay for it, and the cost of developing the technology. Since the demand for technology is derived from the demand for hospital and physician services, the method of provider payment affects the demand for technologies. The change in hospital payment to fixed prices per admission, selective contracting among hospitals, and the development of capitation-based systems (whereby medical providers receive a fixed payment per enrollee regardless of the quantity of medical services delivered), is changing the demand for new technologies. The emphasis is on cost reducing rather than just quality-enhancing technology. A substitution in the type of halfway technology being demanded is also occurring, from caring for the patient in a hospital to being able to provide the treatment in an outpatient setting and in the patient's home.

The circular relationship between technology and insurance ultimately affects investment in technology, the type of technology developed, the demand for insurance, the cost of that insurance, as well as the rise in medical expenditures.

Economic variables, price and income, the tastes of the individual toward risk aversion, and the size of the probable loss thus affect the demand for health insurance.

It is interesting to speculate on the welfare implications of this theory of demand for insurance. In attempting to maximize their utility, consumers will allocate their income so that the marginal benefit from each of the goods and services they consume equals the prices they must pay for those goods and services.

If the price (which represents the marginal cost of producing those goods and services) exceeds the marginal benefits to them, they will be worse off by purchasing those goods and services. They can increase their utility by cutting back on those goods and services for which the marginal benefit is less than the price that must be paid and using the funds saved to purchase other goods and services whose marginal benefits (per dollar) are greater. In this manner they will achieve a higher level of utility than by any other allocation process. If, however, consumers are *forced* to purchase a good whose price is greater than its marginal benefit, they clearly end up worse off than before. Forcing consumers to pay a price for a good that is higher than its marginal benefit is a situation that can occur in the health field if all consumers are required to have complete comprehensive insurance coverage against all of their medical expenses.

As shown in Figure 6-4, there are two situations in which the price of insurance will exceed the amount above the pure premium that the consumer is willing to pay. The first is for medical losses that have either a very high or a very low probability of occurring. In Figure 6-4, the area to the right of P_2 represents medical losses that have a high probability of occurring; these routine medical expenses are for such purchases as physician office visits, a dental visit, and over-the-counter drugs. Comprehensive insurance coverage to include such routine medical expenses would necessitate a price (loading charge), perhaps in the form of a tax on the consumer, that would exceed what they would be willing to pay above the actuarial value of those losses. Requiring consumers to pay that price by law clearly leaves them worse off than if they could self-insure for those losses.

A second situation in which a consumer is made worse off by being required to purchase complete insurance coverage is when there are small medical losses. The price of insurance for that coverage (line BB) is greater than the amount above the pure premium (the solid curved line) the consumer would be willing to pay.

It might be argued that since the price of insurance is less than the aggregate amount consumers would be willing to pay in all situations, requiring insurance coverage for even those medical expenses that they would prefer not to insure against would, on an aggregate basis, still leave them better off with insurance than without. However, as long as the different forms of coverage are divisible and do not have to be sold together, consumers would be better off with *some* coverage than with either complete coverage or none at all.

The welfare implication of mandatory insurance coverage that covers all medical losses, no matter how small or routine and expected they may be, is that some consumers will be worse off than if they had a choice and could self-insure in those situations.

AN APPLICATION OF THE THEORY OF THE DEMAND FOR HEALTH INSURANCE

The theory of the demand for health insurance can now be used to explain why we observe some people insuring against certain types of medical loss (e.g., hospital care) and not others (e.g., dental care). (When the concept of moral hazard is introduced later, it will be shown that although people may buy insurance for hospital services, they still may not insure against all hospital expenses, preferring to bear some of the costs themselves.) Also, since not everyone is "risk averse" (their expected utility curve may be equal to or greater than their actual utility curve with respect to wealth), some people would decide not to buy *any* health insurance. They would prefer to self-insure, not out of ignorance or irrationality, but because they are not risk averse (i.e., for the same reason that some people gamble).

Previously, when the price of health insurance was not greatly reduced as a result of being widely available as a fringe benefit, a sizable percentage of the uninsured, 37 percent according to a survey conducted in the mid-1950s, indicated that they felt they were just as well off without health insurance (9). The potential market for health insurance at that time was less than 100 percent of the population. As the price of medical care increased over time (i.e., the size of the potential medical loss became larger), and as personal income also increased, the demand for health insurance also grew. More recently, only about 10 percent

of the uninsured believe they are just as well off without health insurance.

To determine how well the foregoing model of demand for health insurance predicts the type of health insurance found in the population, we examine the purchase of insurance coverage by type of medical expense. Costs for hospitalization and for surgery would seem far more likely to qualify as high expected losses with a relatively low probability of occurrence than would medical losses such as physician office visits, optometric services, drugs, and dental care, all of which involve relatively smaller medical expenses and are considered by families to be more routine and budgetable.

In examining the period before the tax subsidy for health insurance greatly stimulated the demand for insurance, we find that the economic theory of demand for health insurance is able to explain the type of health insurance observed in the population quite well. Using data from a 1957 to 1958 household survey of the U.S. population, medical expenses by type of service were classified according to whether they had a high or a low probability of occurring and whether they had a high or a low potential loss if they did occur. Low probability of occurrence was arbitrarily defined by whether 20 percent of the population incurred an expense for that medical service during the past year; high potential loss was also arbitrarily defined by whether the average cost incurred by persons using that medical service was greater than $40. This data is shown in Table 6-1, together with the actual percentage of expenditures covered by insurance for each of the medical services examined.

According to the data, the prevalence of insurance was generally consistent with what the economic theory of demand for health insurance would lead us to expect. Those medical services that have a low probability of occurrence and a high expected loss are more likely to be covered by insurance than those expenses with either a high or a low probability of occurrence and low expected loss.

The costs of a medical event have greatly increased over time, leading to an increase in the demand for insurance. Also contributing to an increase in demand was the growth in incomes and the rise in inflation

Table 6-1. Classification of Medical Services by Probability of Occurrence, Potential Loss, and Insurance Benefits, 1957–1958

Type of Medical Service	Probability of Occurrence	Magnitude of Expense	Percent of Expenditures Covered by Insurance	Expenditures on This Type of Service as a Percent of Total Medical Expenditures
Hospital care	Low	High	58	23
Physician charges for:				
Surgery	Low	High	48	7
In-hospital visits	Low	High		
Office visits	High	Low	7	24
House calls	High	Low		
Drugs and medicines	High	Low	1	20
Other medical services	Low	Low	1	8
Dental care	High	Low	—(a)	15

Sources: R. G. Rice, "Some Health Insurance Implications of the Economics of Uncertainty," unpublished paper presented before *The American Public Health Association,* October 6, 1964. Columns 1 and 2 based on data published in O. W. Anderson, P. Collete, and J. J. Feldman, *Changes in Family Medical Care Expenditures and Voluntary Health Insurance: A Five Year Resurvey* (Cambridge, MA: Harvard University Press, 1963).

(a) Less than one-half of 1 percent.

throughout the 1960s and 1970s. As incomes and inflation increased pushing more employees into higher tax rates, more employees preferred to receive additional income in the form of health insurance, which was not subject to personal income taxes. Thus, although the percentage of medical expenditures covered by insurance has greatly increased since the period covered by the data cited above, we would still expect to observe a difference in the distribution of medical expenses covered by health insurance. Those medical services having a lower probability of occurrence and a high potential loss are still more likely to have a higher percentage of their expenses covered by insurance than those services considered to be routine and/or have a relatively lower potential loss. The same relationship holds for more recent data as well.

Aggregate data for 2002 supports the finding that where the probability of use is low and the expected cost is high, the percent of the bill paid for by insurance is highest. Consumers pay only 3 percent of total hospital expenditures out of pocket, with the remainder being paid for by private insurance and government programs. For physician services, approximately 10.5 percent of total expenditures are out of pocket; the out-of-pocket percentage for dental care is 43.3 percent, 47.8 percent for eyeglasses (and other medical durables), and 30.2 percent for drugs (10).

In summary, the model of demand for health insurance suggests that a measure of the adequacy of health insurance should *not* be the percentage of aggregate medical expenses covered by health insurance, with anything less than 100 percent being considered inadequate. Instead, the adequacy of health coverage should be examined separately for each type of medical service. Even if everyone were risk averse, people would not buy insurance for all of their medical expenses. The price of insurance (i.e., the amount above the pure premium) for some medical expenses would exceed the amount some people were willing to pay. Requiring everyone under such circumstances to purchase health insurance for *all* of their medical expenses would make people *worse off,* since the costs of the coverage for some expenses would exceed the benefits.

BIASED SELECTION IN HEALTH CARE MARKETS

Adverse Selection

The earlier discussion of demand for health insurance assumed that the insured population belonged to the same risk group, that is, that they all had the same probability of incurring an illness. The pure premium was based on the average expected loss of that group. An individual, however, is more knowledgeable about his or her own health status than is the insurance company. High-risk individuals therefore have an incentive to purchase insurance at a premium that is based on a lower risk group. The insurance company's concern that this difference in information will lead to high-risk individuals purchasing insurance based on a lower risk group's premium is referred to as "adverse selection."

Insurance companies realize that population groups have differing levels of risk. However, if the insurance company is unable to distinguish between high and low risks, the insurance premium will reflect the average risk of the two groups. In this situation, the high-risk group will purchase insurance since a premium based on the average risk of the two groups is still lower than a premium based solely on their own risk group. Low-risk individuals may not purchase insurance since a premium based on the average of the two risk groups would be greater than their own risk-based premium. Adverse selection would result in a biased sample of those who purchase health insurance; predominately more higher-risk individuals would purchase insurance at a premium that is based on a lower risk group. (Insurers' concern with adverse selection would also occur if they were unable, because of legal prohibitions, to use certain risk factors for determining a premium.)

When adverse selection occurs, the insurance company loses money. To remain in business, the insurance company must raise its premium to reflect the proportionately greater number of high-risk individuals. As the premium is increased, however, more low-risk individuals drop out. To prevent their losing the less risky subscribers, insurance companies are reluctant to raise their premiums without also imposing restrictions on use at the higher premium (11).

The above discussion is illustrated in Figure 6-5. Assume the following: both high- and low-risk individuals have the same relationship between total utility and wealth; they each have $10,000; and if an illness occurs, the loss is $8,000. Low-risk individuals have only a 0.2 probability of incurring an illness, while high-risk individuals have a 0.8 probability. It is further assumed that there are an equal number of low- and high-risk individuals.

The pure premium for the low-risk group is $1,600 ($8,000 multiplied by 0.2) and a resulting wealth position of $8,400. For high-risk individuals, the pure premium would be $6,400 ($8,000 multiplied by 0.8) and a resulting wealth position of $3,600.

The straight line AB shows the expected utility of an $8,000 loss occurring at different probabilities. If health insurance were sold at the pure premium to

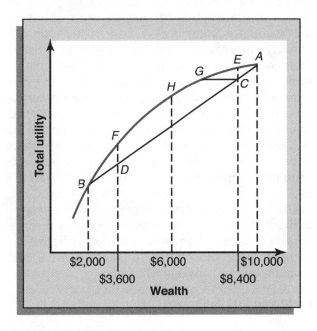

Figure 6-5. Adverse selection.

each risk group, both risk groups would be willing to purchase insurance. The low-risk individual would be at a higher utility level, E, which is greater than their expected utility, C. The low-risk individual would also be willing to pay distance CG in excess of the pure premium. (High-risk individuals would also be willing to purchase insurance sold at the pure premium since their actual utility, F, is above their expected utility, D.)

If the insurance company cannot distinguish between high- and low-risk individuals, the pure premium will be based on the average risk of the two populations. The pure premium for everyone would then be $4,000 ($8,000 multiplied by 0.5). High-risk individuals would purchase the insurance because they would be at a higher utility level, H instead of F. Low-risk individuals, however, would not buy insurance since their utility level with insurance, H, would be lower than G, which is the maximum amount above the pure premium they would be willing to pay.

The approaches used by insurance companies to protect themselves against adverse selection attempt to redress the information imbalance. Excluding from insurance coverage pre-existing conditions (up to one year) which the individual may be aware of but not the insurance company, is one such approach. Similarly, the insurance company may require the individual to have tests performed in order to have the same information as the individual. Insurers may require a minimum waiting period before certain services are covered, e.g., 10 months for obstetrics care. Low-risk individuals may "signal" their lower risk status by their willingness to accept insurance policies that contain high deductibles and co-insurance. Open enrollment periods are also a method to decrease adverse selection. By requiring individuals to choose their health plan once a year, an individual who is ill cannot switch to a more comprehensive, less restrictive health plan just when they become ill, otherwise the more comprehensive plan would receive an adverse risk group.

Preferred Risk Selection

"Preferred risk selection" may occur when insurers receive the same premium for everyone within a group, but the risks within that group vary. The insurer may try to select the lower-risk individuals while receiving a premium that is based on the average risk of the group. Preferred risk selection results when there is a difference between the group premium and the risk level of the individual. As shown in Figure 6-5, the average premium received by an insurer would be $4,000, which would cover both low- and high-risk members of that group. The insurer, however, would be able to increase their profits if they could receive that average premium and attract just the low-risk members of that group.

Approaches used by insurers to attract low-risk individuals include offering benefits that low-risk individuals would find appealing (such as well baby services and sports medicine clinics), while de-emphasizing services that would be attractive to high-risk individuals, such as having a cancer center, cardiac care specialists, and transplant services.

When an employer offers two different health plans at the same price to its employees and the employees differ in their risk levels, both adverse and preferred selection can occur. For example, assume one health plan is an HMO with a restrictive provider network, no deductibles or co-payments, and additional benefits to appeal to young healthy enrollees; the second health plan offers a broader choice of providers, including the most reputable medical centers, self-referral to specialists, and includes a small deductible and co-payments. Low-risk employees will be attracted to the HMO with its additional benefits and no out-of-pocket payments, while those who have a health condition (higher risk) will choose the second health plan. The HMO will have a preferred risk group while adverse selection will impact the second health plan. The problem in both cases is that the premium is the same for both health plans.

When HMOs were first offered as an option to those receiving Medicare in the 1980s, the HMO received a premium for the aged based on their age and sex within a geographic area. That premium was based on 95 percent of what those aged were expected to have cost the government if they remained in the traditional Medicare program. Since the premium was based on the average medical expenditures of the aged within that risk group, the HMO had an incentive to select the healthier aged within each risk group. In recruiting aged to join their HMO, the HMOs did not enroll the aged by mail for fear that the bedridden might join up. Instead, the aged are invited to meetings. Also (up until 2003) the aged were permitted to leave the HMO with 30 days notification. Thus it has been alleged that some HMO physicians informed an enrollee who required expensive surgery that the HMO can perform it but if they were to disenroll they could be cared for at the university hospital, which has better specialists and facilities.

Studies have been conducted to determine whether the government saved money when they paid HMOs 95 percent of the average cost for the aged enrolling in an HMO. These studies indicate that the government *lost*, on average, 6 percent; in other words, if the aged who enrolled in HMOs remained in the traditional Medicare program, the government would have spent 11 percent less on those aged (12). Therefore, the HMOs enrolling the aged received, on average, a preferred risk group; those aged receiving traditional Medicare were more likely to have a chronic illness and therefore less willing to change their provider relationships to join an HMO. The risk adjustment factors used by the government accounted for only about half of the risk selection of new Medicare HMO enrollees. Over time, the longer the aged remained in the HMO their medical costs rose.

The importance of preferred (and adverse) risk selection to an insurer could be seen by the data presented in Table 6-2. One percent of the population incurs 27 percent of total medical expenditures (as of 1996). The top 5 percent of the population incurs 55 percent of total medical expenditures, and 10 percent of the population incurs 69 percent of total expenditures. If an insurer were able to enroll the remaining 90 percent while receiving a premium based on the average, it would make a great deal of money. The problem of preferred risk selection is important for Medicare because 46 percent of those in the top one percent of those with the highest expenditures are over age 65 (13). (The increase over time in medical expenditures for those in the highest expenditure categories is likely due to the development and availability of new medical technologies.)

Concluding Comments on Risk Selection

Adverse selection with respect to the individual insurance market would be reduced if all individuals were required to have health insurance. Individuals would then have no need to join a health plan only when they became ill.

Health insurers also compete on their ability to select low risk groups. An insurer may therefore be more profitable, not because it is more efficient, but because it is better at attracting a preferred risk group.

Table 6-2. Distribution of Health Expenditures for the U.S. Population, by Magnitude of Expenditures, Selected Years, 1928–1996

Percent of U.S. Population Ranked by Expenditures	1928	1963	1970	1977	1980	1987	1996
Top 1 percent	—	17%	26%	27%	29%	28%	27%
Top 2 percent	—	—	35	38	39	39	38
Top 5 percent	52	43	50	55	55	56	55
Top 10 percent	—	59	66	70	70	70	69
Top 30 percent	93	—	88	90	90	90	90
Top 50 percent	—	95	96	97	96	97	97
Bottom 50 percent	—	5	4	3	4	3	3

Source: Adapted with permission from M. L. Berk and A. C. Monheit, "The Concentration of Health Care Expenditures, Revisited," Exhibit 1, *Health Affairs*, 20(2), March/April 2001: 9–18. Copyright © 2001 Project HOPE-the People-to-People Health Foundation, Inc., All Rights Reserved.

To limit preferred risk selection, each group should have a *risk-adjusted premium*. In this way, insurers would no longer have an incentive to select low risk groups; each risk group would have a premium that reflects its risk. Insurers would then have to compete on price (premium) for each risk group. The more efficient insurers would be those who are better able to manage risk. Accurate risk-adjusted premiums would change the nature of insurance competition from risk selection to risk management. Unfortunately, developing risk-adjusted premiums under the Medicare program have not yet met with much success. A great deal of research is devoted to developing better risk adjusters for the aged besides age and sex. (Biased selection is further discussed in Chapter 8, "The Market for Health Insurance.")

THE DEMAND FOR HEALTH INSURANCE UNDER CONDITIONS OF MORAL HAZARD

The previous discussion demonstrated that even when the demand for medical care is assumed to be completely price inelastic, people would still not demand completely comprehensive health insurance because of selling and transactions costs (loading charge). In this section, the concept of moral hazard is introduced to show that its existence also results in a demand for health insurance coverage that is less than 100 percent of a person's medical expenses (14).

If demand for medical care were inelastic with respect to price, the individual's demand curve in the event of illness would look like D_1 in Figure 6-6; that is, the individual would demand Q_1 units of medical care. In the case of moral hazard, when a person has health insurance their consumption of medical care will increase because it is subsidized. It is possible for the insured patient to affect the size of his or her loss when there is some price elasticity to the individual's demand curve. Thus, if an individual became ill, the quantity of medical care that he or she would demand would depend, in part, on the price that had to be paid for that care. If insurance covered the entire cost of the illness episode, the individual represented by

demand curve D_2 would demand Q_2 units of medical care. The presence of some elasticity in the individual's demand curve indicates that the individual will demand different quantities of medical care depending upon how much the individual must pay for that care. Since insurance lowers the price of medical care to individuals, they will consume more care than if they had to pay the entire price themselves. It is this behavior of individuals that is termed "moral hazard."

To the individual consuming medical care under these circumstances, it is perfectly rational behavior—he or she is equating the marginal cost of purchasing that care with the marginal benefit of additional units. Since the marginal benefit of additional units of medical care decreases as the quantity of medical care consumed increases, the individual will continue to consume additional units as long as the marginal benefit of those additional units exceeds their additional cost. Insurance coverage that reduces the price of care to zero under these circumstances results in an inefficient use of medical resources. Since the individual with insurance consumes medical care until the marginal benefits and marginal costs of the last units are equal, this will be at a point where the "true" marginal costs (the costs of *producing* those units) are greater than the marginal benefits. "Too much" medical care will be consumed, and the value of those additional units will be less than the costs of their production. This is illustrated in Figure 6-6 at the point where Q_2 units of medical care are consumed by an individual with 100 percent insurance coverage, with the costs of producing each unit indicated by the supply curve (S).

Another implication of the existence of moral hazard is that although individuals with insurance will consume Q_2 units of medical care if they become ill, they may be unwilling to purchase an insurance policy that provides such extensive coverage. As both consumers of medical care and purchasers of insurance, individuals are expected to consider the price involved in both cases: as consumers of medical services, greater utilization resulting from having insurance will result in their having to pay a higher premium for it. Instead of paying that higher premium, an individual may

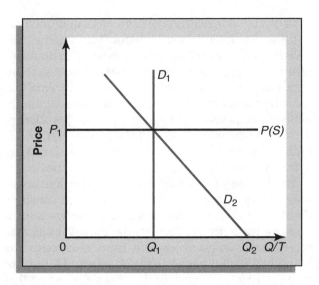

Figure 6-6. The demand for medical care under conditions of moral hazard.

well prefer to self-insure or to purchase a less comprehensive insurance policy. For example, with reference to Figure 6-6, assume that an individual has both a 0.5 probability of not incurring any medical illness during the year (in which case his or her demand for medical care would be zero units), and a 0.5 probability of requiring medical care for an illness during that year. If the individual required medical care, with a corresponding demand curve of D_1, the individual would consume Q_1 units (which represents 100 units) at a cost of $10 per unit. The pure premium in this situation would be 0.5(0) + 0.5($1,000) = $500 per year. If, however, the individual's demand curve were D_2 (where Q_2 represents 200 units of medical care), the pure premium under these circumstances would be 0.5(0) + 0.5($2,000) = $1,000 per year.

These differences in premiums resulting from the price elasticity of the demand curve may be great enough for some individuals to prefer self-insurance, in which case the expected loss to them would be $500 per year [0.5(0) + 0.5($1,000)]. They would consume Q_1 units of medical care if they became ill because, even though their demand curve may be represented

by D_2, they would have to pay P_1 dollars per unit (which is the intersection of D_2 and S) and would consequently consume Q_1 units of care.

Individuals differ in their demands for medical care. If Figure 6-6 represents different demands for medical care and one individual's demand is D_1 while the average demand among the rest of the population is D_2, then a premium for comprehensive insurance to the individual represented by demand curve D_1 would be based upon a utilization level indicated by Q_2 multiplied by a price of P_1. Under these circumstances, an individual may well prefer self-insurance, which would mean a 0.5 probability (as in the previous case) of being ill and, if so, paying a price P_1 multiplied by Q_1 units of medical care. In both of these examples, *requiring* the individual to purchase comprehensive insurance that is the same as that which is purchased by the rest of the population will make the individual worse off (the marginal costs of the premium for the comprehensive coverage will exceed the marginal benefits of that insurance).

Several approaches have been used to limit utilization as a result of the existence of moral hazard. One unsuccessful approach was to rely on internal hospital utilization review committees. As long as hospitals were reimbursed for their costs, physicians were paid separately by Blue Shield, and the patient was not responsible for any part of the bill (under a service benefit policy), none of the participants had an incentive to use the utilization review committee to impose a cost on any of the other participants.

More successful approaches dealing with moral hazard relied on changing either the physician or patient's incentives. Under managed care systems such as health maintenance organizations, the physician is likely to have an incentive (e.g., bonuses at the end of the year) if the organization's expenditures are less than their premium income. Other managed care systems use utilization review. The utilization review organization is separate from the providers being reviewed, and failure to follow the utilization review guidelines results in financial penalties to either the patient or their physician.

Another incentive approach for reducing utilization occurs when deductibles and co-insurance are included as part of the health insurance package. When purchasing insurance, some persons might prefer intermediate choices between the extremes of comprehensive coverage or self-insurance. Deductibles and co-insurance enable consumers to bear some of the risk themselves and pay a smaller premium than if all their medical costs were covered by insurance.

In Figure 6-7A, the pure premium for comprehensive insurance would be represented by utilization level Q_2 multiplied by price P_1 (multiplied by the probability of 0.5). The cost of self-insurance would be P_1 multiplied by Q_1 (0.5). The cost of an insurance policy with a co-insurance feature that lowered the price to the patient from P_1 to P_2 would cost P_1–P_2 multiplied by a utilization level of Q_3 (0.5). The pure premium for a policy with a co-insurance feature would be in between the premiums of the other two alternatives. The availability of co-insurance makes insurance more attractive to some people who would prefer no insurance if their only other choice were comprehensive insurance.

Pauly, in his article on the economics of moral hazard, also discusses the use of deductibles to reduce the costs of insurance premiums. Using only deductibles results either in the consumption of the same amount of care as in the case of no insurance, or conversely, in consumption of the same amount of care as in the situation of complete insurance coverage. This effect of deductibles on utilization is illustrated in Figure 6-7B. Without insurance, the individual represented by demand curve D_1 would, in the event of illness, consume Q_1 units of medical care. With complete insurance coverage, the same individual would consume Q_2 units of medical care. If a deductible were instituted for the individual with complete coverage, then before the insurance would pay the medical costs, the individual would have to use and pay for Q_3 units of medical care at a cost of P_1 times Q_3. After that amount had been paid, the price of additional care (assuming no co-insurance feature) would be zero, and he or she would consume Q_2 units of care.

If the individual decides not to consume up to the deductible (which is P_1 times Q_3 units of medical

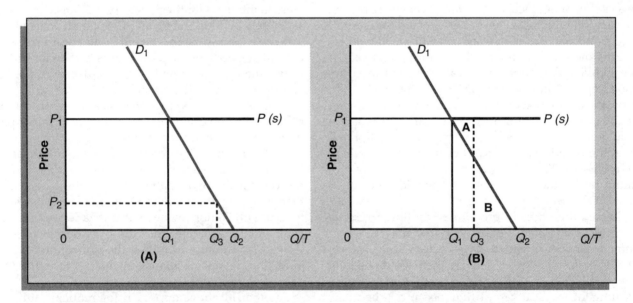

Figure 6-7. The effect of (A) co-insurance and (B) deductibles on the demand for medical care.

care), he or she will merely act as though he or she has no insurance and use Q_1 units of care. Whether or not the individual will pay the deductible ($P_1 \times Q_3$) and then consume up to Q_2 units of medical care depends upon whether the excess amount that must be paid for the deductible (area A in Figure 6-7, which is above the individual's demand curve), is less than the "consumer surplus," represented by area B. The consumer surplus is the area under the demand curve that consumers would be willing to spend but do not have to since it would be at no cost if they first bought Q_3 units of care. If area B exceeds area A, consumers will then pay the deductible and consume Q_2 units of medical care.

Just as the effect of co-insurance on utilization will depend upon the price elasticity of demand and the amount of the co-insurance, the effect the deductible has will also depend upon its size and the price elasticity of demand. In our discussion of deductibles and co-insurance, differences in income have been ignored; it is obvious that any co-payment feature that is unrelated to income levels will have a more important effect on lower-income than on higher-income persons.

The existence of moral hazard thus has two effects. The price of health insurance (total premium) is increased because utilization is greater when the consumer does not have to pay anything out of pocket (the moral hazard issue). Second, there is a decrease in the demand for health insurance when the insurance premium is increased because of the previous increase in utilization. Although the existence of moral hazard results in "overuse" and a consequent increase in the premium, at renewal time the higher premium results in a lower quantity demanded of insurance. Both of these behaviors are rational given the consumer's demand curve for medical services and for insurance and the prices of each.

The conclusion to be drawn from the discussion of the demand for health insurance, whether moral hazard is assumed to exist or not, is that even if all individuals were risk averse, insurance coverage for 100 percent of all of their medical expenses should not be required for all persons. When there are transactions costs for administering claims and when people have different demands for medical care, no single insurance policy is best for everyone. Some persons will prefer to have only some types of medical expense covered; because of the existence of moral hazard, others will prefer to have some cost-sharing features.

SUMMARY AND CONCLUDING COMMENTS

The preceding discussion on the demand for health insurance offers an approach to answering the following questions: How much health insurance should the population have (i.e., what percent of total health expenditures should be covered by insurance), and what components of medical services should health insurance cover? The answers would indicate the degree to which the provision of health insurance in the population is economically efficient. Government intervention to increase or to change the type of health insurance in the population can then be evaluated in terms of whether such action moves the population closer to or further from what would be an optimal quantity and type of health insurance.[6]

To discuss the efficient amount and type of health insurance in the population, it is necessary to have criteria to evaluate what is efficient and what is inefficient in the purchase of health insurance. Assuming competition in the provision (supply) of health insurance, the price at which health insurance is sold will equal the marginal costs of providing it. In a competitive market, the suppliers will also respond to demands for different types of health insurance coverage and provide such coverage at a price that reflects the cost of producing it (these two assumptions are discussed in Chapter 8, "The Market For Health Insurance").

The condition for economic efficiency on the demand side is that consumers purchase the type and

---

6. This discussion assumes no redistribution of medical services; when national health insurance proposals are discussed later, this assumption will be changed. Another assumption, which will subsequently be discussed, is that there are no externalities in the provision of personal medical services. Since redistribution of medical care to low-income persons may in fact have external effects, the efficient distribution of health insurance coverage may necessitate a different amount and type of insurance to low-income groups.

quantity of health insurance coverage to the point where its price equals the marginal benefit to them from additional insurance coverage. Since the demand curve indicates the marginal benefit to be derived from the purchase of health insurance, if the cost of additional insurance exceeds its marginal benefit, consumers will be better off purchasing less coverage. When the quantity of health insurance demanded is equal to the cost of providing that insurance, the individual will purchase the appropriate quantity; that is, the conditions of economic efficiency are met. At that point, the marginal cost of producing health insurance equals the marginal benefit to the consumer of that additional coverage.

The demand for health insurance was analyzed under two assumptions: first, that no moral hazard existed, in that the price of medical care did not affect its utilization or the quality of care demanded; and second, that moral hazard did exist, meaning that there is some price elasticity with respect to the demand for quantity and quality of medical care. In the first situation, it was shown that individuals would *not* want to insure against all events. Insurance would be more likely for those medical services where there is a greater expected loss and the probability of the event occurring is neither extremely high nor rare. Requiring insurance for all losses and all probabilities of it occurring, as well as for all individuals, would be economically inefficient. The cost of the insurance would exceed the marginal benefits to the consumer of additional coverage.

Based on this discussion, what percentage of the distribution of health expenditures should be covered by health insurance? The distribution of health expenditures is skewed, as shown in Figure 6-1: many people have relatively small expenditures, and a smaller percentage of the population have larger expenditures. We would expect large expenses with a low probability of occurrence to be covered by insurance, therefore suggesting that the curve shown in Figure 6-1 should be modified. At a *minimum*, the tail of the distribution (relatively large expenditures for a small percentage of the families) should be covered by insurance through major medical or catastrophic

insurance as shown in Figure 6-8. Further, since the administrative costs of handling small claims are likely to exceed the amount above the pure premium that people that are willing to pay for relatively routine, smaller expenses, a deductible might be included for such expenses, as represented by the shaded portion of the curve in Figure 6-8.

When the demand for health insurance under conditions of moral hazard was discussed, it was shown that given the differences in preferences among people in their demands for medical care, it would be preferable to offer people more than an all-or-nothing choice. People might prefer some co-payment, which would reduce the size of the medical expense in the middle area of Figure 6-8. Insurance, in this instance, would cover less than 100 percent of medical expenditures (different components of the distribution of medical expenses would be covered at different percentages), and the premium for such insurance would be much lower than if it covered the entire distribution of medical expenses.

In discussing other factors affecting the demand for health insurance, the tax deductibility of employer-paid premiums was mentioned; as incomes increase and people move into higher tax brackets, they have a greater incentive to have their employer purchase in-

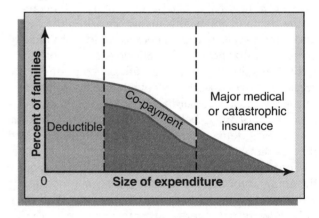

Figure 6-8. The effect of health insurance on the expected distribution of medical expenses among families.

surance on their behalf against more, though smaller, medical expenses. The effect of the tax deductibility of health insurance premiums is a movement *away* from economic efficiency in the demand for health insurance. The "true" cost of health insurance has not been lowered, but its price to higher-income consumers has been. They will, therefore, be purchasing "too much" health insurance. The tax treatment of health insurance premiums has reduced the price of insurance against smaller, more predictable, medical expenses to higher-income people to a point that may be *below* the actuarial value of those expenses. If the tax deductibility of health insurance premiums were no longer allowed, there would be less distortion in the purchase of health insurance because the decision to purchase would more closely correspond to the cost of the insurance and the perceived marginal benefits to the consumer of that additional coverage. (The tax subsidy for the purchase of health insurance is discussed more technically in Appendix 2.)

An important question raised by the discussion of the demand for health insurance is which components of medical care should be covered by health insurance? When only one component of medical care, such as hospital services, is covered by insurance, the price of hospital care to the consumer relative to the prices of other forms of care has been distorted. The decision to use the different forms of care is based, in part, on the relative prices the patient must pay for such care. Inasmuch as these relative prices will not reflect the relative costs of care, moving toward greater economic efficiency in the use of medical care will require the patient to face prices proportional to the costs of such care. An example of insurance coverage that distorted the use of medical components by distorting the relative prices of medical care faced by the consumer was the Blue Cross service benefit policy. A service benefit policy provided very complete coverage for just hospital care while it excluded non-hospital care; this led to an inefficient (more costly) form of treatment when services that could be performed on an outpatient basis were instead performed in a hospital. Competitive pressures forced Blue Cross to provide coverage for non-hospital services.

Certain types of health insurance do not distort the relative prices faced by the patient when seeking care. One example is indemnity insurance, which reimburses the patient a fixed dollar amount or the same percentage co-insurance on all services. Patients and/or their physicians therefore have an incentive to minimize the cost of a medical treatment, and the relative prices of the different components of medical services are not artificially distorted.

A second approach is the use of capitation payments (by or on behalf of patients) to an organization to cover the cost of medical services. Under these arrangements a decision maker, generally a physician, prescribes that combination of services so that the relative costs of different medical services used by the patient equals their relative marginal benefits. HMOs are organizational arrangements whereby the patient is covered by a capitation payment system.

Finally, the method of provider reimbursement affects economic efficiency in the demand for health insurance. The previous method of cost-based hospital reimbursement resulted in higher medical costs. These higher costs increased the size of the probable loss, thereby resulting in a greater demand for health insurance than if other, more efficiency-oriented payment mechanisms had been used.

An important reason for understanding the demand for medical care, as well as the demand for health insurance, is to be able to determine whether or not the quantity (and quality) of medical care consumed is optimal. The optimal rate of output of medical care will be achieved when the price of that care (which is presumed to equal the costs of producing that care under a competitive system) is equal to the marginal benefit of that care. As has been shown, the type of insurance coverage that existed (service benefit coverage) and the current tax treatment of health insurance premiums are reasons why the prices paid by patients have been (and still are) distorted, thereby resulting in consumption of a non-optimal amount of medical care.

To determine whether the price of medical care to the patient reflects the minimum cost of producing that care, it is necessary to turn to an analysis of the supply side of the medical care market.

APPENDIX 1: THE TAX ADVANTAGE OF HEALTH INSURANCE AS A FRINGE BENEFIT

Employees may receive increased income from their employer in either cash or as a fringe benefit in the form of health insurance. The cost to the employer of either choice is the same. To an employee in a high tax bracket, however, employer-paid health insurance may be worth more than an equivalent payment in cash.

If an employee receives an income of $1,000 a week, then, as shown in Figure 6-9, the employee's budget line is I_1M_1. If the employee spent his or her entire income on other goods and services, the employee could purchase quantity OI_1 of other goods and services each week. If she chose instead to purchase just health insurance with her weekly income, the employee could purchase a maximum of OM_1 quantity of health insurance each week. The slope of I_1M_1 represents the relative prices of health insurance and all other goods and services. The combination of health insurance and other goods and services that the employee will actually purchase depends on the employee's tastes and preferences.

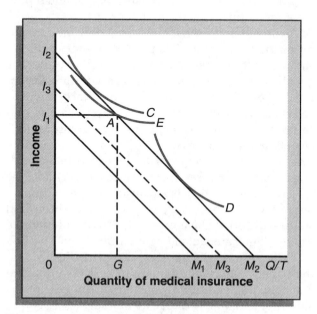

Figure 6-9. Fringe benefits versus money income.

Assume that the employee receives a raise of $200 a week. If the employer gave the raise to the employee in cash, the employee's budget line would increase to I_2M_2. In addition to being able to purchase more health insurance, the increased cash would enable the employee to purchase more of other goods and services.

If the employee has to pay income (as well as social security and Medicare payroll) taxes on a cash raise, then the after-tax value of that cash raise is reduced and is shown by the budget line I_3M_3. The after-tax budget line would depend upon the employee's marginal tax bracket. The higher the marginal tax rate of the employee, the lower will be the new budget line.

If, instead of cash, the employer uses the money to purchase health insurance for the employee (which is not considered as taxable income), the employee's budget line changes to I_1AM_2. The budget line becomes horizontal from I_1 to A. The employee receives OG quantity of health insurance while retaining her current income. (The cash amount of the raise divided by the price of health insurance equals quantity OG.) Thus the employee receives OG quantity of health insurance and still has a budget line of I_1M_1. The employee can still purchase OI_1 of other goods and services (if she spent her entire income) or can purchase GM_2 of additional health insurance (for a total quantity of OM_2 if she spent her entire income on health insurance).

An employee who prefers more of other goods and services rather than additional health insurance would, with a cash raise, be on indifference curve C. An employee who prefers additional health insurance would move to indifference curve D after receiving a cash raise. If the cash raise is then taxed so that the new after-tax income is budget line I_3M_3, those employees could no longer be on indifference curves C and D; they could only be on an indifference curve that is tangent to the budget line I_3M_3. With a fringe benefit, however, both employees could move to higher indifference curves. The employee preferring additional insurance can attain indifference curve D. Indifference curve C is still unattainable under fringe benefits; the highest indifference curve achievable by that employee is indifference curve E.

However, E is still preferable to any indifference curve on budget line I_3M_3.

Employer-paid health insurance is in the employees' interest. As long as employees pay taxes on their cash income but not on employer-purchased health insurance, they have an incentive to receive additional income in the form of fringe benefits. The higher the employees' marginal tax bracket, the greater is their incentive for more comprehensive insurance, such as first-dollar coverage, as well as new types of coverage, such as vision and dental benefits. If health insurance fringes were taxed at the same rate as cash income, employees would demand less health insurance (15).

APPENDIX 2: THE EFFECT ON THE INSURANCE PREMIUM OF EXTENDING COVERAGE TO INCLUDE ADDITIONAL BENEFITS

As insurance companies compete with one another, it becomes important for them to be able to provide a given set of benefits at the lowest possible cost. Benefit design is important in a price competitive market. Since a treatment for an illness can be provided using a combination of settings (e.g., hospital, physician's office, and home care), insurance companies are adding less costly substitutes to their policies. Similarly, as a consequence of its hospital service benefit policy, Blue Cross has broadened its coverage to include out-of-hospital care. The hoped-for effect of adding additional coverage is that substitution away from the hospital toward lower-cost substitutes will occur and the insurance premium can be reduced.

To determine whether or not adding coverage for a non-hospital benefit will reduce the total costs of care (i.e., the premium), the following information is needed:

1. the price elasticity of demand for the newly covered benefit;

2. the co-payment percentage for the new benefit;

3. the cross-price elasticity of demand between hospitalization and the new benefit;

4. the cross-price elasticity of demand between the new benefit and any complementary components of care; and

5. the relative prices of hospital care, the new benefit, and any other complementary components affected.

This information would be used in the following manner to determine whether adding a new insurance benefit would lower the insurance premium. Assuming that the demand for hospital care is as it appears in Figure 6-10A, then without any insurance the patient would have to pay the full cost of a hospital episode if he or she became ill; the patient would have to pay P_{H1}, and, according to his or her expected demand, would use Q_{H1} days of hospital care. The consumer's total expenditures for hospital care would be $(P_{H1} \times Q_{H1})$. With an insurance policy that provided complete coverage for hospital care but not for substitutes to the hospital, such as the Blue Cross service benefit policy, the price of hospital care to the patient would become "zero," and the expected utilization in the event of illness would be Q_{H2}. The total expenditure for hospital care in this case would be $(P_{H1} \times Q_{H2})$.

Including home health visits in the insurance contract with a co-insurance feature will reduce the price of home health visits to the patient, from PM_1 to PM_2, and increase utilization, from QM_1 to QM_2, as shown in Figure 6-10B. The increase in the quantity demanded of home health visits will depend upon the price elasticity of demand for home health visits and the size of the co-insurance payment. The cost to the insurance company of covering home health visits is that part of the actual price that the insurance company will have to pay $(P_{M1} - P_{M2})$ multiplied by the number of home health visits, Q_{M2}. (The patient would pay the remainder, $P_{M2} \times Q_{M2}$.)

If the new benefit acts as a partial substitute for hospital care, then with the reduction in the price of home health visits, patients (through their physicians) will demand less hospital care. How much less hospital care will be demanded will depend upon the cross-price elasticity of demand between hospital utilization and the price of home health visits, which is equal to the percent change in hospital utilization divided by the percent change in the price of home health visits. This is shown in Figure 6-10A by a shift in the demand for hospital care to the left, indicated by demand curve D_2. Since the price of hospital care to the patient with the initial insurance policy was assumed to be "zero," the new quantity demanded will be Q_{H3}. The size of the shift in demand for hospital care will depend upon the magnitude of the cross-price elasticity of demand and the size of the reduction in the price to the patient of the new benefit.

The savings in hospital expenditures to the insurance company of including coverage for a non-hospital service would be the difference in hospital utilization (Q_{H2}–Q_{H3}) multiplied by the price of hospital care, P_{H1}. If the savings in hospital expenditures were greater than the cost to the insurance company of adding the new benefit, the total cost (the premium) would be reduced.

In actuality, other services might be affected by the provision of a new benefit (i.e., subsidizing home health visits). If there are medical services that are complementary to the use of home health visits, there will be an increase in use of these complementary services (a shift to the right in their demand curve). These additional costs may be borne by the patient rather than by the insurance company if the complementary service is not insured.

Following is a numerical example of a change in benefit design illustrating whether or not insuring a non-hospital service will reduce the total cost of an insurance premium. Let us assume the following values for each of the data required in our example:

1. Hospital utilization (Q_{H2}) when home health visits are not covered by insurance is 800 patient days per 1,000 population.
2. The price of hospital care is $400 per day.
3. The price of a home health visit is $40.
4. Home health visits are 600 per 1,000 population.
5. The price elasticity of demand for home health visits is –1.0 (a 10 percent decrease in price leads to a 10 percent increase in home health visits).
6. The cross-price elasticity of demand between hospital patient days and the price of home health visits is +0.2 (a 10 percent decrease in the

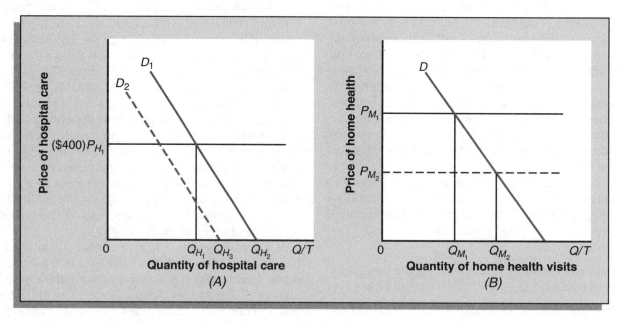

Figure 6-10. The effect on hospital utilization of insuring out-of-hospital services: (A) hospital utilization; (B) home health visits.

price of a home health visit leads to a 2 percent decrease in hospital patient days).

7. After home health visits are included in the insurance coverage, the co-insurance rate is 20 percent; that is, the patient has to pay only 20 percent of the price of home health visits. (It is also assumed that the price of home health visits remains at its previous level.)

With this information we can now calculate the change in the cost of the premium as a result of including home health visits with a 20 percent co-insurance feature.

The total cost of the premium per 1,000 population before the new benefit is added to the coverage is

$$\frac{TC}{1,000} = P_{H1} \times \frac{Q_{H2}}{1,000}$$

$$\frac{\$320,000}{1,000} = \$400 \times \frac{800}{1,000}$$

or $320 per person. The total cost of the premium *after* home health visits are covered at a 20 percent co-insurance rate is

$$\frac{TC}{1,000} = P_{H1}\left(\frac{Q_{H3}}{1,000}\right) + 0.8P_{M1}\left(\frac{Q_{M2}}{1,000}\right)$$

which is

$$\frac{\$303,360}{1,000} = \$400\left(\frac{672}{1,000}\right) + 0.8(\$40)\left(\frac{1,080}{1,000}\right)$$

or $303.36 per person.

The difference is computed as follows:

1. The increased expenditure on home health visits is

$$0.8(\$40)\left(\frac{600}{1,000}\right)(1.8) = \frac{\$34,560}{1,000}$$

This is the percentage of the home health price paid by the insurance company (0.8), multiplied by the price of home health visits ($40), multiplied by the number of home health visits per 1,000 population (600/1,000), multiplied by the percent increase in home health visits as a result of the 80 percent reduction in home health prices to the patient (a -1.0 price elasticity multiplied by an 80 percent reduction in price) leads to an 80 percent increase in utilization, hence, 1.8.

2. Subtract the saving on decreased hospital utilization, which is

$$\$400\left(\frac{128}{1,000}\right) = \frac{\$51,200}{1,000}$$

This is the price of hospital care, multiplied by reduction in patient days as a result of a lower price of home health visits. (The cross-elasticity of +0.2 when multiplied by an 80 percent reduction in the price of home health visits is equal to a 16 percent reduction in hospital utilization; this is then multiplied by 800/1,000.)

3. The net effect of the savings on hospital expenditures less the increased home health expenditures is

$$\frac{\$51,200}{1,000} - \frac{\$34,560}{1,000} = \frac{\$16,640}{1,000} \text{ or } \$16.64 \text{ per person}$$

Given the data and assumptions used in this example, the effect of insuring home health visits would be a net decrease of $16.64 per person in the total cost of the premium ($303.36 versus $320 per person).

In the preceding example, insuring an out-of-hospital service would further reduce the insurance premium if: the price of hospital care increased faster than the non-hospital service, the substitutability between the two services (cross-price elasticity) increased, and the price elasticity of demand for the non-hospital service were reduced.

Adding insurance coverage for an out-of-hospital service is more likely to reduce hospital utilization when this service is used *in conjunction with* hospital care in treatment of an illness episode. An example of this is case management for catastrophic care. If, however, home health visits are covered by insurance and used separately (not as part of the treatment for an illness), there may be a large increase in home health utilization without any consequent lowering of hospital utilization (16). A major medical policy which covers all the medical services used in treatment (after a sizable deductible has been paid) is more likely to result in substitution away from more costly components.

REVIEW QUESTIONS

1. How would you use utility analysis to analyze the following statement?

   Consumers should purchase health insurance policies that cover 100 percent of all medical care expenses. Anything less than 100 percent coverage reflects either irrational consumer behavior or market failure in the insurance industry. (Organize your discussion around diagrams.)

2. Explain why health insurance is more common for hospital expenses than for outpatient expenses.

3. How will a change in the price of medical care affect the demand for health insurance?

4. Discuss each of the factors affecting the demand for health insurance. Indicate the effect that each has on demand.

5. What are the welfare implications of having everyone purchase the same (very comprehensive) health insurance coverage?

6. What is "moral hazard?" How does its existence affect the demand for health insurance? What approaches do insurance companies use to control its existence?

7. What is adverse selection? How does its existence affect the market for health insurance? What are some ways insurance companies protect themselves from adverse selection?

8. What information would you need to know (and how would you use it) to determine whether expanding benefit coverage (e.g., covering hospice services) would lower the cost of an insurance premium?

9. In what way do technological innovations, such as an inexpensive new drug that would replace the need for cardiac surgery or the development of organ transplants, affect the demand for health insurance?

10. Trace through each of the medical markets the effects of making employer-paid health insurance premiums taxable to the employee.

11. It has been proposed that employer-paid health insurance be taxed as part of an employee's income. Evaluate this proposal in terms of economic efficiency, equity (be sure to define efficiency and equity in your answer), and who do you think would be likely to favor and oppose this proposal?

12. Evaluate Blue Cross' hospital service benefit policy in terms of economic efficiency. If the service benefit policy was inefficient, how could Blue Cross survive in a competitive insurance market? Why were hospitals in favor of it?

REFERENCES

1. The discussion in this section borrows heavily from an unpublished article by J. J. German, "A Note on the Economic Theory of Insurance with Implications for Health Insurance," mimeographed, January 1967; and the article by Dennis Lees and Robert Rice, "Uncertainty and the Welfare Economics of Medical Care: Comment," *American Economic Review*, 55(1) March 1965, 140–154. The comment by D. Lees and R. Rice (as well as the comment by M. Pauly in the next section of this chapter) were written in response to Kenneth J. Arrow, "Uncertainty and the Welfare Economics of Medical Care," *American Economic Review*, 53(5) December 1963, 941–973. Arrow claimed that the market for health insurance requires government intervention because there are gaps in consumers' health insurance coverage, and that this is evidence that the market is not producing certain services that consumers are willing to purchase. Lees and Rice argued that Arrow's claims are not evidence of market imperfections but rather are a result of transactions costs. For example, "the transactions cost to the individual of completing and filing applications and forms, paying premiums, keeping records, etc., as well as possible costs of obtain-

ing information, may be of sufficient magnitude to make insurance policies against certain losses not worthwhile." Arrow replied that individuals who cannot take advantage of the economies of group health insurance will face too high a transactions cost (i.e., the price of insurance is greatly in excess of its pure premium) and thus may not purchase health insurance.

2. M. Friedman and L. Savage, "The Utility Analysis of Choices Involving Risk," *Journal of Political Economy*, 56(4), 1948: 279–304.

3. On this last point, see the discussion by Jan Mossin, "Aspects of Rational Insurance Purchasing," *Journal of Political Economy*, 73(4) July/August 1968, 553–568.

4. http://www.cbo.gov/bo2001/bo2001_showhit1.cfm?index=REV-12.

5. Susan M. Marquis and Stephen H. Long, "Worker Demand for Health Insurance in the Non-Group Market," *Journal of Health Economics*, 14(1), May 1995, pp. 47–63, and Jonathan Gruber and James Poterba, "Tax Incentives and the Decision to Purchase Health Insurance: Evidence from the Self-Employed," *Quarterly Journal of Economics*, 109(3), August 1994, pp. 701–733. In a review article Pauly concludes, "The results generally support the view that the impact of loading . . . on insurance purchases is significantly negative. The actual numerical estimates of the elasticity of insurance with respect to the loading 'price,' however, vary considerably, ranging from about –0.2 . . . to numbers greater than unity . . ." (p. 644), Mark V. Pauly, "Taxation, Health Insurance, and Market Failure in the Medical Economy," *Journal of Economic Literature*, 24(2), June 1986: 629–675.

6. Jon R. Gabel and Gail A. Jensen, "The Price of State Mandated Benefits," *Inquiry*, 26(4), Winter 1989, 419–431. This article includes results from studies also conducted by Gail A. Jensen and Michael Morrisey. Another study finds that state mandates have very little effect on the rate of insurance coverage of small firms, see Jonathan Gruber, "State-Mandated Benefits and Employer-Provided Health Insurance," *Journal of Public Economics*, 55(3), November 1994, 433–64.

7. The discussion in this section is based on Burton A. Weisbrod, "The Health Care Quadrilemma: An Essay on Technological Change, Insurance, Quality of Care, and Cost Containment," *Journal of Economic Literature*, 29(2), June 1991: 523–552.

8. *Ibid*, p. 540.

9. E. Friedson and J. Feldman, *Public Attitudes Toward Health Insurance*, Research Series 5 (New York: Health Information Foundation, 1958).

10. Centers for Medicare and Medicaid Services, Office of the Actuary, National Health Statistics Group, [Online information, 2004], http://www.cms.gov/statistics/nhe (accessed on January 8, 2004.)

11. M. Rothschild and J. Stiglitz, "Equilibrium in Competitive Insurance Markets: An Essay on the Economics of Imperfect Information," *Quarterly Journal of Economics*, 90(4) 1976: 629–649.

12. Randall S. Brown and Jerrold W. Hill, "The Effects of Medicare Risk HMOs on Medicare Costs and Service Utilization," in Harold S. Luft, ed., *HMOs and the Elderly*, (Ann Arbor, Michigan: Health Administration Press), 1994.

13. Marc L. Berk and Alan C. Monheit, "The Concentration of Health Expenditures, Revisited" *Health Affairs*, 20(2), March/April 2001, Exhibit 1, p. 12 and p. 15.

14. The discussion in this section is based on the article by Mark Pauly, "The Economics of Moral Hazard: Comment," *American Economic Review*, 58(3), June 1968, 531–537. In Pauly's comment to Arrow's reply to Lees and Rice, he argues that even if there are certain economies in government provision of health insurance that would lower transactions costs, other costs may more than offset such possible savings. In addition to a loss of consumer choice, the existence of "moral hazard" would cause consumers to demand less insurance "at the premium its behavior as a purchaser of insurance and as a demander of medical care under insurance makes necessary." In other words, the existence of moral hazard would result in higher prices for insurance and, consequently, a decreased demand. The lack of complete health insurance coverage in the private market can also be explained by moral hazard, which would not be lessened even if government were somehow able to reduce the transactions costs of insurance to individuals.

15. The reader is referred to the following articles for a more complete discussion of the welfare loss of excess health insurance coverage. Mark V. Pauly, "A Measure of the Welfare Costs of Health Insurance," *Health Services Research*, 4(4), Winter 1969, 281–292, Martin S. Feldstein, "The Welfare Loss of Excess Health Insurance," *Journal of Political Economy*, 81(2), March–April 1973, 251–280, Roger Feldman and Bryan Dowd, "A New Estimate of the Welfare Loss of Excess Health Insurance," *American Economic Review*, 81(1), March 1991, 297–301, and Joseph P. Newhouse, "Medical Care Costs: How Much Welfare Loss?" *Journal of Economic Perspectives*, 6(3), Summer 1992, 3–21.

16. A study of Medicare's home health care program found that such visits did not substitute for inpatient admissions and were used primarily to provide long term care. H. Gilbert Welch, D. Wennberg, and W. Pete Welch, "The Use of Home Health Care Services," *The New England Journal of Medicine*, 335 (5), August 1, 1996, 324–329.

CHAPTER

The Supply of Medical Care: On Overview

KEY TERMS AND CONCEPTS

- Competitive markets
- Optimal rate of output
- Determinants of market structure
- Economies of scale in relation to market size
- Firm versus industry demand curves
- Product market definition
- Geographic market definition
- Monopolistic markets
- Market power
- Market performance

Learning Objectives

Upon completing this chapter, the reader should be able to:

- Explain how supply elasticity is affected by an industry's market structure.
- Describe how, for a given demand curve, different supply elasticities affect price and output.
- Understand the characteristics of production functions and their effects on industry supply.
- Appreciate the effects on prices and output of different market structures.
- Explain why firm demand curves are different from industry demand curves.
- Discuss why competitive markets are the yardstick for evaluating market performance.

DETERMINANTS OF SUPPLY

The concept of economic efficiency is relevant to both the demand and the supply side of an industry. When evaluating economic efficiency, we are concerned that the rate (and type) of output be "optimal." Economic efficiency in demand is related to economic efficiency in supply through prices. The optimal rate of output occurs when the marginal benefit of the last unit equals the price of that unit, which in turn equals the marginal cost of producing that last unit. Several reasons were given why economic efficiency does not occur on the demand side. For example, since employer-purchased health insurance is not included as part of employees' taxable income, the price of insurance is lowered, resulting in more comprehensive coverage than if employees had to pay the full price (with after-tax dollars). Also, the limited information available to patients on prices, physician quality, their diagnosis, and treatment needs have made it possible for some physicians to manipulate patient demands for medical services.

In our examination of the supply side of the medical care sector, the criterion of economic efficiency is also important. If the various markets within the medical care sector are not economically efficient, the cost of medical care is higher than it should be. By examining the reasons for deviations from economic efficiency, we can make policy recommendations to improve the efficiency of the market and reduce the rise in the cost of medical care.

The economic efficiency of the supply side of the medical care sector also has important implications for redistributive policies. If the suppliers of medical services and health insurers are inefficient (resulting in a relatively inelastic supply curve), large price increases would be required to bring forth an increase in medical care output; large price increases—and consequently greater government expenditures—will influence the type of redistribution programs proposed on the demand side, specifically, redistributive programs to disadvantaged population groups. The cost of a national health insurance program would be greater and the availability of services diminished when supply is more inelastic. Because of greater total expenditures, higher prices, and less out-put, the political feasibility of instituting such a program, as well as its comprehensiveness, will be reduced.

Greater price inelasticity will benefit providers by resulting in higher prices, wages, and incomes for providers of medical services. These price increases will be financed by the rest of the population, resulting in lower incomes for the working population.

As shown in Figure 7-1, a relatively inelastic supply curve represented by S_1, would, with an increase in demand from D_1 to D_2, result in a greater price rise and a smaller increase in services provided than if the supply of medical services were more elastic. A more elastic supply schedule could produce the same level of output (Q_1), but at a lower cost. Or for the same increase in demand, provide Q_2–Q_1 more services at a smaller increase in price, P_2 rather than P_1. Total cost after the increase in demand would be $P_1 \times Q_1$ in the inelastic case versus $P_2 \times Q_2$ in the situation where supply is more elastic. In the latter case, more of the increase in total expenditures would go for increased medical services, whereas in the former there would be more rapid price increases with a smaller increase in services.

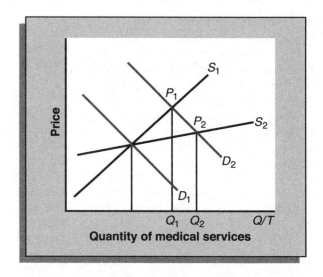

Figure 7-1. The effect of different supply elasticities on the price, quality, and cost of national health insurance.

The elasticity of an industry's supply is affected by the nature of the production function for producing its output, supplier incentives to use the least cost combination of inputs, the industry's market structure, and the degree to which the industry is price competitive. Each of these topics is examined with regard to their effect on supply elasticity and appropriate public policy, if indicated.

PRODUCTION FUNCTIONS AND COST MINIMIZATION

Characteristics of Production Functions

Underlying the supply of any good or service is the production function, which describes the technical relationship between the output of that service and the resources (inputs) used to produce it. If the output were nursing care per patient, then included in the inputs would be the number of and type of nurses on the nursing unit. This technical relationship between nursing care per patient and the types of nurses may be expressed in the following general form:

$$Q_{npc} = f(RNs, LPNs, NAs, UN)$$

where Q_{npc}, which represents quantity of nursing patient care, is functionally related to the number of registered nurses (RNs), licensed practical nurses (LPNs), nursing aides (NAs), and the type of nursing unit (UN).

Certain characteristics of medical production functions are important to understand since they affect the cost and quantity of care provided. First is that the various inputs (e.g., types of nurses) are, to some extent, *substitutable* for one another in the production of nursing care. The substitutability is not one-to-one (i.e., one LPN cannot substitute for one RN). RNs presumably have more skills as a result of their additional education, and therefore LPNs can substitute for some but not all of the tasks performed by the RN.

The second characteristic of production functions is *the concept of marginal productivity* of each input, which is the additional output achieved by increasing

each input by a small amount (holding the other inputs constant). As more of one input is increased (the quantity of other inputs being held constant), its marginal productivity declines. Thus there is a change in the relative marginal productivity of inputs when one input is increased; its marginal productivity declines relative to those inputs that have not been increased. The marginal productivity of each input, together with information on the relative prices (wages) of different inputs, determine which combination of inputs is less costly (since they are substitutable) for producing a given level of output or for meeting an increase in output.

The relative marginal productivities of any two inputs should be equal to their relative prices or wages. When this condition occurs, then the cost per additional output produced (the marginal product) of those inputs are equal. Even though their wages and marginal productivities are unequal, when their ratios are equal the additional output achieved per dollar spent on each input is equal. For example, if an RN costs twice as much as an LPN, then, at the margin, the RN should be twice as productive as the LPN. An increase in RN wages, without any change in RN and LPN productivities, would require a decrease in the number of RNs (which would mean moving up the marginal productivity curve of RNs) so that the ratio of RN wages and marginal productivity is again equal to those of the LPN. Similarly, if RNs' wages were four times greater than those of LPNs but their marginal productivity were only three times greater, then it would be less expensive to achieve an increase in nursing care by increasing LPNs rather than RNs, assuming no change in quality.

A third characteristic of production functions is the distinction between the *short run* and *long run*. Not all the inputs can be varied simultaneously at each point in time. In the short run, one input is fixed and cannot be varied. At any time, the decision-maker can vary the combination of nurses and their numbers on the nursing unit. To change the type of nursing unit itself by enlarging it or improving it through greater use of monitoring mechanisms would take longer. The "long run" is that period of time in which the administrator can vary not only the number and type of nurses, but also the size and character of the nursing unit. The "short run" is that period of time in which the administrator can vary the other inputs but not make changes in the nursing unit itself. Another example of the short versus the long run is with regard to physician services. In the short run, an increase in physician services can be achieved by having the physician work longer hours or by hiring additional personnel. In the long run, medical schools may increase the number of physicians, which are the fixed input in the short run.

When one input is fixed in the short run, this gives rise to the "Law of Variable Proportions" (commonly known as the law of diminishing returns), which states that after some point, continued increases in the variable input (RNs) will result in the marginal productivity of that input declining.

The Law of Variable Proportions is the reason why the industry supply schedule in the short run (the sum of each firm's marginal cost curve) is rising. To increase output, the firm increases its variable inputs whose marginal productivity eventually declines, consequently the marginal cost of additional output rises. (Marginal cost is equal to the wage divided by marginal productivity.) If there is an increased demand for the industry's output, more resources must be drawn into production, and it will be necessary to pay higher wages to bid these resources away from their current use. Thus, in addition to the rising marginal cost curve (because of the Law of Variable Proportions), the marginal cost curve will shift up (or to the left) as the price of inputs rise. In the long run, when all the inputs in the production function can be varied, the supply schedule will become more elastic (i.e., it will require less of an increase in cost to increase supply).

These distinctions between the short and long run are important for determining the extent of economies of scale in producing nursing and other types of medical care. The concept of "Returns to Scale" is another characteristic of production functions. With an increase in the demand for nursing care (derived from an increased demand for medical and hospital care), all the inputs, including the nursing unit, can be increased in the long run. When the nurs-

ing unit is expanded by increasing all of its inputs and the output increases by a larger percent, then economies of scale are said to exist; the cost per unit of output will decline (the long run average cost curve is falling). Constant (and decreasing) returns occur when output expands by a similar (lesser) percentage. Returns to scale (consequently the long run average cost curve) determine which size of unit or facility is less costly, i.e., lower cost per unit of output.

One further aspect of the production function is worth mentioning. Technical change typically results in a greater output being produced with the same or fewer inputs. One example of technical change that has led to a decrease in inputs for treatment of heart disease is the use of new drugs, which has decreased the use of more expensive hospital care. However, in medical care, technical change has usually meant that illnesses that formerly could not be treated can now be cared for. Further, current illnesses will have a higher probability of a successful outcome or a shorter recovery period. Such technical change often expresses itself through a change in medical care *output*, (i.e., an increased probability of recovery) and may result in increased rather than decreased use of inputs, such as improved diagnostic imaging equipment. Thus, both types of technical change have occurred in medical care. It is important to hold the effects of technical change constant when analyzing the production function for medical care.

These characteristics of production functions, input substitutability, marginal productivity of each input, the Law of Variable Proportions, returns to scale, and the least cost method of using inputs (according to their relative wages and marginal productivities) determine the nature of costs, and consequently supply of medical services in the short and long run.

Assumptions Underlying Medical Services Production and Cost Functions

Several important assumptions underlying production functions and cost minimization may not be fulfilled in certain medical markets, resulting in economic inefficiency in producing medical services.

First, *legal restrictions* on the tasks that various health professionals are permitted to perform will affect the decision-maker's ability to substitute inputs to produce a given output. Even if a nurse is capable of performing certain tasks that are reserved solely for the physician, the nurse may not be permitted to perform them because she would be violating the state practice acts. Similarly, attempts by nursing organizations to require the use of fixed input ratios, such as a minimum number of RNs per inpatient day, results in a more costly output because an increase in RN wages relative to those of other personnel would otherwise change the least cost combination of inputs, thereby reducing the ratio of RNs per inpatient day.

Legal restrictions limit the extent to which inputs may be substituted for one another in producing a given level of output. When legal restrictions prevent substitution from occurring when it would not result in a diminution of the quality of care, the legal restrictions have increased the cost of producing that care. The "costs" of restrictive practices, therefore, are the additional resources required to produce a given level of care for a given level of quality.

Second, in determining the least cost combination of inputs it is assumed that *the relative prices of the inputs are not distorted.* For example, if the government subsidizes certain inputs, such as hospital capital or educational programs for health manpower, then the relative price of the subsidized input has been lowered and relatively more of it will be used in production. From a societal perspective, subsidizing just one input results in economic inefficiency in producing that output. If it is desired to increase production of that output, it would be less costly to subsidize the output itself rather than any one input used in producing that output.

Lastly, it is assumed that decision-makers are desirous of *minimizing the cost of producing their output.* This last assumption is particularly important when non-profit hospitals, Blue Cross Blue Shield health plans, and medical schools are examined.

Economic efficiency in production requires decision-makers to use information on the marginal productivity and the relative prices of their inputs to produce the output at minimum cost. Decision-makers of non-profit organizations, however, may have goals other than cost minimization. To the extent that the decision-makers' goals differ from cost minimization and they do not compete in a price-competitive market and/or that the provider payment mechanisms enable them to pursue these other goals, the supply curve of medical care will be less elastic. In other words, it will take larger price increases to produce an increase in services than it would if the objectives and constraints were similar to those of a competitive industry. The objectives of non-profit hospitals, health insurers, and medical schools will be examined to determine the effects of such objectives on industry performance.

Production Functions at All Levels of the Medical Sector

The example of the production function used earlier (nursing care), the information required to be able to minimize costs (marginal productivity and relative prices), and the assumptions underlying the behavior of the decision-makers (a desire to minimize costs), can be applied equally well to other levels of the medical sector. For example, with regard to medical services, the physician faces a production function in providing an office visit which includes such inputs as the physician's own time, time of one or more types of assistants, diagnostic tests and equipment, and the size and layout of the physician's office.

How the delivery of medical services should be organized—namely, the combinations of institutional settings that are least expensive for producing patient care—is essentially a discussion of a production function and cost minimization at a very aggregate level. For example, within an HMO or managed care organization, the primary care physician faces a production function in providing treatment for an illness of a particular diagnosis and of a given level of severity. The inputs are the different institutional settings, such as a hospital, a physician's office, or the patient's home.

To determine the least expensive approach (production function) for providing a patient's treatment, information is needed on the marginal productivities and the relative costs of the different institutional settings, as well as an understanding of the objectives of the decision-makers and the incentives they face. As will be discussed, changes in financial incentives and removal of certain legal restrictions have had important effects on changes in the organization of medical care.

MARKET STRUCTURE

Markets can be characterized by their "structure"; that is, by the number of purchasers and suppliers within that market. Markets that have a large number of buyers and suppliers are considered to be competitive; no individual buyer or seller has influence over the market price. Monopoly occurs when there is only one supplier of a service. Input markets can also be characterized by whether they are competitive or monopolistic. (While firms are suppliers in the services market, these same firms are demanders in the input market.) Again, monopoly can occur in either the services market and/or the input (health manpower) market. (A single purchaser in a market that may have few or many sellers is a monopsonist [discussed in Chapter 16, "The Market For Registered Nurses"]).

Many economists believe that there is a relationship between the structure of a market and its conduct or behavior and ultimately to how well that market performs. Markets that are characterized by many buyers and suppliers are believed to result in greater economic efficiency (lower prices relative to costs and greater output) than markets characterized by fewer suppliers. Such generalizations, however, must be tested against each particular market, its conduct, and hence its performance, since some markets with few firms can be very competitive and achieve economically efficient outcomes.

There are two important determinants of the number of firms in an industry; the extent of economies of scale in relation to the size of the market, and barriers to entry. Economies of scale occur when the average cost of production declines as the size of the firm is increased. The relationship between average cost and

size of firm is U shaped; average cost falls, reaches a minimum (which may be over a wide range of output rather than only one size of firm), and then if the firm size is increased further, average cost increases. The extent of economies of scale differs by industry; the minimum cost-size relationship for health insurers will occur at very large sizes, while for physician groups it may be at a relatively smaller size.

To determine the number of competitors in a market, it is necessary to know the size of the market in addition to economies of scale. For example, if the lowest average cost per unit occurs when a firm produces 200 units per day, then the industry will consist of ten firms when demand is 2,000 units per day. If industry demand were 600 units per day, then the industry would consist of only 3 firms.

Barriers that prevent entry by new firms when demand is increasing will limit the number of competitors in a market, thereby benefiting the existing firms. There are several types of entry barriers; the most permanent being those that are legally granted, such as licensing (e.g., health manpower and Certificate of Need for facilities, and patents to promote technological innovation). An entry barrier can also occur when industry suppliers or their inputs are either directly or indirectly subsidized (through tax laws), thereby providing existing firms with a cost advantage over other firms.

The Demand Curve Facing a Single Firm

The demand curve facing an individual firm is not the same as the industry demand curve. Studies that estimate the market demand for physician or hospital services are typically price inelastic, meaning that there are not very good substitutes to all physician or all hospital services in a given market. (See previous Table 5-1.) The demand curve facing the individual firm, however, is price elastic since there are good substitutes to that firm, other firms in that industry. The difference between the industry demand curve (DD) and firm demand curve (dd) is shown in Figure 7-2. Typically, a competitive market consisting of ten firms will have firm demand curves that are more price elastic than if those ten firms merged into three firms, in which case each firm's demand curve would be less price elastic. When there is only one firm in an industry, then the firm demand curve is the same as the industry demand curve. If all the individual firms were able to collude by acting as one firm, thereby facing the less price elastic industry demand for their services, they would be able to increase their prices. It is this type of collusive behavior that is anti-competitive according to the anti-trust laws.

Most industries are characterized by a market structure that is intermediate between competition and monopoly. Oligopoly markets are dominated by a few firms and each is aware that their actions (such as the price they set) will be matched by their competitors. Because firms in oligopoly markets recognize their interdependence with their competitors, collusion is more prevalent in these types of markets.

Monopolistic competition is characterized by a large number of firms (similar to a competitive industry) that produce an output that is differentiated from the other firms. These output differences may be a result of real or perceived differences in the types of services offered, patient location, quality, or reputa-tion. Since the products or services are somewhat different, monopolistically competitive firms face a slightly downward sloping demand curve, and therefore have some influence over the pricing of their services (similar to the monopoly model). The prices set by such firms, however, cannot differ too greatly from their competitors; otherwise they would suffer large losses in their market share. Monopolistically competitive markets are similar to competitive markets in terms of economic efficiency.

Defining a Firm's Product and Geographic Market

An important part of determining the number of firms competing in a market is correctly defining *the relevant product and geographic market*. For example, anesthesiologists are a separate product market from orthopedic surgeons. Similarly, inpatient acute hospital services are a distinct product market from other facility services, such as outpatient surgi-centers. Defining the product market involves determining how close a substitute certain services are to one another. If products or services are considered to be close substitutes, namely, a significant number of patients are willing to shift to a substitute service if the price of the initial service is increased (cross-price elasticity is high), then both services would be included in the same product market definition.

The geographic market is determined by patients' willingness to travel to a competitor, that is, how close does another hospital have to be for it to be considered a good substitute to a particular hospital. If a significant number of patients are willing to travel to another facility, then the facilities should be considered as being in the same geographic market. Patient willingness to travel depends on the urgency of their medical needs; the geographic markets for obstetric services are smaller than for transplant services.

The number of competitors in a market, however, is inadequate by itself for determining market competitiveness since it does not indicate *potential entry* into that industry by other firms. Although a market may be highly concentrated, entry by other firms may

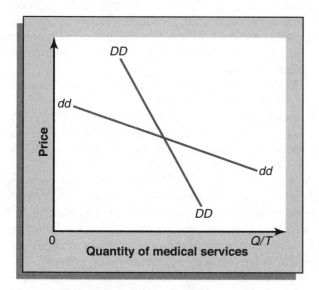

Figure 7-2.   Price elasticity of industry and firm demand curves.

not be very costly, thereby leading the firms in the market to act competitively. For example, although there may be only two health insurers in a large metropolitan area, other health insurers in that state may easily enter that market if premiums are increased resulting in above-normal profits. Similarly, large employers may decide to become self-insured if their premiums exceed their employees' medical and administrative costs. Potential entry makes existing firms' demand curves more price elastic.

An analysis of the determinants of market structure will be undertaken for each of the medical care markets examined. Based on that analysis, it should be possible to determine whether there are sufficient numbers of purchasers and suppliers for that market to be competitive.

COMPETITIVE BEHAVIOR

Market structure influences competitive behavior in an industry. In markets where there are a large number of firms, there is typically intense price competition. Firms in competitive markets do not engage in collusive pricing strategies because of the difficulty of coordinating such behavior among a large number of firms and the incentive of each firm to cheat. Instead, prices approximate the costs of providing the service. (Competitive industries with a large number of suppliers often seek legislation to enable them to achieve what a competitive market does not permit, namely higher prices through limits on entry.) In highly concentrated markets, the costs of negotiating collusive prices among competitors are lower and therefore more likely to occur. More highly concentrated markets (and markets where consumer information is limited) are also characterized by a pricing strategy that results in price discrimination whereby different prices (unrelated to cost) are charged to different purchasers.

Product strategies also differ by market structure. The products and services produced in markets where there are a large number of suppliers are often relatively similar. More highly concentrated markets often invest in research and development to develop new services. Such firms also spend more on advertising with the purpose of differentiating their services from those of their competitors, thereby enabling them to raise their price and increase profits. While the likelihood of collusive arrangements is greater in more concentrated industries (and therefore must be monitored), so is the likelihood of innovation and change.

Characteristics of Medical Markets

There are several distinctive characteristics of medical markets that have affected competitive behavior. Patients lack information on their treatment needs and on provider quality. The physician is the patient's agent in determining treatment needs, specialist referrals, and the settings for providing treatment. And the patient's type of heath insurance (either private or government) affects both patient and provider incentives on use and cost of services.

The patient's lack of information results in each provider's demand curve being less price elastic since the patient is unaware of how good a substitute another provider is. Health insurance that pays all or most of the provider's charges makes the patient less concerned with their use of services and the prices charged by different providers. In such circumstances, providers have less incentive to compete on price and to use other, non-price strategies in competing for patients.

As the patient's agent, the physician can influence the patient's use of services (including their own), as well as determining which other providers are used. Thus, under these circumstances and fee-for-service insurance, providers (such as hospitals) engage in non-price competition for physician referrals.

Depending on how private and government (Medicare and Medicaid) health insurance is structured (that is, the degree of patient cost sharing and method of provider payment), there will be incentives on the part of both patients and providers that will affect the price elasticity of their demand curves.

When physician, hospital, and health insurer competitive behavior is examined, it is important to distinguish changes in their competitive behavior over different time periods. Medicare and Medicaid were enacted in 1965, and provider payment under these programs has been changing. Similarly, there has been an expansion in the population with private health insurance, new forms of health insurance have developed (such as managed care), and the role of private insurers have changed. These changes in insurance coverage, the types of health insurance offered, and the role of insurers, have had an important effect on how physicians, hospitals, and health insurers compete. For example, over time hospital payment has changed from cost based to competing on price to be included in an insurer's provider network; consequently, their competitive behavior changed from non-price to price competition, as their demand curves became more price elastic. Thus the competitive behavior of firms in the different medical markets will also be analyzed with respect to these different time periods.

MARKET PERFORMANCE

Each medical market's performance will be evaluated in terms of whether it approximates economic efficiency. In highly price competitive markets, each firm is both technically (maximum output for given inputs) and economically (least cost combination of inputs used) efficient. Although most medical markets can be characterized as being monopolistically competitive (having a downward sloping demand curve), it is useful to illustrate the outcomes of a competitive market assuming a perfectly competitive industry; the consequences would be similar under price competition. In a price competitive market, as shown in Figure 7-3, the industry price is determined by the intersection of demand and supply (industry supply in the short run is the summation of each firm's marginal cost curve). And, in equilibrium, since each firm sells at the industry determined price, price approximates marginal cost and average total cost, and each firm is producing at the minimum point on the long run average cost curve, thereby taking advantage of economies of scale. Consequently each firm is efficient—otherwise they could not survive—and the 'right' number of firms exist in the industry. The long run industry supply curve (not shown) is determined by entry of new firms, which in a constant cost industry (input prices and productivity unchanged) will be horizontal.

The rate of output in a competitive industry is considered to be optimal since price, which reflects

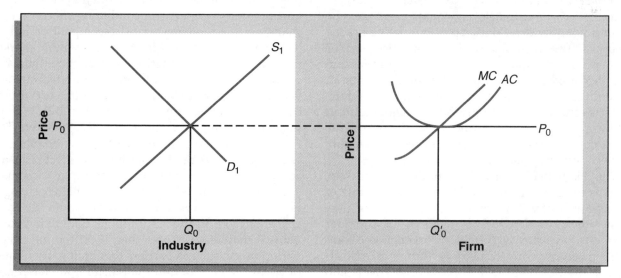

Figure 7-3. The industry and the firm under long-run competitive equilibrium.

marginal benefit, is equal to marginal cost (assuming no externalities). Profits are normal in that price equals average total cost, and included in cost is a normal rate of return on capital and the opportunity cost of the owner's efforts. While profits may be above normal in the short run, over time entry by new firms would bring profits back to a normal rate of return.

Price-to-cost ratios are used to indicate the extent to which prices are competitively determined in an industry. The higher price is relative to cost, the greater is the firm's market power. Firms with market power have less price elastic demand curves for their services. If the competitive industry characterized in Figure 7-3 were to become monopolized, for example, by all the firms merging into one (or by all the firms acting as a cartel), then the remaining firm would have as its demand curve the industry demand curve. The new firm's demand curve would be less price elastic than the (horizontal) demand curves faced by the earlier competitive firms. Previously, each competitive firm faced a highly elastic demand curve because the services provided by the other firms were good substitutes. With only one firm in the industry, the price elasticity of the firm's demand curve would be determined by how good a substitute other industries' services are to its own.

A firm with market power has greater discretion in setting prices, its output, level of quality, and the type of service it provides. (Market power is defined as the ability of a firm to profitably increase its price (and/or decrease quality and access to services) and sustain that increased price for a period of time without an offsetting loss of volume.) Market power, therefore, distorts efficient outcomes; prices are higher, output is lower, profits are greater, and responsiveness of the firm to purchasers is less than would occur in a highly price competitive market.

The distinctive characteristics of medical markets, such as the patient's lack of information, the role of the patient's physician, and the comprehensiveness of health insurance and its methods of provider payment, have affected provider market power, competitive behavior, and industry performance. Also affecting market performance have been ownership differences among firms, such as non-profit hospitals, health insurers (Blue Cross and Blue Shield plans),

and medical schools. In addition, government regulations, subsidies, and tax exemptions have provided some firms with cost advantages over their competitors.

When each of the medical markets is examined, the distinctive characteristics of that market (and how they may have changed over time) and its effect on performance will be examined. Appropriate public policies to improve market performance will also be discussed.

Competitive markets should not be evaluated on whether those who are uninsured or who have low incomes receive access to medical services. It is not the function of competitive firms to subsidize the poor and sick. To ensure that the poor and sick do receive care, government must provide them with subsidies. Competitive markets can then be evaluated in terms of how efficiently they provide those subsidized services. (Alternative approaches for subsidizing those with low incomes and the uninsured are discussed in the chapter on National Health Insurance.)

PUBLIC POLICIES

Although few industries approximate the competitive ideal and long-run equilibrium may never be attained because underlying conditions are constantly changing, the tendency of price-competitive industries is to move in the direction of desirable market performance. The competitive model, more than any other model, is better able to predict the effect on market performance of changes in demand, cost of producing services, supply, and changes in the assumptions underlying a price-competitive market. The usefulness of the competitive model, therefore, is with regard to its predictions and the effect of its assumptions on performance. For example, each market will be examined to determine whether changes have occurred over time in supply and demand conditions and in the assumptions underlying competitive market structures that affect the industry's performance, such as barriers that limit entry of new firms, availability of information, and purchaser and provider incentives, each of which affect competitive behavior and, consequently, performance.

Market performance can presumably be improved through alternative approaches. First, the actual market can be restructured to more closely approximate a competitive industry and greater reliance placed on competitive pressures to achieve the goal of economic efficiency. An example of this approach is the applicability and enforcement of the anti-trust laws that seek to prevent monopolization of an industry. Alternatively, greater emphasis can be placed on regulation and centralized decision making to achieve the desirable outcomes of a competitive market. Under either of these public policy approaches, a comparable set of measures by which to evaluate the performance of each market is required. Unless there is agreement on the desired outcome measures, regulatory and market competitive approaches cannot be compared. The two approaches suggested for improving market performance—increased regulation versus greater reliance on market pressures—will be analyzed according to the economic criteria of economic efficiency.

A competitive market will result in a more elastic industry supply curve than if, for example, the industry were subject to entry barriers. With increased demand, a competitive industry will produce a greater output at a lower price. However, even in a competitive industry, the industry supply curve may be less elastic than is economically feasible because of the nature of the production function and possible restrictions on the use of various inputs.

SUMMARY

In evaluating the performance of each of the medical markets in the remaining chapters of this book, the first step will be to examine the market structure for each of the separate markets, beginning with the insurance market, then the institutional settings in which care is provided, proceeding to the manpower markets, and ending with the education markets. Each market will be compared to a hypothetically competitive medical market. The competitive market is used as the yardstick for comparison since it is inclusive of the conditions necessary for economic effi-

ciency. The performance that might be expected under a competitive market will then be compared with what is observed in the particular medical market. Any divergence in performance between what is expected theoretically and what is observed will be analyzed in terms of differences in the structure and assumptions underlying the hypothetically competitive and actual markets.

To the extent that there are indications of inadequate performance in any particular market, the assumptions that underly a competitive industry will be examined: Is entry by other firms permitted? What are the payment and incentive mechanisms in that industry? And what are the goals and objectives of the suppliers? Nonprofit firms dominate major segments of the medical sector, such as many Blue Cross and Blue Shield health plans, hospitals, and medical schools. Do their objectives, which differ from those of for-profit firms, lead to either desirable or undesirable differences in performance? Finally, what have been the effects on performance of barriers to entry that have been advanced on the grounds of consumer protection?

REVIEW QUESTIONS

1. The following affect the supply of medical care: price of medical care, the prices of inputs, and technological or scientific knowledge. Explain how an increase in each of the above, while the effect of the other two are held constant, will cause changes in supply.
2. Economists claim that there are and have been several causes of economic inefficiency in medical care. List three basic causes, and for each describe why it results in economic inefficiency and poor performance in medical markets.
3. How has the lack of information affected the structure of the medical care market?
4. Contrast the differences in technical versus economic efficiency with respect to the provision of medical services.
5. What information does a decision-maker need to minimize their costs of production?
6. Would a decision maker use an input if it is subject to diminishing returns?
7. Apply the concept of a production function and the idea of "marginal rate of substitution" to an HMO. Show

how this knowledge may be used for deciding upon the settings to be used in providing a medical treatment.

8. Assuming a price-competitive medical market, what is the likely effect on the relative proportion of hospital and physician services used in providing a treatment of the large increase in the supply of physicians?

9. How has the elasticity of supply of medical services affected the government's cost of expanding health care to the poor and uninsured?

10. Why is a competitive market used as a yardstick for evaluating the performance of the different medical care markets?

CHAPTER
8

Market Competition in Medical Care

KEY TERMS AND CONCEPTS

- Certificate of Need legislation (CON)
- Per se anti-trust violations
- Rule of reason anti-trust violations
- Capitation
- Free choice of provider
- Diagnostic Related Groups (DRGs)
- Cost containment programs
- Any Willing Provider (AWP) laws
- Report cards
- HEDIS and CAHPS quality measures

Learning Objectives

Upon completing this chapter, the reader should be able to:

- Explain why market competition occurred in medical services.
- Describe how the anti-trust laws have increased market competition.
- Explain the performance of managed care with respect to its effect on rising medical expenditures.
- Understand whether market competition had an adverse effect on quality of care.
- Describe current employer and insurer efforts to measure and improve quality of care.

THE EMERGENCE OF COMPETITION IN MEDICAL CARE

The delivery of medical services changed dramatically starting in the 1980s. In the late 1970s, the trend appeared to be toward increased regulation. An increasing number of states were moving toward hospital rate regulation, both the state and federal government enacted regulations on hospital investment (Certificate of Need legislation—CON), and granting hospitals public utility status was being proposed by hospital associations and others. Yet, rather than moving in the direction of increased regulation, market competition became the dominant force affecting hospitals and health professionals. This change was not anticipated.

The emergence of market competition was not the result of any legislative objective on the part of Congress or the Administration. How it evolved is instructive for understanding the reasons for change in the medical sector.

Lack of Efficiency Incentives and the Rise in Expenditures

When Medicare and Medicaid were enacted in the mid 1960s, incorporating efficiency incentives was not a political priority. Hospitals were reimbursed their costs plus 2 percent, physicians were paid fee-for-service (FFS) according to their usual and customary fees, and neither capitation payments to HMOs nor selective contracting with specific providers were permitted since the AMA insisted that "free choice" of provider be available to all Medicare and Medicaid beneficiaries. The price constraints facing Medicaid patients were removed and were greatly reduced for Medicare patients. The government was committed to paying for the medical services of the aged and poor, regardless of the cost of those services. Given the methods by which providers were paid, providers had minimal incentives to be concerned with efficient delivery of services or expenditures under these programs.

As a consequence, government expenditures for Medicare and Medicaid greatly exceeded their original projections. Medicare's actuaries stated that Medicare would cost only $2 billion a year. However,

as an entitlement program, the law defined Medicare's benefits and beneficiaries; no limit was placed on its overall expenditures. Federal expenditures under both of these programs rapidly increased from $3 billion in 1966, to $31 billion by 1975, to $111 billion in 1985, to $304 billion by 1995, and to $439 billion currently (2003). State and federal expenditures under Medicaid also increased sharply, from $4 billion in 1966 to $277 billion in 2003.

Rising inflation in the late 1960s stimulated the demand for employer-paid health insurance, which was not considered taxable income to the employee.[1] As incomes increased due to inflation, employees moved into higher income tax brackets (as high as 70 percent), and unions bargained for increased health benefits. With increased insurance coverage in both the private and public sectors, consumer concern with rising health costs declined. Health care providers were able to increase their prices with little fear of decreased demand. In a growing economy with rising inflation and little import competition, business firms were able to pass on their higher labor costs by increasing the prices of their goods and services. Health care expenditures in the private sector went from $28 billion a year in 1965 to $68 billion in 1975 to $769 billion currently.

These massive increases in medical expenditures by both the public and private sectors were equivalent to a huge redistribution of wealth, from the taxpayers to those working in the medical sector.

---

1. During World War II (as demand for labor increased and wage and price controls were in effect), the government, to forestall a possible strike by unionized workers on the West Coast for higher wages, ruled that employer health insurance contributions on behalf of employees would not be considered as taxable income to the employee. The 1954 Internal Revenue Code removed any uncertainty than may have existed among firms regarding this tax exclusion for employer-purchased health insurance. In a recent study of this change in the 1954 IRS code, Thomasson states, ". . . the tax subsidy led to a shift from individual to group insurance and increased the amount of health insurance coverage purchased by households, especially households with high marginal tax rates. Based on an analysis of the change in coverage that occurred during this period, the author estimates a price elasticity of demand for health insurance of –0.54. Melissa A. Thomasson, "The Importance of Group Coverage: How Tax Policy Shaped U.S. Health Insurance," *The American Economic Review*, 93(4), September 2003, p. 1382, 13731382.

Initial Cost Containment Efforts

Early attempts at reducing the rise in medical expenditures came from the federal government. Each time Medicare hospital expenditures were about to exhaust the Medicare Trust Fund, the Medicare payroll tax and its wage base were increased. (Medicaid and the physician portion of Medicare are funded from general tax revenues, and increases in these programs assumed greater importance in subsequent years when the federal deficit became a political issue.) As it became politically difficult to continually increase Medicare payroll taxes, successive Administrations developed a concentrated interest in halting Medicare's rapidly escalating expenditures.

Few options were available to any Administration for limiting Medicare expenditures. Attempting to reduce Medicare benefits or to have the aged pay more would have cost any Administration a great deal of political support from the aged and their supporters. If taxes were not to be continually increased nor benefits reduced to the aged, then the only alternatives for limiting the increase in Medicare expenditures (which were rising by approximately 15 percent a year), were to either limit payments to providers or to place controls on utilization of services.

The Federal government started chipping away at the cost-based reimbursement of hospitals in 1969, when it removed the plus 2 percent from the cost plus formula. In 1971, because of rising inflation, President Nixon placed the entire U.S. economy under a wage and price freeze (the Economic Stabilization Program). After one year, wage and price controls were removed from all sectors of the economy except health care, which remained under price controls until April 1974. Once these controls were removed, physician and hospital expenditures increased very rapidly.

Additional regulatory approaches were tried, but each one either failed to limit rising expenditures or had unintended consequences. Although the Medicare Fee Index limited physician fee increases under Medicare, an increasing number of physicians declined to participate in Medicare, thereby reducing the aged's access to care. In 1974, Congress attempted to limit rising expenditures by enacting the National

Health Planning and Resources Development Act (CON); each hospital's capital expenditures was subject to review by regional planning agencies. Not only did CON fail to limit hospital expenditure increases, existing hospitals used the controls on capital investment to limit competition by preventing new hospitals from entering their market and from free-standing outpatient surgery centers being established. Utilization review (Professional Standard Review Organizations) for hospitalized Medicare patients was legislated by the Congress in 1972. Again, empirical studies failed to find significant savings in hospital use or expenditures as a result of these programs. FFS physicians had no incentive to limit patients' use of the hospital.

In 1979, President Carter made hospital cost containment his highest legislative priority—and Congress, a majority of whom were of the same political party—rejected it. His proposed legislation would have placed limits on the annual percent increase in each hospital's expenditures.

Anti-Competitive Efforts Limiting Choice and Efficiency

From the mid 1960s through the 1970s, medical providers did not compete on price. There was little demand side pressure for providers to engage in price competition. Patients had little incentive to be concerned with medical prices since they had comprehensive health insurance either from the government, Medicare and Medicaid, or from their employers. Free choice of provider was mandated under public programs, information on provider prices (or on any other provider attributes) was unavailable (and in many places such price information was prohibited by medical societies), and physicians, through their medical societies, colluded on their prices when negotiating with insurance companies. Further, large employers and their unions (particularly in the auto and steel industries) were not concerned over rising insurance premiums since they could increase their product prices with little fear of import competition.

Given the size of the U.S. population, differences in income, willingness to pay for health care, etc., it would be expected that a variety of payment and delivery systems, in addition to indemnity insurance and FFS provider payment, would have emerged. However, the number of HMOs and their growth was, for many years, very small. In a competitive medical services market, a demand for such organizations would have existed, particularly if HMOs could be price competitive and provide medical care of a quality comparable to that of the fee-for-service system. Since HMO and managed care growth did not occur for many years, this inadequate supply response should be examined to determine whether it was due to insufficient demand and/or supply side reasons.

One way to determine the potential demand for HMOs is to examine what percentage of the population enrolled in an HMO when it was offered in competition with traditional fee-for-service insurance. Several HMOs, such as Kaiser, required that potential enrollees have a choice between their plan and an alternative, such as Blue Cross-Blue Shield. Based on studies where consumers have had this dual choice option, 20 to 60 percent of the subscribers chose the HMO. It would therefore be expected that a larger percentage of the general population would have been enrolled in such plans. To determine why the growth in such plans during the 1960s and 1970s did not keep up with their potential demand, it is necessary to examine the supply side of this market.

Unless HMOs were as efficient as the FFS delivery system, they would not be expected to increase their market share. However, comparative data of HMO premiums relative to those in traditional fee-for-service insurance indicated that HMOs could compete effectively on price.

The reasons for the very slow growth of HMOs must therefore be found in anti-competitive barriers that inhibited their development. The first such barrier were attempts by state medical associations to deny hospital privileges to HMO-participating physicians, thereby denying HMOs access to hospitals. If an HMO could not provide its potential subscribers with access to hospital care, the plan could not effectively compete with fee-for-service physicians in the community. According to Kessel, HMOs represented a lower-priced substitute to fee-for-service physicians

because the premium was the same for all persons regardless of their income. Since fee-for-service physicians attempted to price discriminate according to a patient's income, a plan that charges all patients the same premium is a form of price cutting for those with high incomes (1).

State and county medical associations had successfully prevented the growth of many HMOs by revoking the membership of or refusing to grant membership to physicians who desired to join them; such memberships had been prerequisites for hospital privileges. To survive, an HMO such as Kaiser had to have its own hospitals. Although various medical societies subsequently lost anti-trust suits, their anti-competitive actions were sufficient to raise the cost to potential HMOs to prevent their large-scale development.

In addition to the above actions, state medical societies were successful in having legislation enacted at a state level that placed additional barriers on HMO development and on an HMO's ability to compete with fee-for-service practice. HMOs were subject to strict regulation by the state department of insurance requiring physicians to be a majority of the controlling board of an HMO, requiring HMOs to permit the participation in its network of any physician in the community, requiring HMOs to be organized on a non-profit basis, and prohibiting HMOs from advertising their benefits and premiums.

Prohibiting an HMO from advertising erects a major barrier to its growth. Prior to the 1980s, consumer ignorance of HMOs was an important reason why potential subscribers did not join. Further, HMOs are subject to greater economies of scale than are solo practitioners. An HMO must have certain minimum facilities, an organization to enroll members, and possibly its own hospital. Unless an HMO is able to enroll a sufficient number of subscribers, it will be forced to operate at relatively higher premiums (i.e., the declining portion of its long-run average-cost curve). If an HMO were prevented from advertising, it would take longer to reach the number of enrollees required to make its premium competitive with fee-for-service insurance. The time and losses required were too great an obstacle for many HMOs.

Restricting the HMO to non-profit status further removed any incentives that might have existed for non-physicians to risk their talents and capital to start on HMO.

The development of market competition was not anticipated. There were, however, a number of events that provided the preconditions for market competition, but only one that made it possible to occur (2).

Federal Initiatives

The Increased Supply of Physicians: For approximately 15 years, through the 1950s and early 1960s, the supply of physicians in relation to the population remained constant at 141 physicians per 100,000. During this period, physicians' incomes were rising (relative to those of other occupations), as were the number of applicants to acceptances to medical schools (see Table 13-1, Table 13-2, Table 13-3, and Table 13-4). As the demand for physicians' services continued to grow, stimulated by the passage of Medicare and Medicaid and the growth of private health insurance, an increased number of foreign medical graduates (FMGs) came to the United States.

During this period there was constant talk of a shortage of physicians. Many qualified U.S. students who could not gain admission to the limited number of medical school spaces went overseas to receive a medical education. Many middle-class families were concerned that their sons and daughters could not become physicians while, at the same time, there was increased immigration by FMGs. The Congress responded to these constituent pressures and passed the Health Professions Educational Assistance Act (HPEA). Senator Yarborough stated the reasons for the passage of the HPEA in 1963. "It was when we were trying to give more American boys and girls a chance for a medical education, so that we would not have to drain the help of other foreign countries." And again, "To me it is just shocking that we do not give American boys and girls a chance to obtain a medical education so that they can serve their own people" (3).

It took a number of years before the full magnitude of this Act took effect. New medical schools were built, and existing medical schools increased their spaces. (The same occurred for other health professions.) By 1980, the supply of physicians had expanded to almost 200 per 100,000, almost a 50 percent increase from the early 1960s. The ratio continued to expand so that by 1990, the physician-to-population ratio reached 230 per 100,000. It is currently (2001) 285 per 100,000 (2001), double what it had been in 1960.

In response to their constituent interests and over the objections of the American Medical Association, Congress enacted legislation that eventually created excess capacity among physicians. It was not Congress' intention to create competition among physicians. However, their actions in passing the HPEA set the stage for it.

The HMO Act: In the early 1970s, President Nixon wanted to enact an inexpensive (to the federal government) health initiative. He proposed stimulating the growth of prepaid health plans, renamed health maintenance organizations (HMOs).[2] Paying health plans a capitated amount per enrollee in return for delivery of comprehensive medical services was not new; the Commission on the Cost of Medical Care first proposed it in the 1930s. Early examples of such organizations are the Kaiser Foundation Health Plan and the Group Health Association. Under capitation, the HMO and its physicians have a financial incentive to minimize the cost of medical care provided to its enrollees.

When Congress passed the HMO Act in 1973, it included two provisions helpful to the development of HMOs and one that was a hindrance. First, employers with 25 or more employees had to offer their employees an HMO option if there was a federally qualified HMO available in their area. Second, federally qualified HMOs were exempt from restrictive state practices described earlier. These provisions reduced the marketing expenses of HMOs and removed restrictions hindering their development. Unfortunately, to become federally qualified, the HMO was required to

---

2. The originator of the term health maintenance organization is Paul M. Ellwood, Jr. See his "Health Maintenance Strategy," *Medical Care*, 9(3) May/June 1971, pp. 291–298.

offer a benefit package that was more expensive than those offered by competing insurance plans.

The benefit requirements necessary to become a federally qualified HMO discouraged many HMOs from taking advantage of federal qualification. It was not until several years later that this benefit requirement was changed following complaints from HMOs that these requirements increased their premiums so that they could not compete with regular health insurance plans. (Also, as part of the 1979 Health Planning Act, large HMOs with enrollment greater than 50,000 persons were exempted from the CON process. Rather than this being pro-competitive legislation for all HMOs, however, the main beneficiaries were the larger, established HMOs.) Once these restrictions were relaxed, HMOs took advantage of the beneficial provisions of the HMO Act. As enrollment in HMOs increased, the lower hospital use by HMO enrollees contributed to hospitals' excess capacity.

The 1979 Amendments to CON Legislation: The initial CON legislation established planning agencies whose purpose was to limit the increase in hospital capital expenditures. HMOs needed access to a hospital to provide a full range of medical services. Hospitals affiliated with HMOs wanted to be able to expand, while other HMOs wanted to construct hospitals. HMOs complained to the Congress that the CON legislation was being used by existing hospitals to block their growth. HMOs represented a competitive threat to existing hospitals and physicians in a community. "HMOs were subjected to more extensive controls than fee-for-service providers. Although financing plans and provider organizations of other kinds could be established without government approval, establishment of an HMO was subject to planning agency review" (4).

In 1979, Congress amended the CON legislation so that the Act should not be used to inhibit competition. However, these amendments did not grant all HMOs a complete exemption from the CON Act; it merely loosened the restrictions.

Except for the change in the CON legislation and the enactment of the HMO Act and its amendments, Congress could not develop a consensus with the various health interest groups as to what legislative approach, if any, should be used to limit the rise in federal health expenditures.

Political Opposition to a Competitive Strategy: In the late 1970s, opponents of President Carter's cost-containment legislation, such as Representatives Gephardt and Stockman, began to propose an alternative approach, the use of market competition. Various academicians, such as Enthoven, wrote on the virtues of market competition (5). However, if market competition had to depend upon congressional action, it would not have occurred. Too many powerful interest groups were opposed to organizing the delivery of health services along competitive lines (6).

Organized medicine correctly foresaw that its members would be worse off under competition. Physicians would have to accept changes in their style of practice, restrictions would be placed on their behavior by utilization review, and price discounting would emerge. Hospitals also did not support a competitive approach. HMOs would decrease the demand for hospital care, and competition would force hospitals to reduce costs and compete on price. Many hospitals preferred the security of a regulatory system. Commercial health insurers also opposed the concept of market competition. They were unsure of their future role in a system of competing HMOs. Instead, insurance companies preferred some form of all-payer hospital rate regulation (same price to all insurers) so that the Blue Cross discount would no longer place them at a competitive disadvantage. Blue Cross was also reluctant to favor a change to market competition. Blue Cross plans with high market shares and good provider relations would have had little to gain from such a change.

Business groups (who might be expected to favor competition) were, at most, lukewarm supporters of health care competition. Many companies believed that they had preferred risk groups and did not want to incur increased administrative costs by offering multiple health plans to their employees.

Unions were among the most vocal of the groups opposing a competitive delivery system. Although unions had been strong supporters of Kaiser, those same unions had a basic distrust of competitive markets. They preferred not-for-profit health plans and wanted the government, rather than markets, to be the regulator of provider and insurer performance. Unions also opposed legislative proposals to make their members more price sensitive by placing a limit on the amount of employer-paid health insurance that was exempt from taxes. Large unions, such as the UAW, had comprehensive health insurance benefits and a tax limit on their members' health benefits would have made their members worse off.

The beneficiaries of a competitive market are consumers. Their interest in pro-competitive legislation, however, is diffuse; the potential benefits of competition were unknown and not viewed as being sufficiently large to warrant their involvement in the political process.

Elimination of "Free Choice" of Provider Under Medicaid: It was not until 1981, under President Reagan, that additional cost-containment legislation was enacted. In return for reducing federal Medicaid expenditures, Congress amended Medicaid so as to provide states with greater flexibility in how they pay for their medically indigent (7). States were no longer required to offer their medically indigent "free choice" of medical provider. This meant that states could take bids and negotiate contracts with selected providers to care for their Medicaid patients. Although the law was a potentially powerful force for using market forces in the Medicaid program, many states moved slowly.

New Hospital Payment System Under Medicare: Starting in September 1983, the Reagan Administration introduced a revolutionary method for paying hospitals under Medicare: fixed prices per admission according to diagnostic related groupings (DRGs), and an annual update index to limit increases in the DRG payment. The hospital and medical associations were powerless against a Republican Administration intent on reducing Medicare expenditures for hospitals. As the incentives facing hospitals changed from per-day retrospective to per-admission prospective payment, lengths of stay for the aged declined, and hospital occupancy fell. Hospital administrators became con-

cerned with physicians' practice styles since it affected the cost of producing a DRG, for which they received a fixed price. However, by the time hospitals began to experience the effect of Medicare DRGs on their occupancy rates, the move toward market competition had already started in the private sector. DRGs reinforced the downward pressure on hospital occupancy rates.

Private Sector Initiatives

Approximately two-thirds of the population has private health insurance coverage, and most private health insurance (85 percent) is purchased through the workplace. The stimulus for competition started in the private sector.

In 1981, the nation entered into a severe recession. In addition, the automobile and steel industries faced increased import competition from foreign producers. These same industries also had the most comprehensive health insurance programs for their employees. The recession led to unemployment, loss of income, and a decrease in health insurance benefits resulting in a decline in elective hospital admissions. The recession also lowered tax revenues for states. Consequently, many states cut back on their Medicaid benefits, decreased the numbers of eligibles, and instituted cost containment measures such as prior authorization for admission. These factors, which led to a decline in the hospital admission rate for those under 65 years of age, started in late 1981.

Once the recession ended, those industries engaged in competition with foreign producers found that the strength of the U.S. dollar relative to other currencies forced them to further reduce their labor costs to remain competitive.

President Reagan's tax cuts in 1981, which reduced the high marginal income tax rates for employees from 70 percent to the mid-30s, provided employees with an incentive to reduce their medical expenditures. A greater portion of any savings from lower insurance premiums could be used to increase their take-home pay.

As a result of these events, industry began to examine ways in which they could contain the rise in their employees' health insurance costs.[3] Business began to pressure health insurers to limit their premium increases and to institute new cost-saving programs. Also, an increasing number of firms started their own self-insurance plans. These firms believed that they, rather than insurance companies, would be better able to control their employees' health care use. Businesses also added deductibles and co-insurance to their employees' health plans, thereby increasing their employees' price sensitivity. A survey of 1,185 companies found that the percentage of firms requiring deductible payments for their employee's inpatient care rose from 30 percent in 1982 to 63 percent in 1984; similarly, the percentage of firms requiring pre-authorization for hospital admission increased from 2 percent to 26 percent over that same period (8).

One of the most important changes firms (or insurers acting on their behalf) introduced was a change in the benefits package. Insurance coverage for lower-cost substitutes to hospitals was introduced. Previously, even though it was less costly to perform surgery in an outpatient setting, if this service was not covered by insurance, it became less costly *to the employee* to have the surgery performed in a hospital. Thus by adding outpatient surgery to the benefit package, the insurance premium paid by the firm could be reduced.

Private-sector initiatives had two effects. First, as purchasers of health care benefits, employers demonstrated their concern with rising health care costs which was transmitted to their health insurers who in turn included low-cost substitutes to hospital care in

their benefit packages and began to undertake hospital utilization review. Prior authorization for admission, concurrent review, and second opinions for surgery were instituted as a means of reducing insurance premiums. Insurers, particularly the Blues, began to change their relationship with providers and became more adversarial. They began to place greater pressure on hospitals to limit their cost increases.

The second consequence of business' concern with their employees' medical costs was that hospitals developed excess capacity. Efforts to reduce hospital utilization, such as utilization controls, the growth of HMOs, and coverage of care in non-hospital settings were succeeding. Occupancy rates in short-term general hospitals declined from 78 percent in 1980 to 64.8 percent by 1985. As excess capacity increased, hospitals were willing to participate with and become part of alternative delivery systems to receive more patients.

The Enforcement of Anti-Trust Laws

Demand side pressures for lower health care costs and the excess capacity among hospitals and physicians were important preconditions for competition. However, had it not been for the application of the anti-trust laws, it is unlikely that market competition would have occurred.

Medical societies and state practice acts inhibited market competition by erecting barriers to the development of competing delivery systems and the corporate practice of medicine. Advertising and fee splitting were also prohibited, and medical societies engaged in boycotts.

Unless the anti-trust laws were applicable to the health sector, physician and hospital boycotts and other anti-competitive behavior could have prevented market competition from once again occurring.

Up until 1975 it was believed that the anti-trust laws did not apply to "learned professions," which included the health professions. In 1975, the U.S. Supreme Court ruled against the Virginia State bar association, who established a minimum fee schedule for lawyers believing that lawyers were not engaged in "trade or commerce." The Supreme Court thereby denied any sweeping exclusion for the learned pro-

---

3. Employers are concerned with overall labor compensation rather than with its components. Therefore, increased health insurance costs typically result in reduced wages. However, union resistance in the auto industry against reduced health benefits together with negotiated multi-year union contracts meant that firms could not immediately shift higher insurance costs back to the employee in the form of reduced wages. Further, a number of major industries, such as the automobile industry, were responsible, as a result of wage negotiations, for paying their retirees' medical costs. Thus any decrease in the rate of increase in medical expenditures decreased the firm's liability and increased its profitability. Consequently, firms (and their unions) had an incentive to control rising health insurance premiums.

fessions from the anti-trust laws. In another important precedent, in 1978 the Supreme Court denied the use of anti-competitive behavior by the National Society of Professional Engineers, even if it was to prevent a threat to either the profession's ethics or to public safety. Encouraged by the Supreme Court decisions, the Federal Trade Commission (FTC) began to vigorously enforce the anti-trust laws in the health field. In 1975, the FTC charged the American Medical Association and its constituent medical societies with anti-competitive behavior. In a 1978 decision, the FTC prevailed. The AMA appealed the verdict to the Supreme Court but was again unsuccessful.

The Supreme Court's decision, rendered in 1982, was a clear signal to health providers that they would now be subject to the anti-trust laws. The FTC subsequently brought suit to prevent physician and dentist boycotts against insurers (Michigan State Medical Society and the Indiana Federation of Dentists), medical societies were prevented from denying hospital privileges to physicians participating in HMOs (Forbes Health System Medical Staff), permitted advertising to be used (FTC versus AMA), and enabled preferred provider organizations and HMOs to compete (9).

Per Se and Rule of Reason Anti-Competitive Behavior: Anti-competitive behavior is illegal on either per se grounds or by virtue of the rule of reason. Per se violations need not be demonstrated to harm the consumer; these activities are believed to be obviously anti-competitive and their effects are clearly harmful to consumers. The government must merely prove that the violation occurred. Price fixing, economic boycotts, tying arrangements, and division of horizontal markets are per se violations. Price fixing occurs when two or more competitors agree on a price at which their service will be sold. An example is when a Medicaid agency requests bids, and two providers agree to submit similar prices. It does not matter whether the fixed prices are minimums or maximums, they are both illegal. A boycott occurs when, for example, a medical society threatens to "departicipate" from Blue Shield or other third-party payer if their payment demands are not met. (Individual firms/physicians acting independently can refuse to participate with an insurer, but a boycott occurs when independent firms coordinate their refusal to join with an insurer). "Tying" occurs when a purchaser who wants to purchase one product is also required to buy a second product (e.g., operating room and anesthesiology services as well). When competitors agree to divide up geographic markets, consumers, or services and not compete with each other, it is illegal.

Other forms of anti-competitive behavior are analyzed according to the rule of reason, which attempts to determine whether the anti-competitive harm to consumers caused by the restraint exceeds the pro-competitive benefits of not permitting the particular activity. Examples of cases brought under the rule of reason are hospital mergers (whether competition among the remaining hospitals would be lessened), staff privilege issues (as when a cardiologist claims that they were denied privileges thereby depriving them of the right to compete against current cardiologists on staff), and the formation of PPOs (whether the PPO includes such a high percentage of the physicians in the market that it becomes a form of price fixing).

Activities by professional associations that provide increased information on the quality and characteristics of health care providers, such as specialty certification, are not anti-competitive since they do not limit either entry or choice of provider. Such actions often improve market performance by providing the consumer with more information. In the past, however, professional regulation resulted in limits on entry and on choice of provider, as well as other forms of anti-competitive behavior.

The application of anti-trust laws to the health field is based on the belief that price competitive markets have desirable outcomes. As new delivery and payment systems emerge in the health field, anti-trust questions will be raised as to whether these new arrangements are pro-competitive (e.g., take advantage of economies of scale) or whether they are a means of lessening competition among competitors. An appreciation of the economics of competitive markets is essential for understanding the probable anti-trust implications of these new arrangements.

The Changing Role of Health Insurers: After the removal of anti-competitive restrictions on HMOs, rapid growth in both the number of HMOs and in their enrollment occurred during the mid 1980s. Employers and others believed HMOs were the solution to rising medical expenditures and achieving quality medical care. It was unfortunate that HMOs became synonymous with the concept of market competition, since many HMOs did not initially engage in price competition.

Early research found that HMOs did not experience lower rates of growth in their premiums. There was a lack of price competition among HMOs and other insurance plans until the late 1980s. Employers offered their employees a choice of health plans, however employees did not have a price incentive to choose a lower-cost health plan since their employer either paid the full premium or the employee contribution was unrelated to the plan selected.

Initially, employers found that they were not saving money by offering HMOs to their employees. HMOs and indemnity insurers competed on nonprice factors, such as the comprehensiveness of the benefits and ease of access to providers. Employers also became concerned that HMOs were enrolling employees who were of lower risk while receiving a premium based on the average risk of the entire employee group.

As employees began to choose health plans based on their co-premiums, the lower employee premium contribution for an HMO led to large numbers of employees switching to HMOs. As HMOs began to increase their market share at the expense of the indemnity plans, insurers began instituting managed care techniques such as utilization review. As a result, inpatient admissions and length of stay declined. Hospital occupancy rates dropped and, with their growing excess capacity, hospitals began to engage in price competition to increase their volume.

Traditional insurers also began to compete against HMOs by starting their own HMOs. In this manner insurers were able to offer different insurance products to consumers who differed in their price elasticities of demand. The least price sensitive subscribers continued to purchase traditional FFS insurance, with the highest premium; those with the most price elastic demands purchased the more restrictive health plans, such as HMOs.

The role of the health insurer changed as a result of employer demands for lower premiums. Previously, insurers had a passive role (marketing, enrollment, and paying claims). Under employer pressure, insurers became involved in decisions affecting the physician's practice. Through utilization management, the insurer determined whether the patient should be admitted to a hospital and how long to stay. Insurer drug formularies limited physician decisions on drug prescribing. Insurer approval was required for patient referrals to specialists. By covering low-cost substitutes to the hospital, insurers determined in which setting the patient was to be treated. And by having hospitals and physicians compete on price to be included in their provider network, the insurer limited the patient's choice of provider.

By not recognizing the demand for cost containment, physicians and hospitals lost an opportunity to perform these functions themselves. Instead, new firms such as HMOs, utilization management companies, and PPO organizations entered the market, decreased medical costs, and transferred revenues from the traditional providers to themselves.

The Change in Managed Care: In the early to mid-1990s, restrictive managed care plans that limited access to specialists and required patients to receive permission from their gatekeepers for referrals grew rapidly. Employees had to choose between competing plans that would contract with physicians and hospitals willing to discount their prices and agree to observe medical practice guidelines. These managed care practices led to a slower growth in premiums and greater takehome wages. However, strong economic growth and a tight labor market in the late 1990s changed employee health plan choices.

Employers, competing for employees, offered health plans with broader provider networks and fewer restrictions on access to care. At the same time, a backlash against managed care occurred. Managed care decreased physician incomes and reduced their autonomy; medical societies lobbied for relaxation of HMO cost control methods and were successful in many states in having "Any Willing Provider" laws enacted. Opposition to managed care also came from consumers who had been forced into tightly managed care plans. Consumer complaints were publicized by the media, which attracted politicians. Managed care was also opposed by those who favored a single-payer system and believed the success of managed care in reducing costs would lessen their case for a single-payer system.

The tight labor market, opposition from physicians, dissatisfied consumers, and those favoring a single-payer system led to a weakening of managed care's cost containment methods. As a result, health insurance premiums rapidly increased.

Moral Hazard and the Development of Managed Care: Managed care was a response to certain market failures in the U.S. health care system. There was a lack of purchaser, patient, and provider incentives in both the use of medical services and with regard to the cost of care. Insurers simply paid claims and passed the higher costs onto employers and employees in the form of higher premiums. Patients with insurance had little incentive to use fewer services (moral hazard) and physicians, paid FFS, had a financial incentive to provide additional care and tests (demand inducement) to the point where the marginal costs of that additional care exceeded their marginal benefits. These lack of efficiency incentives led to rapidly rising medical expenditures. Managed care was designed to address these problems (10).

Managed care's very rapid growth was the result of its greater efficiency in overcoming the lack of both patient and physician incentives to be concerned with the use and cost of care. If managed care was not more efficient or responsive to purchaser preferences, it could not have increased its relative market share.

The market is currently searching for other cost control methods, given the movement away from tight managed care plans. Any new health plans will have to solve the problem of moral hazard on the part of consumers and demand inducement by providers.

CHARACTERISTICS OF MANAGED CARE PLANS

Managed care includes a number of different mechanisms; the use of these mechanisms has changed over time, and different managed care plans use different combinations of managed care techniques. Thus managed care plans encompass a wide spectrum of health plans.

At the least restrictive end of the spectrum are managed fee-for-service (FFS) indemnity plans. Enrollees in such plans pay the insurer a premium and are then responsible for a deductible and coinsurance up to a maximum out-of-pocket expenditure each year. The insurer includes a utilization management component to the traditional (FFS) plan. Patients are responsible for receiving pre-authorization from the insurer for elective hospital admissions (and for outpatient surgeries) and the insurer, once the patient is admitted, reviews the patient's length of hospital stay. If the patient fails to receive pre-authorization, they can be financially liable for the hospital expense. The patient can use any provider and can self refer to a specialist. These types of plans typically have the highest premiums. The cost control mechanisms used by the insurer are primarily patient financial incentives, deductibles and co-payments, and utilization management.

A more restrictive managed care plan is the above-managed indemnity plan with a preferred provider organization (PPO). PPO providers are paid FFS, are not exclusive to any one insurance plan, and are selected based on whether they are willing to provide the insurer with a discount on their fees and are more appropriate users of medical services. If the patient uses PPO providers, then their deductible is lower as well as their coinsurance rate, e.g., 10 percent (or $20) versus 30 percent for a non-PPO provider. Again, it is the patient who has the financial incentive to use fewer services from less costly providers. Not all insurers create their own PPO network; they may "rent" one from another organization.

Indemnity plans often use "catastrophic case management" as an additional cost control mechanism. Once a patient's medical expense reaches $25,000, the insurer assigns a case manager to that patient to try and limit that patient's medical costs. The case manager has authority to provide additional benefits, e.g., installing medical equipment together with nursing care in the patient's home as a means of limiting the length of the hospital stay and reduce the patient's medical costs.

The most restrictive form of a managed care plan is an HMO. HMOs, however, also differ in their restrictiveness. Early HMOs were primarily based upon the staff or group model whereby the HMO either employed physicians (e.g., Group Cooperative of Puget Sound) or contracted with a group of physicians who had an exclusive arrangement with the HMO (e.g., Kaiser Permanente Medical Groups in California). These HMOs were vertically integrated organizations with their own physicians and hospitals. Patients were not required to pay deductibles and only minimal co-payments, e.g., $5 a visit. The HMO's benefits were typically more comprehensive than those offered by the indemnity plan. In addition to lower co-payments, HMOs provided preventive services and covered outpatient prescription drugs based on a formulary that included drugs considered to be cost effective and those drugs on which the HMO was able to negotiate discounted prices. HMO patients that used non-HMO providers or non-formulary drugs were liable for 100 percent of the bill. Staff and group model HMOs relied upon a "gatekeeper" primary care physician who provided primary care and who decided whether to refer the patient to a specialist or to a hospital.

Group and staff model HMOs used the primary care physician to control use of services. Physicians were typically paid a salary plus bonus at the end of the year. Hospitals, which were owned by the HMO, were paid their costs.

Staff model HMOs lost market share to non-staff model HMOs in the 1980s for two reasons: patients wanted to have greater choice of provider and, second, HMOs found it easier to expand by contracting with community physicians and hospitals. This approach reduced the need for many patients to give up their physician if they join an HMO.

Non-staff model HMOs either contract (usually on a non-exclusive basis) with two or more independent groups (network model), directly with physicians in independent practices, and/or one or more multi-specialty groups (Independent Practice Association, IPA). (Community physicians formed IPAs to serve as contracting organizations with HMOs and insurers. An IPA contracts with solo and small groups of physicians on a non-exclusive basis to serve an HMO's or

insurer's enrollees.) Providers in the above models may be paid in various ways: discounted FFS, negotiated rates (perhaps with a small risk-sharing pool at the end of the year), fixed prices per admission, or capitation.

Capitation is a risk-sharing arrangement in which the provider group receives a predetermined fixed payment per member per month (PMPM) in return for providing all of the contracted services. A capitated provider group is at risk for all the contracted services by their enrolled population. The provider group has an incentive to accurately assess their enrollees' risk (actuarial accuracy becomes essential) and to provide care in a cost-effective manner for less than the capitation payment.

The responsibility for cost control under non-staff model HMOs depends upon which entity bears the risk. Early HMOs paid their providers discounted fees and/or a fee schedule; the HMO bore the risk that the cost of medical services would be less than their capitation payment. The HMOs therefore undertook the utilization management function themselves. As more medical groups formed, increased in size, and gained experience in managing patients in a capitated environment, they began accepting capitation payments for medical services. The medical groups then became responsible for utilization review, quality assurance, appropriateness of care studies (including physician profiling, information feedback to their member physicians, and dropping over-utilizers), and payment of their physician members, either fee-for-service or sub-capitation.

As more medical groups, including IPAs, accepted capitation, they negotiated risk-sharing arrangements for reduced hospital utilization. A capitated medical group and a capitated hospital group shared a part of the hospital's capitation payment. The medical group then had an incentive to reduce hospital use, with both groups sharing in the savings.

One variant of the above model (particularly in California) was a large medical group that contracted with an HMO and received 85 percent of the HMO's premium. The medical group then incurred the risk for all of the enrollees' medical services; the group contracted with other providers, such as hospitals, for the services it did not provide. The HMO no longer had any financial risk; it was all shifted to the medical group. The medical group had an incentive to innovate in improving the enrollee's health status as well as reducing their medical costs.

Unfortunately, many medical groups that accepted capitation risk did not understand capitation; they lacked the managerial and actuarial expertise to manage the insurance risk involved in capitation and failed to set aside appropriate reserves. As a result, many medical groups went bankrupt. Few medical groups currently accept capitation payments.

The last type of managed care organization is an HMO with a Point of Service option (POS). A POS plan is similar to an HMO except that the enrollee is allowed to see a non-HMO provider but must pay a significant out-of-pocket expense, e.g., 50 percent of the bill. The advantage to the enrollee of this option is that they are not locked into the HMO. Although POS plans have increased in popularity, out-of-plan use is low because of the high cost sharing.

The premium in a typical HMO is allocated as shown in Figure 8-1. The HMO receives, for example, $100 PMPM. They retain $15 PMPM for administration (including enrollment and customer service), marketing, for care received by enrollees outside the HMO's service area, stop loss insurance for certain catastrophic medical expenses, and profit. About $10 PMPM is used to pay for pharmacy benefits; the HMO

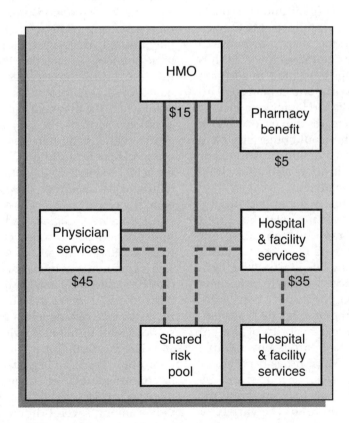

Figure 8-1. Allocation of HMO premiums.

is typically at risk for this benefit. Approximately $40 PMPM goes for medical services, including primary care, specialty care, and ancillary services, such as laboratory tests. And $35 PMPM is for hospital and other facility services (e.g., outpatient surgery). Risk sharing pools between the medical group and hospital are shown by the dotted lines.

Providers within these budgetary allocations may be paid in a variety of ways as discussed above. Within a medical group, many arrangements have been tried and they are continually changing; primary care physicians may be capitated or paid discounted FFS, similarly for specialists. When capitation is not used, then there is usually a withhold of part of the fee to insure that there are sufficient funds at the end of the year.

Managed care organizations (MCOs), as discussed above, encompass a variety of organizational models and a variety of managed care products. MCOs currently offer a diversified product line. In response to employer demand for more employee choice, HMOs have expanded their offerings to include, in addition to an HMO option, a POS plan and a managed indemnity plan, including a PPO. (Having one insurer offer a spectrum of plans decreases the cost of adverse selection to an employer who would otherwise have to contract separately with an indemnity insurer.) For the same reason, indemnity insurers also offer HMO and other options to large employers.

That part of the MCO industry that was primarily HMOs has been changing over time (11). For-profit HMOs have grown more rapidly than non-profit HMOs. For-profit entrepreneurs have been quicker to see the profit from reducing hospital costs in high-use areas and have been more willing to enter new geographic areas, while non-profits have been more concerned with serving a regional hospital system. IPA model HMOs now have a majority of the enrollees and have increased their enrollments relative to staff and group model HMOs. It has been easier for an HMO to expand and to enter a new area by contracting with local physicians than investing the time and money to develop a group. The variety of products offered by HMOs, discussed above, has increased.

The Incentives Underlying Capitation Versus Fee-For-Service

Traditionally, physicians (and hospitals) were paid fee-for-services. Under FFS, providers had an incentive to undertake only those services that were reimbursed. Further, given that physician time and effort were scarce, that effort was allocated according to those activities and services whose price-to-cost ratio (as determined by fee schedules) were highest. Services not reimbursed by the insurer, such as preventive care (changing a patient's lifestyle or instituting a smoking cessation program), received little or no physician effort. Thus medical resources were primarily devoted to acute care services covered by insurance.

FFS payment also has several other incentive effects. When physicians and hospitals are paid to deliver services, their revenues and profits increase by providing more services. Patients, both privately and governmentally insured, are less price sensitive and will demand more services. Thus, given the benefits to physicians from providing more services and increased patient demand for services, providers will deliver services to the point where the marginal benefit to the patient of those additional services are very small. FFS payment, together with price insensitive patients, results in the marginal benefit of additional services being lower than the actual resource costs of those services. Overuse is a natural consequence of FFS when patients are not financially responsible for the cost of those services.

The Benefits of Capitation: The movement from FFS to capitation per enrollee changed provider incentives; capitation incentives are opposite that of FFS. The capitation payment, hence the insurance risk, may be at the HMO level or it may be shifted (all or in part) to one or more provider groups. The extent of the insurance risk depends upon whether the HMO sub-capitates different providers or not.

When the capitation payment remains with one organization, then that organization has an incentive to be concerned with the efficient coordination of all the medical services provided. When the risk is subdivided among several different providers, e.g., medical groups and hospitals, then the financial incentives of the different groups are not aligned and will likely result in inefficiency and conflict. Capitation was intended to increase coordination and decrease inefficiency in the provision of medical services.

Several of the positive incentives that result from capitation are as follows. When each provider (e.g., physicians) is paid separately under FFS and they are not fiscally responsible for costs they impose on other providers (e.g., hospitals), there are no financial incentives to use the least costly setting for patient treatment. Under capitation, the capitated organization has an incentive to provide care in the least costly manner. When medically feasible, there will be greater use of outpatient services, fewer hospital admissions, and shorter hospital stays, with the remainder of the patient's convalescence provided for in another setting or in the patient's home. The emphasis is on minimizing the cost of a treatment (without reducing quality or patient satisfaction).

Capitated organizations also have an incentive to be concerned with the costs of their enrollees' hospital use. The HMO has an incentive to contract with those hospitals that offer lower prices, are located near their enrollees, and have a better reputation for quality. To be competitive, hospitals must be efficient, take advantage of any economies of scale that exist, and eliminate unnecessary and duplicative facilities. Hospitals must first compete on price to be included in the organization's provider network before it can compete for physician referrals.

Capitation provides the medical group with an incentive to increase their physicians' productivity. An increase in demand for nurse practitioners and physician assistants would be expected to perform tasks currently undertaken by physicians. As long as the revenue produced by the additional auxiliaries exceeds their cost, it is in the medical group's interest to substitute less costly personnel as long as quality of care and patient satisfaction are not diminished. Delegation of tasks might (eventually) be based on the training and experience of individuals rather than, as under current state practice acts, whether a profession has a monopoly on the performance of those tasks.

To the extent that preventive care delivered to an HMO's enrollees decreases future demand for more costly medical services, the capitated organization would be expected to provide a greater amount of those services than is provided under fee-for-service. Similarly, to the extent that enrollee health habits can be improved (such as through smoking cessation programs), future demands for medical care could be reduced. (The capitated organization is more likely to undertake preventive-type programs whose payoff is relatively soon rather than further in the future since, given the amount of switching between health plans, it is not clear how long that enrollee will be with the organization.)

It is in the economic interest of HMOs, assuming they are at risk for their enrollees' medical expenses, to prescribe less costly drugs. The HMO has an incentive to evaluate different prescription drugs to determine whether the marginal benefit of a more expensive drug exceeds its additional costs. Similarly, to the extent that prescription drugs decrease hospitalizations, the organization has an incentive to monitor its patients' drug usage. This is particularly true for the aged in Medicare HMOs.

Perhaps the most important incentive under capitation is to innovate in the delivery of medical services. Innovations threaten current providers since they may substitute for existing personnel and facilities, hence decrease their demand. Previously, such innovations have been inhibited either by legal protections for the threatened providers or by anti-competitive actions by the professional associations. A capitated organization, however, has a strong financial incentive to be innovative in methods that reduce costs, improve outcomes, or increase patient satisfaction. Innovation is likely to occur in systems to aid patient diagnosis, improve treatment, better patient compliance, prevention, and adopt management techniques and information systems for decision-making. Increased profit and/or increased market share provide capitated organizations with an incentive to seek out and quickly adopt (when economically feasible) new techniques with both medical and management applications.

Concerns With Capitation: Incentives in a capitated system can be a cause for concern. When providers receive a lump sum per enrollee, their financial incentive is to do as little as possible for the patient since spending fewer resources means greater profits. Similarly, increasing the number of capitated enrollees without increasing the number of providers to serve them will result in decreased access to care. When HMOs (or their providers) receive the same capitation payment for enrollees regardless of their risk levels, providers (or HMOs) have an incentive to seek out lower risk groups. Under FFS, a high-risk patient would receive more services since the provider is paid according to the number and type of services provided.

Capitation of hospitals and physicians, which initially expanded, has since sharply contracted. Few medical groups and hospitals currently rely on capitation payments. Provider capitation mainly failed due to providers' inability to manage risk, to receive risk adjusted capitation payments from insurers, and because of conflict within medical groups regarding physician payment. Some medical groups capitated their primary care physicians (PCPs) and paid specialists discounted FFS. Others paid their primary care physicians discounted FFS and capitated specialists; some medical groups capitated both types of physicians. (When providers are paid discounted FFS, they may share in a bonus if funds remain at the end of the contract period.) In addition to conflict over the size of the capitation and FFS payments, it was difficult to align physician incentives within the group. When PCPs were capitated for all medical services, they had an incentive to provide more specialist services; if PCP capitation excluded specialist care, then they had an incentive to refer too frequently to specialists. Further, under the gatekeeper model, PCPs demanded a greater share of revenues from specialists. Conflict over physician incomes was a major reason for the dissolution of capitation payments.

Both FFS and capitation systems have incentives that either reward overuse or underuse of medical services. It thus becomes essential under both types of payment systems that purchasers monitor insurers and providers for how well patients are served regarding access, quality of care, treatment outcomes, and patient satisfaction.

PERFORMANCE OF A COMPETITIVE MANAGED CARE MARKET

In a relatively short time, managed care has come to dominate the health insurance market. In doing so, it has received its share of criticisms. Limits were placed on patient access, and physicians have seen their incomes reduced and their autonomy eroded. An examination of the effect that managed care plans have had on market performance should therefore examine the following indicators of performance: First, has managed care increased efficiency? If managed care was successful at reducing medical costs, how did it achieve it—was it through decreased prices paid to providers, lower use of medical services, a change in the introduction of new technology, or was it because managed care was able to select healthier enrollees and therefore efficiency was not increased even though costs were reduced? Further, does managed care result in a one-time saving or does it lower the medical expenditure growth rate? Lastly, has price competition adversely affected quality? Did managed care reduce costs by lowering patient satisfaction and patient health outcomes?

Reduction in the Rate of Increase in Medical Expenditures

Although the growth in HMOs and managed care started in the 1980s, it did not spread throughout the United States immediately. Managed care's penetration rate was much greater in certain sections of the country than in others. California was the home to several new HMOs, and the growth in managed care was more rapid than most other states. The effect of these health plan changes is shown in Figure 8-2, which shows the annual percentage change in employer-paid health insurance premiums nationally and in California, along with the annual percentage change in the Consumer Price Index (CPI). Managed care began having a noticeable effect on slowing the ‚rise in insurance premiums by 1993, with continuing reductions for the next 5 years. Premiums increased less rapidly than the CPI. Thus on a national level, inflation-adjusted premiums decreased during 1995 to 1997.

In California where the managed care effect was greatest, annual premium increases were much lower than the national average. For four years, 1994 to 1997, the annual rate of increase was actually *negative*; premiums declined in absolute terms. Further, from

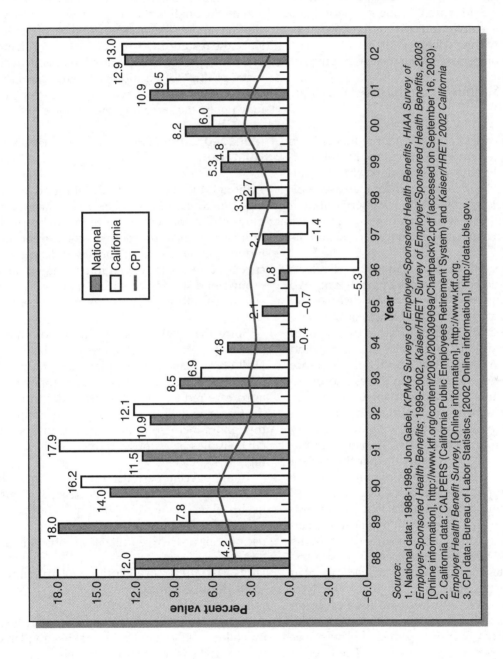

Source:
1. National data: 1988-1998, Jon Gabel, *KPMG Surveys of Employer-Sponsored Health Benefits*, HIAA Survey of *Employer-Sponsored Health Benefits*; 1999-2002, Kaiser/HRET Survey of *Employer-Sponsored Health Benefits, 2003* [Online information], http://www.kff.org/content/2003/20030909a/Chartpackv2.pdf (accessed on September 16, 2003).
2. California data: CALPERS (California Public Employees Retirement System) and Kaiser/HRET *2002 California Employer Health Benefit Survey*, [Online information], http://www.kff.org.
3. CPI data: Bureau of Labor Statistics, [2002 Online information], http://data.bls.gov.

Figure 8-2.   Annual percentage increase in health insurance premiums for the U.S., California, and the CPI, 1988–2002.

1993 to 2001, premiums increased more slowly in California than in the rest of the nation.

The consequence of lower premium increases meant that employee wages increased during this period as a greater portion of employee compensation went toward increased wages. (Chapter 19 discusses who bears the burden of increased insurance premiums.)

Managed Care Savings Through Lower Provider Prices

One of managed care's approaches for reducing costs is to pay discounted prices to providers. By contracting with a limited number of providers who are willing to discount their prices in return for increased volume, insurers seek to provide the same service but at a lower premium. One study determined the source of the savings achieved by managed care and its magnitude (12).

The authors examined how managed care affects treatments and the cost of illness by analyzing two forms of heart disease, ischemic heart disease and heart attacks. They examined differences in spending on care for patients with heart disease in two types of health plans, traditional indemnity insurance and managed care. Further, to decompose this difference in spending between differences in prices and quantity/quality of care, it was important to adjust for quality differences between health plans since the managed care plan might contract with lower-quality physicians to reduce its costs. Two measures of adverse outcomes were examined, whether the patient died and whether the patient was readmitted to the hospital with complications from the heart attack.

The authors found no evidence that health outcomes were worse for patients with managed care insurance. Further, in both types of insurance plans, the treatments for the two diseases studied were similar.

It was also determined that the managed care plan was able to achieve substantial savings which resulted from differences in prices paid for a common set of procedures rather than from differences in the quantity or quality of services provided. The prices paid differed by as much as 40 percent. The rates of procedure use and adverse outcomes were relatively similar in the two plans.

The authors conclude that these results are good news since ". . . (they) . . . suggest that medical care costs can be substantially reduced with little or no effect on the quality of care . . ." However, they express caution about the generalizability of these results since the results are based on just one indemnity and one managed care plan located in Massachusetts, and that "profits" of cardiologists and cardiac surgery units in the hospital have been profit centers, which may not be the same for other disease treatments.

Managed Care Savings Through Reduced Utilization

Although the above study did not find any cost savings due to use of fewer services, managed care employs utilization review for reducing hospital utilization and surgical procedures, concurrent review for reducing inpatient length of stay, gatekeepers to limit specialist referrals, capitation payment to medical groups, and shifting care from more expensive to less expensive settings, such as greater use of outpatient surgery.

Since the 1980s, a large number of studies have been conducted on differences in utilization between HMO-type managed care plans and traditional plans (13). Although study results vary, it appears that managed care reduced hospital utilization through both decreases in length of stay and in admissions (although an increase in outpatient utilization may occur). Studies have found reductions in utilization as high as 40 percent.

In more recent periods, differences in use between types of health plans has decreased as almost all health plans have adopted similar utilization management techniques, and HMOs have relaxed their use of their restrictive utilization control measures.

Does Managed Care Produce a One-Time or Continuous Savings?

Although studies have shown that managed care is much less costly than traditional health plans, an important issue is whether these savings are a one-time savings or does managed care also have a lower rate of increase in its costs.

Managed care's cost containment approaches, which include negotiating discounted prices from providers and decreased inpatient utilization, should be considered a one-time cost saving since it is unlikely that such large cost reductions could continue indefinitely. Lengths of stay are monitored but can only be reduced so far. Hospital use can be further reduced through greater use of substitutes, such as outpatient surgery, but again further decreases in hospital use are limited.

To the extent that managed care has a slower rate of diffusion of new technology, which is an important determinant of medical expenditure growth rates, then managed care would be able to achieve continual cost savings compared to traditional health plans.

The Adoption of New Technology By Managed Care: Traditional health insurance plans had limited, if any, incentive not to introduce new technology even though its benefits relative to existing technology were minor. Patients with little or no cost sharing, FFS physicians, hospitals attempting to maximize the prestige of their institution, and hospitals competing for specialists all had an incentive to adopt and use the latest technology. In many hospitals, the volume of surgical procedures based on the latest technology was so low as to result in higher mortality rates.

Unless managed care evaluated and subsequently adopted new technology based on its relative effectiveness in treatment, managed care would be unable to significantly reduce medical costs over time.

Cutler and Sheiner estimated whether a high managed care penetration rate results in a slower diffusion of technology (14). The authors studied five groups of technology (with specific technologies within each group): cardiac technologies, radiation therapy, diagnostic radiology, transplantation services, and other (extracorporeal shock wave lithotripter). They found that high HMO penetration was associated with a slower diffusion of new technologies in the two time periods studied, 1990 and 1995. Further, this effect, less rapid diffusion of new technologies, increased over time. States with high managed care enrollment were technology leaders in the early 1980s; however, by the 1990s these same states were among the average in adoption of new technologies.

The Competitive "Spillover" Effect of Managed Care

Important for public policy was the issue whether HMOs and managed care competition were reducing the rate of growth in indemnity health insurance premiums. In debates over health care reform in the early years of the Clinton Administration, the Congressional Budget Office (CBO) was responsible for costing out the various reform proposals. CBO's cost estimates were crucial to the acceptability of various health reform proposals. As part of its analysis, CBO assumed that HMOs would not affect the future rate of growth in health care costs. This was the conventional wisdom at the time.

More recent evidence, however, determined that increased HMO competition, measured by HMO penetration in a market, reduces the rise in health insurance premiums among non-HMO plans (the "spillover" effect). HMO and non-HMO insurers are substitutes for each other. As employees are given a price incentive to choose lower cost plans, higher-cost indemnity plans lost market share. To reduce the rise in their premiums and recover their market share, indemnity plans adopted managed care methods. Utilization management by indemnity plans was a response to the HMOs' lower hospital use rates. Negotiating large provider discounts by establishing Preferred Provider Organizations (PPO) was also their response to HMOs' closed provider panels.

Several studies found that indemnity-insured groups located in markets with higher HMO penetration had lower rates of growth in their insurance premiums. Using data for the period 1985 through 1992, Wickizer and Feldstein found that employee groups located in areas with low HMO market penetration had annual premium increases of 8 percent per year (inflation adjusted) compared to 4 percent per year among employee groups with indemnity insurance located in areas with high HMO penetration (15). In another study, Cutler and Sheiner estimated that a ten percent increase in HMO enrollment reduced the total cost growth in that market by four percent (16).

Unless the competitive effect of HMOs on moderating the growth rate of traditional plan premiums is taken into account, simply comparing managed care's premiums to premiums in the traditional plan understates managed care's impact on total health expenditures.

Did Managed Care Achieve Its Savings Through Risk Selection?

An important concern with studies that find HMOs and managed care insurers have lower costs and a lower growth in spending than traditional indemnity plans is that HMOs attract a healthier risk group, younger enrollees, and fewer chronically ill patients. If subscribers with low utilization patterns selected an HMO, differences in utilization rates between HMOs and traditional health plans could not be considered the result of the HMO, nor would it be possible to extrapolate the potential savings if a much larger segment of the population enrolled in HMOs. HMO performance may be more the result of risk selection than a different practice style.

A large number of studies have documented the favorable risk selection by HMOs, providing managed care insurers with as much as a 20 to 30 percent lower utilization rate than non-managed care plans (17). For example, one recent study found that people who switched into an HMO plan from a non-HMO plan used 11 percent fewer medical services in the period prior to switching compared to those that did not switch, and that this lower use continued while they were in the HMO. Those who switched from the HMO to a non-HMO plan used 18 percent more medical services in the period before switching than those who remained in the HMO (18).

Preferred risk selection has also occurred among Medicare HMOs (19). Medicare HMO enrollees had better functional status and were less likely to report their health status as fair or poor compared to Medicare FFS enrollees. Further, Medicare enrollees entering an HMO had costs 37 percent below average, while those leaving the HMO had costs 60 percent above average. Persons who are ill or who have chronic conditions are generally reluctant to leave their physician and switch to an HMO. Under such circumstances, the HMO will enroll those aged who are healthier and have lower expenditures. The government pays for the high-cost aged in the FFS sys-

tem, while HMOs enrolled, at 95 percent of the average cost, those aged with lower average costs. It has been estimated that the government overpays the HMO by 6 percent on average. Research continues to be conducted on developing a better risk adjustment measure.

The most well-known study to determine whether the performance of HMOs was due to biased selection or to the HMO's style of practice was a controlled experiment by RAND Corp. (20). Also included in the study was the amount of out-of-plan use by enrollees in the HMO since favorable HMO performance could be a result of high out-of-plan use. Individuals were assigned to one of three groups: two fee-for-service (FFS) groups, in one all services were free whereas in the other co-payments were required, and a third group was assigned to the HMO (referred to as the HMO experimental group). The study also examined a group that already belonged to the HMO, referred to as the HMO control group. Expenditures were imputed for use of services in the HMO so that comparisons could be made to those in FFS.

Imputed expenditures between those in the HMO experimental and control groups were very similar, although the experimental group had a slightly higher out-of-plan expenditure. Both HMO groups, however, had much lower expenditures (including out-of-plan) than those of the free FFS group (23 to 28 percent less). The size of the expenditures in the HMO groups were comparable to those in one of the FFS plans, which had a 95 percent co-payment up to a family maximum of $1,000 a year. Although expenditures for these groups were comparable, those assigned to the FFS 95 percent co-payment group had fewer face-to-face visits than did the two HMO groups.

The large differences between the HMO enrollees and the free FFS group occurred in their hospital use rates, which were approximately 40 percent lower for the HMO group. The authors attributed this lower use rate to the "style of practice" at the HMO, which is less hospital intensive.

An important determinant of lower hospitalization rates in HMOs is the method by which physicians are compensated. Based on a review of studies that examined physicians' financial incentives and patient utilization, Hellinger states: "Some of the studies . . . compared the utilization on enrollees with the same disease across health plans, some studies compared the utilization of patients in HMOs and in the fee-for-service sector treated by the same physician, and one study investigated utilization in HMOs that reimbursed physicians on a fee-for-service basis to utilization in HMOs that reimbursed physicians on a per capita basis . . . in virtually every study, measures of utilization adjusted for available information on differences in type of enrollee, physician, and health plan were lower when physicians faced incentives to control their use of resources" (21).

When interpreting the results of studies on HMO cost savings, it is important to determine whether enrollees into the HMO and the traditional plan were based on random assignment to control for favorable selection in the HMO. Based on a number of studies that have corrected for selection bias, it appears that total managed care costs were about 10 to 15 percent lower than costs in traditional health plans.

Risk selection is a problem for competitive markets. When the employer or the government pays premiums unrelated the risk of the enrollee, health plans have an incentive to compete for lower risk groups. Biased selection can result in employers and government spending more money when enrollees have a choice of health plans than if everyone enrolled in a single plan.

Paying health plans risk-adjusted premiums limits biased selection. Further, risk-adjusted premiums provide health plans with an incentive to seek out high-risk individuals since the plan could profit by innovating in the management of their care.

Hypothesized Effect of Competition on Quality

There is concern that market competition will reduce quality, particularly when for-profit firms compete. Many believe that for-profit organizations will sacrifice quality for-profit. When non-profit providers do not perform well, it is said that they at least meant well. However, non-profit status by itself does not ensure high quality. It was found that tissue committees in non-profit hospitals did not perform as they should have; county nursing homes are not necessarily noted

for their high quality of care; state mental institutions and Veterans Administration hospitals are not centers of excellence. Outside the health field, non-profit status does not necessarily lead to higher quality, nor is their sensitivity to the public interest greater than that of for-profit competitors. All public schools are not necessarily of higher quality than private schools; municipal governments are often greater polluters than for-profit firms; and when non-profit unions manage their own pension funds, they do not often receive as high a rate of return as received by for-profit funds.

It would be unfortunate if legislation restricted for-profit health plans. For-profit plans responded quickly to demands of the market for HMOs and managed care. They have been innovative and have forced the large non-profit (Blue Cross-Blue Shield) health plans to respond to preserve their market share. Non-profit status, per se, does not guarantee ethical behavior, patient satisfaction, high quality outcomes, or efficiency.

Rather than attempting to regulate for-profit plans or restrict innovations in medical practice, greater emphasis should be placed on health plan and provider outcome measures and accountability.

Non-profit status alone should not relieve us of a concern for quality. Quality should be monitored directly. Consequently, it should not matter that for-profit providers compete. These quality review mechanisms should then apply equally to all providers. (For a debate on whether health providers should be expected to be different from "purveyors of other goods and services," the reader is referred an exchange of letters on this subject between Relman and Reinhardt) (22).

It might be argued that under capitation and competitively determined prices, for-profit HMOs, insurers, and providers might be tempted to provide minimal medical services so as to retain as much of the fee as possible. Although such a situation is possible, several safeguards exist to minimize its occurrence.

Business coalitions, such as the Pacific Business Group on Health (PBGH) and employers require health plans and their providers to collect data by which the health plans can be evaluated on the quality of their care and outcomes. The greater selectivity of better informed groups benefit less-informed subscribers. (All automobile purchasers are not equally knowledgeable, yet automobile companies compete on the basis of quality (e.g., increased warranty periods) as well as on price and styling, because part of their market is knowledgeable and willing to shift their purchases. The same occurs in the markets for other durable goods.) If several large employers no longer offered a particular insurer to their employees because of quality concerns, the insurer would have to change its benefits, accessibility, quality, or premiums if it is not to lose market share. Competition among health plans for the better-informed, large purchasers, those who are more likely to switch plans if quality deteriorates, helps those who are less well informed.[4]

The expected long life of large organizations leads them to behave differently than small firms or those in business for a short time. Whereas an individual entrepreneur may go into business, mislead consumers, produce a poor product, and then quickly move on to another area, it is more "costly" for a large corporation to undertake those business practices that will maximize its present income at the expense of future business. Reputation is an asset, and providing little or no service adversely affects the reputation of the organization and decreases its future business. Poor business practices are more likely to be expected of smaller organizations, for which the costs of entering and leaving a market are lower. This is as true in the medical field as it is for corporations in general. The market disciplines poor quality suppliers.

---

4. When it is costly for purchasers to gather information, suppliers are likely to respond by developing brand-name recognition for their products. The consumer purchases two things when they buy a brand-name product, the product itself and information on the company's reputation as to the quality of the product. Consumers with little information are willing to pay a higher price for a product that contains both of these components than a lower price for just the product itself. In the health field, it is likely that health plans, physician groups, and multi-hospital systems will develop brand-name advertising for their products. (The purchase of university teaching hospitals by investor-owned hospital chains was intended to have the chain's reputation enhanced by the quality reputation of the university hospital.)

Just as the permanence of an organization leads to efforts to maintain or increase quality, so does the size of an organization. In a for-profit organization or in large medical groups, the quality of care practiced by any one physician in the group affects the reputation, hence the incomes, of the other physicians. This spillover effect results in greater use of monitoring mechanisms of participating physicians. Under the previous traditional fee-for-service delivery system, physicians did not have any financial incentives to monitor one another or to impose sanctions against those physicians whose performance, when examined by utilization review and tissue committees, were revealed to be unacceptable. Quality of care is expected to be higher when physicians practice as part of a group than when they remain financially unaffected by the actions of an incompetent or unethical colleague.

Empirical Evidence on Quality of Care

A great many studies have been conducted on the effect that HMOs and competitive markets have had on quality of care. Several studies examined quality of care provided for patients in different disease categories, such as cancer and heart disease. Other studies compared HMO and non-HMO plans on mortality and morbidity outcomes, while others examined quality-of-care process measures. The results of these studies have varied, some finding that HMOs have had more favorable effects while others finding unfavorable effects. Miller and Luft have reviewed the quality literature over different time periods in three articles and conclude that quality-of-care findings are generally similar for both HMO and non-HMO plans (23).

HMOs have a less favorable performance with frail elderly patients and those who are chronically ill.

Generally, patients in HMOs are less satisfied than non-HMO patients, although HMO enrollees are more satisfied with their lower premiums and out-of-pocket costs. Access to care measures, such as difficulty in receiving an appointment, are also lower in HMO plans.

HMOs consistently perform better than non-HMO plans on providing preventive care, such as cancer screening.

Given the wide variation in study findings on each of the above measures, the variety of health plans, differing organizational structures, and geographic location, along with different provider incentive systems, the performance of each health plan needs to be continuously monitored.

Report Cards and Quality Information

An important imperfection in medical markets has been the lack of information on access, patient satisfaction, and on quality of care. Until such information becomes available and it is used together with premiums in choosing health plans, the public will be unable to make informed choices, and providers who deliver higher quality of care will be at a competitive disadvantage.

Most of the privately insured (more than 85 percent) receive their health benefits from their employer. In competitive labor markets, employers would be expected to act as their employee's agent when purchasing health insurance. Unless employers reflected their employee's preferences with regard to the premiums charged, the benefit package, and the quality of the health plan, employers would have to compensate their employees with higher wages. Thus it is in the employer's interest to be an efficient agent on behalf of their employees.

When employers offer their employees a choice of health plans, studies generally indicate that for some (but not all) employees there is a relationship between an employee's choice of health plan and its quality ranking (24).

That many employees do not use quality information in choosing their plan may not be significant as long as the employer uses quality information in deciding which health plans to offer to their employees. Further, many employers only offer their employees a single health plan. Thus, for employers to be efficient agents when employees have no choice of plan, the employer would be expected to use quality information in deciding which plan to select for all of their employees.

Employers have taken the lead in requiring health plans and their participating hospitals and medical groups to provide performance data. Report cards are based on standardized data and are collected by independent organizations. The two most commonly accepted measures of health plan and provider performance are based on data from the Health Plan Employer Data Information Set (HEDIS) and the Consumer Assessment of Health Plan Survey (CAHPS). HEDIS measures, such as preventive measures and physician certifications, are gathered from administrative records of health plans and their participating providers. CAHPS data, which measures enrollee satisfaction with participating providers, is based on surveys of health plan enrollees.

A recent study that examined the health plan choices of large employers and whether they used HEDIS and CAHPS measures of health plan performance in deciding which health plans to offer to their employees found that the large employers disproportionately chose high-quality plans (25). Large employers appear to have been acting as their employees' agent in using quality criteria as well as premiums and other measures in deciding which health plans to offer to their employees.

Although the study only examined the health plan choices of large employers, in a separate analysis the authors also found that health plans that had better quality rankings also had higher market shares.

Large employer groups are also beginning to provide direct financial incentives for improved quality and patient satisfaction. The Leapfrog Group consists of 140 members representing 33 million lives and $70 billion in annual health care expenditures. Their agenda is to publicize data measuring quality, safety, and efficiency. They believe that by providing information on performance, the public will use its purchasing power to create incentives for improvement and will lead to "leaps" in quality and efficiency.

Six California health plans have launched a new initiative to reward physician groups that improve quality of care and service to its members. The plans will pay a total of $150 million annually to medical groups that excel on a number of standardized measures, and they will publish a statewide scorecard starting in 2004 comparing all participating medical groups.

Just as not all purchasers in a market have to be price sensitive for a demand curve to have a downward slope and not all purchasers have to be knowledgeable about the quality of TV sets and computers for ill-informed consumers to also benefit, not all purchasers of health plans need be knowledgeable of plan quality for health plans to compete on quality measures. As long as health plans and their participating hospitals and physicians provide the same standard of care to all of their patients, a few large purchasers (generally large employers) will raise the level of health plan (and provider) quality for all health plan purchasers.

The development of report cards should improve consumers' ability to choose among insurers and providers on the basis of quality, outcomes, access, and price.

Continuing Inefficiencies in the Medical Marketplace

Although managed care has improved the medical industry's performance, much inefficiency remains. The most obvious evidence of such inefficiency is the wide variation in procedures performed, with as much as one-sixth to one-third being considered inappropriate. Inappropriate variation in procedures, however, does not occur just in the U.S.; it occurs in other countries as well, such as the United Kingdom.

Newhouse suggests five reasons why the medical industry does not have better performance (26). Consumers are unable to determine whether bad outcomes of medical treatment are due to poor quality or to their disease. Published data on variations in cardiac surgery mortality by hospitals and surgeons have not deterred patients from still using poorly performing providers.

Second, the development of new technologies, including drugs, has been very rapid, and the diffusion of this information to providers is not uniform. New knowledge makes existing surgical techniques and training obsolete. There is a long time lag before new treatment methods are fully adopted by most physicians.

Third, there is widespread use in medical care of administered, fixed prices, such as those paid by Medicare. The profitability of performing a service is related to the difference between its price and its marginal cost. Services are performed more (less) frequently when the difference in price and cost is greatest (least). Legislated prices and the unit to which they apply also affect quality. For example, paying a fixed price per admission will lead to quicker discharges, while paying per day will lead to inappropriately long inpatient stays. Further, paying a fixed price per diagnosis, regardless of severity of illness, will cause providers to shun sicker patients. The same occurs when health plans are paid the same premium regardless of an enrollee's risk level.

Fourth, it has been difficult to develop measures by which the performance of health plans and their participating providers can be evaluated. Until such measures can be developed, superior performance cannot be financially rewarded. Both high- and low-quality physicians are reimbursed similarly.

Lastly, politics and regulation are not directed at enhancing efficiency; many times its effect is the opposite. Although closing certain hospitals may improve both quality and efficiency, their communities may oppose it because of their desire to have a hospital and for the jobs it provides. Regulations also limit entry into markets and define the tasks that health professionals may perform. These regulations are often meant to benefit certain groups rather than have as their objective increased efficiency.

It will be difficult to eliminate all of the reasons for inefficiencies under any type of medical system, whether it is based on competition or government control. However, the greater use of information technology for disseminating information to purchasers and providers, along with developing financial incentives to reward quality, should improve the performance of the medical system.

SUMMARY

Market competition emerged because business and the federal government developed a concentrated interest in holding down the rise in their medical expenditures. As a result of the 1981 recession, severe import competition, and a lowering of marginal tax rates, business pressured insurers to introduce cost-saving innovations in their benefit packages. Low-cost substitutes to traditional providers developed, namely HMOs and outpatient surgery clinics. The federal government changed hospital incentives and created excess hospital capacity when it introduced prospective fixed prices (DRGs).

Excess capacity among physicians and hospitals and the changed incentives in both business and government were important preconditions for market competition. However, it is unlikely that market competition would have occurred had it not been for the applicability and enforcement of the anti-trust laws. The anti-trust laws eliminated anti-competitive barriers to price competition and new types of insurance and delivery systems.

Managed care competition changed the incentives facing the purchaser and suppliers of medical services. Managed care was a response to the problems of market failure and solved the problem of moral hazard on the demand side and demand inducement on the supply side.

The rapid growth of HMOs forced traditional insurers to adopt managed care methods. The development of managed fee-for-service, PPOs, Point of Service plans (POS), and the development of IPAs, was indicative of the market's attempt to match employer and employee preferences by offering them a choice between higher premiums and restricted access to care.

Competitive markets provide for a diversity of preferences among purchasers in the amount they are willing to pay and in types of health plans. Health plan choices, however, can result in biased selection. A concern with competitive health care markets is that health plans will compete on risk selection rather than on how well they can manage medical treatments.

Cost differences among competing health plans may represent enrollment of lower risk groups rather than differences in plan efficiency. Further, biased selection can cause adverse selection among health plans receiving higher risk enrollees, thereby leading to the plan's eventual demise. Risk-adjusted premiums can control biased selection among health plans.

Market competition changed the medical sector. Managed care achieved what it was intended to do, reduce the rise in medical expenditures. It achieved this objective without reducing quality of care. Insurers, physicians, and hospitals are being evaluated, and information is being provided to employees and patients on quality of care, patient satisfaction, and other measures of health plan and provider performance. Insurers and providers are becoming accountable for their performance.

Many impediments to a competitive medical market still exit. Providers are not rewarded financially for superior quality, consumers are unaware of those providers who provide higher quality care, technological advances are not quickly diffused and adopted by providers, administered prices reward providers for performing some services more than others, and regulations restrict entry into markets and the tasks health professionals are permitted to perform.

Although the competitive market can and should be improved, its performance exceeds what occurred previously and what could be achieved through a greater regulatory environment, as typified by the Medicare system. The pre-managed care environment and regulation had a lack of patient and provider incentives, lack of information on quality and outcomes, and rapidly increasing medical expenditures.

Market competition alone cannot solve all of the concerns that many people have with regard to our health care system. Competitive markets improve efficiency and are responsive to consumer demands. It is not the responsibility of competitive markets to provide care for those who cannot afford to pay for care. Redistributing medical services requires government intervention; however, government involvement need not be direct. Government subsidies can be provided through a market mechanism, such as through the use of vouchers used in competing health plans. For a given redistribution subsidy, a market approach to the delivery of services can more efficiently achieve the redistribution objective.

Medical expenditures will continue rising in a competitive market, as they should. Advances in medical technology will continue to increase medical costs as will an aging population. Rising incomes will also increase use and expenditures since medical care is income elastic. Quality is also income elastic. Thus as incomes increase, expenditures on medical care will also increase. Government regulations requiring health plans to include costly benefits and/or mandate how care is provided (either by types of health professionals or in which institutional settings) will also increase health plan costs and premiums.

Thus increased medical expenditures are not an indication that market competition cannot reduce the rise in medical costs. Instead, given the above demographic, economic forces, and regulations, market competition attempts to achieve the "appropriate" rate of increase in medical expenditures.

REVIEW QUESTIONS

1. What are the reasons that the health field changed from a non-price competitive market to a price-competitive industry in the 1980s?
2. If HMOs were such a good idea, why did their growth only start in the mid 1980s and not before?
3. "Free choice" of physician has been interpreted by organized medicine (and dentistry) to mean that a patient's choice of physician should not be restricted to those physicians participating in a particular delivery system. Under what circumstances has this interpretation of "free choice" resulted in anti-competitive behavior by organized medicine?
4. How does managed care solve the problems of moral hazard and demand inducement?
5. What are different cost containment approaches used by managed care firms?
6. Explain the similarities and differences between managed fee-for-service plans, HMOs, POS plans, and PPOs.
7. What are the different incentives to providers of being paid on a capitated basis rather than fee for service?
8. Why are Any Willing Provider Laws considered to be anti-competitive?
9. How can selection bias among health plans affect an employer's total medical premiums?
10. Evaluate the following statement. "A competitive policy for medical care has been a failure be-

cause many of the poor are unable to receive needed care."

REFERENCES

1. See Reuben Kessel, "Price Discrimination in Medicine," *Journal of Law and Economics,* 1, October 1958, 20-53. This article is discussed more completely in the chapter on "The Market for Physician Manpower."
2. For a more complete discussion of the reasons for deregulation in both the medical and non-medical sectors, see Paul J. Feldstein, *The Politics of Health Legislation: An Economic Perspective,* (Chicago, Illinois: Health Administration Press), 2nd ed. revised, 2001, Chapters 5 and 6.
3. "Health Professions Educational Assistance Amendments of 1965," *Hearing Before the Subcommittee on Health of the Committee on Labor and Public Welfare,* U.S. Senate, 89th Congress, 1st Session, September 8, 1965, 39–40.
4. For a complete discussion of CON and its legislative changes, see Clark C. Havighurst, *Deregulating the Health Care Industry: Planning for Competition,* (Cambridge, Mass.: Ballinger, 1982) p. 222.
5. Alain C. Enthoven, *Health Plan,* (Reading, Mass.: Addison-Wesley, 1980).
6. For a more complete discussion of these issues, see: Donald W. Moran, "HMOs, Competition and the Politics of Minimum Benefits," *Milbank Memorial Fund Quarterly,* 59 (2) Spring 1981, 291–296; Alain C. Enthoven, "How Interested Groups Have Responded to a Proposal for Economic Competition in Health Services," *American Economic Review,* 70(2) May 1980, 142-148; and John K. Iglehart, "Drawing the Lines for the Debate on Competition," *New England Journal of Medicine,* 305(5) July 30, 1981, 291–296.
7. *Medicaid Freedom of Choice Waiver Activities,* Hearing Before the Subcommittee on Health of the Committee on Finance, U.S. Senate, 98th Congress, 2nd Session, March 30, 1984.
8. *Company Practices in Health Care Cost Management,* (Lincolnshire, Ill.: Hewitt Associates, 1984).
9. For a review and analysis of health care anti-trust actions in the health field, see Deborah Haas-Wilson, *Managed Care and Monopoly Power,* (Harvard University Press: Cambridge, Mass.) 2003. Also see, *Statements of Anti-Trust Policy in Health Care,* Issued by the U.S. Department of Justice and the Federal Trade Commission, Washington, D.C. August 1996.

10. For an excellent discussion of why managed care evolved and how it has performed, see David Dranove, *The Evolution of American Health Care: From Marcus Welby to Managed Care,* (Princeton: Princeton University Press) 2000.

11. Jon Gabel, "Ten Ways HMOs Have Changed During The 1990s," *Health Affairs,* 16(3), May/June 1997, 134-145.

12. David M. Cutler, Mark McClellan, and Joseph P. Newhouse, "How Does Managed Care Do It?," *RAND Journal of Economics,* 31(3) Autumn 2000, 526–548.

13. Sherry Glied, "Managed Care" in *Handbook of Health Economics,* Vol. 1A, eds. A. J. Culyer and J. P. Newhouse, (New York: North-Holland Press, 2000), 707–753. Also see Robert H. Miller and Hal S. Luft, "HMO Plan Performance Update: An Analysis of the Literature, 1997–2001," *Health Affairs,* 21(4) July/August 2002, 63–86, and Robert H. Miller and Hal S. Luft "Does Managed Care lead to Better or Worse Quality of Care?," *Health Affairs,* 16(5) September/October 1997, 7–25.

14. David M. Cutler and Louise Sheiner, "Managed Care and the Growth of Medical Expenditures," in Alan M. Garber, ed., *Frontiers in Health Policy Research,* Vol. 1, (MIT Press: Cambridge, England) 1998, 77–116.

15. Thomas M. Wickizer and Paul J. Feldstein, "The Impact of HMO Competition on Private Health Insurance Premiums, 1985-1992," *Inquiry,* 32(3) Fall 1995, 241–251.

16. Cutler and Sheiner, op.cit.

17. Sherry Glied, *op. cit.,* Table 2 pp. 729–730 contains a list of selection studies.

18. Sean Nicholson, et al., "The Magnitude and Nature of Risk Selection in Employer-Sponsored Health Plans," Working Paper Series, National Bureau of Economic Research: Cambridge, Mass.) August 2003, Working Paper 9937.

19. Gerald Riley, et al., "Health Status of Medicare enrollees in HMOs and Fee-For-Service in 1994," *Health Care Financing Review,* 17(4) Summer 1996, 65–76, and "Risk Assessment and Risk Adjustment in Medicare," Chapter 15 in *Annual Report to Congress,* (Physician Payment Review Commission: Washington, D.C.), 1996.

20. Willard G. Manning et al., "A Controlled Trial of the Effect of a Prepaid Group Practice on Use of Services," *New England Journal of Medicine,* 310(23), June 7, 1984, 1505–1510.

21. Fred J. Hellinger, "The Impact of Financial Incentives on Physician Behavior in Managed Care Plans: A Review of the Evidence," *Medical Care Research and Review,* 53(3) September 1996, 294–314.

22. Arnold S. Relman and Uwe E. Reinhardt, "Debating For-Profit Health Care," *Health Affairs,* 5(2) Summer 1986, 5-31. This exchange was initiated as a result of the authors' participation in the following report. Institute of Medicine, *For-Profit Enterprise in Health Care* (Washington, D.C.: National Academy Press, 1986).

23. Robert H. Miller and Harold S. Luft, "HMO Plan Performance Update: An Analysis of the Literature, 1997–2001," *Health Affairs,* 21(4)July/August 2002, 63–86, "Does Managed Care Lead to Better or Worse Quality of Care?," *Health Affairs,* 16(5) September/October 1997, 7–25, and "Managed Care Plan Performance Since 1980: A Literature Analysis," *Journal of the American Medical Association,* 271(19), May 18, 1994 1512–1519.

24. Dennis P. Scanlon, et al., "The Impact of Health Plan Report Cards on Managed Care Enrollment," *Journal of Health Economics,* 21(1) January 2002, pp. 19–41, Nancy Beaulieu, "Quality Information and Consumer Health Plan Choices," *Journal of Health Economics,* 21(1) January 2002, pp. 43–63, and Gerald J. Wedig and Ming Tai-Seale, "The Effect of Report Cards on Consumer Choice in the Health Insurance Market," *Journal of Health Economics,* 21(6) November 2002, pp. 1031–1048.

25. Michael Chernew, et al., "Quality and Employers' Choice of Health Plan," NBER Working Paper No. 9847, July 2003, (National Bureau of Economic Research: Cambridge, Mass.).

26. Joseph P. Newhouse, "Why Is There A Quality Chasm?," *Health Affairs,* 21(4) July/August 2002, 13–25.

CHAPTER
9

The Market for Health Insurance:
Its Performance and Structure

KEY TERMS AND CONCEPTS

- Benefit/premium ratio
- Community rating
- Experience rating
- Risk-adjusted premiums
- Underwriting cycle
- Guaranteed issue
- Guaranteed renewal
- Portability
- Pre-existing exclusion

Learning Objectives

Upon completing this chapter, the reader should be able to:

- Describe how the health insurance market evolved over time.
- Understand the reasons why the health insurance market is very price competitive.
- Explain why medical loss ratios are not useful for inferring insurer efficiency or quality.
- Describe the reasons for the underwriting cycle.
- Evaluate the equity and efficiency consequences of mandating community rating.
- Explain how risk selection adversely affects the health insurance market.

INTRODUCTION: ECONOMIC EFFICIENCY

It is important to determine how efficiently each sector of the medical care market performs. If these separate sub-markets do not perform efficiently, then there may be a legitimate role for public intervention to increase the efficiency of the marketplace. Government intervention to increase efficiency is different from, and should be kept separate from, government intervention to redistribute the output of the medical care market. A government policy that attempts to do both simultaneously, either through a government agency or comprehensive regulation, may do neither as well as separate policies directed toward either efficiency or equity.

Economic efficiency with regard to the supply of health insurance typically means that there are no entry barriers; that the number of firms in the market is the "right" number—that is, each firm operates at a minimum point on the long-run average cost curve; that each firm attempts to minimize its cost of production—that is, achieve internal efficiency; and that the firms are price competitive. However, even if the health insurance industry is economically efficient in the supply of health insurance, imperfections may exist in the input market in which insurance companies are demanders (purchasers) of physician and hospital services. Physicians and hospitals are suppliers of these inputs. To the extent imperfections exist in these "input" markets, the price of health insurance will be higher, and there will be less variety in the types of health insurance products sold.

The performance of the health insurance market will be evaluated on how competitive it is and also on whether suppliers of medical services have placed restrictions on an insurer's ability to sell certain types of insurance products. Hypotheses will be offered to explain possible divergence from economic efficiency, since any intervention to improve economic efficiency in this market should be consistent with the reasons for inadequate performance.

BACKGROUND

Blue Cross plans were started, capitalized, and controlled by hospitals as non-profit health insurers. The first Blue Cross plan began in the 1930s, and the benefit package was designed to increase the demand for hospital care. Blue Cross had a service benefit policy, a patient was entitled to 30 days of hospital care (the only benefit Blue Cross provided), and did not have to pay any deductible or co-payment for their stay (1). Regardless of whether the participating hospital had high or low costs, Blue Cross paid their enrollees' hospital bills in full. Thus hospitals did not have to compete on price for patients. Blue Cross reimbursed hospitals according to their charges or their costs.

Blue Cross plans initially offered group insurance in order to avoid adverse selection. They priced their insurance policies using "community rating," whereby all the insured in the same geographic area or "community" (which may be as large as a state) are charged the same basic premium even though a group's claims experience or an individual's risk level differs.

Each Blue Cross plan was required to sign up 75 percent of the hospitals and beds in its area. Blue Cross was thereby precluded from establishing a preferred provider network and forcing hospitals to compete to join Blue Cross' network.[1]

Each Blue Cross plan had a monopoly within its market over its type of service. Blue Cross plans were not permitted to compete with each other as did commercial insurers; each plan served a particular geographic market, and other Blue plans were not allowed to enter another Blue plan's market. If one Blue Cross firm was more efficient and wished to expand its market, it could not do so at the expense of another Blue Cross plan. (The national Blue Cross organization, which owns the Blue Cross trademark and licenses plans to use it, opposed such competitive behavior. However, given the applicability of the antitrust laws to the health field, Blue Cross plans can no longer divide up markets among themselves.) Each plan benefited by being the designated representative

1. Olson claims that "this requirement ensured that no Blue Cross plan could select only the most efficient hospitals in its area. Its effect was to reduce competitive pressures on less efficient hospitals." Mancur Olson, "Introduction" in Mancur Olson, ed., *A New Approach to the Economics of Health Care,* (Washington, D.C.: American Enterprise Institute, 1981), p. 10.

of Blue Cross' reputation and by being the only one to offer the Blue Cross insurance package to subscribers.

Blue Cross is a loose federation of independently operating plans joined together by an interplan system for handling claims incurred in other areas. The national Blue Cross organization provides certain important functions, such as representing all Blue Cross plans in their relations with the federal government and testifying on legislation affecting the health insurance industry.

Blue Shield plans, started by medical societies, provided insurance coverage for physician services and reimbursed participating physicians according to their usual fees (up to a percentile limit), thereby lessening their enrollees' incentive to shop around. Patients whose incomes were below a specified level were insured according to a service benefit; that is, they had their physician fees paid in full by Blue Shield. Patients whose incomes were above the specified limits could be "balanced billed" by physicians for the difference between Blue Shield's physician payment and the physician's customary fee. Over time, as more Blue Shield subscribers' income exceeded the specified income level and were balanced billed, employers threatened to switch insurers if Blue Shield did not eliminate balance billing. To survive, against their medical society's opposition, Blue Shield plans agreed to a service benefit plan for all their subscribers. Blue Shield plans also used community rating for determining its premiums.

Blue Cross and Blue Shield maintained the principle of "free choice" of provider; that is, their enrollees were not given a financial incentive to choose between providers on the basis of price.

The Blue plans were innovators in the health insurance market. These plans demonstrated that by insuring large groups, adverse selection would not bankrupt the health insurer. Given the success of the Blue plans and the growth of private insurance, commercial (for-profit) insurers entered the market in the 1940s. Throughout the 1930s, 1940s, and the early 1950s, the Blue plans were the dominant health insurers. Not until the mid 1950s did commercial insurers grow more rapidly than Blue Cross-Blue Shield (BCBS) and have a greater share of the private insurance market.

Commercial insurers sold indemnity insurance, typically paid the subscriber a certain dollar amount for hospital and physician services, as contrasted to the Blues' service benefits which paid the provider in full for the cost of the service. The commercial insurers also differed from the Blues in that they relied on "experience rating" rather than community rating for pricing their policies. Experience rating relied on the group's prior claims experience (or a new group's risk level) to determine its premium. Thus all groups were charged different premiums based on their own experience. By using experience rating, the commercials were able to attract the lower risk groups from BCBS since the commercials charged lower risk groups lower premiums than did BCBS, which charged those groups an average, or the community rated, premium.

Experience rating increased the market share of the commercial insurers and eventually forced the Blues to abandon community rating; as lower risk groups switched to the commercials, the average risk level of those with the Blues increased, as did the community rated premium.

During the 1980s, the private health insurance market underwent dramatic changes. New types of insurance products were developed, the most notable being Health Maintenance Organizations (HMOs). Commercial insurers and BCBS plans, which previously offered only indemnity and service benefit policies, also offered HMO options to their subscribers. Similarly, independent HMOs offered their group enrollees an indemnity option in addition to an HMO. Another option offered by HMOs was a Point of Service (POS) plan, which allowed an HMO's enrollee to seek care from a non-HMO provider but at a high co-payment, usually 40 percent.

The variety of health insurance products has grown rapidly since the early 1980s, as have the methods of provider reimbursement. In 1980, traditional insurance with unrestricted access to all providers comprised 95 percent of all private insurance. By 1993, only 46 percent of the privately insured were enrolled in traditional insurance, and by 2003 that percentage was down to only 5 percent. Managed care has become the dominant forms of health insurance. See Figure 9-1. Managed care

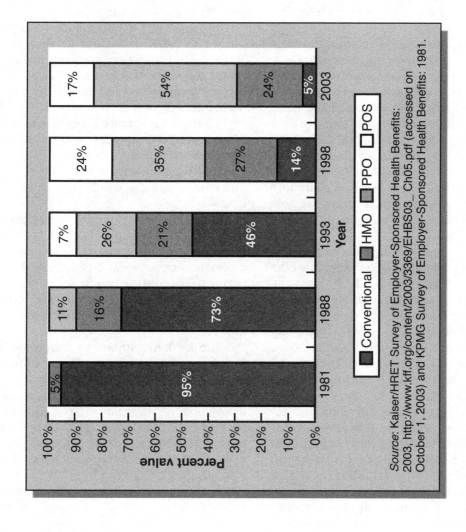

Source: Kaiser/HRET Survey of Employer-Sponsored Health Benefits: 2003, http://www.kff.org/content/2003/3369/EHBS03_Ch05.pdf (accessed on October 1, 2003) and KPMG Survey of Employer-Sponsored Health Benefits: 1981.

Figure 9-1.   Health plan enrollment, selected years, 1981–2003

broadly defined refers to both HMOs and health insurance (both indemnity and service benefit policies) that use utilization management. Appropriate use of medical services, such as prior authorization for a hospital admission or for outpatient surgery, review of the patient's length of hospital stay, case management of catastrophic care, and monitoring physicians' utilization patterns are examples of utilization management.

Health insurers also include a Preferred Provider Organization (PPO) as an option to their enrollees. PPOs are a closed panel of providers who are willing to discount their prices and/or who have lower use rates than other providers. (PPOs are a means of price competition between providers who are part of a PPO and those who are not.) Enrollees who use a PPO provider pay a lower co-payment and much higher co-pay if they use a non-PPO provider. PPO providers hope to receive a greater volume of a firm's employees in return for discounting their prices and/or being more appropriate users of services. PPOs have developed rapidly since the mid 1980s.

A large number of employers have decided to self-insure (whereby they, rather than the insurer, bear the financial risk of their employees' medical expenses). The employer may then contract with an insurer or a Third Party Administrator (TPA) to provide Administrative Services Only (ASO), including claims processing. Smaller companies also consider this option, together with a reinsurance component, to protect themselves against an employee's catastrophic medical expenses. In 1974 (as part of ERISA—The Employment Retirement Income Security Act), Congress exempted self-insured firms from state regulations mandating that insurance include such provisions as hair transplants and in vitro fertilization, as well as the inclusion of certain providers, such as chiropractors and faith healers. By becoming self-insured, these firms are able to reduce their health care costs by excluding state mandates from their coverage.

Thus the health insurance market consists of traditional indemnity-type plans based on fee-for-service payment, service benefit plans (BCBS), HMOs, PPOs, and self-insured companies. Fee-for-service plans are predominately managed care since they include utilization review mechanisms. In addition to their own plans, commercial insurers and BCBS also market HMOs, PPOs, and Administrative Service Only (ASO) contracts to employers who are self insured. There are also independent Third Party Administrators (TPAs), HMOs, and PPOs who market their services directly to employers.

The "product," health insurance, differs both according to "real" characteristics such as type of coverage, patient cost-sharing arrangements, methods of claims payment, the provider panel, as well as according to perceived differences in product, such as reputation for payment of claims. Premium differences between insurance firms would be expected to differ in accordance with these product differences. If the price of insurance between firms differs by a greater amount than what is justified by product differences, groups would be expected to switch insurers.

Thus insurance companies compete on the basis of price as well as in terms of product differences. If insured groups are able to switch insurers according to differences in prices and products, the market will perform in an efficient manner. The "product" will be expected to change over time and also to conform more closely to the preferences of the insured group.[2]

Since 1980, in addition to changes in the types of insurance products being offered, there have also been important organizational changes among the Blue plans. As a result of mergers and acquisitions, the number of Blue plans decreased from 114 in 1980 to 77 in 1990 and to 42 by 2003. In 1987, Congress removed the Blue's federal tax exemption believing that they performed no differently than the commercial insurers. Further, in 1994, the Blue Cross Association permitted its member plans to become for-profit.

---

2. Since there are such large differences in the costs of handling a group and an individual, most individuals in a group would prefer to forego the benefits of individually tailored policies to take advantage of the lower cost of a single group policy.

THE STRUCTURE OF THE HEALTH INSURANCE MARKET

Important in determining the number of competing firms, firm behavior, and the performance of the industry is the industry's market structure. Economies of scale, entry barriers, and whether any firms have cost advantages over other firms determine the market structure of the health insurance market.[3]

Economies of Scale:

Economies of scale, given the size of the market for health insurance, determine how many firms can compete in the sale of insurance. The extent of economies of scale also indicates whether the insurance business is a "natural" monopoly; that is, can the functions performed by insurance companies be performed less expensively by just one firm? (Another aspect of efficiency in production concerns whether each firm is operating in the most efficient manner.)

It has been difficult to separately estimate the extent of economies of scale in supplying health insurance from differences in the firm's (internal) efficiency and the functions it performs. Many companies differ in their administrative functions and they do not perform them equally well. The range of administrative functions, includes marketing and selling policies, processing applications and policies, maintaining the policy file, processing claims, reviewing claims, and paying claims. The variety of contracts offered, each entailing a different cost, and the extent to which the company has group or individual policies (it is more costly to handle individual policies) also differs among firms.

Several studies have attempted to empirically estimate the extent of economies of scale among different health insurers. Using data from the early 1970s, Vogel and Blair examined economies of scale for commercial health insurance companies only since their output mix (e.g., variety of contracts, percentage of

non-group policies, etc.) was very different from that of Blue Cross. The authors determined that economies of scale do exist, and that the administrative cost ratio declines with increased size of operation. When economies of scale were investigated separately for Blue Cross and for Blue Shield (in their non-Medicare business), no economies of scale were found. The authors then included in their analysis BCBS plans that had merged. They observed lower administrative costs for these merged, larger firms. Based on these studies, the authors concluded that economies of scale do exist in the non-profit sector, although the gains from such economies are offset by internal inefficiency ("x-inefficiency") because they were nonprofit firms (2).

In a follow-up study, Blair and Vogel undertook a "survivor" analysis to test for economies of scale (3). In this type of analysis, firms are assigned to different categories according to their size. The growth of firms in each size category is studied over time. If substantial economies of scale exist, then firms in the largest size classes will grow rapidly at the expense of firms in the smaller size categories. Smaller firms will either have to expand their scale of operation (and/or merge), or they will be forced to leave the industry. The authors found that all but the smallest size categories expanded over the period 1958 to 1973. They concluded that economies of scale existed but that they were not as large as originally believed since other size categories also grew.

The authors also attempted to determine whether economies of scale exist in the administration of Medicare Part A (hospital claims payment). They found results opposite of what they expected. Administrative costs per claim increased with the size of the firm. The interpretation of this finding was that the cost-based method used by Medicare to pay intermediaries encouraged higher administrative costs (4). An experiment in which the government awarded Medicare Part B contracts on the basis of a competitive bid found that submitted bids were quite low relative to their historical cost and lower than carriers reimbursed on a cost basis (5). The authors concluded that sizable government savings were possible if Medicare intermediaries were selected and paid

---

3. As will be discussed later, state regulations may affect competition in the individual insurance market.

according to a competitive bid rather than the cost-based payment system.

Also suggestive of economies of scale are the mergers of Blue Cross-Blue Shield plans over the past decade. Smaller Blue plans have found that the size of their market area limits their growth, and they are reluctant to enter and compete in other Blue plan's markets. In addition to the usual reasons for expecting economies of scale, such as lower marketing, claims processing, and administrative costs, larger insurers with subscribers in many different geographic areas are able to undertake analyses of different practice patterns and determine, for given illnesses, which practice patterns result in both lower costs of treatment and improved outcomes. These findings can then be disseminated to participating providers in other geographic areas.

Even though economies of scale exist in the insurance industry and financial requirements exist for becoming an insurer (such as minimum reserve requirements), a firm selling health insurance in one city can easily market its product in another city while centralizing all of its administrative functions. Entry by insurers into profitable markets is relatively low cost. Thus either a sufficient number of insurers exist within a market or can potentially enter that market for the health insurance industry to be competitive. There are more than 1,000 for-profit health insurers and 42 Blue Cross and Blue Shield plans.

Blue Cross-Blue Shield Cost Advantages

Differences in costs between firms, unrelated to their efficiency, have given some types of insurers a competitive advantage over other firms, thereby affecting the industry's structure. Blue Cross and Blue Shield plans received two important cost advantages over commercial insurers that enabled them to increase their market share at the expense of their competitors.

Favorable Tax Treatment: Until 1987, Blue Cross plans were exempt from both federal and state premium taxes because they were believed to behave differently than their for-profit competitors. Commercial insurers, on average, pay a 2 percent state tax on their total premiums. However, since administrative expenses are typically 10 percent of premiums, 2 percent of total premiums is equal to 20 percent of administrative expenses. Thus the Blues' tax exemption was a significant portion of administrative expenses. Studies found that the competitive advantage of the Blues' exemption from state premium taxes enabled Blue Cross to increase its market share between 1 and 6.7 percent (6).

In return for such favorable tax treatment, however, the Blues were subject to greater regulation by state insurance commissioners who approved their premium increases. Several states limited premium increases that the Blues wanted to charge their non-group (individual) enrollees, which the Blues claim caused them to lose money on this line of business. To escape such regulation, a number of Blue Cross plans converted to mutual insurance companies.

The Blues lost their federal (but not state) tax-exempt status under the 1986 tax reform legislation. A Government Accounting Office (GAO) report found that the pricing practices of the Blues were similar to those of the commercials, namely experience rating of large groups; there were few subsidies for high-risk individuals enrolling in the Blues; that the Blues had profit-making subsidiaries; and that "all these activities tend to reinforce the perception that the plans are similar to commercial companies" (7).

The Blue Cross Hospital Discount: The second, and perhaps more important, competitive advantage that Blue Cross had over commercial insurers is the price discount that Blue Cross received from hospitals that was unavailable to other insurers. The size of the hospital discount to Blue Cross was as high as 27 percent in some states. According to one study, the Blues' discount resulted in an average increase in their market share of 7 percent (8).

The competitive consequences of Blue Cross' cost advantages were as follows. A firm in a competitive market with a cost advantage could undercut the prices of other firms and drive them from the market. If this were to occur, the public would benefit from that cost reduction in terms of lower prices. However, researchers found that BCBS plans with a cost advantage were able to increase their market shares, but not to the extent thought possible. The researchers developed several hypotheses as to how Blue Cross plans used their competitive advantage.

Because the Blues were controlled by the hospitals, it was in the hospitals' interest to provide the Blues with a competitive cost advantage, namely, a discount. In this way, the price of Blue Cross coverage was lowered relative to commercial insurance. Hospitals benefited by assisting the expansion of a more expensive type of insurance (only hospital care). Hospitals were consequently able to increase their volume and charges faster than they would have otherwise.

Weller distinguishes between discounts that are pro-competitive (i.e., a firm is a tough bargainer and tries to reach the lowest price possible from its suppliers) and discounts that are anti-competitive (i.e., a supplier gives a favored purchaser a preferential price). Based on the findings that Blue Cross plans were started and controlled by hospitals and that those Blue Cross plans with relatively high market shares were also in areas where hospital costs were relatively high, Weller concluded that the hospital discount could be explained more adequately in terms of anti-competitive behavior on the part of hospitals (9).

Another study concluded that in addition to benefiting hospitals, the Blue plans were less efficient. Thus their cost advantage was also used to benefit their management and employees in terms of higher salaries and internal "slack" within the organization (10).

These cost advantages have provided the Blues with greater market shares than they might otherwise have had, their hospitals with more advantageous benefits, as well as benefiting Blue Cross management. Had it not been for their relatively greater administrative inefficiency and their more costly hospital-only benefit package, the commercial insurers would have suffered even greater lost market shares.

Blue Cross plans are no longer controlled by hospitals. As Blue Cross competes with other insurers, hospitals and Blue Cross have developed an adversarial relationship. However, even though the cost advantages (preferential tax exemptions and hospital discounts) that contributed to such a large market share were removed, the large market share of the Blues still provided those Blue plans with increased market power, hence a competitive advantage (11). A Blue Cross plan that is the dominant insurer in an area is able to extract a discount from hospitals because of its purchasing power than is an insurer with a small market share. The hospital must continue to give a discount to a dominant insurer if it is not to suffer large losses of patients to competitive hospitals.

One study found that the Blues used their large market share (monopsony power) to extract greater price concessions from hospitals and that in the price competitive health insurance market, these reduced input costs were passed on to employer groups as reduced premiums (12).

Current competitive pressures in the insurance market, the consolidation and mergers of BCBS plans, and the need for capital has resulted in a number of Blue plans converting to for-profit status, such as WellPoint and Trigon (13). Several very large for-profit Blue plans have become formidable competitors in the health insurance market and, seeking additional acquisitions, are attempting to become amongst the largest insurers in the industry. The profitability of these plans and their growth strategy suggest that there are large economies of scale in health insurance.

Changes in a Health Insurer's Market Shares

Although there appear to be large economies of scale in the production of health insurance, given the size of the insurance market, a sufficient number of insurers exist to make the health insurance market quite competitive.

Table 9-1 shows the population covered and relative market shares both over time and by type of carrier. While the overall market share of commercial insurers is greater than Blue Cross and Blue Shield, in any one market there are usually several commercial insurers, but generally only one Blue Cross-Blue Shield Plan. Thus, particularly in the northeast and midwest, the Blue Plans have a much larger market share than any one commercial insurer; in a number of states their market share exceeds those of all the commercial insurers. (It was not possible to separate out duplicate coverage between commercials, BCBS, and independent plans. An employer that self-insures, for example, may use an insurance company to administer their claims processing (ASO contract); this would show up as an increase in independent plans as well as part of an insurer's market share.)

As shown in Table 9-1, there have been dramatic changes in market shares by type of insurance company, particularly starting in the mid 1980s. Independent plans, which include HMOs, company self-insurance plans, and administrative service contracts only, have increased their share of the market from 5 percent in 1970 to 30 percent in 1985 to 69 per-

cent in 1996; this increased growth came at the expense of traditional indemnity plans and Blue Cross, which have lost market share. The decline in market shares of BCBS plans has been dramatic.

INDUSTRY CONDUCT AND COMPETITIVE BEHAVIOR

The Components of the Health Insurance Premium

To understand how health insurers price their products, it is useful to examine the components of the health insurance premium, shown in Figure 9-2. The loading charge, which includes administrative and claims processing costs, marketing expense, reserves against losses, and profits, represents approximately 8 percent of the premium when insurance is sold to groups. The loading charge is much higher in the in-

Table 9-1. Enrollment of Persons with Hospital Expense Protection, 1950–1996

Year	Civilian Population (Thousands)	Net Number of Persons Insured		Gross Number of Persons Insured		
		Total Number (Thousands)(a)	Percent of Population	Commercial Insurance Percent of Total(a)	Blue Cross-Blue Shield Percent of Total	Independent Plans Percent of Total(b)
1950	150,790	76,600	50.8	48.3	50.7	5.7
1955	162,967	101,400	62.2	52.8	50.0	6.4
1960	178,140	122,500	68.8	56.5	47.4	4.9
1965	191,605	138,700	72.4	55.9	45.6	5.0
1970	201,895	158,800	78.7	56.5	47.3	5.1
1975	213,789	178,200	83.4	55.8	48.5	7.4
1980	225,621	187,400	83.1	56.3	46.3	17.7
1985	236,219	181,300	76.8	55.4	43.4	30.4(c)
1990	247,763	181,700	73.3	45.7	39.0	47.4(c)
1996	263,943	187,500	71.0	40.2	36.1	68.7(c,d)

Sources: Source Book of Health Insurance Data—1999–2000, (Washington, D.C.: Health Insurance Association of America, 2000), p. 39, Table 2.10; U.S. Bureau of the Census, Statistical Abstract of the United States, 2001, 121st edition, (Washington, D.C.: U.S. Department of Commerce, 2001), p. 8, Table 2.

(a) The data in this column refers to the net total of persons protected, i.e., duplication among persons protected by more than one kind of insuring organization or more than one insurance company policy providing the same type of coverage has been eliminated. Included in the BCBS and commercial percentages are Administrative Services Only (ASO) agreements and their sponsorship of HMOs and PPOs, which are also counted as independent plans.

(b) "Independent plans" include self-insured plans, plans employing third-party administrators, and HMOs.

(c) For 1984 and later, estimates of persons covered by "Independent plans" have been developed by HIAA in the absence of other available data.

(d) In 1996, within Independent plans, the 68.7% is comprised of HMOs, and self-insured. This is an increase from 1990 when the 47.4% was comprised of HMOs, 20% and self-insured, 27.4%.

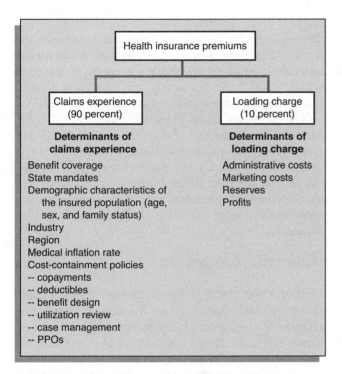

Figure 9-2. The determinants of health insurance premiums.

The price of insurance is the benefit/premium ratio, which is the percent of the total premium paid out in benefits to each insured group. If, for example, the premium for each member in a group was $1,000 per year and the utilization experience of that group resulted in an average payout of benefits equal to $900 per member per year, the benefit/premium ratio would be 0.9. The difference between benefits and total premiums (the "loading charge") goes for administration, claims processing, marketing, and insurer profit. In a price-competitive market, each of the components of the loading charge would be efficiently produced, and a competitive rate of profit would be included.

Another term for the benefit/premium ratio is the *medical loss ratio*. A high medical loss ratio means that the loading charge is a small percentage of the total premium.

When the benefit/premium ratio is close to 1.0, the group is "experience rated," that is, the premium reflects the expected experience of the group (and the loading charge is competitively produced). The benefit/premium ratio becomes closer to 1.0 the more competitive the industry and groups would be expected to change insurance companies when their benefit/premium ratio surpasses the amount they are willing to pay for real or perceived product differences between firms.

One indication of the competitiveness of the industry is the variation in benefit/premium ratios when size of group is held constant; the smaller the variation, the more efficient the market. (Because of economies of scale in marketing and administering different-sized groups, the larger the size of group, the closer the benefit/premium ratio would be to 1.0.)

Table 9-2 shows the ratios of expenditures (benefits) to premiums by different types of insurance plans for the period 1955 to 1996. Of interest in this table are the differences in the benefit/premium ratio between group and individual policies; group policies have lower marketing costs, and the insurer is less concerned about adverse selection. If an individual became part of a group, they would pay a much lower premium for the same coverage.

The use of the benefit/premium ratio as a measure of industry performance has diminished in more

dividual market, reflecting higher marketing costs and higher reserves. The claims expense is affected by the group's risk factors, such as the employees' age and sex, the type of industry (e.g., construction workers or accountants), location (to reflect medical costs in that region), the benefit package desired by the employees, the medical inflation rate in the coming year, and which cost-containment policies (such as the size of the deductible) are included in the benefit package.

The size of the loading charge is related to the various cost-containment options, which increase administrative expense while reducing claims expense. Unless the additional cost of cost containment is less than the savings from reduced claims expense, they would not be undertaken. Thus managed care companies' higher administrative expenses are not an indication of inefficiency.

recent years. Previously, when almost all health insurance consisted of indemnity plans and insurers performed only administrative tasks, the benefit premium ratio was an indication of how much was spent on administration and how much on the delivery of medical services. With the growth of managed care and multiple types of health plans, however, the benefit/premium ratio no longer simply measures the division of medical and administrative expense.

Currently, a low benefit/premium ratio can indicate increased responsibility by the insurer for medical management functions, such as utilization review, quality assurance, and provider profiling, functions that have as their purpose lower medical costs. Further, health plans today offer a variety of products, from indemnity, to closed panels of providers, an HMO option, a Point of Service (POS) plan (where the HMO patient can use non-HMO providers and pay a high co-payment), as well as a variety of pharmacy benefits for the different health plans, life and disability insurance, dental plans, and mental benefits. This greater range of products and benefits has increased the administrative and market-

ing cost to the insurer. (These are not wasteful expenditures since they are in response to purchaser demands.) Similarly, insurers differ in their percentage of individual, small group, and large employer enrollees, which affect their marketing and enrollment costs. (Appendix 1 discusses this subject in greater detail.)

The previous close approximation of the benefit/premium ratio to 1 shown in Table 9-2 suggests that health insurance has been a relatively price-competitive industry. As the industry has changed starting in the mid 1980s, however, measures other than the benefit/premium ratio discussed below are more indicative of the price competitiveness of this industry.

Insurer Price Competition

Until the mid 1980s, price competition among traditional insurers was based on the size of the loading charge. Actuaries estimated the expected claims expense given the above risk factors of the group, the group's location, benefits, and so on. Insurers therefore had an incentive to minimize their loading

Table 9-2. Ratio of Benefit Expenditures to Premium Income, According to Type of Plan, 1955–1996

Year	All Plans	Blue Cross-Blue Shield	Commercial Insurance Companies Total	Group Policies	Individual Policies	Independent Plans(a)
1955	.721	.933	.725	.839	.530	.912
1960	.760	.929	.789	.904	.529	.965
1965	.793	.938	.819	.936	.547	.906
1970	.860	.964	.872	.958	.581	.962
1975	.868	.960	.886	.984	.511	.867
1980	.901	.970	.847	.897	.580	.936
1985	.843	.904	.798	.834	.583	.886
1990	.886	.893	.819	.842	.646	.899
1996	.877	.886	.830	.851	.712	.969

Sources: Numbers for Commercial Insurance Companies and Independent Plans, 1955–1975, were developed from data provided in Marjorie Smith Carroll and Ross H. Arnett, "Private Health Insurance Plans in 1978 and 1979: A Review of Coverage, Enrollment and Financial Experience," *Health Care Financing Review,* September 1981, 3(1), pp. 55–88. The remainder of the data (All Plans, Blue Cross-Blue Shield, and the data for 1980–1996) comes from *Source Book of Health Insurance Data—1999/2000,* (Washington, D.C.: Health Insurance Association of America, 2000), pp. 41, 44, Tables 2.13, 2.18.

(a) "Independent Plans" include plans that offer health services on a prepaid basis and self-insured health plans.

charge. Cost containment measures such as utilization review and PPOs were viewed as an intrusion into the practice of medicine by the medical profession and were not used by insurers.

The introduction of utilization management and the use of provider panels dramatically changed the role of health insurers with regard to the practice of medicine. Insurers no longer passively accepted physicians' treatment decisions. Instead they established practice guidelines and reviewed physicians' medical decisions. Provider panels affected the patient's choice of provider. This change in the insurers' role did not (and was not able to) occur until the antitrust laws became applicable to the medical services industry in 1982.

When HMOs began to enter the group health insurance market in the early to mid 1980s, they set their premiums just below the premiums charged by traditional insurers. This practice was referred to as "shadow pricing." At that time, most (if not all) of the premium was paid by the employer on behalf of the employee. When the employee did pay part of the premium, it was not related to cost differences between different health plans. The employees' choice of health plan was therefore unaffected by differences in prices between health plans. To compete against the traditional plan which offered unlimited choice of provider, HMOs, with their restricted provider panels, offered more benefits. Although the HMO had a lower cost of providing care, it still charged premiums that were only slightly below those of the non-HMO health plans. The difference between their premiums and costs of care were used to provide the employee with greater benefits and increase the HMO's profits.

Employers initially believed that offering an HMO option to their employees would reduce insurance premiums because the HMO's lower cost would be passed on to the employer. However, this did not occur because of the HMOs use of shadow pricing. The rapid growth in HMOs did not occur until employers received some of the savings in the form of lower premiums and/or employees became responsible for paying the difference between the lowest cost plan and the plan they chose.

Another form of competitive behavior engaged in by insurers and HMOs was preferred risk selection.

When an HMO was offered along with a traditional health plan to an employer group, *at similar premiums*, the traditional plan received an adverse risk group. HMOs were able to attract a lower risk group of employees through design of their benefit package, for example, emphasizing well baby care. Also, those who were at higher risk or who were ill wanted to continue with their own physicians rather than switch to the HMO's restricted provider panel. It was for this reason that traditional health plans, when offered along with HMOs, wanted to be assured that they would receive a minimum percentage of the employees in a group (e.g., 50 percent of the employees). Alternatively, the insurer would offer the employer a choice of different plans, managed fee-for-service and an HMO, at the same premium for each age-sex risk group, and the insurer then made the monetary transfers between its own plans. Similarly, to internalize the cost of adverse selection to the non-HMO plan, when a single HMO is offered to an employee group, the HMO also offered a non-HMO product along with their HMO for the same premium in order to provide an employee group with more choice.

There are subtle methods by which a health insurer can achieve a preferred (low) risk group when the premiums of the different risk groups are not risk-adjusted. The plan can contract with new specialists compared to specialists who have been in practice longer (and whose chronically ill patients would remain with them). The health plan can advertise in newspapers rather than keeping brochures in physicians' offices where the population reading them are, on average, sicker than those who read the newspaper. And waiting rooms for pediatric patients can be attractive and waiting times short, compared to waiting times and access to referrals for chronically ill patients.

To date, risk-adjusted premiums have not been widely used by employers (nor have medical groups accepting sub-capitation payments from HMOs used them). Medicare pays HMOs a risk-adjusted premium for those aged who join an HMO. However, the risk factors used by Medicare have been insufficient to fully account for the preferred risk group received by HMOs. Risk adjustment is an area that is receiving a great deal of attention and research funding.

Risk-adjusted premiums would limit insurers' ability to compete on how well they can select preferred risks. Insurers would then have to compete on their administrative expense (loading charge) and on how well they manage risk. Risk-adjusted premiums provide efficient insurers with an incentive to accept high-risk patients. A risk-adjusted premium that fairly reflects the expected expense of high-risk patients provides insurers with an incentive to innovate and to manage the care of such patients. (Appendix 2 discusses how to construct risk adjusted premiums.)

Insurer Price Elasticities of Demand: Consumer Price Sensitivity Among Health Plans

Consumer willingness to switch health plans in response to changes in their out-of-pocket premiums is an indication that insurer demand curves are price elastic, which is characteristic of a very competitive industry. An insurer's demand curve is much more price elastic than the overall market demand for health insurance since there are better substitutes to each insurer than there is to health insurance in general.

Several studies have estimated the price elasticity of demand for a health plan; these results are shown in Table 9-3. The elasticity estimates indicate that in-

surers face very price elastic demand curves, one estimate is as high as –7.9. However, firm price elasticities shown in Table 9-3 are *average* price elasticities that may obscure important variations within the population. Price elasticities are likely to differ according to population characteristics, such as age, health status, income, and how long a person has been in a health plan. To determine the likely effect on a firm's demand as a result of the firm changing its price, it is more useful to estimate price elasticities according to the above population characteristics.

The following discussion provides a more complete explanation of how price elasticity differs by the switching costs of different population groups and how these estimates compare to using average price elasticities presented in Table 9-3.

In a typical large-employer setting, employees have a choice of several health plans and are able to change health plans during open enrollment periods. Once enrolled in a health plan, however, there are switching "costs" of changing plans. The employee has to spend time learning about the other health plans, their provider networks, and possibly establish a relationship with a new physician. A new plan offers greater uncertainty since employees have experience with the quality and access of their current plan. Switching costs are likely to be higher for those who have had a longer relationship with their health plan

Table 9-3. Price Elasticities for Health Insurance Plans

Study	Dependent Variable	Elasticity
B. S. Strombom, T. C. Buchmueller, P. J. Feldstein (2002)	health insurance plans	–0.80 to –5.20, avg. –2.50 (all plans)
B. S. Strombom, T. C. Buchmueller, P. J. Feldstein (2002)		–2.30 to –6.60, avg. –5.30 (managed care)
A. B. Royalty and N. Solomon (1999)		–3.70 to –6.20 (managed care)
D. M. Cutler and S. Reber (1996)		–2.00
B. Dowd and R. Feldman (1994/95)		–7.90
P. F. Short and A. K. Taylor (1989)		–2.60 to –5.30
W. P. Welch (1986)		–2.00 to –6.20

Sources: D. M. Cutler and S. Reber, "Paying for Health Insurance: The Tradeoff Between Competition and Adverse Selection," *Quarterly Journal of Economics,* May 1998, 113(2), pp. 433–466; B. Dowd and R. Feldman, "Premium Elasticities of Health Plan Choice," *Inquiry,* Winter 94/95, 31(4), pp. 438–444; A. B. Royalty and N. Solomon, "Health Plan Choice: Price Elasticities in a Managed Competitive Setting," *The Journal of Human Resources,* Winter 1999, 34(1), pp,. 1–41; P. F. Short and A. K. Taylor, "Premiums, Benefits, and Employee Choice of Health Insurance Options," *Journal of Health Economics,* December 1989, 8(3), pp. 293–312; B. A. Strombom, T. C. Buchmueller and P. J. Feldstein, "Switching Costs, Price Sensitivity and Health Plan Choice," *Journal of Health Economics,* January 2002, 21(1), pp. 89–116; W. P. Welch, "The Elasticity of Demand for Health Maintenance Organizations," *The Journal of Human Resources,* Spring 1986, 21(2), pp. 252–266.

and participating physician, those who are older, and those who are in poorer health.

If switching costs are sufficiently high, employees may remain in a plan even if their monthly out-of-pocket premium (co-premium) increases relative to the co-premiums of alternative plans; they become less price sensitive to price differences among competing health plans. High switching costs make health plan demand curves less price elastic and therefore limit price competition among health plans.

Switching costs are a concern in health insurance markets if they are correlated with health risk. If switching costs are greater for enrollees who have a greater need for medical care, then they will be less likely than low-risk enrollees to switch plans in response to a change in relative prices. If this occurs, then price changes will lead not only to shifts in market share, but also to changes in the cost of providing health care across plans. A plan that loses share due to an increase in relative price will tend to see its average cost increase as younger and healthier enrollees switch to lower-priced plans. If this occurs and premiums are not risk-adjusted, adverse selection will result.

The effect of a change in relative co-premiums on employee switching behavior was recently analyzed (14). The study was based on 5 years (1993 to 1997) of open enrollment data from a large employer (the University of California) comprising more than 100,000 employees at 11 locations throughout California having a standard benefit design. Administrative data on each employee provided information on the employee's age, sex, salary, job tenure, job classification (academic, management, or support staff), and home ZIP code to indicate whether the employee lives in a rural area. Unique to this study was the ability to match employees (and their spouses) with data from other sources to develop measures of health status. Data from the California Cancer Registry (CCR) and from the Office of Statewide Health Planning and Development (OSHPD) were matched to employees (and spouses) for the period 1988 to 1997 (diagnosed cancers) and 1991 to 1997 (hospitalizations by DRG) for identifying those individuals considered to be of "high risk" and who are likely to face higher switching costs due to an

established provider relationship. Given the ability to match employee identifiers with data from the CCR and OSHPD, it was possible to construct the above health status indicators for new enrollees prior to their UC employment, which was not possible for other such studies. Data on cancer diagnosis or hospitalizations should be relevant to employee and spouse health plan choice decisions.

At each location for each year, employees had a choice of an indemnity plan, a PPO/POS plan, and several HMOs.

In 1994, the University of California changed the method by which it contributed to its employees' health plan premiums. At each of the University's nine campuses, there were two fee-for-service plans (a "high option" indemnity plan and a PPO) and several HMOs. Prior to 1994, the University had paid the full premium for most plans and subsidized the cost of the most expensive plans. In 1994, the University limited its contribution to the cost of the least expensive plan; employees had to pay the additional cost (co-premium) of more expensive plans. Given the five years of study data, substantial variation in premiums exist within as well as across health plans.

The following study findings, presented in Table 9-4, are:

- Employees are very price sensitive when choosing a health plan. A 10 percent increase in the relative price of a health plan will cause a decrease in enrollment of between 20 and 80 percent depending upon the employee's age, how long they have been employed, and their health status.

- In each of the health status/age categories, the longer the person has been employed with the company (tenure), the lower their price sensitivity.

- For each health status/tenure category, the higher the person's age, the lower their price sensitivity.

- Within each age/tenure category, the higher the risk level, the lower the price sensitivity.

To illustrate the effect of a change in relative health plan prices when enrollees who differ in age, job tenure, and health risk have different price sensitivities, the study authors conducted a simulation analysis of a $5 and a $25 monthly premium increase. Four competing health plans are hypothesized, each having the same distribution of enrollee characteristics (age, job tenure, and risk level) and market share. The hypothetical health plan before any premium changes is shown in the top section of Table 9-5. The second section of the table illustrates the effects on the plan that increases its premium by $5 or by $25; its market share declines, the average age of its enrollees as well as the percent of its enrollees in the high-risk category increases, and the expected monthly claims cost per household increases. Those plans not increasing their premium, shown in the bottom section of the table, experience an increase in market share, a decline in their enrollees monthly claims cost, a decrease in the average age of its enrollees, and end up with a lower risk group.

Table 9-4. Insurer Perspective Price Elasticities

Age and Tenure	Low Risk	High Risk
Age 30 and younger		
New hire	−8.41	−6.72
Employed 1–5 years	−4.20	−4.68
Employed for > 5 years	−3.42	−3.82
Age 31–45		
New hire	−6.21	−5.54
Employed 1–5 years	−3.68	−3.30
Employed for > 5 years	−3.12	−3.28
Age 46 and older		
New hire	−4.69	−3.23
Employed 1–5 years	−2.66	−2.22
Employed for > 5 years	−2.02	−2.03

Source: Bruce Strombom, Thomas Buchmueller, and Paul J. Feldstein, "Switching Costs, Price Sensitivity and Health Plan Choice," *Journal of Health Economics*, 21(1), January 2002, pp. 89–116.

Table 9-5. Simulation Analysis: The Effect of a Premium Increase on Plan Market Share and Expected Claims Costs

	All Plans (US $)	
	$5 — mo.	$25 — mo.
Premium Increase		
Baseline		
Market share (%)	25.00	25.00
Mean age of enrollees	38.40	38.40
Percent of enrollees in high-risk category (%)	9.96	9.96
Expected monthly claims costs per household (US $)	268.83	268.83
After price change—plan raising premium		
Market share (%)	23.70	19.30
Mean age of enrollees	38.60	39.40
Percent of enrollees in high-risk category (%)	10.13	10.81
Expected monthly claims costs per household (change relative to baseline, US $)	270.95 (+2.12)	279.19 (+10.36)
After price change—other plans		
Market share (%)	25.40	26.90
Mean age of enrollees	38.30	38.10
Percent of enrollees in high-risk category (%)	9.91	9.76
Expected monthly claims costs per household (change relative to baseline, US $)	268.17 (−0.66)	266.36 (−2.47)

Source: Bruce Strombom, Thomas Buchmueller, and Paul J. Feldstein, "Switching Costs, Price Sensitivity and Health Plan Choice," *Journal of Health Economics*, 21(1), January 2002, pp. 89–116.

The study findings have important implications for health plan price competition. Requiring employees to bear the additional cost of choosing a more expensive health plan makes those employees more price sensitive. If a health plan were to increase its relative premiums, *it would suffer a large reduction in market share among newly hired young employees in the low-risk category.* Conversely, the plan would lose a much smaller percentage of older employees in the high-risk category.

The correlation of price sensitivity and health risk implies that changes in relative prices will lead to:

• Changes in the market shares of competing plans.

• Changes in the expected costs of plans due to changes in the average risk profiles of their enrollees.

Health plans that increase their relative premiums will tend to see their risk pools deteriorate as younger, more price sensitive, lower-risk enrollees leave for lower-priced plans.

Because older enrollees who have a higher health risk and who are more costly to insure are less likely to switch health plans in response to premium increases, insurers who increase their premiums (relative to their competitors) will not only lose market share but also experience higher claims cost as the younger, healthier, enrollees switch to lower-cost plans.

In the absence of risk-adjusted premiums, price competition among insurers will increase as insurers compete on price both to gain market share and to attract lower-risk enrollees.

Risk-adjusted premiums would eliminate distortions in health plan choices that arise when premiums differ because of differences in the risk of enrollees across plans.

These findings indicate that the demand curve facing the individual health plan is very price elastic; small relative price increases (co-premiums) will cause much greater percentage decreases in a health plan's enrollment, making such price increases unprofitable.

The Underwriting Cycle

The recurrent underwriting cycle in the group market is another indication of the price competitiveness of the health insurance industry. This cycle is characterized by three years of underwriting losses followed by three years of underwriting profits (15). The underwriting cycle goes back to at least the 1960s; more recent data on the cycle are shown in Figure 9-3.

The underwriting cycle, which results in profits and losses to health insurers, is not caused by large swings in subscribers' claims expenses but is instead a *pricing* cycle. The reasons for the recurrent cycle are as follows: When health insurers are very profitable in their group business (underwriting profits at their peak), they seek to increase their market share (in the group market) by lowering their prices. As the insurer begins to reduce their premiums, their medical loss ratio increases (claims expense as a portion of the decreased premium increases). Given the price competitiveness of the insurance market, groups are able to compare premiums at different insurers, thus all insurers respond to an insurer's reduction in premiums (relative to the claims expense of a group) by reducing their premiums as well. As each insurer lowers its premium to gain market share, and the other insurers follow those price reductions, profitability of the insured groups fall.

During the profitable stage of the underwriting cycle, the insurer's sales force, which is rewarded with bonuses for signing more groups (and not penalized for signing unprofitable groups), is typically given greater authority (relative to the insurer's actuaries) to reduce premiums and sign up higher risk groups.

There is a time lag between when an insurer negotiates a premium with an insured group and when the insurer begins to receive the claims expense originating from that group and is able to calculate its medical loss ratio. The time lag may be between six to nine months. Often before the insurer has a full understanding of its underwriting profit (or loss) on each insured group, it will have to negotiate the following year's premium with that group. Insurers are

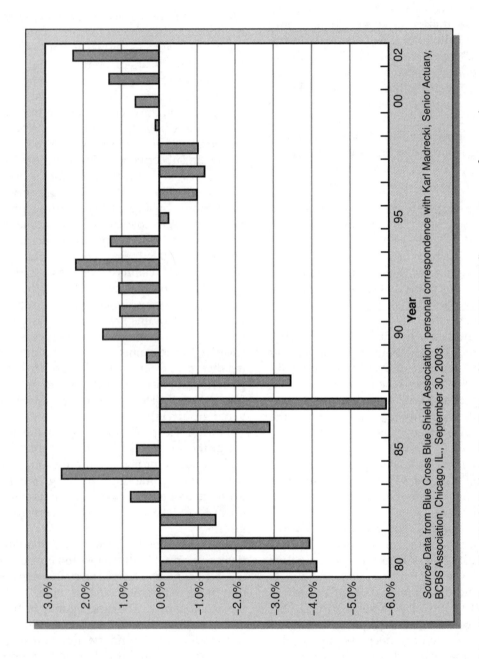

Figure 9-3. Blue Cross-Blue Shield Underwriting Gains and Losses, 1980–2002 (in percentages of revenue).

Source: Data from Blue Cross Blue Shield Association, personal correspondence with Karl Madrecki, Senior Actuary, BCBS Association, Chicago, IL., September 30, 2003.

initially unaware that they are incurring losses, and when they do they cannot immediately change their premiums; they must wait until the next renewal period.

Once the insurer experiences underwriting losses, the actuaries have greater input into each insured group's pricing decision. Premiums are rapidly increased for all groups, particularly those groups with the largest losses. At this point, the insurer is no longer interested in increasing market share; the insurer's goal is to return to profitability.

As the insurer reduces the number of unprofitable groups and increases premiums on other groups, its underwriting profit increases. After a few years, the insurer believes that it could increase profitability further by increasing its market share, and the cycle begins once again.

It is surprising that this pricing cycle continually repeats itself. If, however, at the profitable stage of the cycle several large insurers decide to lower their premiums to increase market share, insurers who do not respond with similar price reductions will lose most of their group business. Thus the insurance underwriting cycle provides evidence of the price competitiveness of the group insurance market.

The underwriting cycle affects the annual rate of increase in premiums, thus it is important for understanding the reasons for short-term changes in premiums. The effects of public policy as well as private cost containment efforts may be minimized or exaggerated because of when those changes occur during the underwriting cycle (16).

The Efficiency and Equity Aspects of Community Rating

A further example of the insurance industry's price competitiveness was the use of community rating as a method for pricing health insurance and how market forces caused a change in that approach. Community rating, as contrasted to experience rating, charges subscribers the same premium regardless of the experience or risk factors, i.e., age and sex, of the group.

An early example of the use (and consequences) of community rating was by Blue Cross. Aged persons (who had much higher hospital use rates than younger persons) were charged the *same premium*.[4] The benefit/premium ratio for aged persons was, therefore, greater than 1.0; the benefits paid on their behalf exceeded the premiums they paid for insurance. Since the average benefit/premium ratio for all groups in a community rating system had to be close to 1.0, this meant that low users of hospital services had benefit/premium ratios much less than 1.0.

When the expected costs of groups differ, the effect of community rating is that a subsidy is provided to high-use groups financed by a (regressive) "tax" on lower-use groups. A large intergenerational transfer would be expected to occur wherein younger age groups subsidize older age groups who have higher use rates (17). Any such "subsidy-tax" system can be evaluated on the basis of two economic criteria: first, its effect on efficiency—namely, does it affect the quantity of health insurance purchased?—and second, its equity—does such a redistribution scheme cause higher-income subscribers to subsidize lower-income subscribers?

With regard to the efficiency aspects of community rating, low-user groups are typically low-risk groups. An individual is willing to pay a certain amount above the pure premium for health insurance. Charging low-risk groups a much greater amount above their pure premium than if they were experience rated results in fewer low-user groups purchasing insurance. Low-user groups might decide that they would be better off if they self-insured (no insurance) rather than pay the community rate. Depending upon the price elasticity of demand for insurance, low-user groups would be expected to demand less insurance under community rating.

Similar to an excise tax that is placed on some goods and services but not others (hence distorting their relative prices), a community rate is a tax on the insurance premium of a low-risk person. The result of such a "tax" is a decreased demand for health insurance coverage. Community rating does not permit

---

4. Even under community rating, however, premiums differed according to whether the individual was married or single and whether or not he or she belonged to a group.

low-risk groups to purchase insurance at its costs of production, which is its actuarial value plus administrative cost.

Community rating is considered economically inefficient. Low-risk groups buy too little insurance; they cannot buy insurance at the cost of producing it (for their risk group). (A similar inefficiency occurs when a monopolist charges a price for a service that exceeds its cost of production.) High-risk groups buy "too much" insurance; since the price of insurance is subsidized, their price is below the cost of producing their insurance, thus the marginal benefits of their additional insurance is less than the marginal costs of producing the additional coverage.

As shown in Figure 9-4, CR is the community rated premium which is the average of the experience rated premiums of high- and low-risk groups, whose experience rated premiums are, respectively, P_{HR} and P_{LR}. Assuming the demand curve for health insurance by both groups is the same and indicated by D, then when both groups are experience rated, they will demand Q_{HR} and Q_{LR} quantity of health insurance, respectively. Their marginal costs, reflected in their experience rated premiums, equals the marginal benefits they receive, namely the quantity demanded of health insurance.

If community rating is mandated, the marginal cost of insurance is increased for low-risk groups and decreased for high-risk groups; low-risk groups move up their demand curve and demand less health insurance, Q_O, while high-risk groups move down their demand curve and demand a greater quantity of health insurance, Q_O. Under community rating, the marginal benefits of insurance to both groups are no longer equal to their respective marginal cost of producing those benefits. The marginal costs are less than the marginal benefits for low-risk groups, while the marginal costs exceed the marginal benefits for high-risk groups. The quantity demanded for each group is no longer optimal.

Community rating is also inefficient because it subsidizes and therefore increases unhealthy lifestyle behavior. As long as there is some price elasticity to unhealthy lifestyles, community rating removes the financial incentive to reduce such activities, such as smoking, being overweight, having high blood pres-

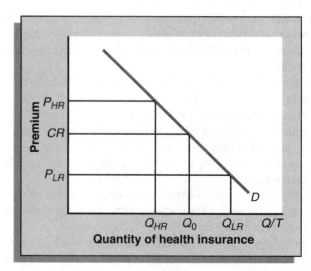

Figure 9-4. The economic inefficiency of community rating.

sure, etc. Further, community rating decreases an employer's incentive to undertake risk-reducing behavior among its employees for the purpose of reducing both the employer's and employees' medical expenses, hence premiums.

Perhaps the main reason for mandating community rating, according to its advocates, is that it would increase the number of insured persons, primarily those who are at higher risk, by being able to afford the lower premiums. Without relying on government subsidies, community rating subsidizes high-risk (presumably low income) persons by taxing low-risk (presumably higher-income persons).[5] However,

---

5. An additional reason suggested for community rating is that it is insurance with a longer time horizon. Since everyone grows old, the young (low risk) who subsidize the aged eventually receive such a subsidy themselves. However, when the premium (based on average risk) exceeds what a low-risk premium would cost, low-risk individuals would buy less insurance. Subsidized high-risk individuals would buy more insurance. This is inefficient (one cannot purchase insurance at the cost of producing it), as well as being an unstable situation; it therefore could not exist in a price-competitive insurance market. Instead, it would be more equitable to vary the insurance premium over time according to age, since age (a proxy for risk) is also correlated with income and assets. Thus an age-adjusted premium would be more equitable over time than community rating.

community rating not only is an inefficient mechanism for redistributing medical care, but it has inequitable redistributive effects.

Using risk factors such as age and sex as the criteria for providing insurance subsidies assumes that all high-risk people have lower incomes than low-risk people. However, many older people have higher incomes than those who are younger. The direction of the subsidy, however, goes from the younger (low risk) to the older (high risk) person, regardless of their relative incomes. Further, the actual subsidy goes to the group that *uses* more medical services, not necessarily to the group that has the highest risk of hospitalization.

Empirical studies document the unintended redistributive effects of community rating (18). A study of Michigan Blue Cross revealed that under community rating the most heavily subsidized group were auto workers. The next most heavily subsidized group was comprised of healthcare professionals—physicians, nurses, and other hospital employees. These subsidized groups had higher-than-average incomes. What occurred under community rating was that the subsidy-tax concept operated in reverse: *those with lower incomes subsidized those with higher incomes.* Similarly, if community rating was to be geographically based, then there would be unintended wealth transfers from poorer, rural communities to wealthier, urban communities that have higher health care expenditures.

If society agreed with the value judgment that subsidies should be provided to lower-income families to increase their purchase of health insurance, this goal could be achieved more efficiently through a system of direct subsidies to those families instead of attempting such redistribution indirectly through community rating.[6]

---

6. Blue Cross' goals did not include being the most efficient welfare agent. Instead, Blue Cross may have attempted to increase its enrollment and in so doing, allocated its taxes and subsidies according to a policy that facilitated the greatest increase in its growth. This policy would result in charging lower premiums to groups whose demands are more elastic (such as large unions) and higher premiums to groups with less elastic demands, instead of matching the subsidy to income level.

Community rating is inefficient because it distorts the price of health insurance to different user groups. It raises the price of health insurance to low-user groups, thereby decreasing their demand for health insurance. Their demand for health insurance was less than if they had been experience rated. Community rating is also an inefficient method of distributing subsidies for the purchase of health insurance.

Community rating cannot survive in a price competitive market (19). Competitive forces cause insurance premiums to become experience rated. This is in fact what occurred. In the mid 1950s, commercial insurers charged low-user groups experience rated premiums. As low-user groups left Blue Cross, the community rated premium to the remaining Blue Cross subscribers increased; this in turn caused additional groups, who were subsidizing others, to switch to commercial insurers. Blue Cross had to abandon community rating in its group market. Even Blue Cross plans, such as Michigan Blue Cross, that had a great deal of market power (because of strong union preferences for a non-profit insurer) had to change its rating practices.

Advocates of community rating have sought legislation to legally mandate it since it could not survive in a competitive market. An example of one such case is provided by the experience of New York State, where community rating was enacted for the individual and small group markets and took effect in April 1993.

New York health insurers were required to offer a community rate regardless of age, sex, or other risk factors, such as medical condition. Initial reports of the effect of community rating were predictable. Large numbers of young healthy people dropped their coverage as their rates sharply increased (20). The insurance pool began to consist of a greater number of older, sicker persons. The average age of policyholders increased, as did the average claim expense, which for some insurers, doubled. (Average claims cost increased 46 percent for the individual market.) The total number of insured persons *decreased*, increasing the number of uninsured by 400,000.

A recent study of New York's community rating legislation arrives at a somewhat different conclusion (21). The authors compared three states, New York (which implemented community rating), Pennsylvania (which did not), and Connecticut (which placed very few restrictions on how insurers could set their premiums). They found that "While coverage rates in the New York small group market did fall, and the age distribution of the covered population did shift towards older persons in a manner consistent with a market-wide death spiral, . . . we find almost identical changes in Pennsylvania and Connecticut. . . ." They further ". . . find evidence that New York's reforms led to an increase in the market share of HMOs in the small group and individual market." The authors conclude that the primary goal of community rating proponents, an increase in the percent of the population with insurance, did not occur.

The major effect of community rating in New York, according to the above study, was a shift away from indemnity insurance to HMOs. If these more restrictive forms of insurance that are better able to control costs were unavailable, it is likely that premiums would have sufficiently risen to result in the predicted adverse death spiral, dramatically reducing the number of insured.

Proposals have been made at both the federal and state level to require "community rating" as a basis for establishing health insurance premiums. Legally mandating community rating eventually results in insurers engaging in preferred risk selection. If the benefit coverage is not mandated along with community rating, then insurers would compete for low-risk groups by structuring their benefits accordingly, e.g., including higher deductibles, emphasizing wellness programs, and de-emphasizing chronic care specialists. It is more likely that along with community rating a standard benefit package would also be mandated. However, insurers could still attempt to enroll low-risk groups according to where they locate their providers, the services they emphasize, and access to referrals for specialists. An additional problem with mandating a standard benefits package is that subscribers have different preferences regarding the benefits they are willing to purchase and the size of the deductible and co-payment desired (both of which determine their premium).

Maintaining a community rate with a single set of benefits when subscribers differ in their utilization experience and in their preference for benefits, cost sharing, and cost containment techniques is highly inefficient. Diversity in consumer preferences can be dealt with most efficiently by a health insurance system that offers a variety of benefits, cost-sharing arrangements, and rate structures. If society desires everyone should have at least a minimum level of health insurance, subsidies can be provided directly to those with low incomes instead of mandating a community rated insurance scheme for all.

The McCarran-Ferguson Act

Enacted in 1945, the McCarran-Ferguson Act provides the insurance industry with a limited exemption from the anti-trust laws (22). The Act states that the anti-trust laws apply to the business of insurance *unless* the insurance companies are regulated by the states. Even though the state may regulate the insurers, insurers are still prohibited from engaging in boycotts, coercion, or acts of intimidation.

Various medical organizations have claimed that the McCarran-Ferguson Act has permitted health insurers to act in an anti-competitive manner; colluding to fix both the prices they charge and to limit how much they pay physicians. Further, that the collusive activities of health insurers contribute to the rising cost of health insurance premiums.

No evidence exists that health insurers collude in setting premiums above the competitive level. The most serious impediment to competitive pricing has been in the state regulated individual market when the state mandates community rating. Further, the structure of the health insurance market is very competitive; there are a large number of insurers, and the costs of entry are relatively low. Even though large economies of scale in the production of insurance exist, low entry costs make insurance markets highly contestable. The ability of groups to become self-insured also limits insurers' ability to engage in anti-competitive pricing. The underwriting cycle is additional evidence of a lack of collusive pricing by insurers, otherwise insurers would not suffer continual periods of large underwriting losses.

The structure of the industry and the number of actual and potential competitors, together with their pricing behavior, indicate that the health insurance market is very price competitive. Shifting the cause of rapidly rising premiums to insurers deflects attention from the actual reasons for rapidly rising premiums, such as greater use of expensive technology, rising input prices, and inappropriate use of services.

THE PERFORMANCE OF THE HEALTH INSURANCE MARKET

Two important aspects of market performance are the extent of price and product competition among insurers. Price competition among insurers reduces the loading charge and eliminates any excess profits; when firms earn normal rates of return, premiums reflect the cost of producing health insurance. Product competition forces insurers to respond to the insured population's preferences for different types of insurance. The health insurance industry has changed over time; from predominately non-profit insurers to mostly for-profits, to new types of health plans, and a change in the role of insurers from merely administering employer health benefits to a more interventionist role with the rise of managed care. The performance of the industry depends upon how competitive it is and how well it responds to consumer demands.

Insurer Profitability

The most relevant time for evaluating the performance of the industry is from the mid 1990s to the present. During this period, managed care became a national phenomenon (previously it was dominant only in certain sections of the country). In more recent years, managed care's restrictive cost controls were loosened and providers, through mergers and market consolidations, were able to exercise market power in their health plan negotiations.

The yardstick for measuring market performance is how close the industry approximates the model of a perfectly competitive market. Several characteristics of the competitive model are price competition, free entry and exit, and in the long run, prices reflect costs of production, and no excess profits exist.

It is difficult to determine whether premiums reflect costs since the divergence between the benefit/premium ratio and 1.0 may be the result of increasing administrative functions related to cost containment programs, the multiplicity of insurance products offered, and so on. Instead, the price competitiveness and profitability of the industry over time are used to indicate the competitiveness of the industry.

Three examples were used to indicate the price competitiveness of the industry: insurer-firm demand curves, the underwriting cycle, and community rating. Firm demand curves were determined to be very price elastic based on studies of the likelihood of employees switching health plans as a result of small changes in their co-premiums. The underwriting cycle occurred because insurers reduced their prices to increase their market share, followed by price increases to recover from severe losses. Community rating disappeared (except in state-regulated individual markets) because of lower prices offered by insurers to groups whose experience rated premium was below the community rate (large groups were also able to self-insure if their claims experience was below the community rate). The market for health insurance was considered to be highly price competitive.

The second indication of competitive markets is whether above normal profits are able to persist over time. Even though some insurers may be able to have higher profits for a longer period than other firms (perhaps due to superior management), the insurance industry, on average, does not exhibit persistent high profits. Again, data on the underwriting cycle support the hypothesis that insurers do not earn continual high rates of return. The net profit margin on insurers' premiums have varied over time from slightly greater than 4 percent to losses almost reaching negative 4 percent. In recent years, the net margin has been profitable. Although insurers also earn interest on their premiums in addition to their underwriting margin, the size of the margins and their variability are indicative of a relatively competitive industry (23).

Product Competition in the Health Insurance Market

The health insurance industry is a supplier of insurance and a demander of medical services; it thus operates in two different markets. As a supplier of health insurance, insurers can be a price competitive industry even though the markets in which they purchase medical services may be monopolistic. To the extent that the *medical services* market is not price competitive, then insurance premiums will be higher since claims expense will be greater than if the input (provider) market were competitive. In addition to increasing input prices, a non-competitive medical services (input) market may also be able to restrict the types of products that health insurers can market, such as cost containment programs and participation in HMOs. Thus the ability of insurers to respond to consumer demands will affect the performance of the health insurance market.

An important development over the past decade has been the introduction of cost containment programs by the health insurance industry. Cost containment methods include utilization review (such as pre-authorization prior to being admitted to a hospital), concurrent review (review of length of stay while in the hospital), second opinions for surgery, drug formularies, as well as Health Maintenance Organizations (HMOs) and Preferred Provider Organizations (PPOs). These cost containment approaches differ from the use of deductibles and cost sharing, which have long existed, in that these newer approaches place the insurer between the traditional patient-physician relationship. The physician's decision-making authority is subject to review.

The Previous Unavailability of Cost Containment Methods: The rapid increases in medical expenditures and health insurance premiums are not a recent phenomenon. Therefore why weren't insurance companies more aggressive in adopting such measures previously in their attempts to control rising costs? One study examining the potential savings to an employer from adopting utilization review found that it was very effective in reducing hospital use and medical expenditures; the savings-to-cost ratio was found to be 8 to 1 (24).

One possible reason for the unavailability of such restrictive cost control insurance products was insufficient demand by the purchasers of health insurance, employers and employees. Employer-purchased health insurance is exempt from federal, state, and Social Security taxes; thus the employee does not bear the full cost of rising medical expenditures. The after-tax value of the savings to employees from more restrictive cost containment methods was too low given the high marginal income tax rates during the 1960s and 1970s. Many employees also believed that health benefits were a hard-won benefit and that restrictions on those benefits would be a "give back." Further, firms engaged in overseas competition were provided with import protection, e.g., the auto companies benefited from "voluntary" quotas being placed on Japanese imports, which made it possible to pass on higher employee costs (in the form of medical care) to consumers in the form of higher auto prices. (With a less price elastic demand curve as a result of decreased availability of foreign substitutes, increased employee health costs (compensation) resulted in higher auto prices; in the 1980s, with more import competition and a more elastic demand curve, increased employee medical costs caused greater decreases in production and employment, thereby increasing employer and employee concern with rising medical costs.)

While it is possible that there might not have been much demand for restrictive cost containment methods among firms, it is unlikely that all firms and purchasers would have been opposed to such measures. It is therefore necessary to examine supply side reasons why cost control measures were not offered.

A second possible explanation for the previous lack of cost control programs is that other insurers would copy an insurer who innovated in developing such programs. The innovator would not gain any competitive advantage and would incur costs if the innovation did not work. Similarly, if an insurance company were successful in changing the practice style of physicians, then the physicians would treat other insurer's patients in a similar manner; the innovating insurer would incur the costs of inducing physicians to change and not receive any competitive advantage (25).

The third, and most likely, explanation for the lack of cost control methods is based on anti-competitive behavior by providers.

Health insurance consists of three components: the pooling of risks, the administration of claims, and the expense of physician and hospital services. In a competitive market, an insurance company will be able to lower its costs (hence increase its profits or lower its premiums) if, in performing the risk function, it selects preferred risks (individuals who are less costly) and if it is efficient in the administration of claims. Insurance companies would be able to reduce their costs for medical services if they are able to purchase hospital and physician services at lower prices or have their subscribers use fewer such services. Health providers have always been more concerned with the prices they received and whether controls were placed on the use of their services than on how insurance companies pool their risks and administer their claims.

Competition among insurance companies on the basis of how well they are able to reduce provider prices or utilization is contrary to the economic interests of physicians and hospitals. Blue Cross and Blue Shield plans, which were developed and controlled by hospitals and physicians, therefore did not engage in such cost control activities. When other insurers did initiate such activities, physicians (and other health providers) engaged in anti-competitive behavior to prevent the insurer from continuing such actions.

Faced with competition during the early 1930s, insurers lowered their costs; insurers in Oregon placed restraints on physician utilization. Preauthorization of services and monitoring of claims were used. Physicians accepted such constraints on their behavior since it was during the depression, physicians did not have as many patients, and they were unsure of their ability to collect from those they did have. Consumers benefited from these cost containment measures through lower insurance premiums.

The response by the Oregon medical society was twofold: first, to threaten physicians who participated in such insurance plans with expulsion from the medical society and, second, the medical society started its own insurance plan, which did not use aggressive utilization review procedures. With the growth of their own insurance plan, physicians were encouraged to boycott other insurance plans. The medical society's sponsored health plan grew, and enrollment in other insurance plans declined. To secure physician partic-

ipation, other insurers had to become less aggressive in their cost containment efforts (26). The medical societies were thereby able to ensure that the type of insurance programs offered to the public were also those that were in the physicians' economic interests.

Additional examples of such anti-competitive behavior were organized medicine's actions against capitated (prepaid) health plans, such as Kaiser and HMOs (27).

Through their anti-competitive behavior, medical organizations precluded certain types of insurance coverage that would have reduced medical expenses from being offered in the insurance market. Co-payments and deductibles have always been acceptable to physician organizations since they did not interfere with physician pricing or decision-making.

The Supreme Court's ruling in 1982 that upheld the applicability of the anti-trust laws to the health professions made such anti-competitive behavior illegal.

Throughout the 1980s, in return for lower premium increases, employer and employee demand for cost containment programs increased. The reduction of federal tax rates in 1981 also served to stimulate demand for such cost containment products by decreasing the tax subsidy for more comprehensive insurance. Free of anti-competitive restraints on the types of insurance products they were able to offer, insurance companies were better able to match their insurance products to the preferences of each employer group.

Recent Developments in Health Insurance Products: Managed care techniques, such as limited provider networks, prior authorization for inpatient care and for specialist referrals, primary care gatekeepers, and negotiated discounts with providers, as well as provider risk sharing through capitation, proved successful. By the mid-1990s, health insurance premiums were barely rising; in California, a state where managed care started early, premiums, in absolute dollars, actually declined during that period.

Rapidly increasing insurance premiums and relatively stable incomes during the late 1980s and early 1990s stimulated the demand for managed care. However, as real incomes began to increase during the late 1990s and employers competed for labor driving wages still higher, employees wanted health benefits with fewer restrictions and greater access to specialists. The demand for tightly managed care plans declined. Managed care firms responded to these changes in consumer demand and broadened their provider networks and eliminated other cost containment techniques, thereby increasing access to care. As health plans relaxed their restrictions, they began to lose their ability to control costs.

At the same time consumer demand was changing, a backlash against managed care occurred. Led by anecdotes of denial of care and physician anger against the interference of managed care in their practices, legislators at both the state and federal level began to place limits on managed care.

With the loosening of managed care's cost control and the continuing growth of technology and new drugs, health insurance premiums once again began to increase rapidly.

To control rising health care costs, employers are increasing deductibles and co-payments and limiting their health plan contribution. Current cost containment approaches impose greater financial incentives on employees to use fewer services and to select less expensive health plans. Insurers and employers are searching for new ways to contain rising health costs.

A relatively new approach being considered by several large employers as a means of reducing rapidly increasing insurance premiums is a defined contribution plan (DCP) (31). Although this approach has received a great deal of publicity, its popularity is uncertain.

The idea of a defined contribution is not new; providing employees with a fixed dollar amount to use in choosing a health plan has been proposed by many as a means of making employees price sensitive to the cost of different health plans and stimulating competition.

The new use of the DCP insurance product reduces the employer's involvement in managing their employees' health benefits, shifting more of the decision-making to the employee. The DCP plan works as follows: The employer allocates a specific (tax exempt) dollar amount for the employee's health benefits. Part of this amount is deposited in an employee account from which the employee can purchase medical serv-ices. The remainder of the employer's contribution is used to purchase a large deductible catastrophic health insurance policy. The employee is responsible for the difference in medical expenses between the amount deposited in their account and the cata-strophic policy deductible level. (Unused funds in the account roll over into the following year and may be taken by the employee if they change jobs). Lastly, the companies marketing such DCPs offer the use of the Internet to assist employees with their decision-making, such as establishing preferred provider networks.

The growth of defined contribution plans, if it were to become widespread, would represent a dramatic shift in the private health insurance system. Instead of employers contracting with large insurers to manage their employees' health benefits, the employee becomes responsible for their medical expenses until their catastrophic insurance limit is reached. Employees would need the appropriate information to make informed decisions on their medical needs and choice of provider.

Federal and State Health Insurance Regulation

Federal Legislation: In 1996, health insurance regulatory reforms were enacted at the federal level. The Health Insurance Portability and Accountability Act (HIPAA) removed certain health insurance market imperfections. Included in the legislation was *Guaranteed Issue,* whereby health insurers have to offer group health insurance to groups willing to purchase it. Thus insurers would not be able to deny coverage to groups they believe would be high risk. *Guaranteed Renewal* requires health insurers to renew all health insurance policies, precluding them from dropping individuals or groups who incur high medical costs. Consistent with the concept of insurance, a person who purchases insurance should not lose it once they incur a serious illness. *Portability* is important because employees are often reluctant to leave their jobs because they cannot take their health insurance with them. Under the new legislation, employees are able to continue their insurance coverage if they move to another employee group or if they become self-employed. *Limitations on Pre-Existing*

Exclusions means that once an individual has met the (usual 12 month) pre-existing exclusion limit for any illness, an insurer cannot re-impose another 12-month waiting period if the employee changes jobs. Employees are thus more likely to be able to change jobs without fear of being without health insurance if they or a family member have an illness.

In addition to the above, the new law expanded the tax deductibility of health insurance premiums (up to 80 percent from the current 30 percent) for the self-employed by the year 2006. This will begin to eliminate an inequity that exists between the self-employed and those employed by groups, who currently receive 100 percent tax deductibility of their premiums.

State Health Insurance Regulation: States have also enacted health insurance legislation; state high-risk pools have enabled those who are uninsurable to purchase insurance at subsidized rates. However, other state legislation has impeded the efficient functioning of the insurance market, such as mandated community rating, reduced limits on pre-existing exclusion waiting periods, mandated benefits and providers, rate regulation of insurance premiums, and Any Willing Provider (AWP) laws. These laws have adversely impacted the market's efficiency.

Any Willing Provider laws require insurers to accept all out-of-network providers that agree to abide by the plan's contract terms. About 25 states have enacted AWP laws. Traditionally, HMOs have been able to negotiate lower payments by assuring providers that their direct competitors would be excluded from the network, thereby guaranteeing them a larger volume of patients. But because AWP laws prevent HMOs from making these promises, providers have little incentive to offer discounted prices. These government restrictions reduce the options available for those consumers who are unwilling to pay for such open provider networks; their premiums are increased. A recent study, for example, found that AWP laws reduce the cost savings effect of HMOs, particularly with regard to physician expenditures; providing an economic rationale for physician support for such laws (29).

State requirements regarding rating methods and maximum premiums, particularly with regard to the *individual market,* have resulted in a decline in competition as the number of insurers participating in the individual insurance market decreased. For example, in 1995 the insurance commissioner in Washington State decreed that for a given period of time the 12-month waiting period for pre-existing conditions would be eliminated, and after that the pre-existing waiting period should only be three months and that insurers serving the individual market could not increase their premiums (30). Adverse selection began. Those who were sick purchased insurance—some from their hospital beds. Those with chronic conditions left the state's high-risk pool to purchase less expensive private coverage. The demand for insurance declined because low-risk individuals believed that they could buy insurance once they became ill, given the short waiting period.

Insurance companies filed lawsuits seeking large rate increases as their claims increased. Individuals who had insurance began to drop their coverage as the courts permitted insurers to increase their rates. Given the losses incurred by the insurers and the uncertainty over future rate increases, the number of insurers participating in the individual market decreased.

Washington State provides an example of the equity and efficiency consequences when the individual health insurance market is regulated. Insurers will exit markets and others will not enter when government regulation creates uncertainty whether profits can be earned. Consequently, few insurers will compete, and choice of insurers and products will be limited.

SUMMARY

The market structure of the health insurance industry was examined with respect to the extent of economies of scale, whether barriers to entry existed, and whether any insurers had any cost advantages over other insurers. Although there appear to be large economies of scale in the production and sale of health insurance, there are a large number of insurers and few barriers to entry. The market structure for insurance is considered to be competitive.

Blue Cross was established by hospitals and grew at a rapid rate because it was able to see the vast potential demand for coverage of health care costs. The commercial insurance companies entering the market after Blue Cross also grew because of their product and pricing innovations. They offered a benefit coverage (major medical insurance) that differed from that offered by Blue Cross, they offered indemnity payments rather than a service benefit policy to subscribers and providers, and they priced their premiums according to the experience of the group, which led to the demise of community rating. The newest entrants, HMOs and PPOs, were a response to market demand for lower premiums that was not being met by traditional insurers. Unless competition were possible, it is unlikely that consumers would have been offered a greater choice in benefits, cost-sharing arrangements, premiums to match their own experience, and types of insurance products.

The applicability of the anti-trust laws to the health field removed restrictions on the types of products insurers are permitted to sell. Previously, medical societies had been able to act anti-competitively to restrict an insurer's sale of cost control programs that interfered with physicians' decision-making authority. The previous role of providers in limiting the sale of cost control products by insurers illustrates the importance of competition in provider markets on the price and quantity of medical care. The demand for medical services and the supply of those services are linked together by the health insurance market. Thus, even if the health insurance market were competitive, restrictions in provider markets (either anti-competitive or legal) can have adverse effects on consumers.

The health insurance market is very price competitive, as indicated by the estimated high-price elastic firm demand curves, the recurring underwriting cycle, and inability of the Blues to maintain community rating.

The use of benefit/premium (medical loss) ratios as a measure of efficiency has lost its relevance given the wide variety of policies and functions performed by different insurers.

The performance of the health insurance industry has improved as employees (or employers acting on their behalf) have become more price sensitive in their choice of health plans and a large variety of types of health plans are now available. Indicative of the competitiveness of the industry is its lack of excess profits and cyclical periods of underwriting losses.

Competitive markets force insurers to minimize their administrative costs and to respond to insured groups demands for different types of insurance coverage. The incentives inherent in such competition are more effective for achieving economic efficiency in the demand and supply of health insurance than having one large firm administer a standard insurance policy for everyone. Innovations in benefit packages and in cost minimization are more likely to occur when there are strong competitive pressures than when firms, whether they are for-profit or non-profit, are protected from such competition.

A growing concern with regard to efficiency and equity, however, are regulations enacted by some states and those being considered by other states. These regulations, such as shorter waiting periods for pre-existing conditions, community rating, and state mandates, decrease the demand for insurance by allowing people to wait until they are ill before they buy insurance (shorter waiting periods), impose a regressive "tax" on low-income groups to subsidize the care of those who are older and at higher risk (community rating), and increase the cost of health insurance (state mandates), thereby decreasing the demand for insurance (31).

APPENDIX 1: THE USE OF MEDICAL LOSS RATIOS AS A MEASURE OF HEALTH PLAN PERFORMANCE

Critics of private health insurers have pointed to their high administrative costs and the correspondingly lower portion of claims payout (low medical loss ratio) as an indication of poor performance. These critics claim that it would be in the public interest if a greater portion of the premium dollar were paid out for medical services than retained for administration and profits. "Single Payer" advocates have used Canada's higher medical loss ratios to justify a Canadian-type system. Medical societies have (self-interestly) proposed limits on insurers' administrative expenses to increase physician payments.

Superficially it would appear that the lower the administrative costs (as a percentage of premiums) the more efficient the insurer, and that the insurer is less likely to skimp on quality of care. Further, the greater the proportion of the premium being returned in the form of medical services, the more apparent value the enrollee receives from buying health insurance.

A for-profit insurance company would only undertake those administrative functions that have a favorable cost-benefit ratio, otherwise they would be foregoing profit. If administrative expenses were wasteful, a competitive insurer could enter the market, have lower administrative costs, consequently charge lower premiums, and increase their market share. That this does not occur suggests that administrative costs are not a sign of inefficiency.

Can any validity be attached to either a high or low medical loss ratio?

The Absolute Size of the Premium

Concentrating on the administrative expense portion of the premium ignores the absolute size of the premium. Any health care system, whether it is Canada's or this country's Medicare system whose administrative costs are a small percentage, such as 3 percent for Medicare, may have *higher premiums* than a managed care firm offering the same benefits but whose administrative cost are a higher percentage of premiums. Medicare, which may simply pay for all claims submitted by health care providers, will have low administrative costs but also spend more in medical claims because it does not adequately check for fraud and abuse. Medicare may pay for services not performed, services may be up-coded, unnecessary services may be provided, and services are provided in more expensive settings when the patient could be cared for in an outpatient facility or in their own home.

The U.S. Government Accounting Office has claimed that Medicare's administrative costs are too low; that Medicare could save money (reduce their medical expenses) if they used some of the private sector's managed care techniques.

There are also a number of other reasons why medical loss ratios should not be used to indicate an insurer's efficiency, quality of care provided, or the value received by its enrollees.

Insurance Products Offered

The greater the variety of health insurance products offered by an insurer, the greater their administrative cost. An insurer that offers an indemnity product as well as a PPO, an HMO, pharmacy benefit plans, vision benefits, dental plans, life and disability insurance, and different combinations of deductibles and co-payments with each of the above plans is going to have a higher administrative cost than an insurer than offers fewer products and co-payment options.

Insurers that offer a wide variety of health plans have joint marketing, enrollment, and administrative costs that can be allocated in various ways to the different health plans. Depending upon how these joint costs are allocated, some health plans may show higher administrative costs than others.

Similarly, insurers that operate in different states may report different medical loss ratios based on how the insurer allocates joint costs across its state plans. For example, the insurer may centralize the marketing and enrollment costs of a large corporate account that has enrollees in multiple states.

Differences in the Types of Insurance Purchasers

Insurers that enroll a higher proportion of small groups and individuals will have higher marketing (hence administrative) costs than insurers that concentrate on large employer groups. It is much less costly to market to a single corporate headquarters for thousands of employees than to advertise and sign up a few employees at a time. Large employers will also perform some of the enrollment functions themselves. Insurer concern with adverse selection (hence monitoring costs) is greatly reduced when a large employer group is enrolled than when the same number of self-employed individuals seek to buy insurance.

Large employer groups typically have more comprehensive benefits than those enrolled in the individual market. Thus the medical loss ratio will also be higher among large groups for no other reason that the number of medical claims and cost of those claims will be higher among those with more comprehensive benefits.

The Functions Performed By the Insurer

Insurers differ in the functions they perform, which affects their administrative cost ratio. An insurer that undertakes utilization management rather than simply paying all claims submitted will have higher administrative costs (as a percentage of premiums) but lower premiums. These insurers will be more efficient as well as offer enrollees greater value for their premiums.

Similarly, an insurer that emphasizes preventive services to its enrollees, tracking enrollees by their age and the last time they had certain preventive services, will have higher administrative costs. Further, an insurer that collects data from both its enrollees and its providers on quality of care, patient waiting times for services, and patient satisfaction will have higher administrative expense than other types of insurers.

Relationships Between the Insurer and Its Providers

Administrative costs will be higher in those insurers that perform all the administrative functions themselves than when those same functions are the responsibility of their contracted providers. For example, an insurer that capitates a medical group in effect delegates various administrative functions, such as medical management and physician quality reviews, to the medical groups. The administrative costs for these functions are included in the medical group's negotiated capitation payment and are not visible; the insurer will appear to have a very high medical loss ratio compared to an insurer who does not delegate these functions.

Insurers who have a large provider network will have higher administrative costs than insurers that contract with fewer hospitals and physicians. In this case the size of the network, consequently the insurer's administrative cost, are determined by enrollee preferences as to how much provider choice and travel distance to a provider they are willing to accept.

Variability of Medical Loss Ratios

The use of medical loss ratios as an indication of insurer efficiency, quality, or to justify restricting for-profit insurers is inappropriate. Medical loss ratios among insurers can vary for many reasons. Some non-profit insurers have higher medical loss ratios than for-profit insurers, while some for-profits have higher medical loss ratios than non-profits. There is no consistent pattern. Even for the same insurer (whether it is for-profit or non-profit), its medical loss ratio varies greatly across different states.[7]

Rather than relying on such a flawed measure as an insurer's medical loss ratio, it would be more appropriate for those interested in health care reform to directly compare insurer performance according to quality of care provided, patient satisfaction, benefit structure, and overall premiums. While more difficult to do, such comparisons are more meaningful than relying on a simple medical loss ratio.

APPENDIX 2: DEVELOPING RISK-ADJUSTED PREMIUMS

Risk-adjusted premiums are based on various proxies for employee risk factors, such as age and sex. In the following example, for simplicity, age is used as the measure of risk for incurring medical expenditures (32).

Assume an employer group has ten employees that differ in age. As shown in Table 9-6, column 1 describes the four age levels of the employees. Column 2 indicates the risk factor associated with each age group. The "average" employee is assumed to be age 40 and to have a risk factor of 1.0. Each of the other age group's risk factors is calculated relative to the average employee whose risk factor is 1.0. For example, if a 30-year-old person, on average, incurs $800 med-

---

7. Robinson's article on which this discussion is based includes a table showing the medical loss ratios for a number of for-profit and non-profit insurers in the different states in which they operate. James C. Robinson, "Use and Abuse of the Medical Loss Ratio to Measure Health Plan Performance," *Health Affairs*, 16(4) July/August 1997, 176–187.

Table 9-6. A Hypothetical Example of Risk-Adjusted Premiums

Age	Risk Level	Number of Employees	Total Risk Level
30	0.8	3	2.4
40	1.0	2	2.0
50	1.3	3	3.9
60	1.6	2	3.2
Total		10	11.5

Average risk level per employee = 1.15, which is (11.5/10).

ical expenses in a year and the average employee who is a 40-year-old incurs $1,000 medical expenses, then the risk factor for the 30-year-old person is 0.8. Similarly, if 60-year-old employees incur, on average, $1,600 of medical expenses each year, then their risk factor, relative to those who are 40, is 1.6. The risk factors for each employee group can be calculated using past medical claims data.

(Another risk factor such as sex can be incorporated by simply expanding the rows (to eight) in the table above so that for each age group there is a risk factor for males and one for females.)

The third column in Table 9-6 lists the number of employees in each age group with their corresponding risk factor. Column 4 is a calculation of the total level of risk by age group. In the 30-year age group there are 3 employees, each with a 0.8 risk factor, for a risk total of 2.4. Summing up the total risk by each age group equals 11.5. Dividing the total risk level (11.5)

by the 10 employees results in an average risk factor per employee equal to 1.15.

Assume first that the employer does not use risk-adjusted premiums and pays $100 per member per month (PMPM) to each of two competing health plans. As shown in Table 9-7, each health plan enrolls five employees, who differ in their risk factors. Plan A enrolls two 30 year olds (total risk factor is 2 × 0.8 = 1.6), two 40 year olds (2 × 1.0 = 2), and one 50 year old (1.3), for a total risk level of 4.9. Plan B enrolls one 30 year old (0.8), two 50 year olds (2 × 1.3 = 2.6), and two 60 year olds (2 × 1.6 = 3.2) for a total risk level of 6.6.

Both health plans receive a total of $500 for five employees, but Plan A's risk level for those employees is 4.9 compared to 6.6 for Plan B. Plan A will make a profit based on preferred risk selection, while Plan B will lose money because it received a higher risk group. Plan B will eventually have to exit the industry, not because it is less efficient than Plan A but because it received a higher risk group.

If the employer used a risk-adjusted premium, then the average monthly premium per employee ($100 PMPM) is divided by the average risk level of the employees (1.15), which equals $87 PMPM.

Assuming the same employees went to the same health plan as in the previous example, then Plan A would receive

2 × 0.8 × $87. = $139.2 plus 2 × 1.0 × $87. = $174. plus 1 × 1.3 × $87. = $113.1 for a total amount of $426.30

Table 9-7. Risk Levels in Two Hypothetical Health Plans

	Plan A					Plan B				
Age	Risk Level	Number of Employees	Total Risk Level	PMPM $100	PMPM $87	Risk Level	Number of Employees	Total Risk Level	PMPM $100	PMPM $87
30	0.8	2	1.6	$200	$139.20	0.8	1	0.8	$100	$69.60
40	1.0	2	2.0	$200	$174.00	1.0	0	0	0	0
50	1.3	1	1.3	$100	$113.10	1.3	2	2.6	$200	$226.20
60	1.6	0	0	0	0	1.6	2	3.2	$200	$278.40
Totals		5	4.9	$500	$426.30		5	6.6	$500	$574.20

PMPM is Per Member Per Month

Plan B would receive $574 for its five employees who are at higher risk.

The above example assumed the employer paid the entire premium for each employee. The next example assumes an employer uses risk-adjusted premiums but that an employee choosing a more expensive health plan pays the additional cost of the more costly plan.

Each health plan competes for employees based on a demographically neutral premium (DNP); the premium is based on an average employee with a risk factor of 1.0. For example, an HMO offers a DNP of $100 PMPM. A competing PPO offers a DNP of $110 PMPM. As shown in Table 9-8, a 40 year old choosing the HMO pays no premium, and the employer pays the HMO $100. A 40 year old choosing the PPO would pay $10 per month and the employer would pay $100, with the PPO receiving its DNP of $110 PMPM. The PPO enrolling a 30 year old receives $88, which is the DNP multiplied by the employee's risk factor ($100 × 0.8 = $88.); that premium is split between the employee who pays $10, which is the additional amount of the more costly health plan, $DNP_{PPO} - DNP_{HMO}$ ($110 − $100), and the employer who pays $78 ($88 − $10). A 50 year old choosing the PPO would pay $10 ($DNP_{PPO} - DNP_{HMO}$, $110 − $100), and the employer would pay $133 (1.3 × $100 − $10).

When a health plan is paid a risk-adjusted premium, the plan is paid more for enrolling higher-risk employees and therefore has an incentive to compete for such enrollees. Further, high- and low-risk employees enrolling in the same plan pay the same amount.

REVIEW QUESTIONS

1. Describe the types of competitors in the health insurance market.
2. What components determine the size of a premium?
3. Does a benefit-to-premium (or medical loss) ratio close to 1.0 necessarily mean that the insurer is being efficient and is minimizing the cost of providing medical services?
4. What determines the price elasticity of demand for an individual insurer? Why does the price elasticity of demand facing the individual insurer differ from the overall market demand for health insurance?
5. What is the difference between "experience" rating and "community" rating? Under which pricing system do insurers have an incentive to engage in preferred risk selection?
6. Discuss whether or not community rating is economically efficient and equitable.
7. Explain why an insurer's pricing strategy of reducing its relative co-premium charged to an employee group would also reduce the average risk level of its subscribers.
8. What would be the effect of "risk-adjusted" premiums on insurers' engaging in preferred risk selection strategies?
9. Do All-Payer systems whereby the state regulates hospital charges so that every purchaser pays the same price for hospital care enhance competition among insurers? Who do you believe would be for and against All-Payer systems?

Table 9-8. Risk-Adjusted Premiums with Employees Paying the Additional Cost of a More Expensive Health Plan

Age	Risk Factor	DNP = $100			DNP = $110		
		Total Premium	Employee Co-Premium	Employee Payment	Total Premium	Employee Co-Premium	Employee Payment
30	0.8	$ 80	0	$ 80	$ 88	$10	$ 78
40	1.0	$100	0	$100	$110	$10	$100
50	1.3	$130	0	$130	$143	$10	$133
60	1.6	$160	0	$160	$176	$10	$166

DNP is Demographically Neutral Premium

10. Explain how managed care plans (such as HMOs) and defined contribution plans are alternative approaches for controlling moral hazard.

11. Why are Any Willing Provider laws anti-competitive?

12. How have previous anti-competitive restrictions by medical societies affected the types of health insurance products offered?

REFERENCES

1. Louis Reed, *Blue Cross and Medical Service Plans,* (Washington, D.C.: U.S. Public Health Service), 1947. Also see Robert Eilers, *Regulation of Blue Cross and Blue Shield Plans,* (Homewood, Ill.: Richard D. Irwin), 1963.

2. Ronald J. Vogel and Roger D. Blair, *Health Insurance Administrative Costs,* Social Security Administration, Office of Research and Statistics Paper 21, October 1975.

3. Roger D. Blair and Ronald J. Vogel, "A Survivor Analysis of Commercial Insurers," *Journal of Business,* 51(3), July 1978, 521–529.

4. Roger D. Blair, Jerry R. Jackson, and Ronald J. Vogel, "Economies of Scale in the Administration of Health Insurance," *Review of Economics and Statistics,* 57(2), May 1975: 185–189. In another study of the performance of Medicare (Part A) processing costs, H. E. Frech found lower cost per dollar processed, lower average processing time (in days), and fewer errors per $1,000 processed in for-profit as compared to not-for-profit firms. H. E. Frech III, "The Property Rights Theory of the Firm: Empirical Results from a Natural Experiment," *Journal of Political Economy,* 84(1), February 1976, 143–152.

5. Stephen T. Mennemeyer, "Effects of Competition on Medicare Administrative Costs," *Journal of Health Economics,* 3(2), August 1984: 137–154.

6. H. E. Frech, "Blue Cross, Blue Shield, and Health Care Costs: A Review of the Economic Evidence," in Mark V. Pauly, ed., *National Insurance: What Now, What Later, What Never?* (Washington, D.C.: American Enterprise Institute, 1980): 251–252, and Killard Adamache and Frank Sloan, "Competition Between Non-Profit and For-Profit Health Insurers," *Journal of Health Economics,* 2(3), December 1983: 225–243. The importance of the state tax exemption as a Blue Cross competitive cost advantage has diminished as more firms have become self-insured and, because of ERISA, are not subject to such premium taxes.

7. *Health Insurance: Comparing Blue Cross and Blue Shield Plans with Commercial Insurers,* Report to the Chairman, Subcommittee on Health, Committee on Ways and Means, House of Representatives (Washington, D.C.: U.S. General Accounting Office, July 1986): 20.

8. Adamache and Sloan, *op. cit.*

9. Charles D. Weller, "On 'FTC Sings the Blues' and Its Respondents," *Journal of Health Politics, Policy and Law,* 7(2), Summer 1982, 547–558.

10. H. E. Frech and Paul Ginsburg, "Competition Among Health Insurers," in Warren Greenburg, ed., *Competition in the Health Care Sector: Past, Present, and Future* (Germantown, Md.: Aspen Systems Corporation, 1978).

11. Mark V. Pauly, "Competition in Health Insurance Markets," *Law and Contemporary Problems,* 51(2), Spring 1989: 237–271.

12. Stephen E. Foreman, John A. Wilson, and Richard M. Scheffler, "Monopoly, Monopsony and Contestability in Health Insurance: A Study of Blue Cross Plans," *Economic Inquiry,* 34(4), October 1996, 662–677.

13. For a recent update on the Blues, see Robert Cunningham and Douglas Sherlock, "Bounceback: Blues Thrive As Markets Cool Toward HMOs," *Health Affairs,* 21(1) January/February 2002, 24–38.

14. Bruce A. Strombom, Thomas Buchmueller, and Paul J. Feldstein, "Switching Costs, Price Sensitivity, and Health Plan Choice," *Journal of Health Economics,* 21(1) January, 2002, 89–116.

15. For an early article discussing the underwriting cycle, see Jon Gabel, et al., "Tracing the Cycle of Health Insurance," *Health Affairs,* 11(4), Winter 1991, 48–61.

16. The disappointment of many observers over the apparent ineffectiveness of cost containment techniques during the late 1980s and early 1990s may have been the result of its effects being overshadowed by the underwriting cycle. Paul J. Feldstein and Thomas M. Wickizer, "Analysis of Private Health Insurance Premium Growth Rates: 1985–1992," *Medical Care,* 33(10), October 1995, 1035–1050.

17. For a more extensive discussion of community rating, see Pauly, "The Welfare Economics of Community Rating," *Journal of Risk and Insurance,* 37(3), September 1970, 407–418. See also, David F. Bradford and Derrick A. Max, *Intergenerational Transfers Under Community Rating,* (Washington D.C., American Enterprise Institute), 1996.

18. *Health Care Insurance Regulation Program: An Assessment of Effectiveness,* Executive Office of the Governor, Lewis Cass Building, Lansing, Mich., March 1973: p. 11. Also see, Dana P. Goldman, Arleen Leibowitz, Joan

Buchanan, and Joan Keesey, "Redistributional Consequences of Community Rating," *Health Services Research*, 32(1), April 1997, 71–86.

19. For a discussion of the adverse selection death spiral, see Michael Rothschild and Joseph E. Stiglitz, "Equilibrium in Competitive Insurance Markets: An Essay on the Economics of Imperfect Information," *Quarterly Journal of Economics*, 90(4) November 1976, 630–649.

20. "New York Finds Fewer People Have Health Insurance a Year After Reform," *The Wall Street Journal*, May 27, 1994, p. A2. See also Karen Pallarito, "Commissioner Berates Actuarial Report," *Modern Healthcare*, 24(43), October 24, 1994, p. 40.

21. Thomas Buchmueller and John DiNardo, "Did Community Rating Induce An Adverse Selection Death Spiral? Evidence from New York, Pennsylvania, and Connecticut," *American Economic Review*, 92(1), March 2002, 280–294.

22. Patricia M. Danzon, "The McCarran-Ferguson Act: Anticompetitive or Procompetitive?," *Regulation*, 15(2) Spring 1992, 38–47.

23. For a discussion of HMO profitability, see Mark V. Pauly, et al., "Competitive Behavior In the HMO Marketplace," *Health Affairs*, 21(1) January/February 2002, 194–202.

24. Paul J. Feldstein, Thomas M. Wickizer, and John R. C. Wheeler, "Private Cost Containment: The Effects of Utilization Review Programs on Health Care Use and Expenditures," *New England Journal of Medicine*, 318(20), May 19, 1988, 1310–1314.

25. Mark V. Pauly, "Paying the Piper and Calling the Tune: The Relationship Between Public Financing and Public Regulation of Health Care," in Mancur Olson, ed., *A New Approach to the Economics of Health Care*, (American Enterprise Institute for Public Policy Research: Washington, D.C.) 1981: 67–86.

26. Lawrence G. Goldberg and Warren Greenberg, "The Emergence of Physician-Sponsored Health Insurance: A Historical Perspective," in Warren Greenberg, ed., *Competition in the Health Care Sector*, (Germantown, Md.: Aspen Systems Corporation, 1978).

27. For early examples of such activities, see "The American Medical Association: Power, Purpose, and Politics in Organized Medicine," *Yale Law Journal*, 63(7), May 1954, 938–1022.

28. Jon B. Christianson, Stephen T. Parente, and Ruth Taylor, "Defined-Contribution Health Insurance Products: Development and Prospects," *Health Affairs*, 21(1) January/February 2002, 49–64.

29. Michael G. Vita, "Regulatory Restrictions on Selective Contracting: An Empirical Analysis of 'Any Willing Provider' Regulations," *Journal of Health Economics*, 20(6), November 2001, 955–966.

30. "Embers Glow Through Ashes of Washington State's Reform," *Medicine and Health Perspectives*, (Washington, D.C.: Faulkner and Gray), April 1, 1996, and Bill Richards, "Perils of Pioneering: Health-Care Reform in the State of Washington Riles Nearly Everyone," *The Wall Street Journal*, April 5, 1996, p. A1.

31. Gail Jensen and Michael Morrisey, "Employer-Sponsored Health Insurance and Mandated Benefit Laws," *Milbank Memorial Fund Quarterly*, 77(4) December 1999, 425–459.

32. The following article discusses the results of using different risk adjustment models. Wynand P.M.M. Van De Ven and Randall P. Ellis, "Risk Adjustment in Competitive Health Plan Markets," in *Handbook of Health Economics*, vol. 1A, eds. A. J. Culyer and J. P. Newhouse, (New York: North-Holland Press, 2000), 755–845.

CHAPTER

10

The Physician Services Market

KEY TERMS AND CONCEPTS

- Economies of scale in medical practice
- Survivor analysis
- Market power of medical groups
- Physician industry consolidation
- Monopoly model of physician pricing
- Monopolistic competition
- Supplier-induced demand
- Target income hypothesis
- Medicare physician assignment
- Resource-Based Relative Value Scale (RBRVS)
- Balance billing
- Income-related Medicare Part B premiums

Learning Objectives

Upon completing this chapter, the reader should be able to:

- Explain the reasons for the growth of medical groups.
- Understand physician pricing behavior.
- Discuss why the physician services market is charactrized as "monopolistic competition."
- Describe the theory and evidence supporting "Supplier Induced Demand."
- Explain why variations exist among physicians in their use rates.

INTRODUCTION

The emphasis of this chapter is on the efficiency with which physician services are produced, how those services are priced, and how well the physician services market performs. The physician services market is comprised of physician firms, either physicians in solo practice or medical groups. Although physicians are the most important input used in producing physician services, other inputs (both labor and non-labor, such as nurses, other personnel, medical supplies, and capital), are also used in producing physician services. Different combinations of these inputs, including physicians, can be used to produce physician services. Determination of the number of physicians and the market for medical education are discussed in separate chapters. Although these markets are closely related to the market for physician services, the rationale for discussing these subjects and the pricing and provision of physician services separately is that the determinants of the number of physicians are not identical to the factors that determine the quantity of physician services or how they are priced.

Overview of the Physician Services Market

The demand and supply of physician services and the inter-relationship between this market and the physician manpower and education sectors are more easily visualized with reference to Figure 10-1. This diagram is also useful for understanding different types of public policies that may influence the physician services market.

The demand for physician services is determined by factors such as those discussed previously. There are non-economic factors, such as need and cultural-demographic factors; the economic factors are the patient's income, the price the patient must pay for physician services (as well as the price of substitute and complementary services), the type and comprehensiveness of insurance coverage, and any time costs that are involved in the purchase and use of physician services.

The price of physician services as shown in Figure 10-1 is determined by the interaction of both supply and demand factors. Price, in turn, influences patient demand and the amount of services providers are willing to provide.

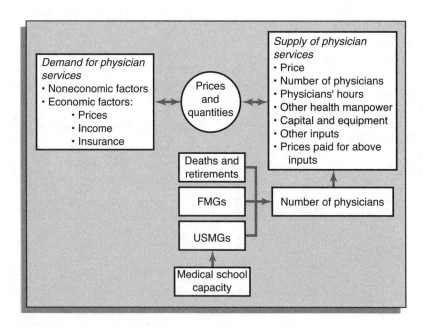

Figure 10-1. The market for physician services.

The supply of physician services is affected by the price received for physician services (a movement along the supply curve of physician services) and by the cost of producing those services (changes in those costs result in shifts in the supply curve). The cost depends upon input productivities and input prices. These are affected by the number of physicians, the number of hours they work, their use of auxiliaries, the capital and equipment available, and other inputs and expenses necessary to the provision of physician services, such as malpractice coverage. The number of physicians combined with other inputs determines the available supply of such services. Physician services may be provided using different combinations of physicians and other health manpower. Physicians may undertake to perform all of their tasks themselves, or they may delegate varying amounts of those tasks to auxiliaries. With a greater degree of task delegation, physicians will be able to increase their productivity. The extent to which physicians delegate their tasks will affect not only the quantity and type of physician services available, but also their cost.

In the short run, the firm producing physician services (whether it is the solo practitioner or large multi-specialty medical group) can increase its output by increasing all of the inputs except physicians. Physician hours, which can also be varied, are determined by the labor-leisure trade-off; the extent to which the physician is willing to vary their hours of work as both the price received per hour of work and his or her income changes. Namely, do physicians reduce (increase) their hours of work as their prices increase (decrease)? The sum of all the physician-firm supply curves is the industry supply curve of physician services.

The long run is that period of time in which the fixed input (the number of physicians) can be changed. Changes in the number of physicians result from deaths and retirements, immigration of foreign-trained medical graduates and physicians, and increases in the number of U.S.-trained medical graduates (USMGs). The number of USMGs is determined by the demand for and supply of medical education. The demand for a medical education is influenced by a number of factors, among which is the relative rate of return to such an education; as shown in Figure 10-1, the price and quantity determined in the physician services market (which is equivalent to gross physician income) is one component of that rate of return.

As shown in Figure 10-1, medical education is an important determinant of the number of physicians and, consequently, the supply of physician services. Separate chapters are devoted to an analysis of both the physician manpower and medical education markets, to include the development of their structural characteristics, their consequent effect on performance, and the relevant public policies within each market.[1]

Government policies have intervened at several points in physician markets. With respect to the demand for services, Medicare and Medicaid have served to stimulate the demand for services among specific population groups. In addition to the direct effects of these two programs, there were also indirect consequences: persons not subsidized by Medicare and Medicaid faced higher prices for physician services as demand by Medicare and Medicaid patients increased; price controls imposed by Medicare and Medicaid on the price of physician services affected the availability of services to both Medicare and Medicaid patients as well as privately insured patients. The hours physicians were willing to work and the time Medicare and Medicaid patients had to wait to receive such services were also affected. Examples of government price controls on physicians' fees were the imposition of federal price controls on all medical services between 1971 and 1974, the Medicare Economic Index (limits on physician fees) enacted in the 1970s, and the 1992 Medicare physician payment system known as the Resource Based Relative Value Scale (RBRVS), together with its annual updates, which controlled annual percent increases in physician fees.

---

1. Quality-assurance mechanisms are placed, primarily, on medical inputs, such as on the training requirements for physicians, and not on the services provided. The development of such "process" quality measures has had important effects on the structure of health manpower and health education markets. Alternative approaches to achieving quality assurance and their effect on performance are therefore discussed in chapters dealing with the manpower and education markets.

Government policies on the supply side have, in the past, resulted in increased numbers of physicians by providing subsidies for both the construction of new medical schools and for existing schools to increase their enrollments. Government loans and scholarships were provided (through the medical schools) to medical students which, by lowering the cost of a medical education, increased its demand. Government policy has affected the inflow of foreign-trained medical graduates and physicians through changes in immigration policies. State legislation limiting who can practice medicine and defining the tasks that may be performed by various categories of health manpower also affected the supply of physician services.

Objectives of the Physician-Firm

In other markets, firms set prices and output to maximize profit subject to the constraint of market demand. These assumptions are important for predicting supplier behavior, namely that firms will attempt to minimize their costs, set price and output according to their demand and cost conditions, and how the firm's price and output would change when demand and costs change.

While these assumptions may be sufficiently accurate at an aggregate level when analyzing the physician services market (such as predicting the effect on prices when insurance increases patient demand or the supply of physicians increase), its usefulness at the level of the individual physician-firm has been questioned (1).

There has been a great deal of debate in the health economics literature whether physician-firms have as their objective maximization of profits and, second, whether they are constrained by market demand; physicians may "create" demand for their services. Further, in the heavily regulated Medicare and Medicaid markets, physicians do not set prices, but instead face government-determined prices. The validity of the profit-maximization assumption, the ability of physicians to set their own price and output, and whether physicians are constrained by limited demand, has changed over time. Previously, physicians were less constrained by government-regulated prices and by managed care organizations. It is likely that when physicians had more market power (greater ability to set prices and manipulate patient demand), they did not seek to maximize profit but instead to maximize their utility, which consisted of some combination of profit and what was best for their patient.

In more recent years as managed care organizations instituted utilization management and selected physicians for their networks based, in part, on physician performance, physician market power declined, and the assumptions of profit maximization subject to the constraint of market demand have become more useful. The role of the physician as the patient's agent, however, continues to be important and, given extensive insurance coverage and imperfect patient information, provides physicians with some market power. As will be discussed further, this model of the physician-firm as a competitor with some market power (monopolistic competition) is used when analyzing their pricing behavior.

When evaluating the performance of the market for physician services, observed measures of performance will be compared with what might be expected to occur in a hypothetical competitive market. The reasons for any possible divergence between the observed and hypothetical outcomes will then be analyzed, and policies to improve the market will be proposed.

THE STRUCTURE OF THE PHYSICIAN SERVICES MARKET

In a price-competitive market, the number of competitors is determined by the extent of economies of scale and whether there are any entry barriers. In describing the structure of the physician services market, it is important to determine the extent to which there are cost savings to be gained by practicing in large medical groups; there are few restrictions on physician mobility into different markets. As will be discussed in the chapter on medical education, there have been (and still are) barriers to entry into the medical profession. Physicians must be licensed, they must graduate from an approved medical school, and the number of spaces in medical schools has been restricted. However, given the large number of practicing physicians even if entry into medicine is limited, it is still possible that the market for physician services could be competitive.

For more than 100 years, the predominant form of medical practice was solo practice with fee-for-service reimbursement. Given the large number of physician-firms in a market, the structure of the physician services market could have been characterized as competitive, however there was very little price competition. Various restrictions limited price competition among competitors, such as limits on both physician advertising and on insurance companies' ability to negotiate discount prices among physicians. The applicability of the anti-trust laws to the health field in the early 1980s eliminated physician-imposed restrictions on advertising and price competition. As competitive restrictions were removed and the number and size of managed care organizations increased, physicians began to compete on price to be included in HMO and insurer provider networks. Price competition changed the structure of the industry.

Economies of Scale in Medical Practice

To survive and profit in a price-competitive market, firms must minimize their costs of production. Thus one explanation for the shift from solo to group practice is that physicians could increase their productivity and lower their costs if they were to take advantage of any economies of scale in group practice. The average cost of providing physician services is expected to decline from sharing inputs such as aides, equipment, and offices and from volume discounts on supplies.

Studies on economies of scale attempt to determine which size practices have the lowest average cost for producing physician services. Further, it is possible to estimate the amount of inefficiency that exists among physician practices by calculating the increase in productivity that would occur if existing sized groups were equal to the size that is estimated to be of lowest cost. It is important, however, to separately analyze physician practices in urban and in rural areas, otherwise the extent of inefficiency for rural practices will be overstated. The optimal (least cost) size of practice in a rural area will be smaller since patient travel costs are higher given the lower population density. *The optimal size of a practice should consider not only practice costs, but also patient travel costs.* The larger the group size in a rural area, the greater is patient travel costs. The optimal size practice, therefore, is one that combines both practice costs and patient travel costs, which would result in smaller practices in rural than urban areas (2).

A problem in estimating economies of scale in medical group practice is the definition and measurement of outputs and inputs. Large medical groups provide a greater variety of outputs than do small groups or solo practices. Larger groups are also more likely to own laboratories and x-ray facilities and have different types of contractual arrangements with HMOs and health plans, thereby requiring additional administrative personnel. Unless outputs and inputs are measured accurately and adjustments made for differences in outputs, the results of studies may incorrectly conclude that large groups have higher costs and are therefore less efficient.

Detailed information on the quantity and mix of each of the services provided in a physician's office is generally unavailable. Empirical studies must therefore use proxy measures for physician services, such as annual gross patient revenues. Although this measure may reflect differences in quality and service mix among practices, it contains a serious problem in that higher patient billings may not reflect differences in output but may result from higher prices being charged for similar services.

Another often-used proxy for the output of a physician's practice is the weekly number of office visits, which implicitly assumes that quality does not vary by size of group. Physician productivity studies also generally assume that the mix of patient visits among different physician practices is similar. Over time, however, the physician output mix has changed; for example, specialists perform a greater proportion of all physician services.

The measurement of manpower inputs, with differing relative productivities, in production function studies can bias the results unless different manpower categories are separately measured. Physician extenders, such as physician assistants and pediatric nurse practitioners, are the closest substitutes for the physician and are more productive than are allied health workers (e.g., registered nurses), medical technicians (e.g., x-ray and lab technicians), and nonmedical assistants (e.g., clerical and administrative persons).

Also important in interpreting studies on economies of scale is whether there are selection biases in the types of physicians that join group practices. If, for example, less productive physicians are more likely to join one form of medical practice than another, then differences in productivit (hence cost per unit of output) may be more a result of the type of physician than the size of the practice.

Two types of studies have been undertaken to determine the extent of economies of scale in medical groups. The first examines whether patient revenues and/or visits per physician are higher in larger than in smaller practices. The second is a "survivor" analysis, which assumes that the fastest growing size of group is the most efficient.

According to empirical studies, the cost-size relationship appears to be U shaped; small groups appear to be more productive than solo practitioners, but very large groups are less productive (per physician) than smaller groups. For example, using data from the late 1960s, Reinhardt concluded that physicians in groups generate about 5 percent more patient visits and billings than those in solo practice (3). The average number of weekly patient visits for general practitioners (GPs) in groups was 16 percent higher than for solo GPs. Two other studies, one using data on physician office visits from a 1978 national survey of group practice, the other using practice revenues, found that group size had a negative effect on the physician's hourly patient load and revenues; the larger the group, the lower the physician's productivity and/or office revenues (4).

Pope and Burge calculated the optimum size of a medical group by various categories, such as for single specialty groups, e.g., primary care, cardiology, surgery, and also for multi-specialty groups. They found that the optimal size group varies by these categories, being largest for multi-specialty groups with the other groups having about five physicians each. The amount of inefficiency that exists for each of these types of groups (which is the difference between their actual and optimal size and the increased productivity of being larger) varies, but generally being less than 10 percent (5).

Several of these studies attempted to determine whether the finding of economies of scale is due to physicians in different sizes of groups using the optimal number of aides. Early studies concluded that physicians hired less than the optimal number of aides. Using 1965 to 1967 data, Reinhardt determined that the average solo physician could profitably employ twice as many auxiliaries. Employing four rather than two auxiliaries, which was the average during 1965 to 1967, would have resulted in a 25 percent increase in the number of patient visits per physician (6). Reinhardt calculated the optimal number of aides for a solo physician based on the price received per visit, the marginal productivity of an aide, and the weekly wage of the aide. (The marginal productivity of the aide, which is the additional number of visits produced by the aide multiplied by the price received per visit is the marginal revenue product of the aide, or the additional value of that aide. The physician should be willing to pay a weekly wage—assuming no additional costs—equal to the additional value generated by that aide.) The employment of aides should increase as the price of the visit increases and decrease as the cost of aides increase.

Using 1976 data on office-based physicians, Brown re-estimated the production analysis performed earlier by Reinhardt and found that physicians in group practice were 22 percent more productive than those in solo practice (7). Brown concluded that solo and group physicians used nurses efficiently but overutilized non-nurses, such as clerical and secretarial help. The increased productivity of group physicians was primarily due to greater use of physician assistants.[2] Brown found that the overall use of aides by physicians declined after 1978, attributing the decline to the rapid increase in the supply of physicians after 1980 (with a consequent change in their wage relative to aides) and the changing specialty distribution of physicians (using a different number of aides).

As shown in Table 10-1 (which is an update of Brown's table), the per-physician use of aides increased more than 40 percent, from 1.72 to 2.45, since 1985. It is likely that this is the result of both the increase in number of physicians practicing in groups as well as increases in the size of groups in response to the more competitive managed care environment.

The second type of study on economies of scale relied on survivor analysis, which is based on the premise that as a result of competitive market pressures, the most efficient size practice would expand while less efficient practices will contract. Survivor-type analyses implicitly incorporate patient travel costs since patients would prefer to pay higher prices to go to smaller, higher cost practices than traveling to larger, lower cost practices located further away.

Marder and Zuckerman examined changes in the size distribution of medical practices for three periods,

---

2. For a group practice to determine whether they are over or under utilizing aides, it is necessary to have the following information: first, an estimate of the marginal productivity (MP) of each of the inputs used in producing a physician visit. (The marginal product of each input is derived from a production function for a physician office visit.) Next, the marginal product of each input is divided by its cost per hour. The resulting ratio is then compared for each of the inputs. For example, assume that the MP of a physician is 2.8 visits per hour, and the MP of an aide is 0.8 visits per hour, their respective costs (wage) per hour are $75 and $18, and their ratios (MP/physician wage and MP/aide wage) are 0.037 and 0.044 respectively. Comparing the MP per dollar spent on physicians to the MP per dollar spent on aides indicates that aides (in this example) have a higher MP per dollar spent and are therefore being underutilized. Hiring an additional aide would increase the total number of physician visits produced but cause a decrease in the MP of that new aide (because of the law of diminishing returns) from (for example) 0.8 visits to 0.67. Given their respective MPs and the same relative costs per hour, the use of aides is now optimal since the MP per dollar spent on physicians (0.037) is equal to the MP per dollar spent on aides (0.037). (For a given output level, the optimal use of inputs could have been achieved if the group practice reduced the use of the physician input, thereby moving up the physician's MP curve and raising the ratio of the MP/physician's wage.) Aides would have been overutilized in the earlier example if their initial MP was 0.5 visits per hour instead of 0.8, in which case their ratio would have been 0.027 compared to 0.037 for the physician input. Thus, to determine optimal use of inputs, it is necessary to know both the relative MPs and relative wage rates of each input used in the production of a physician visit.

Table 10-1.   Physicians and Aides Employed in Offices of Physicians, 1970–2001

	1970	1975	1980	1985	1990	1995	2001
(1) Total Employment in Offices of Physicians (thousands)	477	618	777	894	1,098	1,512	1,774
(2) Office-based Practicing Physicians (thousands)	188	213	271	329	360	427	514
(3) Aides = (1) – (2)	289	405	506	565	738	1,085	1,260
(4) Aides/Physicians = (3) / (2)	1.54	1.90	1.87	1.72	2.05	2.54	2.45

Source: U.S. Department of Health and Human Services, *Health, United States,* various issues: *1983–1986:* Table 96, p. 217, and *2002:* Table 99, p. 269; American Medical Association, Division of Survey and Data Resources, *Physician Characteristics and Distribution in the U.S., 2003–2004 ed.,* (Chicago: AMA, 2003), Table 5.1, p. 320.

Note: Totals exclude persons in health-related occupations who are working in nonhealth industries, as classified by U.S. Bureau of the Census.

1965 to 1969, 1969 to 1975, and 1975 to 1980 (8). The authors concluded that in the period up to 1975, solo practices (one to two physicians) were less efficient since all other size groups grew. In the later period, 1975 to 1980, solo practice continued to decline but by a very small amount, and there was very little change in the other single specialty size groups. For multi-specialty groups, only large multi-specialty groups (100 or more physicians) increased significantly and were therefore considered to be efficient. For single specialty groups, small sized groups appear to be most efficient.

These findings of economies of scale appear to be confirmed by more recent (available) data indicating that more physicians are joining group practices. As shown in Table 10-2, in 1969, 21.7 percent of physicians were in group practice; by 1980, this had increased to 32.8 percent, and by 1996 to 46.2 percent. The fastest-growing form of group practice during the 1980s was the single-specialty form of practice, increasing from 10.9 to 19.6 percent of physicians between 1980 and 1996. It is interesting to note that while there are three times as many single-specialty groups than multi-specialty groups, multi-specialty groups are much larger in average size, 23.4 versus 6.4.

As shown in Table 10-3, the group size that has increased most rapidly has been the largest, those with more than 50 physicians. Such groups now include about 36 percent of all physicians in group practice.

Table 10-2. Number, Average Size, and Distribution of Office-Based Physicians by Group Affiliation, Selected Years, 1969–1996

Type of Practice	Distribution of Physicians According to Type of Practice			Number of Group Practices			Average Size of Physician Group		
	1969	1980	1996	1969	1980	1996	1969	1980	1996
Total Office-Based Physicians (Nonfederal)(a)	100.0	100.0	100.0	—	—	—	—	—	—
Individual Practice(b)	78.3	67.2	53.8	—	—	—	—	—	—
Group Practice	21.7	32.8	46.2(c)	6,371	10,762	19,658(d)	6.2	8.2	9.3
Single-Specialty Group Practice	7.1	10.9	19.6	3,169	6,156	13,934	4.1	4.8	6.4
Multi-Specialty Group Practice	13.2	20.1	24.9	2,418	3,552	4,396	10.1	15.2	23.4
Family or General Group Practice	1.5	1.8	1.7	784	1,054	1,328	3.5	4.5	5.4

Sources: National Center for Health Statistics, *Health, United States, 1986*, DHHS Publication (PHS) 87-1232, Public Health Service (Washington, D.C.: U.S. Government Printing Office, December 1986), p. 163. J. N. Hung and G. A. Roeback, *Distribution of Physicians, Hospitals, and Hospital Beds in the United States, 1969*, vol. 2, Metropolitan Areas Center for Health Services Research and Development (Chicago: American Medical Association, 1970). P. L. Havlicek, *Medical Groups in the United States: A Survey of Practice Characteristics*, (Chicago: American Medical Association, 1999), pp. 41–45.

(a) "Total office-based physicians" includes all patient care physicians except residents, interns, and full-time hospital staff. In 1996 there were 445,765 office-based physicians, which excluded 153,159 residents and interns as well as full-time hospital staff who provided patient care.

(b) The AMA defines a "group" as three or more physicians. Therefore, "Individual Practice" includes offices with a single physician and offices with two physicians.

(c) Excludes 477 physician positions in groups with unknown specialty composition.

(d) Excludes 162 groups whose specialty composition was unknown.

Table 10-3.   Distribution of Groups and Group Physicians by Group Size

	Distribution of Groups			Distribution of Physicians		
Group Size	1969	1980	1996(a)	1969	1980	1996(b)
Total number	6,371	10,762	19,468	40,093	88,290	206,557
			Percent Distribution			
3–4	65.0%	55.3%	45.9%	34.6%	22.7%	15.0%
5–15	30.3	37.5	44.2	34.2	32.9	30.7
16–25	2.4	3.6	4.8	7.6	8.7	9.0
26–49	1.5	2.2	2.8	8.2	9.1	9.1
50 +	0.8	1.4	2.3	15.4	26.6	36.2
Total	100.0	100.0	100.0	100.0	100.0	100.9

Source: Steve G. Vahovich, *Profile of Medical Practice, 1973 ed.,* (Chicago, IL: American Medical Association, 1973): Table 11; Sharon R. Henderson, *Medical Groups in the U.S., 1980* (Chicago, IL: American Medical Association, 1982): Table 3-2; Penny L. Havlicek, *Medical Groups in the U.S.: A Survey of Practice Characteristics, 1999 ed.* (Chicago, IL: American Medical Association, 1999): Table 3-1.

(a) Excludes 352 groups with unknown size.

(b) These figures represent physician positions. These figures were obtained by asking groups to report the number of physicians in their groups. Because physicians may practice in more than one group, some physicians may be counted more than once. Thus, these figures may overstimate the number of group physicians.

Note: In 1980, 100+ group size totaled 18,899 (21.4%) physicians.
In 1996, 100+ group size numbered 59,179 (28.7%) physician positions.

The percent of physicians in the other group sizes have either declined (the smallest groups), or have remained constant.

Based on the above empirical studies, the observed increase in the number of physicians in group practice and the increase in size of each group suggests the following: group practice is a more efficient form of organization; the optimal size of group varies according to specialty practice; and the extent of inefficiency between actual and optimal size is relatively small, less than 10 percent. Thus the trend toward group practice must be examined for reasons other than lower average costs resulting from economies of scale.

Additional Reasons for the Growth of Medical Groups

There are several reasons, unrelated to increased physician productivity, why both the size of medical groups and their number have increased.

Informational Economies of Scale: A distinguishing characteristic of the medical market is the lack of purchaser information on physicians, their accessibility, quality, bedside manner, and prices. Getzen uses this lack of patient information as an explanation for the formation of medical groups (9). Physicians are better able than patients to evaluate other physicians. There are therefore "informational economies of scale" to medical groups; it is less costly for the medical group to evaluate and monitor their member physicians than for consumers to do so. The higher patients' search costs, the larger is the optimal size of the group. Being a member of a medical group conveys information to patients regarding the quality of its members; it is equivalent to a "brand name" for physicians in that group.

A new physician entering a market is at a disadvantage compared to established physicians in that it takes time to develop a reputation and to build their practice. (An established physician, relative to a new physician with an unknown reputation, would have a less price elastic demand curve, hence able to charge a higher price relative to marginal cost.) By joining a medical group, the group's reputation is immediately transferred to the new physician. The new group physician is able to receive patients from other, busier physicians in the group; they become a better substitute to established physicians. In return for transferring the reputation of a group to a new physician, the group usually extracts some of the new physician's income and places them on probationary status for two to four years before they become a partner in the group.[3]

The reputation of the group is more important to the patient for those physician services that are less frequently used and that are more difficult for the patient to evaluate. It is for this reason that specialists are more likely to be part of a group than family practitioners. Patients are better able to evaluate the manner or style of a physician than the physician's technical ability. Finding a specialist involves greater search costs on the part of the patient (as well as by an insurer or employer contracting for physician services). Multi-specialty groups offer greater informational economies of scale than do groups comprised of family practitioners.

Reduction of Risk and Uncertainty: The desire by physicians to reduce uncertainty and share risk is an additional reason for their participation in medical groups. When physician compensation in a group is not directly related to productivity, the physician's risk is reduced. Solo practitioners are likely to experience greater variation in workload and income than are members of a group practice who share the workload. Risk-averse physicians are more willing to trade off the greater incentives of solo practice (whereby they receive the full return from their work effort and do not have to share their revenues) to become part of a group. The larger the size of the medical group, the smaller the uncertainty (variation) over one's annual income.

The trade-off with less risk is that productivity incentives decline as the physician receives less of his or her own marginal revenue. Gaynor and Gertler estimate that more risk-averse physicians are willing to sacrifice about 11 percent of their gross income compared to less risk-averse physicians (10).

Large groups with greater sharing of revenues will be less productive than smaller groups whose compensation is more directly related to their productivity. Disputes among group physicians over compensation are an important reason why many physicians have not joined groups and why groups have dissolved. Further, when physicians in a large group share the costs of inputs, each physician has an incentive to increase their use of inputs if the benefit they receive from the additional input use exceeds their share of the additional costs (11). And, as the size of the group increases, each physician's incentive to monitor the behavior of others in the group decreases since the benefits of monitoring must be shared among more physicians while the individual bears the costs of monitoring. To provide productivity incentives and to limit inefficiencies, large groups rely on physician committees and management to determine compensation and resource allocation, a source of dissatisfaction and conflict among group physicians.

The difficulty of closely matching productivity and efficiency incentives to physician compensation as the size of the group increases is an important reason for diseconomies of scale that limit the size of medical groups.

Increased Market Power: Large medical groups have greater market power than smaller groups, which enables them to increase their market share and/or receive higher prices from health plans. Large groups are better able to market their services directly to health plans and hospitals. It is less costly (both administratively and in evaluating performance) for an insurer to contract with a single large group than with many individual physicians. Health plans are also able to shift the responsibility of utilization management to large medical groups. Further, large medical groups were more willing than smaller medical groups to accept capitation contracts from HMOs since they were better able to spread the risk of large medical expenses over a larger patient population. The HMO was thereby able to shift its risk to the large group. (Unfortunately, many large medical groups were unable to manage their capitation contracts and lost money; consequently few medical groups currently accept capitation contracts.)

Large medical groups also have greater leverage over hospitals because they can decide to which hospitals they will admit their patients. They are therefore

---

3. The group would be expected to add new physicians up to the point where the marginal revenue product of the last physician equals the average revenue product of the group. When MRP = ARP, then average income, which is equivalent to average revenue product, would be at a maximum.

better able than smaller groups to negotiate preferred arrangements with their selected hospitals, from having the hospital share some of its revenue with the group ("risk-sharing pools") to having the hospital invest capital to increase the group's productivity.

Difficulties in Developing Large Medical Groups

Although large medical groups are able to spread overhead expenses over a greater volume of patient visits thereby reducing per-unit costs, it takes time to build the personnel and data infrastructure to manage the complex clinical and financial needs of a large medical group. Access to capital for developing the necessary infrastructure and for expansion has also been a constraint on the growth of groups. Further, many large medical groups that accepted capitation and risk-based contracts failed to develop the necessary actuarial expertise and information systems. As a result, these groups were forced to file for bankruptcy.

Perhaps the most difficult aspect of building a large medical group is bringing together physicians who have a common vision and group culture. Developing a common group culture among physicians previously in independent practice often takes years. Disagreements among group physicians over governance, compensation, and productivity incentives have led to the breakup of many medical groups. Smaller groups have been better able to perform continuous peer monitoring and productivity-based payment.

Monopolistic Competition

The market structure for physician services can be characterized as monopolistic competition. This market structure has elements of a competitive market in that there are many competitors and no entry barriers. Physicians can move into more profitable areas or areas having less managed care penetration. Monopolistic competition is characteristic of a monopoly model in that the firm has a downward sloping demand curve. Each of the many physician-firms has some market power in that it provides a service that is somewhat differentiated from its competitors.

Each physician-firm's monopoly power is derived from the fact that other physician-firms are not perfect substitutes. Neither physicians nor their services are homogeneous; they differ not only in the variety of physician services offered but also in the manner in which each physician provides that service. There are real as well as perceived differences in their quality, perhaps reflected in the medical school they attended and where they had their residency; they differ in their age and sex, in how they communicate with their patients, in how long patients must wait and the value the patient places on waiting time, the location of the physician's office, etc.

The industry demand curve for physician services is less price elastic than the demand curve facing the physician-firm. As shown in Figure 10-2, there are two demand curves. DD is the overall market demand for physician services, and dd is the demand curve facing the individual physician; dd has a more gradual slope (more price elastic) than DD since there are better substitutes for each physician than there are for all physicians' services. Thus empirical findings that the demand for physicians' services is price inelastic would refer to the overall market demand curve (DD) and not the demand facing the individual physician firm (dd).

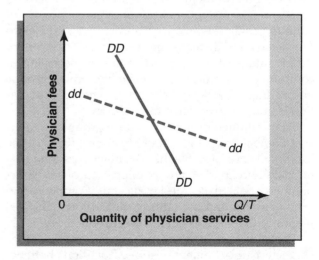

Figure 10-2. Monopolistic competitive market for physician services.

Table 10-4. Price Elasticities of Demand for Physician-Firms

Study	Dependent Variable	Elasticity
T. R. McCarthy (1985)	physician services	−3.07 to −3.32
R. H. Lee and J. Hadley (1981)		−2.80 to −5.07
R. A. McLean (1980)		−1.75 to −2.16

Sources: R. H. Lee and J. Hadley, "Physicians' Fees and Public Medical Care Programs," *Health Services Research,* Summer 1981, 16(2), pp. 185–203; T. R. McCarthy, "The Competitive Nature of the Primary-Care Physician Services Market," *Journal of Health Economics,* June 1985, 4(2), pp. 93–117; R. A. McLean, "The Structure of the Market for Physicians' Services," *Health Services Research,* Fall 1980, 15(3), pp. 271–280.

Estimates of physician-firm price elasticities of demand are shown in Table 10-4, indicating that physician-firm demand curves are price elastic. The price elasticity of demand for primary care physician services has been estimated to be about −3.0, meaning that a 1 percent increase in price will result in about a 3 percent decrease in the quantity of services demanded (12).

In summary, the structure of the physician services industry has changed over time. It is consolidating. The image of the physician in solo practice has disappeared. More physicians are part of a larger economic entity, and the average size of groups is increasing.

The advantages of group practice include economies of scale, (to include the sharing of managerial expertise, technical personnel, claims processing, physician recruitment, utilization management, and marketing), informational (reputation) economies of scale to purchasers, reduced uncertainty and risk to physicians, and increased market power. The primary disadvantage of group practice lies in the lack of a common group culture among newly formed groups and reduced efficiency incentives when compensation is not directly related to productivity.

The continued growth of medical groups and their size, some in the hundreds of physicians (in multiple locations), indicates that the advantages of economies of scale and market power appear to offset diseconomies related to designing fair compensation arrangements and monitoring other physicians' behavior with regard to quality and productivity.

The physician services market is believed to be characteristic of "monopolistic competition" both because of the large number of competitors within a market and because each physician has a somewhat differentiated service, thereby providing each physician with a downward sloping demand curve.

A monopolistic competitive market structure can be used in the following ways to explain differences in physician fees. When variations in prices and increases in prices are observed, a competitive model relies on differences in costs (e.g., physician office expenses) to explain these price changes or differences. When these variations in prices cannot be explained by just differences in costs, then an economist explores whether differences in price elasticities of demand among firms or changes in price elasticities are the reason for changes in prices; this is the monopoly explanation. To determine whether price elasticities have changed, an economist would examine whether consumers have become more or less price sensitive, such as by having more comprehensive insurance coverage.

The next section discusses how physician-firms set price in a monopolistically competitive market and their responses to factors that have changed the price elasticity of physician demand curves over time.

MARKET CONDUCT

Firms in different market structures exhibit different patterns of economic as well as political behavior. Firms that are in a monopolistic competitive industry are characterized by their ability to price their services as would a firm with some monopoly power. Also, the greater the number of firms in a market, the more difficult it is for the firms to collude on methods to maintaining their monopoly power by limiting price competition; it is costly for the firms to negotiate and agree on prices and to monitor each others' pricing behavior. Also, such pricing agreements would be in violation of the anti-trust laws. Thus firms in monopolistic competitive industries are also characterized by political behavior to limit price competition. Consequently, firms in a monopolistic competitive industry compete in two markets. The first is the economic marketplace where each firm competes against the other firms. The second is the political marketplace where competing firms are allies seeking beneficial economic legislation, such as through enactment of State Practice Acts or imposing sanctions on physicians for engaging in "unethical," that is, competitive behavior.

The Period Prior to Medicare and Medicaid

Prior to the passage of Medicare and Medicaid in the mid 1960s, patients paid more than 60 percent of physician fees out of pocket, government paid 7 percent, and private insurance paid for 32 percent of physician expenditures. See Figure 10-3 (page 228).

Insurance coverage for payment of physician fees was not uniform among all physician specialties; it was primarily for in-hospital physician services. Hospital-based specialties, such as radiology and anesthesiology, as well as surgeons (whose services were considered to be more costly), had the largest percent of their revenues covered by private insurance. As insurance paid a greater portion of the surgeon's fee, the decline in the patient's price sensitivity lowered the price elasticity of demand for surgeons' services. (For a discussion of this point, see Chapter 5, "The Demand For Medical Care" Appendix: The Effect of Co-Insurance on the Demand for Medical Care.) Those medical specialties that required less use of the hospital (such as primary care physicians, pediatrics, and psychiatry) had the smallest percent of their revenues covered by private insurance. Thus the demand curve for primary care physician services was much more price elastic than that of the surgeon.

Not surprisingly, members of those specialties with the largest percent of their revenues paid by insurance also had the highest incomes.

A Monopoly Model of Physician Pricing: The effect of having insurance coverage for surgical services as compared to primary care services is shown in Figure 10-4 (see page 229). The initial demand and marginal revenue curves are D_1 and MR_1. The physician's marginal cost curve is MC which, for simplicity, is assumed to be constant. The resulting price is P_1.

Increased insurance coverage for physician services makes the demand for surgical services less price elastic; it shifts from D_1 to D_2. The marginal revenue curve also shifts rightward. Thus, even though marginal costs have not changed, the intersection of the steeper MR_2 with MC results in a higher price, P_2, on the demand curve.

The surgeons' price markup (their fee relative to marginal cost) was higher than those physicians whose patients did not have insurance coverage.[4]

Surgeons did not compete directly for patients; they competed amongst themselves for patient referrals from primary care physicians. Given the surgeon's high price-to-cost ratio and excess capacity among many surgeons, it might be expected that in a price-competitive market, surgeons, seeking a greater number of referrals, would be willing to share their fee with the referring physician. To prevent price competition among surgeons (which would have reduced their incomes), medical societies, under the greater control of surgeons, declared "fee splitting" to be unethical behavior.

The Effect of Prohibiting Advertising on the Demand for Physician Services: Until the Supreme Court decision in 1982, advertising was prohibited by state codes

---

4. Assuming profit maximization, the estimate of price elasticity of demand can be used to determine the price markup or price/cost ratio for the firm. For example, if the firm knows its price elasticity of demand and marginal cost, the firm can determine its profit-maximizing price using the following formula:

$$Price = MC/(1 + 1 / -Pe). \text{ When } Pe = -3, \text{ then}$$

P = MC / (1 − 1 / 3), = MC / (2 / 3), = MC (3 / 2), = 150 percent (MC). If MC were $100, then price would be $150. The higher the price elasticity, the smaller the markup.

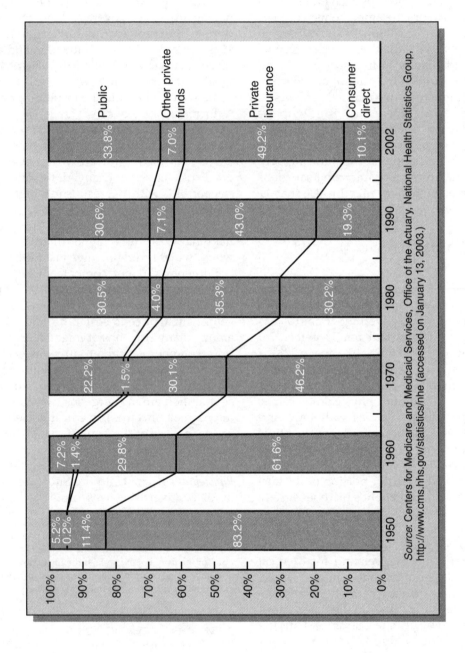

Figure 10-3.   Distribution of expenditures on physicians' services by source of funds, selected years, 1950–2002.

Source: Centers for Medicare and Medicaid Services, Office of the Actuary, National Health Statistics Group, http://www.cms.hhs.gov/statistics/nhe (accessed on January 13, 2003.)

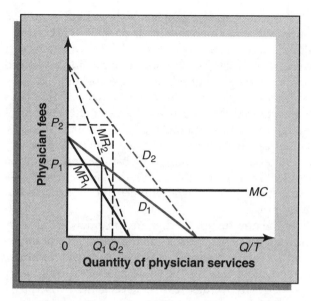

Figure 10-4. The impact of insurance on physician services.

Advertising of medical services performs three functions. First, it reduces the patient's search costs. When price information is unavailable, wide variations in prices will exist since it will be up to the patient to search out the firms with the lowest prices. Since search is costly, patients will not keep searching until they find the firm that sells its services at the lowest price. Search will continue until the marginal benefit of increased search (lower prices) equals the marginal cost of additional search.[5] When information is disseminated through advertising, travel and other costs are lowered. Differences in prices, as well as differences in quality and other attributes of the service would continue to exist, but these differences would be smaller than previously.

(In a world of perfect information, prices charged for what is perceived to be the same product would be the same, and differences in prices would reflect differences in their costs of production.)

"Price-dispersion is a manifestation of—and indeed it is a measure of—ignorance in the market" (13). Without provider information, the consumer may first have to purchase the service to determine its attributes as well as its price.[6] Although advertising is less effective when services are directly experienced, provider information on prices and qualifications still contributes to the information the consumer needs to make a choice. The consumer might then have to resort to additional sources, such as employee satisfaction surveys, provider report cards, and consumer groups, for additional information on the provider.

that regulated ethics in the health professions. The penalties for violating such codes were severe, including suspension of the practitioner's license. Prohibitions on advertising were in physicians' economic interest. Had medical societies permitted advertising, the effect would have been to lower the average price of physician services.

During the period when there was limited private and public insurance for physician visits (hence a greater financial incentive to shop for lower prices), physicians competed on both price and non-price factors. Patients, however, had little information on competing physicians' prices, quality, and accessibility. To determine the attributes of different physicians and the price of their services, the patient had to spend time and money searching. Patients who place a high value on their time will search less and will be willing to take a chance on paying higher prices. This lack of information on competing physicians made other providers poor substitutes for the patient's current physician; consequently, physician-firm demand curves were less price elastic than if such information were more readily available.

5. The optimal search time is determined by both the costs and benefits of searching for lower prices. The benefits of search are greater the more expensive the service, the more frequently it is used, the greater the out-of-pocket price paid by the patient, and the less emergent the need for the service. The costs of search are greater for those with higher incomes (who are also more likely to have insurance). The above suggests that less price dispersion should be observed for visits to a family practitioner than for the services of a surgical specialist.

6. Nelson classified goods into two categories: search goods and experience goods. Search goods are those for which adequate information concerning their desirability exists prior to purchase (e.g., an airplane trip). Experience goods need to be purchased to be assessed (e.g., a dinner in a restaurant). Philip Nelson, "Advertising as Information," *Journal of Political Economy,* 82(4), July/August 1974: 729–754.

Second, advertising that provides patients with information on the similarity and differences of services sold by different providers enables patients to evaluate the degree of substitutability of competing providers. The demand curves of the different providers are made more price elastic.

The effect of advertising on prices can be shown with reference to Figure 10-5. With little information available to patients to judge other physicians, the physician's demand curve is less elastic, shown as D_1. Assuming that the physician-firm wishes to maximize its profits, it will set its price at that point on the demand curve where the marginal revenue (MR_1) and marginal cost curves intersect. The resulting price will be P_1. With advertising, patients have more information by which to evaluate substitute physicians, such as physician qualifications, accessibility in terms of location and hours, and so on. Other physicians now become better substitutes to one another. As this occurs, the physician's demand curve becomes more elastic (the closer the substitute, the more elastic the demand curve). The new, more price elastic demand curve is D_2. For the sake of simplicity, the marginal revenue curves in Figure 10-5 were drawn so that they intersected the marginal cost curve at the same point. With the same marginal cost curve, a more elastic demand curve results in a lower price, P_2 instead of P_1.

The cost of advertising is not shown in Figure 10-5 since it does not increase the firm's marginal costs; instead, advertising increases the firm's average cost curve. Advertising costs should be considered a fixed cost since they are unrelated to the cost of producing additional quantities of the particular service. Thus the cost of advertising itself does not affect the price charged by a firm attempting to maximize its profits. The price would be determined by the price elasticity of demand and the marginal cost of producing that service. By causing the firm's demand curve to become more price elastic, advertising is expected to *lower* prices.

In the non-health field, many products are already viewed by consumers as being relatively homogeneous. One firm's soap or aspirin is considered to be a good substitute for the same product produced by another firm. In these cases, advertising is used by a firm to differentiate its product from that of its competitors. As shown in Figure 10-5, if a firm is selling a relatively homogeneous product (demand curve D_2), it advertises to make consumers believe that other products are less substitutable for its own, thereby hoping to change its demand curve to D_1.

Third, a firm's inability to advertise has been used as a barrier to entry in a market. For example, large organizations such as HMOs are subject to economies of

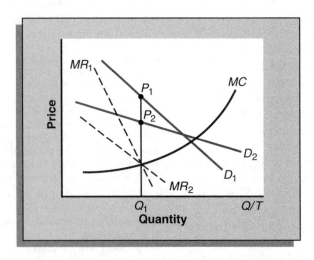

Figure 10-5. The effect of advertising on the elasticity of demand and on the firm's pricing strategy.

scale; that is, they must achieve a minimum enrollment size before their premium can be competitive to those of traditional insurance plans. Their previous inability to advertise required such plans to incur large losses; they had to price their premiums competitively, but since they had such small enrollments, their costs per enrollee exceeded their premiums. Advertising enables such plans to increase their enrollments quickly so that they can take advantage of economies of scale.

The strongest empirical evidence on the effects of advertising in healthcare has been based on studies of optometrists (14). The Federal Trade Commission (FTC) attempted to determine what happens to prices and quality of services among providers who advertise compared to those who do not. Data was collected from three types of optometrists: optometrists in cities where advertising of eye examinations and eyeglasses was prohibited, optometrists who did not advertise even though advertising was permitted in their areas, and optometrists who did advertise. The FTC used seven individuals with similar visual conditions who "were trained at two schools of optometry with regard to the components of an optometric examination. They obtained examinations, recorded price, time spent, and details on the various tests and procedures performed" (15).

The findings of this study were that "the presence of advertising causes substantial and significant declines in the prices of eye examinations offered by all types of optometrists." Prices were reduced, but not by as much, even for optometrists who did not advertise but who were located in markets where advertising occurred. Further, non-advertising optometrists in advertising markets spent more time with their patients (a proxy for quality) than did advertising optometrists and even more time than did non-advertising optometrists in non-advertising markets.

The author concludes that advertising does not reduce quality by all practitioners in a market. In fact, enough non-advertisers remain in advertising markets so that the overall market quality is higher. The removal of advertising restrictions was estimated to result in a 20 percent decrease in price without any decline in overall quality. Non-advertisers in advertising markets compete on price and quality, and apparently consumers are able to choose and differenti-

ate between providers on the basis of prices and quality of service (16).

Another indication of quality—patient satisfaction—was based on a survey of retired persons undertaken after price advertising began in Florida. One of the test questions was: "All things considered, the next time you buy eyeglasses or contact lenses, would you return to the same place where you bought your last pair?" The responses were then matched to another question that asked if the place of last purchase advertised prices. The issue, "Are consumers more dissatisfied with opticians who advertise?" was thus answered. "The results show that while 58 percent of the customers of non-advertising opticians indicated a willingness to give the seller repeat business, 86 percent of the advertisers' customers indicated they would return . . . only 8 percent of the customers of advertising opticians said that they 'probably' or 'definitely' would not go back. A full 25 percent of the customers of non-advertising opticians gave the same answer. . . . In brief, if there is a quality problem, it is not with advertising opticians. Rather it would appear that it lies with those who refuse to advertise their prices" (17).

The strong desire health (and other) professions have had to maintain codes of ethics that prohibit advertising can be explained by the fact that professional control over information leads to higher prices.

Physician Pricing Under Private and Public Insurance

The conduct of the physician-firm after the mid 1960s was affected by the expansion of private and public insurance coverage and the physicians' continuing role as the patients' agent. As a result, physicians' market power increased, enabling physician-firms to increase their prices and volume of services, as well as engaging in price discrimination between private and public insurance programs.

Both private and public insurance for all physician services increased during the mid 1960s to the 1980s. Medicare and Medicaid were enacted for the aged and poor, and private insurance also became more prevalent. The method of reimbursement preferred by physicians has always been fee-for-service according to their "usual, customary, and reasonable" (UCR) fees. Such a pricing strategy enables physicians to set what they believe is the profit-maximizing price. With the growth in private insurance for physician services and the passage of Medicare and Medicaid, the amount the patient had to pay out of pocket for such services was reduced (the demand curve facing physicians whose patients had private insurance became less price elastic). As shown in Figure 10-3, by 1980, only 32 percent of physician expenditures were paid out of pocket by patients. As the patients' responsibility for payment of physician fees declined and physicians charged third-party payers according to their UCR fee, the usual market constraints, such as patients' seeking lower prices, disappeared; physician fees increased rapidly.[7]

The lower out-of-pocket prices caused by the expansion of public and private insurance led to an increase in the quantity demanded of physician services. Consequently, moral hazard became a financial concern to third-party payers. It was rational for patients, whose price was decreased, to use additional services to the point where their (reduced) marginal costs (out-of-pocket price plus time costs) equaled the (lower) marginal benefit from increased physician visits. Physicians, paid fee-for-service, had little, if any, incentive to limit patient demand. Patient and physician financial incentives increased the cost of private and public insurance.

---

7. One explanation for rising physician fees has been the rapid increases in malpractice premiums. Malpractice premiums, however, are a fixed cost; they do not vary according to the number of deliveries or the number of surgical procedures performed. If a physician sets a profit-maximizing price (i.e., marginal revenue equal to marginal cost), changes in fixed cost should not have any effect on the physician's price. If physicians were able to pass on increases in their fixed costs, it is unlikely that they would spend their time in marches on their respective state capitols seeking legislative relief. Only in the long run in a competitive industry would increased fixed costs result in higher consumer prices. Since there is evidence that physicians were receiving above-normal rates of return during this period (Chapter on Health Manpower Shortages and Surpluses), the long-run explanation is not applicable. Increased malpractice premiums may be used as a reason for increasing prices by physicians even though the more accurate explanation was a lessening price elasticity of the patient's demand curve; higher costs are a more palatable explanation than increased ability to pay.

Physician Price Discrimination—Accepting Medicare Assignment: Even in the period before extensive public and private insurance for physician services, physician-firms were able to demonstrate their monopoly power by engaging in price discrimination. Patients were segmented according to their price elasticity of demand, namely ability to pay. Surgeons charged higher prices to their wealthier patients than their lower-income patients for the same service. The different demand and marginal revenue curves (and same marginal cost) in Figure 10-5 also illustrates the physician-firm charging different prices to patients having different elasticities of demand. (Charging each patient the maximum amount they are willing to pay for a surgical procedure is an example of "first degree" price discrimination.)

The growth of private and public insurance (particularly for those with low incomes) did not eliminate physicians' desire to price discriminate. The following example explains how physicians were able to price discriminate between privately and publicly insured patients.

When Medicare began, participating physicians had the option of accepting or rejecting assignment for payment of a beneficiary's claim. A physician accepting Medicare assignment was paid 80 percent of their approved fee by Medicare, and the patient was responsible for the remaining 20 percent co-payment (in addition to a small annual deductible), which had to be paid directly to the physician. A physician not accepting assignment billed the patient for the entire fee, which was greater than the Medicare-approved fee. The patient then paid the entire fee directly to the physician and was reimbursed by Medicare for only 80 percent of the approved fee. Thus the patient was responsible not only for the 20 percent co-payment of the approved fee, but also for the difference between the approved fee and the physician's charge. This difference was referred to as "balance billing." In addition, the patient had the increased burden of submitting the claim for payment before being reimbursed by Medicare for 80 percent of the physician's approved fee.

The percentage of physicians accepting Medicare fees as full payment has varied over time, its low was about 50 percent in 1976. The closer Medicare-approved fees were to fees in the private sector, the higher the assignment rate. (In the 1980s, the increasing supply of physicians, the growing competition among physicians for patients, and an increase in Medicare fees to participating physicians led many physicians to decide that it was in their economic interest to accept assignment.) The assignment rate also varied according to region of the country, which reflected the market for physician services, and by physician specialty, which reflected the risk to the physician of not being paid by the patient. For example, surgeons, who had larger total charges, were more likely than primary care physicians to accept assignment. Also, the patient was more likely to have to return to their primary care physician.

The following is an analysis of how Medicare reimbursement has in the past affected physician assignment. Assume that physicians have three types of patients: private-pay patients, which includes those with private insurance as well as Medicare non-assigned patients; Medicare-assigned patients; and Medicaid patients. It is further assumed that the physician's fee is highest for the private-pay patients, lower for Medicare-assigned patients, and lowest for Medicaid patients. To maximize their income, physicians will serve patients paying the highest fees before serving other patients. How many patients in each category the physician will serve will depend on the size of each market and the physician's marginal cost schedule.

The Medicare assignment problem can be described with reference to Figure 10-6 (18). The demand curve for physician services is D_1. The marginal revenue curve associated with that demand curve is MR_1. The downward-sloping demand curve assumes that physicians have some monopoly power. For private pay patients, the physician is a "price setter." Medicare is such a large purchaser of physician services (accounting for about 20 percent of total physician expenditures), that it is a monopsonist, that is, Medicare is a price setter because it can set the price it pays for physician services. The Medicare price is a horizontal line at P_M. The physician is thus a "price taker" in the Medicare (and Medicaid) markets.

The physician will start by serving the private market. If the physician's marginal cost curve (MC) intersects the downward sloping MR curve at a point

above P_M, such as A, this will determine the quantity of physician services to be produced and the price charged (the price charged will be that point on the demand curve directly above point A, which is where MR = MC). A physician in such a situation would not serve any Medicare-assigned patients. If, however, the physician's MC curve intersected MR at a point below the Medicare price (P_M), the physician would serve that number of private patients given by the intersection of MR and P_M (shown by Q_1). The physician would also serve Medicare-assigned patients up to the point where MC equals P_M.

As shown in Figure 10-6, the physician would serve OQ_1 private patients and Q_1Q_2 Medicare-assigned patients. The marginal revenue of both private pay and Medicare patients would be equal at that point. (If the physician served more than OQ_1 private patients, the foregone revenue from Medicare patients, PM, would exceed the MR of additional private patients.) The price for private patients would be P_1, while the Medicare price would be P_M. The physician's MR curve is changed so that it becomes MR up to the point of intersection with P_M, and then it is horizontal (P_M). (In this example, the physician would not serve Medicaid patients assuming that Medicaid pays a price less than P_M.) A physician would enter the Medicaid market if the number of both private and Medicare patients is relatively small so that the physician's MC curve intersects the Medicaid price (which would be horizontal) as is the Medicare price, but presumably at a lower level.)

Several important factors affected the physician's assignment rate. These may be classified as demand factors, supply factors, and Medicare policies. For example, an increase in private insurance that increased the private demand for physicians' services would shift the demand and MR curves to the right. If MC were unchanged, then MC would intersect MR at a point to the right of Q_1. The physician would serve more private patients and accept fewer assigned patients. The reverse would occur if an increase in the supply of physicians led to a decrease in private demand per physician, thereby increasing assignment. A change in the factors affecting the physician's MC curve, such as increased wages for personnel working in the physician's office, would also affect the assignment rate. With an increase in MC, the new MC curve would intersect P_M to the left of Q_2. There would thus be a decrease in the number of assigned patients. Similarly, a decrease in MC would increase assignment.

Medicare policies also affect assignment. An increase in Medicare's price would raise P_M. The higher P_M would intersect the MR curve at a point to the left and higher than the previous point. Assuming that the higher P_M intersected MR at point A, there would be a decrease in private-pay patients served (as well as an increase in their price), and an increase in the number of assigned patients. Other Medicare policies may have an effect on P_M without explicitly changing it. For example, if Medicare makes it more (less) difficult for physicians to collect their fees for assigned patients (such as by delaying or speeding up payment), this would be similar to a decrease (increase) in Medicare's net price. The consequence would be an increase (decrease) in the number of private patients served and a decrease (increase) in the number of assigned patients.

The above theoretical model for understanding assignment also contradicts the belief that physicians "cost shift," that is they charge private-pay patients more when government pays physicians less. This is unlikely to occur because it would not be a profit-maximizing strategy. Empirical evidence supports the above theoretical discussion that physicians *lower* (raise) their prices to private patients when physicians' fees for Medicaid patients are *reduced* (increased) (19).

Physician Behavior: Supplier-Induced Demand

Given the patient's lack of knowledge regarding their diagnosis and treatment needs, the patient must rely upon the physician for advice on both. Thus, an agency relationship exists between the patient and the physician. When the physician acts as a "perfect" agent for the patient, then the physician's recommendation would be similar to what the patient would decide if the patient had the physician's expertise. The physician would consider the patient's medical condition, income, insurance coverage, out-of-pocket prices for different treatment settings, preferences, etc., when making a treatment recommendation.

The physician, however, is a supplier of both advice and a service. As such, there is a concern that because the physician has a financial interest in supplying services, the information provided to the patient could be biased. The lack of patient information, together with extensive insurance coverage, reduces patients' sensitivity to physician prices. When the physician modifies the diagnosis and treatment rec-

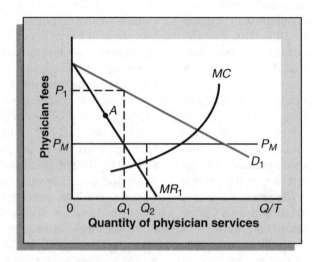

Figure 10-6. Physician decision whether to accept Medicare assignment.

ommendation to include a favorable effect on his or her own economic wellbeing and a well-informed patient would not want those services, then the physician is an "imperfect" agent. In a fee-for-service payment system, this imperfect agency relationship has been referred to as "supplier induced demand" (SID).

In its simplest form, demand inducement is an extreme example of monopoly power in that the physicians can both induce their own demand and set their own price.

The amount of demand that an "imperfect" agent physician will induce has been hypothesized to be a trade-off between increased income and the disutility of providing unnecessary care. The physician is assumed to be a utility maximizer; the physician receives utility from additional income and from practicing good medical care. The greater the quantity of induced demand, the greater the physician's income, hence utility. However, when the physician induces demand, it is assumed that the physician incurs a "psychic" cost or disutility. If the physician's income were to fall either because of an increase in the supply of physicians or because of government limits on fees, the psychic cost of inducing demand is less than the marginal utility of the additional income it generates. At low levels of demand inducement, this psychic cost may be low in that additional follow-up visits might be justified and certainly not result in harm to the patient. At higher levels of induced demand, the increased psychic cost to the physician of additional treatment (e.g., unnecessary surgery) exceeds the marginal utility of the additional income. The quantity of SID that the physician is presumed to induce is where the psychic cost of additional care equals the value of additional income.

Demand inducement is wasteful in that the expected costs to the patient from the additional care are greater than the expected benefits. Since the expected costs exceed the expected benefits, the physician—as the patient's (imperfect) agent—would be expected to induce demand only when they face declining fees and/or decreased demand for their services.

One variant of how much demand a physician will induce is based upon what "target income" the physician desires. The target income is assumed to be determined by the local income distribution, particu-

larly with respect to the relative incomes of other physicians and professionals, such as dentists and lawyers. According to this theory, to forestall a decrease in income physicians will either increase their fees or induce demand (shift the demand curve to the right) to enable physicians to maintain a target income.

Figure 10-7 shows the effect on physician fees and quantity of services of an increase in the supply of physicians using traditional economic theory as well as the target-income hypothesis. If market demand and supply were originally D_0 and quantity S_0, respectively, equilibrium will be at price P_0 and quantity Q_0. An increase in the number of physicians in an area would shift supply to the right, to S_1, which would, under traditional economic theory, result in a *lower* equilibrium price, P_1, and an increase in the quantity demanded (a movement down the demand schedule for physician services). The effect of an increased supply on physician incomes will be based on whether the market demand curve for physicians is price elastic or inelastic. If the market demand curve were price inelastic (consistent with empirical

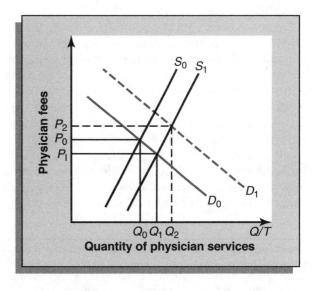

Figure 10-7. An illustration of the target-income hypothesis.

evidence), then total physician incomes would decline with an increase in the number of physicians. According to traditional economic theory, physicians would be unable to increase price or shift demand because as profit maximizers they have already set their fees to the maximum allowed by the market.

Under the target-income hypothesis, with an increase in the number of physicians in the community to forestall a decrease in their demand and incomes, physicians induce an increase in their demand to D_1. The effect is an increase (or no change) rather than a decrease in physician fees. Proponents of SID do not necessarily believe that physicians can increase their fees and demand indefinitely. Because they are utility rather than profit maximizers, physicians are presumed to be to the left (not on) their market demand curve, thereby able to increase demand as their incomes fall.

Empirical Evidence: The literature on physician-induced demand is extensive (20). The hypothesis is based upon empirical evidence indicating use of physician services is positively related to increases in the supply of physicians, to reductions in Medicare physician fees, or to facilities in which physicians have an ownership interest, after adjusting for other variables.[8]

There has been a great deal of debate over the validity of the empirical evidence on supplier-induced demand. Both the logic and the empirical work underlying many SID studies have been criticized. Critics contend that supply follows increases in demand rather than demand following increased supply (which would be induced demand). For example, the empirical finding of a positive association between physician fees and physician/population ratios is the result of inadequately adjusting for omitted demand factors, such as differences in the physician visit, namely patient time and quality of a physician visit, as well as in-patient information. As the number of physicians in an area increases, travel and waiting times to see physicians decrease; this results in an increase in the quantity of visits demanded as the patient's time costs are lowered. Similarly, as the quality aspects of a physician visit are increased (as measured by the amount of physician time per visit), the patient would be willing to pay a higher price for a physician visit. Critics of SID believe that if it were possible to adjust many of the studies for omitted demand factors, increased use was the result of increased demand (increased supply follows increases in demand—not the reverse) and there would be a negative relationship between physician/population ratios and physician fees.

Using a traditional economic framework, Pauly and Satterthwaite attempt to explain the observed relationship between an increase in the number of physicians and fees in terms of a decline in consumer information, consequently, an increase in search costs (21). They analyze the situation among primary care physicians where the patient's insurance coverage is less than for surgeons, and therefore price incentives still exist. In choosing a physician, consumers depend on the recommendations of others rather than shopping as they typically do in other markets. When there are few physicians in an area, each physician's reputation is known throughout the community. Consumers are likely to know people who have gone to each physician. However, when there are a large number of physicians in a metropolitan area, the consumer's knowledge of each physician's reputation is less. There is also less information on each physician's qualifications and prices. An increase in the number of physicians in an area, therefore, increases the consumer's difficulty in finding out about each physician. As the consumer's cost of search increases, the consumer becomes less price sensitive, and the physician's demand curve becomes less elastic. Physicians (or firms in monopolistically competitive markets) will then raise their prices.

The following are brief descriptions of supplier-induced demand studies based on the positive association of physician supply to use of services and, second, physician responses to decreases in their fees.

---

8. Note that an increase in the physician/population ratio—a rightward shift in supply—and an observed increase in utilization would not, by itself, be indicative of SID since the observed increased utilization would be caused by a movement down a demand curve. In the traditional case, however, fees and incomes would also decline.

In an early study on SID, Victor Fuchs found that a 10 percent increase in the surgeon/population ratio resulted in a 3 percent increase in per capita utilization. Also, opposite to what would be expected using traditional economic analysis, he found that prices were increased in this situation of induced demand. Thus, although the average surgeon's workload decreased by 7 percent, income per surgeon declined by a smaller amount. The extent of demand inducement, even among surgeons, is, however, limited since "the average number of operations per surgeon . . . is far below the level that surgeons consider a full workload . . . and below the quantity that surgeons would be willing and able to perform at the going price" (22).

A number of studies have found limited, if any, demand inducement. For example, Rossiter and Wilensky using 1977 data distinguished between patient-initiated ambulatory visits (57 percent of all visits) and physician-initiated ambulatory visits (43 percent of all visits), thereby permitting separate estimates of the impact of the physician/population ratio on each type of visit (23). The authors concluded that an increased physician/population ratio had no impact on patient-initiated visits, although it did have a positive impact on physician-initiated visits; the effect, however, was very small; that is, a doubling of the physician/population ratio, which would be a huge increase, would lead to only an 11 percent increase in physician-initiated visits.

For physician-initiated visits, the study found that the out-of-pocket money price and time price (time in the physician's office) had the expected negative effect on number of physician-initiated visits. That is, either patients or physicians or both are somewhat sensitive to the out-of-pocket price of services, while patients are sensitive to time prices.

McCarthy, using data from a 1974 American Medical Association Survey of 187 individual primary care physician firms in large metropolitan areas, did not find evidence of induced demand for primary care physician services (24). He found that the physician-to-population ratio (squared) had a negative impact on the number of physician office visits. Patients were found to be sensitive to both time (in-office waiting) and money prices, both of which had negative relationships to office visits. Time and price both had price elasticities greater than −1. Moreover, the number of organized outpatient departments and emergency rooms per 100,000 population, which are measures of substitute sources of care, also had large negative impacts on physician office visits. (These results also support the premise of a monopolistically competitive market for physician services.)

While concluding that there is an absence of physician-induced demand *at the margin*, McCarthy acknowledges that there may have been demand inducement in the past. Reinhardt underscored this qualification, emphasizing that if an increase in the physician/population ratio leads to a decline in visits per physician, this simply indicates that physicians cannot *at the margin* induce demand to raise their incomes (25). This finding says nothing about what physician-induced demand occurred in the past and, therefore, how much money is currently being spent on physician-induced visits and tests.

It should be kept in mind that McCarthy studied primary care physicians, where the lack of patient information is not as great as when patients use specialists who are used much less frequently; also, insurance coverage for primary care physicians is not as great as it is for specialists.

A second set of studies on SID examined whether physicians, to maintain their incomes, prescribed more services when Medicare reduced physicians' fees. Rice examined a change in the Medicare payment system in Colorado between 1976 and 1977, which resulted in a relative decrease in fees paid to urban physicians (their reimbursements rose by less than 5 percent) and a relative increase in fees paid to non-urban physicians (their reimbursements rose by approximately 20 percent) (26). He found that the lower the reimbursement rate for different services (medical, surgical, laboratory, and radiology), the greater was the intensity of the service provided. For example, a 10 percent decrease in the reimbursement rate for medical services led to a 6.1 percent increase in medical service intensity.

Studies have examined the effect of fee-for-service versus capitation payment the number and type of surgeries performed. Patients are least able to judge whether or not a surgical procedure is necessary. The patient may be able to determine whether additional home and office visits are providing any benefits, but in the case of surgery, the consequences to the patient of being mistaken may be more serious. The types of surgery that were likely to result from demand creation are tonsillectomies, appendectomies, and hysterectomies. The physician might have rationalized that these surgical procedures were beneficial and did not affect the patient's ability to function. The patient would have no way of determining whether such surgery was useful since his or her wellbeing would probably be unchanged after recovering from it.

The rate of surgical procedures was higher when the physician was paid fee-for-service even though the population groups being compared had similar characteristics and similar physician and hospital coverage (27). In one group, Health Insurance Plan of Greater New York (HIP), the physician was reimbursed on a capitation basis (an annual payment per enrollee regardless of the number of procedures performed); for the other group of patients, covered by Group Health Insurance in Washington, D.C. (GHI), the physician was paid fee-for-service. The rate of hospitalized surgical procedures for HIP (capitated) enrollees was 4.38 per hundred persons per year; for GHI it was 7.18.

In another study of GHI and HIP populations, no significant difference was found in surgical procedures between adult males, but they were found between adult females—6.56 in GHI and 4.97 in HIP. In a third comparative study of physician reimbursement under capitation (Kaiser) and fee-for-service (Blue Cross-Blue Shield and commercial insurance), when patients had identical benefit coverage under all three plans, it was found that the hospitalized surgical procedure ratios per hundred persons per year were 3.3, 6.9, and 6.3, respectively. A fourth comparison was of two groups of federal employees with the same benefits, where one group belonged to a capitation plan, while the other group belonged to a fee-for-service system. It was found that the rate of hospitalized surgical procedures was 3.9 in the capitation plan and 7.0 in the fee-for-service system. One-third of this difference in the rate of surgical procedures was a result of differences in the rate of surgical procedures for appendectomies (1.4 versus 2.6), tonsillectomies (4.0 versus 10.6), and "female surgery" (5.4 versus 8.2).

When Medicare instituted a new physician payment system in the 1990s (discussed below), surgeons were expected to suffer sharp reductions in their fees, consequently in their incomes. Yip tested whether the fee reductions resulted in increased volumes of services by thoracic surgeons (28). She found that thoracic surgeons increased their volumes to both Medicare and privately insured patients so that they were able to recover 70 percent of their lost income.

The above finding can be illustrated with respect to Figure 10-6. A reduction in Medicare fees will affect the physician's Medicare as well as their private patients. As described earlier, a lower Medicare fee (indicated by a downward shift in a perfectly elastic, horizontal demand curve) will intersect the marginal revenue curve of private patients at a lower point, thereby leading to a lower price for private patients and an increase in the number of private patient visits. The physician will see fewer Medicare patients (a "substitution" effect—a lower Medicare price is a movement down the physician's supply or marginal cost curve). However, if the reduction in Medicare fees results in a large (negative) income effect on the physician, the physician might induce demand to offset the loss of income. By decreasing their marginal cost curve, such as by reducing the time spent per patient, the physician will be able to see more Medicare patients; the lower marginal cost curve will intersect the horizontal Medicare price further to the right than with the previous marginal cost curve.

The concern that physicians would induce their demand in response to a fee reduction caused Medicare's actuaries to propose a 6.5 percent fee reduction when the new Medicare physician payment system was introduced. They estimated that for each one percent reduction in fees, volume would increase by one-half percent. The increase in volume did not occur in aggregate, although as Yip showed, it did for some specialties.

Another test of the demand inducement hypothesis is whether physicians refer patients for treatment and/or testing to ancillary facilities where they have an ownership interest. Proponents of these types of joint ventures claim that quality is enhanced through improved monitoring of ancillary care providers. Critics of such joint ventures claim that unnecessary care and higher health care costs result from such self-referrals. Various studies have shown that physician ownership in each type of facility was associated with higher utilization of laboratory tests, diagnostic imaging, patient use of radiation therapy, and physical therapy per patient (29). The empirical evidence on demand inducement is the basis for federal legislation prohibiting physicians with an ownership interest in a clinical laboratory or diagnostic center referring Medicare and Medicaid patients to those facilities. A number of states have enacted similar laws.

Supplier-Induced Demand and Traditional Theories: Different theoretical models have been developed to explain the empirical evidence of a positive association between physician/population ratios and higher fees and/or use rates. At one end of the spectrum there is the SID theory which assumes that the physician is a utility maximizer not an income maximizer, and at some point the disutility to the physician of providing unnecessary care exceeds the marginal utility of the additional income they earn; this limits the extent of their demand inducement. At the other end of the spectrum are proponents of traditional theories (physicians as profit maximizers with limited or no ability to induce demand) who claim that much of the empirical work supporting SID is based on faulty research.

Rather than assuming demand inducement does or does not exist, McGuire and Pauly present an alternative approach for examining the issue. Whether or not the physician will induce demand depends upon whether the income effect dominates the substitution effect of a price change (30). If a fee reduction has a sufficiently large impact on the physician's income, it will outweigh the substitution effect of the price reduction, which is for the physician to supply less as the price goes down. When the income effect is stronger, the physician's behavioral response will be to attempt demand inducement to increase their income. It is difficult to generalize on the issue of demand inducement since the income effects of price changes may be larger for some payers than others, it will vary by physician specialty, and the ease by which physicians are able to reduce their cost curves. Further, while some induced demand is acknowledged by many, the amount of SID is not limitless; it

is uncertain that physicians are able to induce still more demand.

The SID and traditional theories lead to quite opposite predictions. Under the traditional view, continued increases in the physician/population ratio are likely to result in a lower rate of increase in both physician fees and incomes (assuming the overall market demand for physicians is price inelastic).

Supplier-induced demand would predict that the consequences of an increase in the physician/population ratio would be a shift to the right in the demand for physician services and a faster increase in physician fees and use of services than in the past as more physicians attempt to attain their target income. Expenditures on physician services (with doubtful effects on health status) would be expected to increase rapidly.

The policy prescription by several SID proponents has been to impose arbitrary government limits on both the number of physicians and on expenditures for physician services. The expenditure limit approach is currently part of Medicare's physician payment system.

Alternatively, concerns over physician-induced demand and moral hazard can be alleviated by greater reliance on market forces. The movement to private sector market forces starting in the 1980s demonstrated the success of this approach.

Managed Care and Physician Price Competition

Managed care methods (utilization review) and organizations (HMOs) arose in the 1980s as a cost control mechanism in the private sector. Increased insurance coverage for physician services combined with fee-for-service physician payment, an increasing supply of physicians, and supplier-induced demand led to overuse of services and rapidly increasing health insurance premiums. Under pressure from large employers to limit premium increases, health insurers developed a more adversarial relationship with providers, and new types of insurers (HMOs) entered the market.

The introduction of managed care dramatically changed the market for physician services. Premium competition among insurers provided them with a financial incentive to reduce their input costs. To limit the rise in physician expenditures, insurers sought to reduce the two components of expenditures, physician fees and utilization. Insurers were able to reduce fees by forming Preferred Provider Organizations (PPOs), a small network of physicians to care for their enrollees. To become part of a PPO and thereby have access to the insurer's enrollees, physicians, who had excess capacity, had to discount their fees. Insurers viewed all physicians within a specialty as being close substitutes and selected physicians according to their willingness to discount their fees. Demand curves facing physician-firms became highly price elastic.

Insurers used several methods to control utilization. Insured enrollees were required to pay the full costs of care if they used non-PPO physicians. Insurers also instituted utilization review for hospital admissions and second opinions on surgery to reduce inappropriate care. In addition, insurers monitored and selected their participating physicians according to the appropriateness of their practice behavior.

The success of managed care organizations in reducing physician expenditures depended on the relative bargaining power of insurers as compared to physicians in a market. Insurers had a great deal of leverage over physicians when there was a large number of competing physicians and there were few insurers, each having a large number of enrollees. Empirical evidence found that competitive physician markets (larger number of physicians per capita) and concentrated insurance markets led to lower fees. (31). (Insurers were less successful in reducing physician expenditures in those markets where the insurance markets were more competitive and there were fewer physician-firms per capita among whom they could choose.) Under managed care, the outcome of competitive physician markets was consistent with traditional economic theory, namely higher physician/population ratios led to lower, not higher, fees.

The change in purchaser (insurer) behavior led to changes in the market structure for physician services. Unable to induce demand to increase their incomes and moral hazard limited by utilization management, physician-firms had to become more price competitive to participate in PPOs and to develop market power in other ways. There was an increase in both the number of physician groups and in the size of groups. (See Tables 10-2 and 10-3). Physician-firms increased in size. These trends were to take advantage of economies of scale and to better compete for insurer contracts. By undertaking functions performed by the insurer, such as utilization review, and reducing the negotiation cost of insurers having to contract with many independent physician-firms, large physician groups were more likely to be designated by the insurer as PPO providers and receive an increased number of enrollees. Large physician groups were also able to negotiate profit-sharing arrangements with hospitals (that were capitated by the insurer) in return for referring their patients to those hospitals and for reducing hospital use.

Large physician groups, particularly in California, also negotiated capitation contracts with insurers, thereby shifting the risk from the insurer to the physician group (32). These medical groups believed that greater physician control over their enrollees' care would increase both patient quality and physician profitability. Unfortunately, many of these physician groups did not have adequate management expertise and were unable to manage the financial risk associated with capitation, resulting in the group's bankruptcy.

As the physician services market became more price competitive in the 1980s and 1990s, some physicians resorted to anti-competitive approaches. In some areas, physicians formed very large physician groups, incorporating a large percentage of the physicians in the market area with the intent of negotiating on behalf of all of their members with health insurers. In effect, these physician organizations were simply an attempt to monopolize the market for physician services. By including most of the community's physicians in their group, the group's demand curve became less price elastic; insurers had fewer substitutes among whom they could choose. Similarly, in some communities all the specialists, such as anesthesiologists, formed a single group to negotiate their fees with insurers. (The demand curve for all the specialists became the industry demand curve for those specialists, hence less price elastic.) The Federal Trade Commission (FTC) ruled that large physician groups (comprising more than 30 percent of physicians) and groups containing all or most of the specialists in a market would be prosecuted as being anti-competitive (33).

Competitors also often resort to political behavior to eliminate price-competitive markets. Unable to form illegal cartels, medical associations sought legislation permitting them to achieve what the FTC was prohibiting. However, the American Medical Association was unsuccessful in having federal legislation enacted allowing non-employee physicians to collectively bargain with insurers. At the state level, however, many medical societies were successful in having Any Willing Provider (AWP) legislation enacted. AWP laws effectively decrease price competition since any physician is able to participate in an insurer's PPO. Physicians no longer have an incentive to discount their fees in return for a greater volume of patients if other, non-PPO physicians could also have access to those same patients.

PERFORMANCE OF THE PHYSICIAN SERVICES MARKET

When evaluating the performance of a market, the yardstick by which to judge each market's performance is the competitive market. Each firm must be internally efficient and take advantage of economies of scale if it is to be price competitive. In the long run, there are no excess profits since there are no entry barriers; consequently, in the long run prices approximate production costs, and output is greater than under other market structures.

How does the performance of the physician services market compare to the theoretically ideal competitive model?

When evaluating the performance of the physician services market, one must be aware that there have been changes in both its structure and in its conduct, consequently its performance. The industry has somewhat consolidated; physicians are more likely to practice in groups, and the size of groups, particularly multi-specialty groups, have increased. Physician-firms have had a downward sloping demand curve because patients relied upon them for their diagnosis and treatment needs and were unable to judge the ac-

curacy of their recommendations and substitutability of physicians. The large number of physician-firms in a market (each having a downward sloping demand curve) is characteristic of a monopolistic competitive industry.

Physicians' market conduct exhibited monopoly power, as evidenced by monopoly pricing and induced demand. Lack of patient information and subsequently extensive health insurance for physician services enabled physicians to engage in price discrimination and supplier-induced demand. Physicians were able to charge different types of patients (and/or their insurers) different prices for the same services. Physicians operated in two markets, the private and governmentally insured markets. The physician–firm was a price setter in the private market and a price taker in the Medicare and Medicaid markets. With small co-payments for physician services, patients had little concern with physician fees. Moral hazard was a concern to insurers, but neither providers nor patients had a financial incentive to limit use of services. In this environment, physicians were able to induce demand for their services in both the public and private markets.

Physician Expenditures, Prices, and Incomes

During the 1960s, 1970s, and most of the 1980s, the market for physician services did not perform well. Expenditures for physician services rose rapidly, as did physicians' fees and incomes. The quality of physician services was unknown since little information was available on outcome measures and, until the early 1980s, medical societies prohibited the publication of physician quality measures (or any other competitive information).

As shown in Figure 10-8, after the passage of Medicare and Medicaid in 1965, physician fees and expenditures (adjusted for inflation) increased rapidly. By the early 1970s, expenditures were increasing more rapidly than fees (the difference being higher utilization). The reason for this divergence was an increase in the economy-wide inflation rate, which began to rise in the late 1960s as President Johnson used an "inflation tax" to finance the Vietnam War. (Inflation moved more wage earners into higher marginal tax brackets,

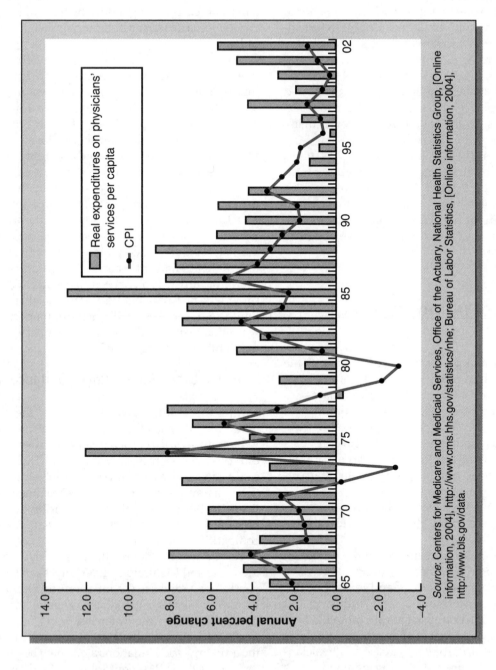

Source: Centers for Medicare and Medicaid Services, Office of the Actuary, National Health Statistics Group, [Online information, 2004], http://www.cms.hhs.gov/statistics/nhe; Bureau of Labor Statistics, [Online information, 2004], http://www.bls.gov/data.

Figure 10-8. Annual rate of change in physician's expenditures per capita and the CPI for physicians' fees, adjusted for inflation, 1965–2002.

the highest being 70 percent, thereby increasing federal tax revenues.) President Nixon imposed price controls (referred to as the Economic Stabilization Program—ESP) on the economy in 1971 and removed it the following year; however, it was kept in place for the medical sector until 1974. Price controls slowed the rate of increase in physician fees, but not expenditures. Following the removal of those controls in 1974, physicians' fees and expenditures increased sharply.

The rate of increase in real physician fees and expenditures diminished in the late 1970s and early 1980s because of rapid increases in the rate of inflation and then the economy went into a recession. By the mid 1980s, expenditures increased much more rapidly than fees as use of services increased. Managed care began to have its impact on fees and expenditures by the mid 1990s.

The performance of the physician services market changed with the introduction of managed care. Under pressure from employers to reduce their employees' health insurance premiums, insurers developed managed care techniques and new, innovative insurers such as HMOs entered the market. As insurers engaged in premium competition for employer business, they sought to reduce their input costs by reducing use of services and providers' fees. Insurers, not the patient, became the purchaser of physician services. Physician-firm demand curves became more price elastic as knowledgeable insurers were able to gather data on physician prices and use rates and compare physician performance. By monitoring physician behavior, managed care insurers also reduced physicians' ability to induce demand for their services. Insurers were willing to *shift their enrollees* to those physician-firms offering the lowest prices. Before physicians could compete for an insurer's patients, they first had to compete on price to be included in the insurer's provider network.

Managed care changed the performance of the physician services market. Physician supply was increasing rapidly during this period, and their excess capacity made physicians more willing to discount their fees for an increase in patients. Expenditures and fees rose less rapidly. Managed care and the increased physician supply also led to a gradual decline in physician incomes.

As shown in Figure 10-8, it was not until the early 1990s that annual increases in physician fees and expenditures became smaller. Managed care began to affect more physicians during the 1990s, and the new Medicare physician payment system also became more stringent.

When the annual percent increase in total expenditures is compared to the percent increase in physician fees, it appears that during different time periods, fee increases have accounted for between one-half and two-thirds of the increased expenditures. (Part of these fee increases represents different types of visits. When physician fees are adjusted both for inflation and by the decline in the out-of-pocket price as a result of third-party coverage, the physician fee, *in constant dollars faced by the average patient*, actually declined over the last 30 years.) The composition of office visits and surgical procedures have likely changed over time. Thus, part of the increase in physician fees is due to more costly visits and procedures, including more specialty services as well as additional services per visit.

The decline in physician fees during the 1990s was likely the result of increasing competitive pressures occurring among physicians. (In the more recent period, driven by increased use of services, physician expenditures are again increasing rapidly.)

Comparing physician incomes over time also illustrates the impact of the new competitive environment; physicians' monopoly power has been eroded.

With the growth of private and government payment for physician services starting in the mid 1960s, the demand for physician services increased more rapidly than supply. As a result, physician incomes increased rapidly. Between 1965 and 1975, physician incomes increased by more than 100 percent, which was a more rapid rate of increase than that of dentists, lawyers, and most likely, any other profession. Except for psychiatry, the annual rate of increase in physician incomes exceeded that of the CPI, as shown in Figure 10-9.

By the late 1970s, inflation was increasing rapidly (annual rate of increase between 1976 and 1985 was 7.2 percent) and the supply of physicians was expanding more rapidly than demand for physician services. Consequently, the rate of increase in physi-

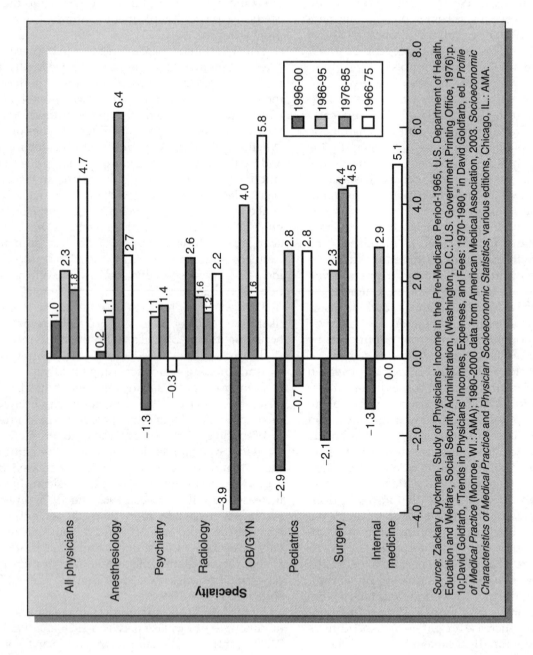

Source: Zackary Dyckman, Study of Physicians' Income in the Pre-Medicare Period-1965. U.S. Department of Health, Education and Welfare, Social Security Administration, (Washington, D.C.: U.S. Government Printing Office, 1976):p. 10;David Goldfarb, "Trends in Physicians' Incomes, Expenses, and Fees: 1970-1980," in David Goldfarb, ed. *Profile of Medical Practice* (Monroe, WI.: AMA); 1980-2000 data from American Medical Association, 2003. *Socioeconomic Characteristics of Medical Practice and Physician Socioeconomic Statistics*, various editions, Chicago, IL.: AMA.

Figure 10-9.   Average annual percent change in real net income from medical practice by specialty, 1965–2000.

cians' real incomes (adjusted for inflation) declined. However, real incomes for hospital-based physicians and surgeons continued to increase. Incomes for primary care physicians were, in part, limited by Medicare fee controls, while technological advances permitted specialists to perform more procedures at higher fees. In the period 1986 to 1995, physicians' real (adjusted for inflation) incomes once again increased, with the largest increases occurring for OB/GYN physicians. The new Medicare physician payment system implemented in 1992 (discussed below) benefited PCPs by raising their fees at the expense of specialists.

In the most recent period, 1996 to 2000, managed care became more pervasive with its emphasis on paying discounted fees to physicians. The average annual percent increase in physician incomes slowed, with PCPs, surgeons, and OB/GYN physicians having the lowest annual increases.

The effect of managed care and the increased supply of physicians is also illustrated in Figure 10-10, which shows the annual percent change in median physician incomes from 1981 to 2000. While there is variability in year-to-year percent changes in incomes, a definite downward trend in physician incomes is visible by the 1990s.

By the end of the 1990s, most of the privately insured population was enrolled in one of several types of managed care plans. However, the managed care industry began to undergo changes that affected insurers' ability to control physician expenditures. The 1990s were characterized by a growing economy and an increasing demand for labor. As their incomes increased, employees demanded health plans that had broader provider networks and fewer restrictions on referrals to specialists. A consumer and political "backlash" against managed care plans also occurred. Further, managed care plans lost large sums of money in several lawsuits regarding denial of experimental treatments to enrollees. As a consequence of these events, managed care plans weakened their cost control measures. Many states also enacted Any Willing Provider (AWP) laws, which had the effect of broadening provider networks, thereby limiting price competition among physicians to be included in health plan networks.

During the period that managed care revolutionized the private health insurance market, Medicare continued to use fixed prices, paid physicians fee-for-service, and relied on expenditure limits to control total Medicare physician payments. Except for a small portion of Medicare patients enrolled in Medicare HMOs, Medicare did not use managed care techniques. Physicians were still able to induce demand in the Medicare market. Medicare remains an unmanaged, fee-for-service, payment system.

An important consequence of managed care was an increased emphasis on data for measuring quality of care. Under pressure by large employers, insurers began to collect data that could be made available to enrollees during the open enrollment period for choosing a health plan. Medical groups began to be rated according to various quality and patient satisfaction measures. The availability of this information will enable employees to make more informed choices, thereby making different physicians and medical groups closer substitutes to one another, and consequently, their demand curves more price elastic.

Small Area Variations in Use Rates

An important aspect of the performance of the physician services market, in addition to the competitiveness of the market as indicated by the rate of growth in expenditures, prices, and incomes, is whether the appropriate output is being provided.

A disturbing aspect of physician practice behavior is the wide variations in treatment patterns for patients with the same diagnosis. Stimulated by John Wennberg's early research, numerous studies have documented wide variations in use rates for hospital admissions and in surgical procedures among different communities, as well as for the same specialties. For example, the rate of coronary bypass operations in Utica, New York, was 45 percent greater than in Syracuse (0.83 per 1,000 versus 0.57 per 1,000); were people in Utica being overtreated, or were those in Syracuse being undertreated? Again, C-sections as a percent of all births were 38 percent in Oneida, New York, while they were only 18 percent in Rochester (34). Attempts to explain these variations examined whether they were the result of differences in demand. However, after adjusting for

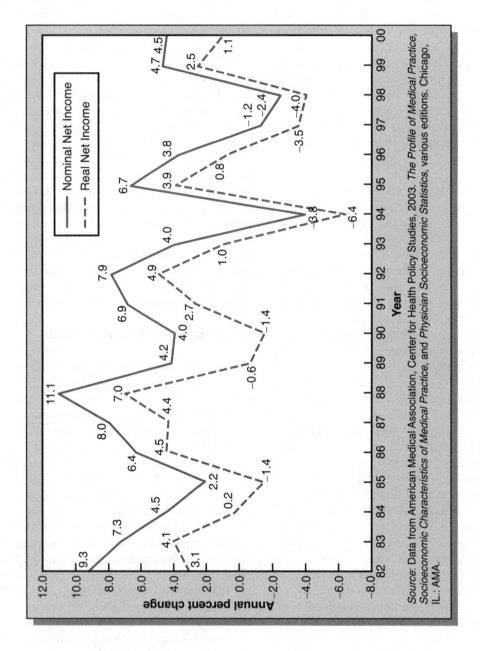

Figure 10-10. Annual percent changes in median physician net income after expenses and before taxes, 1982–2000.

age, sex, and health status, as well as differences in insurance coverage and incomes, the large variations in use rates remained.

Similarly, there are wide variations in use rates in other countries, such as Canada and England. The demand inducement hypothesis is also not helpful in explaining these wide variations. When supply factors that could influence demand as well as economic factors that might provide physicians with an incentive to induce demand were held constant, community variations in use by specialty still persist. Further, there are no incentives for physicians to induce demand in Canada or England, yet similar variations exist within each of those countries.

The inability of traditional supply and demand factors to explain the wide variations in use of medical services is cause for concern in terms of patient health outcomes, as well as for economic efficiency. If, after adjusting use rates by procedure for the relevant demand factors variations still exist, then some patients are receiving too much treatment while others may be receiving too little. Some patient's lives are endangered, and favorable medical outcomes could be achieved with fewer resources.

For example, the number of carotid endarterectomies has increased from 15,000 per year in 1971 to 85,000 in 1982 to an estimated 108,000 in 1994 and, most currently (2000), 124,000. The purpose of the procedure is to reduce the risk of stroke or death in patients with extracranial vascular disease. In one study, it was determined that 32 percent of the Medicare patients examined (1,302 Medicare patients randomly selected in three regions in 1981 who had the procedure) had the procedure for inappropriate reasons. Another 32 percent had the procedure for equivocal reasons (35). These procedures carry with it a significant risk of complications and death.

A number of studies have been undertaken showing wide rates of use for particular surgical procedures with no differences in patient outcomes. If low users do not receive low-quality care but have the same outcome as high users, then performance, in terms of expenditures and patient outcomes, can be improved.

It has been hypothesized that variations in use both between communities and even within a hospital for a given specialty are related to the school where the physician was educated, length of time in the community, and community norms. For example, it was determined that in two excellent centers for medical training, Boston had a higher hospital admission rate than New Haven. Further, physician practice styles within a specialty have been found to be more important than patient severity of illness in explaining variations in use rates.

The gains from providing information to physicians in order to decrease inappropriate use is shown in Figure 10-11. Differences in physicians' belief as to the efficacy of treatment is shown by the three

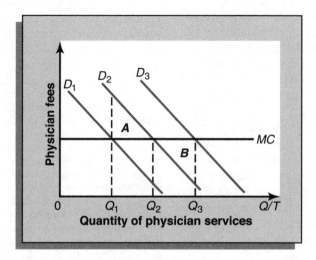

Figure 10-11.   The effect of differences in physicians' practice styles on procedure use rates.

demand curves, D_1, D_2, and D_3; D_2 represents the demand for a particular procedure in a community based on what the fully informed physician would recommend. Social, economic, and demographic factors as well as morbidity between the three communities represented by the different demand curves are assumed to be similar. The only difference between the communities (represented by the different demand curves) are differences in physicians' practice styles and beliefs. The cost of providing that procedure is assumed to be constant and represented by MC. The "appropriate" use rate in the community is Q_2, at which point the marginal value of an additional procedure equals its marginal cost. Communities whose physicians place too great a belief in the treatment value of that procedure would have a use rate Q_3. Similarly, "too low" a use rate is shown by Q_1.

Providing information to physicians whose practice patterns result in demand curves D_1 and D_3 would improve economic welfare in the following manner. Individuals living in communities whose physicians believe the efficacy of a particular procedure is less (D_1) than it actually is (D_2) would be better off if the use rate of that procedure were increased; the marginal benefits of that procedure exceed its marginal cost. This lost value is represented by area A. Similarly, when the use rate is too high, the cost of that procedure exceeds its additional value; this excess of cost over its value is represented by area B.

Studies undertaken by managed care organizations and the federal government are attempting to determine the medical value or appropriateness of specific medical interventions. Such studies and the dissemination of their results can improve physician decision-making and save enormous resources. Inappropriate use and wide variations among communities and physicians within a given specialty are indicative of serious physician information imperfections. Economic efficiency and patient outcomes could be improved if inappropriate use were reduced. Increased physician information on appropriate treatment should, together with appropriate incentives, improve the performance of the physician services market, with a consequent reduction in medical expenditures and improved patient outcomes.

SUMMARY

The structure of the physician services market has changed, from a predominance of solo practice to an increase in the number of physicians practicing in groups. Group size is also increasing. The movement to group practice and larger sized groups is due to economies of scale, reputational economies of scale, physicians' desire to reduce uncertainty and risk (although risk sharing reduces productivity incentives), and greater market power when negotiating with insurers and hospitals.

Although the physician services market is not concentrated, there are certain peculiarities of this market that provide physicians with some monopoly power, namely a downward-sloping demand curve. Patients have limited information on physician practice styles, their fees, and their accessibility. Physicians differ on their technical ability as well as in how they relate to the patient.[9] Patients have had little information by which to choose and judge physicians. In such a market situation, the costs of search are high, and wide variations are able to exist in fees, quality, and practice styles.

Lack of information on competing physicians has made it difficult for patients to determine how good a substitute other physicians are to their own physicians. Also making patients less price sensitive is the growth in third-party insurance. With lower out-of-pocket costs, the patient has a decreased incentive to search for lower-priced physicians; their costs of search, primarily time and travel costs, are likely to exceed the marginal benefits of increased search, namely lower net prices.

9. Perfect purchaser information rarely exists in any market. Many consumers have little or no information on prices and quality of other consumer products, such as appliances, and yet these markets are relatively competitive. This lack of information is resolved in several ways. For example, brand name products often sell at higher prices than non-brand name items since they consist of two goods, a firm's reputation and the product itself. In some markets, those consumers who are informed and are price sensitive give the demand curve for that product its downward slope; even if ten people are not price sensitive with respect to the price of gasoline but several others are, the horizontal summation of all the individual demand curves for gasoline would be negatively sloped.

Physicians' downward sloping demand curves, together with a large number of competing physicians, is indicative of a monopolistically competitive market structure.

Physician conduct is indicative of their monopoly power. Before the anti-trust laws became applicable to healthcare in 1982, physicians engaged in various forms of anti-competitive activities, such as insurer boycotts and bans on advertising. Physicians' pricing and practice behavior were also indicative of monopoly power. With a less price elastic demand curve as a result of lack of patient information and extensive insurance coverage, physicians were able to price as would a monopolist (always in the elastic portion of their demand curve) by setting their fees in excess of marginal cost. (For example, the price elasticity of demand facing individual primary care physicians was estimated to be –3.0, indicating that the physician-firm has market power.)

One form of physician conduct was particularly indicative of monopoly power, namely supplier-induced demand, which is the ability of physicians to shift their demand curves. It is not known how much demand inducement exists, however additional demand inducement in the private sector appears to be limited as a result of managed care. Managed care made physician-firm demand curves more price elastic, with a consequent decrease in physician fees and incomes.

The market for physician services has undergone major changes which have affected its performance. The movement toward managed care resulted in greater oversight of physicians' practice behavior. Utilization review mechanisms, emphasis on appropriateness of care, and physician profiling reduced inappropriate use of services.

An important remaining source of inefficiency in the physician services market is variations in medical services that are due to differences in physicians' practice styles. In coming years as outcomes research expands, information on appropriate care patterns is likely to be used by medical groups, hospitals, insurers, and self-insured firms to improve market performance, reduce expenditures, and improve patients' health.

The expansion of information systems to permit greater monitoring of physicians' practice patterns and the publicizing of these results offers promise that inappropriate care will be reduced. The increase in physician supply has not led to more rapid increases in fees and utilization as would be expected if physicians were attempting to maintain a target income. The strengthening of market forces is likely to improve market performance.

APPENDIX: HOW MEDICARE PAYS PHYSICIANS

In 1989, the Prospective Payment Reform Commission, in response to its Congressional mandate to develop a new method of paying physicians under Medicare and to slow the growth in Medicare physician expenditures, proposed four significant recommendations. The first was to phase in, starting in 1992, a fixed-fee schedule for Medicare physician payment based on a Resource Based Relative Value Scale (RBRVS); the second was to limit "balance billing" among physicians, which is the amount beyond the Medicare payment that a non-participating physician can charge the Medicare patient; third, to establish an overall expenditure target for Medicare physician expenditures, referred to as a Volume-Performance Standard (VPS); and fourth, to fund research on medical effectiveness. These recommendations, which were historic changes in the payment of physicians under Medicare, were enacted by Congress in 1989 (36).

The impetus for changes in physician reimbursement came from two sources. The first, and most important, was the federal government, whose interest was (and still is) in reducing Medicare Part B expenditures, which is funded out of general revenues, and consequently, increases the federal deficit, an important political problem. The government, however, was constrained in achieving this objective by not having a large number of physicians drop their Medicare participation. The second impetus for change came from various physician specialties, third-party payers, and a number of academicians who believed that the previous Medicare payment system was inefficient and also resulted in inequities among physicians.

Background on Medicare Part B Financing

The financing of Medicare Part B and the distribution of expenditures under that program have changed over time. Currently, 73 percent of Medicare Part B expenditures are financed out of the federal government's general tax revenues; 23 percent is paid for by premium contributions from the aged. (The remaining 4 percent comes from interest received from invested funds.) Federal contributions under Part B now represent one of our larger federal programs; Part B expenditures rose from $779 million in 1967 (Medicare's first year) to over $44 billion in 1990, and to $113 billion by 2002. They are expected to reach $191 billion by the year 2010 (37). (Physicians receive approximately 40 percent of all Part B payments (down from 44 percent 5 years ago), the remainder goes to other providers, such as hospital outpatient departments and home health care providers.)

Any reduction in Part B expenditure increases will make a significant contribution toward reducing the federal budget deficit.

Politics has restricted the choices available to the federal government for reducing the rise in Part B expenditures. Each choice imposes a cost on some constituency. Higher costs could be imposed on the aged, providers could be paid less, the non-aged could pay higher taxes (to subsidize the Part B premium, and/or future generations could bear the cost through a higher federal deficit).

The financial burden on the aged could be increased by raising the $100 Part B deductible and the 20 percent co-payment, both of which would reduce the aged's demand for physician services, hence reduce federal expenditures. Similarly, the ageds' portion of the Part B premium, currently 25 percent, could be raised, also reducing federal expenditures. (Unless each of these increased costs to the elderly are income related, they would be equivalent to a regressive tax, which would be particularly severe on low-income elderly.)

Whichever political party proposes shifting a greater portion of the Part B costs to the elderly is likely to pay a political "price." The elderly have high voting participation rates, associations representing their interests are quite active, and members of Congress run for re-election every two years.

Previous attempts to reduce the rate of increase in Medicare expenditures relied on shifting the burden to healthcare providers (lower payments) and to the non-aged (higher taxes) and/or future generations (greater deficits). The aged were not required to pay additional costs. During the Economic Stabilization Program in the early 1970s, provider payments were reduced; it was the basis of the Medicare Economic Index, which placed limits on physician fee increases; it was the method used to control Medicare hospital expenditures, and continues to be the preferred federal approach to slowing the rise in Medicare expenditures.

The federal government is, however, limited in how little it can pay participating physicians since it must ensure that a sufficient number of physicians are willing to participate in Medicare. The loss of a significant number of physicians could cause access problems to the aged in some geographic areas. Once access begins to decline, Congress will be pressured by the aged to increase physician participation.

Fee-for-service results in two types of inefficiencies. First, the (imperfect agent) physician has an incentive to perform more services. Second, physician fees under Medicare were initially based on their fee profiles. As such, insured services were priced higher in relation to cost than other services. (Those services having a higher relative "profit" provide physicians with an incentive to perform a relatively greater number of these services). Also, because of limits on Medicare, fee increases over time, and rigidities in Medicare fees, some services were priced much higher than others in relation to their cost. As procedures became routine and their costs fell with experience and volume, the fee for performing that procedure did not decline. The fee for coronary artery bypass surgery was initially established when the procedure required a great amount of a surgeon's time. As the surgeon's experience with this procedure increased and it became possible to delegate various aspects of the care for this procedure (e.g., pre- and post-care), the price for the procedure should have fallen, but Medicare did not decrease it.

Inequities among physicians also occurred because Medicare paid physicians according to their fee profiles but did not increase them frequently. Thus new physicians were able to establish a higher fee profile than older, established physicians in the same specialty. Further, large differences in fees for the same service between regions existed, unrelated to differences in cost of living. And fees charged by physicians for the same service varied depending upon the physician's specialty.

These inefficiencies and inequities in Medicare payment for physician services caused differences in physician incomes, affected physicians' choice of specialty, and practice location.

Resource-Based Relative Value Scales

The proposed new physician payment system was to serve two groups, each with differing objectives. The federal government wanted to control the rise in Medicare physician expenditures while increasing access by the aged to physicians. A number of academicians and physician organizations wanted a new fee structure to correct the inefficiencies and inequities (among physicians) of the previous system.

Since the main purpose of a relative value scale was to correct the inefficiencies and inequities of the Medicare fee schedules, the following principles should have been followed (38). First, there should be one price for each service regardless of the training and background of the person performing that service. Second, fees should be proportional to the costs of performing each service, so as not to bias the mix of services. Third, the costs of providing the service should be based upon the most efficient method (i.e., lowest level of training required) rather than on averages of costs or charges.

Reimbursement for physician services according to the task performed rather than the level of training of the person performing it will eventually affect the specialty distribution of physicians. If a particular

service can be performed equally well by a family practitioner, a specialist should not receive a higher fee for performing it. If specialists are not as busy as they would like to be and they use their excess time performing services that non-specialists can perform equally well, reimbursing specialists at a higher rate will provide them with a higher income than they would otherwise have.[10]

The relative value scale, developed by Hsaio, et al., attempted to approximate the cost of performing each physician service (39). Its premise was that in a competitive market the price of a service would, in the long run, reflect the cost of producing that service. The cost-based approach to determining relative values is complex (relative values were established for over 7,000 services); it required a great deal of analysis and data, must be continually updated, and involves a number of assumptions which, if different, could change the outcomes. For example, the calculation of the physician's time assumes that the surgeon spends a certain amount of time before and after the operation, and it assumes an average length of time for the various tasks that the physician performs.

The total relative value for a service is divided into three components: First, the physicians' work, including the complexity of the service in order to allow for differences in skill and effort required. Also included is opportunity cost, so that physicians with different training times can earn the same rate of return. Second are practice expenses, to include overhead expenses, such as office payroll and deprecia-

---

10. The principle of establishing payment rates based on the lowest level of training required should apply to physicians and their aides as well as between physicians with different specialties assuming the quality is the same. Under fee-for-service, a financial incentive to delegate is created if the same payment were made for a particular task regardless of whether it was performed by a physician or an aide. If the time of a lesser-skilled individual—a nurse or physician assistant, for example—can be substituted for a physician's time, the allocation of resources is improved. In the short run, the physician's time is freed for more complex tasks; in the longer run, if lesser-trained manpower takes over some of the tasks now performed by physicians, a smaller supply of physicians will be needed. Task delegation should occur automatically under a capitation system since physicians who did so would be able to treat a larger number of patients and earn greater net revenues.

tion on equipment. Third is malpractice insurance, since its cost varies across specialties.

Two methods were used for estimating the complexity of a task: personal interviews, and a modified Delphi technique in which each physician was able to compare his or her own estimate to the average of physicians within that specialty. Many assumptions were required (such as in calculating opportunity cost) that the years required for training in a specialty are the minimum necessary. Further assumptions were made regarding the lengths of working careers across specialties, residency salaries, hours worked per week, and an interest rate to discount future earnings.

The new payment system consisted of two parts. The first part, as described below, assigned values or weights to all services and procedures. Second, a conversion factor was applied to those relative values to translate them into dollars or fees. (The conversion factor was initially determined so that the new payment system would be "budget neutral," that is, payments under the new system would be equal to what payments would have been under the previous system.) Table 10-5 illustrates the calculation of the relative value scale and the conversion factor to determine the fee for an office visit.

Hsiao, et al., performed a very useful service in calculating a relative value scale based on resource costs. In doing so, data requirements and assumptions had to be explicitly defined. A number of criticisms, however, have been made of a cost-based relative value scale (40). For example, unless relative values include

Table 10-5. Calculations of Physician Payment Rate Under RBRVS Office Visits (Mid-Level) NYC (Manhattan)

	Relative Value		Geographic Adjustment	Adjusted Relative Value
Physician work	0.67	×	1.09	0.73
Physician expense	0.69	×	1.35	0.93
PLI*	0.03	×	1.67	0.05
				1.72
		Conversion factor	× 36.20	
		Payment Rate		$62.09

*Professional liability insurance

a quality factor, high-quality physicians will decrease quality. Further, since there are constant changes in technology, equipment, office expenses, residents' salaries, and the time required to perform various services, unless the relative value units are updated, Medicare physician fees will diverge once again from market fees, creating imbalances between supply and demand for physician services and among specialties.

Relative value scales were also meant to redistribute income among the different physician specialties by realigning fees proportional to cost for all services. Fees for cognitive services were increased while fees for performing technical procedures were decreased. Primary care physicians gained at the expense of procedure-oriented specialists. For example, it was estimated that payments to family practitioners increased 37 percent, internists 16 percent, with declines of 21 percent for radiologists, 20 percent for thoracic surgeons, and 17 percent for ophthalmologists. The income redistribution among physician specialties explained their relative political positions on the new fee schedule.

Limits on Balance Billing and Total Physician Expenditures

To achieve the government's goal of increasing access, reducing the cost to the aged of going to the physician, and limiting the growth in physician expenditures, limits were placed on the amount that physicians could balance bill, and a target was set for how fast Medicare physician expenditures were permitted to increase.

Physicians not accepting assignment could not charge more than 115 percent of the approved Medicare fee and are only paid 95 percent of that fee, therefore receiving, at a maximum, only 109 percent of the Medicare approved fee. *Thus even physicians who decide not to participate in Medicare are restricted in how much they can charge for treating a Medicare patient.*

As part of the original RBRVS system adopted in 1992, the government's approach to control physician expenditure increases was an annual update of the conversion factor which, when multiplied by the relative value scale, results in Medicare physician fees for the following year. If the volume of physician services increased faster than expected, the conversion factor would increase less so that expenditures remained within the target. As it turned out, the volume and mix of services increased less rapidly than expected for surgical services. Consequently, to maintain the target rate of Medicare payments for surgical services, their conversion factor increased more rapidly. *These changes in fees were unrelated to any changes in demand or supply for such services.*

In 1997, the annual update formula was changed to achieve a "Sustainable Growth Rate" (SGR) in Medicare physician expenditures. The SGR conversion factor was determined annually and was comprised of four parts: the percent increase in real GDP per capita, a medical inflation rate of physician fee increases, the annual percent increase in Part B enrollees (other than Medicare+Choice enrollees), and the percent change in spending for physician services resulting from changes in laws and regulations, such as expanded Medicare coverage for preventive care. Tying the SGR to GDP per capita represented an affordability criteria; Part B expenditures, which were subsidized by the federal government, were to be based on what the country could afford. As the economy rapidly grew in the late 1990s, physicians received generous Medicare fee increases. However, with the start of a recession in late 2000, there was a decline in the percentage growth in real GDP per capita, with the consequence that physician fees were *reduced* 5.4 percent in 2002. To forestall further fee reductions in 2003 as the economy faltered, Congress agreed (after much lobbying by physician organizations) to repeal the scheduled fee reductions.

Calculation of fee increases based on a formula whose objective is to limit the growth in physician expenditures is incompatible with the government's other objective of maintaining access to physician services by the aged. Fees based on achieving a target of physician expenditures will be unrelated to the supply and demand for Medicare physician services. Medicare fees should attempt to equilibrate the demand and supply of physician services in the Medicare market. However, as occurs with any government-imposed price, Medicare fees will either result in shortages (decreased access) or unnecessary windfalls to physicians. Medicare physician fees differ from mar-

ket-determined prices regionally and by physician specialty. To mimic competitive market prices, fees should account for changes in physicians' input costs and changes in demand. Regulated fees rarely achieve this goal.

As a consequence of the SGR physician fee reductions, a shortage occurred in the Medicare market—price was below the equilibrium level. Fewer primary care physicians accepted new Medicare patients and access to care by the aged declined. As the difference in fees between the Medicare and private markets became larger, primary care physicians shifted more of their time (supply) to the non-regulated (private) market, reducing the supply in the Medicare market. With an increase in supply in the private market, price in the private, non-Medicare market will increase less than it would have otherwise.[11]

One method by which access could be improved is to allow physicians to balance bill (charge the Medicare patient the difference between the regulated and market price). However, under the new system, the maximum amount that can be balanced billed is 109 percent of the Medicare fee. Previously, an increase in the number of physicians who balance billed was an indication that Medicare fees were falling behind fees in the private market. Balanced billing, however, was opposed by organizations representing the aged because it increases the aged's net price for physician services. As a result, balanced billing under Medicare is virtually eliminated.

---

11. The probable effects on the Medicare and non-Medicare markets would be similar to the earlier discussion on Medicare assignment. With reference to Figure 10-6, limiting physician fee and/or payment increases will decrease the Medicare price over time. This lower price will intersect the physician's marginal cost curve to the left of Q_2, thereby reducing the quantity supplied to government-paid Medicare patients. Similarly, as the Medicare fee is reduced, it will intersect the MR curve for private patients to the right, at a lower point. Again, fewer Medicare patients will be served as the physician increases services to the non-Medicare market. Further, the physician's price in the private market should decrease as he or she increases their supply in that market. Whether price decreases or increases in the private market depends upon whether one believes that physicians are limited in their ability to induce demand and increase their price at will (the neoclassical approach), or whether physicians will be able to "cost-shift" and raise fees in the private market (demand inducement or target income theories).

The Congress tried to achieve several contradictory objectives in enacting the RBRVS Medicare physician payment system. These were: first, to limit the growth in Medicare physician expenditures (because it contributed to the budget deficit) by limiting the conversion update factor; second, increase access to care for the aged by having a large number of physicians participate in Medicare (accept assignment); and third, reduce the aged's out-of-pocket expenditures by limiting balance billing. Limits on both balance billing and Medicare fee increases (conversion update) will eventually cause a significant shift of primary care physician supply to the non-Medicare market. If the gap between Medicare and private fees for primary care physicians becomes too large, the aged may find that the only way to increase their access to PCPs is to join a Medicare-managed care plan where there are no restrictions on what the plan can pay physicians.

It is highly likely that Medicare's physician payment policy will continue to change in the years ahead as the conflict in objectives over limiting Medicare physician expenditures and access to care by the aged becomes greater. The federal government need not rely on a single payment method. Having a variety of health plans available for the aged to choose will allow both patients and physicians to move into those systems that are most preferable, and entry and exit from these plans will provide information on how each of these systems performs.

Proposed Changes to the Medicare Physicians' Market

A number of proposals have been made to improve the equity and efficiency of physician services funded by Medicare. The following are two such proposals.

An Income-Related Premium For Medicare Part B: Currently, the aged pay only 25 percent of the Medicare Part B premium, the remainder being funded by general tax revenues. This subsidy is provided to all of the aged, regardless of their incomes or wealth. Making the premium income related would have two effects: first, high-income aged would receive less of a subsidy, thereby decreasing the federal

budget deficit or making the funds available to low-income non-aged. Second, reducing the subsidy to the aged would increase their cost of remaining in the current Medicare fee-for-service system compared to joining a Medicare-managed care plan (Medicare+Choice). This subsidy distorts the relative prices to the aged of their health plan choices. The increase in relative price of remaining in the fee-for-service system would cause more of the aged to switch to Medicare+Choice health plans.

Tax Medi-gap Policies: More than 70 percent of the aged have purchased private health insurance ("Medi-gap" policies) to cover their out-of-pocket medical expenditures. The effect of such policies is to remove most of the cost-sharing provisions of Medicare, which include a 20 percent co-payment for physician services. Removing the co-payment increases the quantity demanded of physician visits with a consequent increase in Medicare expenditures. The premium for Medi-gap policies, however, is based only on the co-payment for those visits, not the Medicare portion of the expenditures. There is, in effect, an externality; those purchasing Medi-gap policies pay only a small part of their additional use of services, the taxpayers pay the remainder.

In addition to decreasing the price of physician services, Medi-gap policies reduce the patient's incentive to shop for lower prices and makes it more difficult for Medicare+Choice plans to compete for Medicare patients; Medi-gap enrollees have less incentive to join these other plans since they have access to an unrestricted choice of providers with almost full coverage at subsidized rates (41). Taxing Medi-gap policies to offset the increase in Medicare expenditures that result from such policies would decrease the demand for such policies, re-institute cost sharing and provide incentives for shopping, and enable managed care plans to better compete for Medicare patients.

REVIEW QUESTIONS

1. There are two contrasting theories of physician behavior. The first is the traditional model, and the second is referred to as "physician-induced demand" or "target income."

a. Explain each model, and describe how each of these models differ in their assumptions regarding physician behavior and patient information.

b. What empirical evidence has been used to support the physician-induced demand theory? What alternative explanations support the observed data?

c. What would be the consequences of an increase in the supply of physicians on the price of physician services, the quantity of physician visits, and total physician expenditures of each of these theories?

2. What are some of the ways in which health insurers seek to compensate for the information advantage physicians have?

3. How do fee-for-service and capitation payment systems affect the physician's role as the patient's agent?

4. The price elasticity of demand for physician services has been estimated to be –0.2; does this mean that each physician is a monopolist with a price inelastic demand curve?

5. What information would you need, and how would you use it to determine whether physicians were over or under utilizing aides in their practice?

6. Large variation in physician fees exist for the same type of service within the same market area. Provide two alternative explanations for this variation, one based on a competitive market model, and the other using a monopoly framework. Do the same for the rise in physician fees over time.

7. What characteristics of the physician market provide physicians with market or monopoly power?

8. Why has the size of multi-specialty medical groups been increasing in the last several years?

9. Explain the advantages and disadvantages to a physician for joining a group practice as compared to being in solo practice.

10. Explain how a resource-based relative value scale is used to determine physicians' fees.

11. Resource-Based Relative Value (RBRVS) fees pay all physicians (within a specialty) the same fee for the same type of service. What are the similarities and differences between RBRVS fees and fees established through a price-competitive market? If relative-value fees and market-determined fees differ, what are the consequences of using relative-value fees?

12. Outline the structure of the physician services market. What features of this market differ from the purely competitive model? What changes, if any, would you suggest to change the performance of this industry?

13. The following statement appeared in the *Wall Street Journal*: "Most people who provide services say they're sorry that they have to raise prices, but they say they have no choice. Doctors say their fees have gone up because of whopping increases in malpractice insurance premiums." How would you use economic analysis to analyze this statement? Be explicit regarding any of your assumptions. (Hint: Are malpractice premiums a variable or a fixed cost?)

14. Explain how physicians decide how many Medicare patients to accept, the price they charge their private patients, and the effect on both of the above of a decrease in the price Medicare pays physicians for Medicare patients.

15. As demand for primary care physicians increase in the private sector, what would be the likely effect of the elimination of balance billing for all Medicare patients on: access to care by primary care physicians, the out of pocket price paid by Medicare patients, the supply of physician services to Medicare patients, and physician fees and supply of visits to the non-Medicare population?

REFERENCES

1. There are several excellent discussions of the physician services market and the applicability of economic models for analyzing physician behavior. See Thomas G. McGuire, "Physician Agency" in *Handbook of Health Economics*, vol. 1A, eds. A. J. Culyer and J. P. Newhouse, (New York: North-Holland Press, 2000), 461–536, David Dranove and Mark Satterthwaite, "The Industrial Organization of Health Care Markets," in *Handbook of*

Health Economics, vol. 1B, eds. A. J. Culyer and J. P. Newhouse, (New York: North-Holland Press, 2000), 1093–1139, and also Martin Gaynor, "Issues in the Industrial Organization of the Market for Physician Services," *Journal of Economics and Management Strategy*, 3(1), Spring 1994: 211–255.

2. For an example of how economies of scale and patient travel costs are used to determine the optimal number and size of obstetrical units for Chicago, see Millard F. Long and Paul J. Feldstein, "The Economics of Hospital Systems: Peak Loads and Regional Coordination," *American Economic Review*, 57(2), May 1967: 119–129.

3. Uwe Reinhardt, "A Production Function for Physician Services," *Review of Economics and Statistics*, 54(1), February 1972: 63 (55–66).

4. Philip Held and Uwe Reinhardt, "Prepaid Medical Practice: A Summary of Recent Findings from a Survey of Group Practices in the United States," *Group Health Journal*, 1(2), Summer 1980: 4–15.

5. Gregory C. Pope and Russel T. Burge, "Economies of Scale in Physician Practice," *Medical Care Research and Review*, 53(4), December 1996: 417–440. Economies of scale are also found in the following study, Jose J. Escarce and Mark V. Pauly, "Physician Opportunity Costs in Physician Practice Cost Functions," Journal of Health Economics, 17(2), April 1998: 129–151.

6. Uwe Reinhardt, *op. cit.*

7. Douglas M. Brown, "Do Physicians Underutilize Aides?," *The Journal of Human Resources*, 23(3), Summer 1988: 342–355. For a more recent production function study, see Norman K. Thurston and Anne M. Libby, "A Production Function for Physician Services Revisited," *Review of Economics and Statistics*, 84(1) February 2002: 184–191.

8. William D. Marder and Stephen Zuckerman, "Competition and Medical Groups: A Survivor Analysis," *Journal of Health Economics*, 4(2), June 1985: 167–176.

9. Thomas E. Getzen, "A 'Brand Name Firm' Theory of Medical Group Practice," *The Journal of Industrial Economics*, 33(2), December 1984: 199–215.

10. Martin Gaynor and Paul Gertler, "Moral Hazard and Risk Spreading in Partnerships," *The RAND Journal of Economics*, 26(4), Winter 1995: 591–614.

11. Joseph Newhouse, "The Economics of Group Practice," *The Journal of Human Resources*, 8(1), Winter 1973: 36–57.

12. Thomas R. McCarthy, "The Competitive Nature of the Primary Care Physician Services Market," *Journal of Health Economics*, 4(2), June 1985: 93–117.

13. George Stigler, "The Economics of Information," *Journal of Political Economy*, 69(3), June 1961: 213–235.

14. In one of the few studies on physician advertising, the authors found that physicians advertised to attract more desirable patients. John Rizzo and R. Zeckhauser, "Advertising and Price, Quantity, and Quality of Primary Care Physician Services," *Journal of Human Resources*, 27(3), Summer 1992: 381–421.

15. John E. Kwoka, Jr., "Advertising and the Price and Quality of Optometric Services," *American Economic Review*, 74(1), March 1984: 211–216.

16. Using data from a previous FTC study in which the FTC trained nineteen professional interviewers to identify the equipment and procedures used in eye examinations, Haas-Wilson found that commercial practice restrictions used in various states in 1977 increased the price of an eye examination and a pair of eyeglasses by 5 to 13 percent, holding constant the thoroughness of the eye exam and the accuracy of the eyeglass prescription. Deborah Haas-Wilson, "The Effect of Commercial Practice Restrictions: The Case of Optometry," *Journal of Law and Economics*, 29(1) April 1986: 165–186.

17. Statement of the National Retired Teachers' Association and the American Association of Retired Persons on the Economics of the Eyeglasses Industry Before the Monopoly Subcommittee of the Senate Small Business Committee, U.S. Senate, May 24, 1977. Cited in Lee Benham, "Guilds and the Form of Competition in the Health Care Sector," in Warren Greenberg, ed., *Competition in the Health Care Sector* (Germantown, Md.: Aspen Systems Corporation, 1978).

18. The discussion in this section is based on Lynn Paringer, "Medicare Assignment Rates of Physicians: Their Responses to Changes in Reimbursement Policy," *Health Care Financing Review*, 1(3), Winter 1980: 75–90.

19. Mark H. Showalter, "Physicians' Cost Shifting Behavior: Medicaid Versus Other Patients," *Contemporary Economic Policy*, 15(2) April 1997: 74–84.

20. For a comprehensive discussion of supplier-induced demand including a critique of the empirical literature, see Thomas G. McGuire, *Handbook of Health Economics*, *op. cit.*

21. Mark V. Pauly and Mark A. Satterthwaite, "The Pricing of Primary Care Physicians' Services: A Test of the Role of Consumer Information," *Bell Journal of Economics*, 12(2), Autumn 1981: 488–506.

22. Victor R. Fuchs, "The Supply of Surgeons and the Demand for Operations," *Journal of Human Resources*, 13, Supplement, 1978: 35–56.

23. Louis F. Rossiter and Gail Wilensky, "A Reexamination of the Use of Physician Services: The Role of Physician-

Initiated Demand," *Inquiry*, 20(2), Summer 1983: 162–72; and "Identification of Physician-Induced Demand," *Journal of Human Resources*, 19(2), Spring 1984: 231–244.

24. Thomas R. McCarthy, *op. cit.*

25. Uwe Reinhardt, "The Theory of Physician-Induced Demand: Reflections After a Decade," *Journal of Health Economics*, 4(2), June 1985: 187–193.

26. Thomas H. Rice, "The Impact of Changing Medicare Reimbursement Rates on Physician-Induced Demand," *Medical Care*, 21(8), August 1983: 803–815.

27. George Monsma, "Marginal Revenue and Demand for Physicians' Services," in H. Klarman, ed., *Empirical Studies in Health Economics*, (Baltimore: Johns Hopkins University Press, 1970).

28. Winnie C. Yip, "Physician Responses to Medical Fee Reductions: Changes in the Volume and Intensity of Supply of Coronary Artery Bypass Graft (CABG) Surgeries in the Medicare and Private Sectors," *Journal of Health Economics*, 17(6), December 1998: 675–699.

29. Jean M. Mitchell and Tim R. Sass, "Physician Ownership of Ancillary Services: Indirect Demand Inducement or Quality Assurance?" *Journal of Health Economics*, 14(3), August 1995: 263–289.

30. Thomas G. McGuire and Mark V. Pauly, "Physician Responses to Fee Changes with Multiple Payers," *Journal of Health Economics*, 10(4), 1991: 385–410.

31. Jack Zwanziger, "Physician Fees and Managed Care Plans," *Inquiry*, 39(2), Summer 2002: 184–193.

32. James C. Robinson, "Physician Organization in California: Crisis and Opportunity," *Health Affairs*, 20(4) July/August 2001: 81–96. Also Lawrence Casalino, "Canaries in a Coal Mine: California Physician Groups and Competition," *Health Affairs*, 20(4), July/August 2001: 97–108.

33. Jeffrey Brennan, David Pender, and Markus Meier, *FTC Anti-Trust Actions in Health Care Services and Products*, (Federal Trade Commission: Washington, D.C.) April 2003. http://ftc.gov/bc/hcupdate030401.pdf.

34. "Patient Data May Reshape Health Care," *The Wall Street Journal*, April 17, 1989: B1. For a review of small area variation studies, see Sherman Folland and Miron Stano, "Small Area Variations: A Critical Review of Propositions, Methods, and Evidence," *Medical Care Review*, 47(4), Winter 1990: 419–465.

35. Constance Winslow, David Solomon, Mark Chassin, Jacqueline Kosecoff, Nancy Merrick, and Robert Brook, "The Appropriateness of Carotid Endarterecomy, *The New England Journal of Medicine*, 318(12) March 24, 1988: 721–727.

36. John K. Iglehart, "The New Law on Medicare's Payments to Physicians," *The New England Journal of Medicine*, 322(17), April 26, 1990: 1247–1252.

37. Department of Health and Human Services, Centers for Medicare & Medicaid Services, *2003 Annual Report of the Board of Trustees of the Federal Hospital Insurance and Federal Supplementary Medical Insurance Trust Funds*, [on-line information, 2003], http://www.cms.hhs.gov/publications/trusteesreport/2003/tabiic5.asp (accessed on May 6, 2003).

38. Uwe E. Reinhardt, "Alternative Methods of Reimbursing Non-Institutional Providers of Health Services," in *Controls on Health Care*, Proceedings of a Conference, January 7–9, 1974 (Washington, D.C.: National Academy of Sciences, 1975).

39. William C. Hsiao, Peter Braun, Douwe Yntema, and Edmund Becker, "Estimating Physicians' Work For a Resource-Based Relative Value Scale," *The New England Journal of Medicine*, 319(13), Sept. 29, 1988: 835–841. Also see in same issue, William C. Hsaio, et al., "Results and Policy Implications of the Resource-Based Relative-Value Study": 881–888.

40. The following book is devoted to an analysis of the Hsiao approach, H. E. Frech, ed., *Regulating Doctors' Fees*, (The AEI Press: Washington, D.C.), 1991.

41. Thomas McGuire, "Paralyzing Medicare's Demand-Side Policies," in *Regulating Doctors' Fees, op. cit.*: 174–192.

CHAPTER
11

The Market for Hospital Services

KEY TERMS AND CONCEPTS

- Hospital economies of scale
- Survivor analysis
- CON as an entry barrier
- Hospital's geographic market
- Industry consolidation
- HHI index
- Product or demand substitutability
- Profit-maximizing model of hospital behavior
- Utility-maximizing model of hospital behavior
- Physician control model of the hospital
- Non-price hospital competition
- Hospital price discrimination
- Medicare Diagnostic Related Groupings (DRGs)
- Cost shifting

Learning Objectives

Upon completing this chapter, the reader should be able to:

- Discuss the different theories why most hospitals are "not-for-profit."
- Contrast the utility maximizing, profit maximizing, and physician control models of hospital behavior.
- Explain why hospitals engaged in non-price competition before the 1980s.
- Describe how hospitals competed under managed care.
- Explain why hospitals in a price-competitive market are unable to "cost-shift."

BACKGROUND

The most important institutional setting to be analyzed is that of hospitals. In 2002, hospital expenditures totaled more than $486 billion, or 36.3 percent of personal health care expenditures and constitute the largest single healthcare expenditure category. Hospitals have been both the object and the beneficiary of much federal and state legislation. A great deal more emphasis is therefore devoted to hospitals than to other institutional settings.

Hospitals are classified according to the major type of service delivered, length of stay, and control or ownership. A short-term hospital is one in which its patients, on average, have lengths of stay of less than 30 days. As shown in Table 11-1, of the 5,801 hospitals listed by the American Hospital Association, 5,170 are classified as short-term hospitals. The major types of services by which short-term hospitals are classified are general, psychiatric, and tuberculosis and other respiratory diseases. The general hospital is the predominant type of hospital; 4,927 hospitals have this service classification. Hospital control or ownership can be categorized as governmental (i.e., federal, state, and local), non-profit (i.e., voluntary or community), or for-profit.

Psychiatric, tuberculosis, and long-term hospitals have generally been public institutions for welfare reasons and because of externalities, such as the contagiousness of tuberculosis which led the state to provide care for such persons in order to protect the rest of the population. The demand for such public institutions has decreased dramatically.

The decline in demand for tuberculosis hospitals has been the result of improved environmental conditions, widespread testing and earlier discovery, and improved treatment techniques. New treatment techniques for mental illness, including drug therapy, have shifted the demand for incarceration in a public psychiatric hospital to a demand for treatment in nongovernment psychiatric facilities with a shorter length of stay. Short-term general hospitals have also developed substitute facilities in the form of psychiatric units; these, together with outpatient treatment, provide psychiatric services that have left only the poor, the senile, and the incurable to the care of mental hospitals which provide care of a different quality at much lower cost.

The decline in demand for long-term hospitals is partly attributable to the development of substitute facilities (i.e., nursing homes), along with increased patient incomes and public insurance to pay for such care.

The demand for care in short-term general and other special hospitals, however, has increased over time, particularly since the 1960s. This increased demand resulted from the growth in health insurance, an aging population, and changes in medical technology which made possible the provision of new services, such as organ transplants. Since the mid 1980s, however, innovations in medical technology have made it possible to perform many surgical procedures in an outpatient setting. And insurance companies' interest in lowering the cost of hospital care shifted the demand for many surgical procedures from the hospital to outpatient surgery centers. Continued advances in medical technology are leaving the hospital with "high tech" type services while shifting the treatment of most other types of services to an outpatient facility.

The analysis of the market for hospital services emphasizes the performance of the short-term general hospital, and within that type of hospital, the voluntary, non-profit institution. The predominant form of control and organization of the short-term general hospital is nongovernmental and non-profit; these hospitals number 2,998. State and local governmental are next in predominance, numbering 1,156; then come the for-profit (investor-owned) hospitals, with 754. When one examines the data in Table 11-1 on admissions and the number of beds, the voluntary non-profit short-term general hospital is even more predominant as the major institution involved in the delivery of hospital services. These institutions have 71 percent of the short-term general beds and admit 70 percent of the patients.

Table 11-1 reveals that the large majority of short-term general hospitals have fewer than 200 beds, with 46 percent having fewer than 100 beds. These same hospitals, however, account for only 11 percent of

Table 11-1.   Selected Data on U.S. Hospitals, 2001

Type of Hospital	Number of Hospitals	Percent Change 1980–90	Percent Change 1990–2001	Beds	Admissions	Percent Distribution of Admissions	Occupancy Rate(a)
Short-term						97.7	
General(b)	4,927	–8.2	–9.1	827,769	33,833,828	94.9	64.5
State and local government	1,156	–18.8	–19.9	132,178	4,634,205	13.0	64.1
Voluntary	2,998	–3.9	–6.0	585,070	24,982,640	70.1	65.8
Investor-owned	754	2.6	0.7	108,718	4,196,744	11.8	57.8
Federal	243	–6.1	–27.9	51,900	1,000,882	2.8	69.8
Long-term(c)	631	27.1	–29.3	107,771	809,730	2.3	81.9
Community	4,908	–7.7	–8.8	825,966	33,813,589	100.0	64.5
Bedsize category							
6–99 beds	2,267	–11.9	–6.5	115,151	3,592,780	10.6	50.7
100–199 beds	1,218	–4.7	–6.7	174,024	6,777,542	20.0	60.7
200–299 beds	635	3.4	–14.1	154,420	6,630,307	19.6	65.5
300–399 beds	348	–1.0	–14.7	119,753	5,328,441	15.8	66.4
400–499 beds	191	–16.5	–14.0	84,745	3,778,746	11.2	68.9
500+ beds	249	–10.1	–12.6	177,873	7,705,773	22.8	72.8

Source: American Hospital Association, *Hospital Statistics,* (Chicago, IL: American Hospital Association), various editions: 1982 ed., table 1, 1991–1992 ed., text table 3, table 5A, 2003 ed., table 2.

(a) Ratio of average daily census to every 100 beds.

(b) "Short-term general" includes community hospitals and hospital units of institutions. Community hospitals group consists of state and local government, voluntary and investor-owned hospitals.

(c) Includes general, psychiatric, tuberculosis and other respiratory diseases, and all others.

admissions. The vast majority of admissions, about 70 percent, occur in hospitals that have 200 beds and more.

Hospitals not only differ in their size and ownership, but also in the services they offer. Hospitals are multi-product firms. The services offered in a 500-bed teaching hospital are different from those found in a 150-bed community hospital. Further, while both institutions will offer some similar services, such as obstetrics, the larger teaching hospital will also have facilities to provide care in greater depth, such as for high-risk pregnancies and neonatal intensive care units.

One indication of the multi-product nature of hospitals is the high rate of technological innovation in new services. Examples of technological innovation over the last 17 years are shown in Table 11-2. The number of hospitals offering organ transplantation

has risen from 244 hospitals in 1984 to 386 hospitals in 2001. (The cost of an organ transplant is approximately $250,000, but it varies by organ. For example, while it is $100,000 for a kidney transplant, it costs $250,000 for a liver, $300,000 for heart and lung, and as high as $470,000 for an intestinal transplant.) The percentage of hospitals with new diagnostic equipment, such as Magnetic Resonance Imaging (MRI) devices, has risen from 3 percent to 56 percent. Thus simple comparisons of hospital costs between hospitals or over time should be used with caution since such comparisons do not allow for the vast differences in services offered or the introduction of new technology.

The picture that emerges of the hospital industry is of many small hospitals, likely located in rural areas, operating at low occupancy rates, and serving a small percentage of the patient population. The growth in medical technology has occurred at the larger-sized

Table 11-2.   Trends in Selected Medical Technologies Provided by Community Hospitals, 1984 and 2001

	1984		2001	
	Number of Hospitals	Percent of Total	Number of Hospitals	Percent of Total
Cardiac catheterization	942	17.7	1,605	38.7
CT scanner	2,555	47.9	3,625	87.3
MRI	166	3.1	2,333	56.2
Open-heart surgery	631	11.8	936	22.6
Organ transplantation	244	4.6	396(a)	9.3

Source: American Hospital Association, *Hospital Statistics*, 1990–1991 ed. and 2003 ed. (Chicago: American Hospital Association), 1990 ed., p. xii, 2003 ed., table 7, pp. 153–162.

Note: Data represents the number of hospitals providing the above services rather than the number of such technologies within the hospital.

(a) Data for transplant services.

hospitals where most patients are treated, and which are located in more urban communities.

The above descriptive data illustrate the changes that have been occurring in the hospital sector. The short-term general hospital has increased in size and in the volume of services delivered; it has changed its product, and in turn there have been very large increases in the cost of its output. The large sums of money spent on hospitals make it important to determine the efficiency with which this market performs.

Also important for understanding the behavior and performance of this industry are its special characteristics, namely, its non-profit ownership status and the role of the hospital's medical staff in controlling the use of the hospital's resources in providing patient treatment that distinguish it from other types of firms.

DETERMINANTS OF MARKET STRUCTURE

The market structure for hospitals can be characterized according to how many hospitals compete with one another. At one extreme is the competitive market where there are many competitors. At the other end is monopoly, with only one hospital in the market. Two important factors determine how many hospitals compete within a given market: economies of scale and barriers to entry. Entry barriers increase the mar-

ket power—hence profitability—of those hospitals currently in the market. Such barriers have, at various times, proven to be significant in determining the number of hospital competitors. For example, Certificate of Need (CON) legislation required that a hospital receive approval from a state agency before the hospital was able to build or purchase facilities or equipment that exceeded $100,000. New hospitals trying to enter a hospital's market were denied a CON. Existing hospitals also used CON legislation to prevent their competitors from adding services to compete with those offered by their own hospital.

Similar to entry controls have been quasi-controls, such as the (previous) refusal of an insurance company (e.g., Blue Cross) to pay for hospital care in certain types of institutions (e.g., for-profit hospitals). The price to the patient of going to a for-profit hospital was thereby increased relative to a non-profit hospital where the patient's Blue Cross insurance paid for everything.

During the period of managed care competition from the early 1980s to 2000, utilization management and the shift to outpatient care created excess capacity among hospitals; entry barriers were not a significant determinant of hospital market structure. More recently, however, excess capacity has declined, in part because of hospital mergers. In the many states not having Certificate of Need legislation, economies of scale is the main determinant of market structure.

The Extent of Economies of Scale in Relation to the Size of the Market

Economies of scale occur when average cost falls as the size of the firm is increased. The theoretical relationship between hospital cost and size is U-shaped. As the size of the facility (and its production) is increased, average cost per unit decreases, reaches a minimum, and then increases. The reasons for this expected relationship are several: with a larger facility there can be greater specialization of labor; further, licensure, as a means of assuring competent personnel in the health field, limits flexibility in delegation of tasks; thus larger institutions are able to more fully use licensed and specialized personnel than can smaller hospitals. Specialized equipment and facilities can also be used to their capacity in larger institutions. Finally, larger institutions are more likely than smaller institutions to be able to take advantage of quantity discounts in purchasing.

Offsetting these advantages of size is the greater proportion of time and effort required to coordinate and control work in large organizations. In general, for sufficiently small outputs, efficiency increases with size because the advantages that accrue from the use of specialized labor and equipment far outweigh the increased cost of management. As size increases, however, the reduction in per-unit cost afforded by greater specialization begins to decline and is eventually outweighed by increased costs of coordination and control. Other things being equal, average hospital costs thus may be expected to decline initially and then rise as size is increased. How rapidly these gains and losses from scale of operation occur is what determines the shape of the long-run average cost curve.

For a given size of market, the larger the firm size required to achieve the minimum costs of production, the fewer the number of firms that will be able to compete. In a price-competitive market, when the most efficient size of firm is large, smaller firms with higher average costs will not be able to survive. Also determining the competitiveness of a market is the size of the geographic market (the larger the geographic market the greater the number of competitors), and the closeness of substitutes.

Determination of market structure and the existence of hospital market power have become important in recent years because of an increase in hospital mergers. The Federal Trade Commission (FTC) and the Department of Justice (DOJ) are concerned that hospital mergers will lessen competition in the merging hospitals' market.[1] Crucial to the prosecution of the resulting anti-trust case are two important elements, both of which determine whether there are close substitutes to the merging hospitals: the definition of the relevant *product market* and the definition of the merging hospitals' *geographic market* (and the relative market shares of the merging hospitals within those markets).

Depending upon the definition of the geographic (and product) market, a market structure can be either monopolistic or competitive. For any least cost size of hospital, the larger the geographic size of the market, the greater are the number of hospitals that are able to compete in that market. The geographic definition of the hospital's market determines which hospitals compete with one another.

When there are no close substitutes and the particular service is the only one in a particular geographic area, then the hospital with that service has market power, that is, it has monopoly power.

Market power is generally defined as a firm being able to act without suffering any economic harm, namely, the firm would not lose a significant amount of sales if it were to raise its price, e.g., 5 percent, or provide less acceptable services. If a firm were to do either of these actions when close substitutes are

---

1. In addition to the argument that the merger does not lessen competition and/or that entry is easy for new firms, the merging hospitals may justify the merger on grounds that efficiency will be increased by taking advantage of economies of scale, the cost savings of which will then be passed on to consumers in the form of lower prices. Another justification used for the merger is to save a failing hospital, thereby preserving its assets for competition. With the merger there will be the same number of firms as if the hospital failed; further, that there are no other potential buyers for that failing hospital. Given the limited empirical evidence on economies of scale, it is difficult to prove large efficiencies as a result of a merger. In the latter case, the failing hospital should be acquired by the least-competitive hospital so as to not be anti-competitive. http://www.ftc.gov/bc/healthindex.htm

available and other competitors are located nearby, their higher prices or less acceptable services could not be maintained; patients would either switch to competitors, to firms that offer close substitutes, or new competitors would enter the market. In a competitive market, price and other attributes of the service would reflect their respective marginal costs. Only with market power would a firm be able to raise its price above marginal cost without fear of competitors' actions.

In merger cases, the relevant product and geographic markets as defined by the FTC are generally narrower than the definitions used by the analysts for the merging hospitals. A very narrow interpretation of the relevant product and geographic markets would find that there are no close substitutes to the hospital's service and that the geographic area served by the hospital is sufficiently small as to find few other competitors. Under this narrow definition, the merging hospitals would be found to have a high market share in both the product and geographic markets, thereby providing the merged hospitals with increased market power. Proponents of the merger typically develop broader interpretations of the geographic and product markets, thereby indicating a smaller market share for the merging hospitals.

Product or demand substitutability depends upon a willingness of purchasers or patients to use alternative services. Alternative services should be reasonable substitutes, i.e., have a high cross-price elasticity. Presumably, adult open heart surgery has low substitutability with other surgical procedures, while inpatient cataract surgery has a high substitutability with outpatient cataract surgery. One indication of how close a substitute two products are is their price differential (assuming the prices are not regulated by government). If the price of one service has a much higher price than the other, then they are usually not close substitutes. Typically, product market definitions have been less controversial in merger cases.

The determination of the relevant geographic market has been more difficult to determine. Conceptually, the relevant geographic market would include suppliers who are currently in the market; second, those firms in the market not currently pro-

viding the service but who could add that service in a reasonable time period; and third, suppliers not in the market but who are capable of entering the market within a reasonable time. Entry by new suppliers into a geographic market is easier for services that are subject to small economies of scale, such as a competitor hospital offering a wellness screening program. More complex and costly programs, such as a transplant program, could only be introduced into a market after a number of years.

The patient's willingness to travel to other suppliers of the service also defines the geographic market. Patients might be willing to travel to a more distant hospital that is less expensive (or higher quality) than be admitted to a local hospital that is more expensive (or of lower quality) when the value of their travel cost and time is less than the higher costs of going to the local hospital. The total price of hospitalization includes the implicit costs of travel and time plus the explicit out-of-pocket cost of the hospital and is the relevant price to the patient, not just the hospital portion of that price.[2] Thus, when a high value is placed on patient travel relative to the cost of the service, such as for emergency care and obstetrics services, then the relevant market is smaller than when the patient is willing to travel further for more costly services, as is the case for elective surgery, such as transplants. One study found that distance has an important effect on hospital admissions for selected surgical procedures; a 10 percent decrease in distance increased admissions by 13 to 14 percent (1).

---

2. In addition to providing information useful for determining hospital market structure, knowledge of hospital economies of scale is also useful for planning regional hospital systems. Planning such systems requires the same information that would produce the outcomes of a competitive market. In a competitive system, economic efficiency is achieved when both implicit as well as explicit costs are minimized. Thus, in addition to economies of scale (explicit costs), there are additional costs, such as patient travel cost and the cost of not having a bed (or service) when needed. For a discussion of the economics of health facilities planning and an illustration with respect to obstetric facilities, see Millard F. Long and Paul J. Feldstein, "The Economics of Hospital Systems: Peak Loads and Regional Coordination," *American Economic Review,* 57(2), May 1967, 119–129.

The relevant geographic market is also affected by the definition of the product market; the market area for wellness and transplant programs are not the same. The relevant geographic market thus depends upon the type of care, with primary care services having a more localized market while tertiary care has a broader geographic market.

Controversy exists as to how the geographic market for hospitals should be empirically defined (2). Several studies have used a specific geographic distance, such as a 5- or 15-mile radius around a hospital (the hypothesis being that the patient's physician is unwilling to travel long distances to admit and treat the patient). Others have used government designations, such as counties or Standard Metropolitan Statistical Areas. (Geographic definitions, such as county, are usually larger than the hospital's actual market.) Other researchers have used patient origination data, defining the market as consisting of those ZIP codes from which a hospital drew a certain percentage of its patients, e.g., 75 to 90 percent of its patients. In such cases, a hospital was defined as a competitor if it admitted a certain percent, e.g., 25 percent, of its patients from that hospital's market.

Within a geographic area, researchers have classified the market as being more or less competitive based on the number of hospitals in that area; others have used the Herfindahl-Hirschman Index (HHI), which is the measure of concentration used by the Department of Justice in its merger guidelines.[3] The advantage of this index is that it is sensitive to both the number of firms and to their relative sizes (e.g., percent of total admissions). Thus for the same number of firms in the market, the index will indicate greater market concentration if a few firms have a high market share than if all the firms had the same share. A merger between large firms will result in a much greater increase in the index than if two small firms merged.

Estimating whether a merger may be anti-competitive involves calculating the market share's HHI index of each of the competitors (within the relevant product and geographic markets) both before and after the proposed merger. If the new HHI exceeds 1,800 under the proposed merger, then the merger is likely to trigger an anti-trust investigation. The HHI, however, is not sufficient by itself to indicate whether the proposed merger will be anti-competitive; it is also necessary to determine the competitiveness of that market, how hospitals compete, and whether competition will be decreased as a result of the merger.

As the number of hospital mergers increase and more anti-trust cases are brought against such mergers, greater effort is being placed on defining hospital geographic markets and whether mergers lessen competition in those markets.

Empirical Findings on the Extent of Economies of Scale in Hospital Services

It has been difficult to empirically estimate the cost-size relationship of hospitals. Hospitals are not homogeneous in size or other characteristics. Hospitals are multi-product firms. In addition to producing inpatient services (which differ in their quality), the type of patient treated, and the severity of the particular case, hospitals also produce outpatient services (education, training, research, and community services). Hospitals also differ in the prices they pay for their labor and non-labor inputs as well as in their efficiency of operations. Studies have found it difficult to estimate the effect of size on average cost while holding constant all the other factors mentioned above.

For example, if larger hospitals are subject to economies of scale but they also treat more seriously ill patients, then it may appear that larger hospitals have *higher* per-unit costs. This problem is illustrated

---

3. The Herfindahl Index is calculated by summing the squared market shares of each firm in the market. For example, if there are five hospitals in an area and each has the same market share, 20 percent, then the HHI is

$$20^2 + 20^2 + 20^2 + 20^2 + 20^2 = 2,000.$$

If the five firms had unequal market shares, the HHI would be

$$40^2 + 30^2 + 10^2 + 10^2 + 10^2 = 2,800.$$

in Figure 11-1. The hospital represented by the short-run average cost curve at point C is on a lower (different) long-run average cost curve than hospital B or A because it provides fewer services. If one were to examine unadjusted (for number of services) data on average cost and size, one would observe data points that represent the relationship between hospitals D and A. It would appear that hospital D (which is smaller) has lower costs than hospital A, and that average costs increase as the size of the hospital is similarly increased.

If the different products offered by these two hospitals can be held constant, then it would be determined that hospital A is producing its output in the least costly facility (it is operating in a facility that is at the minimum point on its long-run average cost curve) on long-run average cost curve $LRAC_3$. Hospital D, however, is not only producing a different product (one that is less costly to produce than the one produced by hospital A), but it is also in a facility that is not least costly; it is at point D rather than point C.

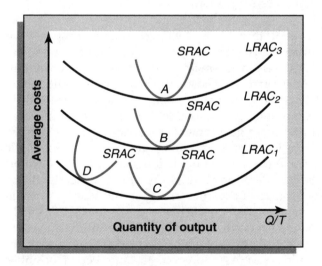

Figure 11-1. Variations in average cost between hospitals.

Researchers have used two general approaches for estimating hospital economies of scale. The first is a multivariate analysis where the different factors affecting hospital costs are included in the empirical analysis so as to be able to determine the net effect of size on average costs per admission or per-patient day (3). Examples of measures that have been included in cost studies are the number and type of facilities and services, patient case-mix measures (the proportion of a hospital's patients classified into various diagnostic categories), quality (mortality rate, non-patient care outputs of the hospital, such as teaching programs, and the impact that interns and residents have on hospital costs), outpatient services (which may share facilities and equipment with inpatient services in the hospital), and differences among hospitals in their physicians' contribution to the hospitals' output (4). For example, teaching and community hospitals differ in their employment of staff physicians. Hospitals that employ physicians will include in their costs the physician's salary and consequently have higher costs than hospitals that do not employ physicians, although there may be no difference in either hospital's output.

To summarize the findings on economies of scale, there appear to be slight economies of scale: hospitals with approximately 200 to 300 beds appear to have the lowest average costs. The shape of this average cost curve is shallow; that is, it does not fall sharply, nor is the minimum point much below that of hospitals on the ends of the curve.[4]

---

4. To determine whether there are economies of scale, the output measure is allowed to be curvilinear; that is, either the variables are transformed into logarithms or a squared term is included for the output measure. For example, if the net effect of beds on average cost per admission is -0.04 BEDS $+ 0.0001$ BEDS^2, then the size of hospital with lowest average costs is determined by taking the partial derivative of AC with respect to BEDS, setting it equal to zero, and solving for BEDS.

$$\frac{\varphi AC}{\varphi BEDS} = \begin{array}{ll} -0.04 + 0.0002 & BEDS = 0 \\ + 0.0002 & BEDS = +0.04 \\ & BEDS = 200 \end{array}$$

Average costs per admission would be at a minimum in hospitals with 200 beds.

For highly specialized services such as organ transplants, the extent of economies of scale can be used to indicate how many such services can be offered in a given area.

Hospital cost studies have found that the mix of patients in the hospital is an important determinant of hospital costs; in some cases, case mix explains more than 50 percent of the variation in average costs between hospitals. Since large teaching hospitals have a sicker mix of patients, unless case mix is held constant, it would appear that they are subject to diseconomies of scale. (Accurate measurement of the hospitals' patient mix and the complexity of the cases is important in paying hospitals under any prospective payment system, such as Medicare and Medicaid).

The second type of study for estimating economies of scale is survivor analyses that examine changes in the size distribution of hospitals over time. Hospitals with the lowest average cost would be expected to gain market share, while those that are either too large or too small would be expected to lose market share. Survivor analyses implicitly include all the factors that affect hospital costs, such as multiple outputs and services offered, as well as patient travel costs, whereas multivariate studies must attempt to include them and develop accurate proxy measures for each.

Survivor-type analyses have found that hospitals with less than 100 beds have lost market share over time. Thus, similar to the multivariate studies, it appears that hospitals with more than 100 beds, up to about 300 beds, have lower average cost (5).

Lending support to the finding of economies of scale is data showing changes in the size distribution of hospitals over time, shown in Table 11-1. In the period before the onset of managed care (which created excess capacity among all size hospitals), the average hospital size had been increasing. The number of hospitals in the smaller bed size categories, less than 100 beds, declined (they expanded in size), while the number of hospitals in the larger bed size categories increased. Since hospitals were reimbursed according to their costs during this period, this change in the size distribution of hospitals was not necessarily due to greater efficiency with increased size. (Since the mid 1980s with the decline in hospital use, part of the

decrease in the number of small hospitals has been a result of their closure rather than increases in their size.)

In the managed care period 1985 to the present, hospitals were no longer paid according to their costs, price competition became more pervasive, there were greater incentives for efficiency, utilization declined as a result of utilization management, and technological advances permitted many types of surgical procedures to be performed in outpatient surgery centers. Many hospitals came under severe financial pressures. As hospitals were forced to close and others to merge, the largest percent declines occurred among the larger sized hospitals, more than 300 beds. The size distribution of hospitals appears to be compressing; hospitals at greatest risk of closure or merger appear to be both very large and small (rural) hospitals. The least-cost size of hospital now appears to be about 200 beds.

Given the above findings regarding economies of scale, it becomes important to examine the geographic size of hospital markets to determine how many hospitals can compete within their markets, hence the type of market structure.

The Extent of Hospital Markets

In 2001 there were 4,907 community hospitals. Of these, 2,741 were located in metropolitan areas, and 2,166 were in non-metropolitan areas. While 56 percent of the community hospitals are located in metropolitan areas, these hospitals contain 79 percent of the beds in community hospitals. Metropolitan Statistical Areas (MSAs) are government designations for geographic areas that represent an integrated social and economic area. A city with a population of at least 50,000 would be considered an MSA. MSAs would not necessarily be indicative of a particular market in which a hospital competes since for some services the travel time might be too great while for other services (those subject to large economies of scale) the market may encompass multiple MSAs. However, the number of hospitals within an MSA provides a general indication of the number of competitors within a hospital's market.

As shown in Figure 11-2, in 2001, 169 MSAs (or 46 percent) have fewer than 4 hospitals, and 63 MSAs (18 percent) have 4 to 5 hospitals. The remaining MSAs (36 percent) have more than 6 hospitals. However, these 36 percent of MSAs with 6 or more hospitals contain approximately 78 percent of the community hospitals that are located in metropolitan areas.

Based on the above calculations, it would appear that for the community hospitals that are located in MSAs (56 percent of all community hospitals and 79 percent of the beds), 46 percent of the MSAs have highly concentrated markets (less than 4 hospitals), and another 18 percent of MSAs are also quite concentrated (4 to 5 hospitals). (It is important to remember that the relevant geographic market for specialized services is likely to encompass more than one MSA.) However, these concentrated markets (64 percent of the MSAs) represent only 22 percent of the community hospitals located in metropolitan areas (MSAs). The large majority of community hospitals (and beds) are in less concentrated MSAs, with more than six hospitals per MSA.

In concentrated hospital markets, the market structure may be characterized as being an "oligopoly," that is, the hospitals are mutually interdependent; each

hospital is aware that they are affected by their competitor's behavior. In the current price-competitive environment and limited measures of hospital quality by which hospitals can differentiate themselves, hospitals in oligopoly markets compete on price to be included in an insurer's provider network. Hospital mergers in oligopoly (concentrated) markets are likely to be closely examined by federal anti-trust agencies.

The market structure of 36 percent of the MSAs, which contains 78 percent of the community hospitals in MSAs, could be characterized as "monopolistic competition." Hospitals in these markets are also engaged in price competition. Mergers and acquisitions are being used to consolidate hospitals in these markets so that the resulting number of hospital systems within a market are representative of oligopoly markets.

The size of most hospital markets for specialized services has expanded, making these markets more competitive. Travel costs for the patient and family are a small portion of total medical costs for complex treatments. The demand for highly specialized services is generally not of an emergency nature; the relevant market in which competition for such services

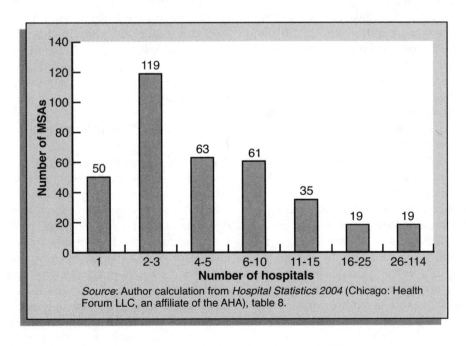

Source: Author calculation from *Hospital Statistics 2004* (Chicago: Health Forum LLC, an affiliate of the AHA), table 8.

Figure 11-2.   The number of hospitals in metropolitan statistical areas, 2001.

occurs is much larger and for some specialized services, such as organ transplants, at a regional. (Thus, it is unlikely that a case can be made for treating them as a natural monopoly.)

The Growth of Multi-Hospital Systems

The structure of the hospital market has changed over time. Until the late 1970s, hospitals were predominately non-profit, independent institutions, generally competing in local markets, and providing inpatient services. Currently, hospitals are part of a larger organization, a multi-hospital system, and provide a broad range of services, such as ambulatory care clinics, inpatient care, outpatient surgery, and home care.

Non-profit multi-hospital systems have made the industry more concentrated and vary in how closely the hospitals within each system are controlled. In some systems, the hospital affiliation agreements are relatively weak. The hospital and its medical staff are able to retain their decision-making authority over expenditures and investments. Weak forms of affiliation enable the hospital to take advantage of some economies of scale, such as joint purchasing arrangements.

In stronger affiliations, hospitals are completely merged into the larger organization; the institution loses its autonomy. The reasons favoring this type of arrangement are also to take advantage of economies of scale, such as lower interest costs and greater access to the capital markets, lower administrative costs, as well as improved cash management and lower malpractice premiums. There are also economies in marketing a large network of providers to an insurer as compared to insurers contracting with separate facilities. Further, merging hospitals in the same market consolidates that market reducing the number of competitors, and increases the combined hospitals' market power; they are able to negotiate higher prices with insurers and HMOs. Each of these reasons requires the institution to be more tightly integrated with the other hospitals in the system. Those hospitals facing declining occupancy rates, more stringent reimbursement policies, and declining profitability are more willing to give up their autonomy to survive.

Multi-hospital systems, which are comprised of investor owned, secular non-profit, religious, and public institutions, represent about 40 percent of the total nonfederal short-term general beds. Although there was an increase in the number of non-profit hospital systems during the 1990s, most of these systems are relatively small, between five to ten hospitals each. While the number of investor-owned systems declined (largely through mergers), the average number of hospitals per system increased to 42 hospitals per system in 2001 (6). The number of hospitals per system, however, varies greatly.

There are fewer hospitals in non-profit systems because these systems attempt to increase their market share within a particular geographic area. Hospital systems have also joined together in voluntary purchasing networks to take advantage of purchasing economies. Several investor-owned systems have concentrated on non-urban markets where there is little competition; they purchase a non-profit hospital that is in financial difficulty and invest capital to add services and attract physicians. These investor-owned systems have been financially successful with this strategy.

To remain independent and profitable, an unaffiliated community hospital must be located in a growing market where a high percent of the population has private health insurance and has a high degree of market power. Not many community hospitals are in such a situation.

Vertical and Virtual Integration

The role of the hospital and its product line has been changing. Before managed care and under fee-for-service payment, hospitals were the center of the medical delivery system. The most modern technology was housed in the hospital, hospitals competed for physicians based on their technology and services, and hospital administrators were concerned with filling their beds. As managed care grew, provider incentives changed, and procedures began to be shifted outside the hospital. It became more profitable for HMOs (as well as hospitals and their physicians) to keep capitated patients out of the hospital. Medical technology reinforced capitation payment incentives by making possible greater use of non-hospital services such as outpatient surgery, diagnostics, sub-acute care, and home care. Hospital utilization decreased. Hospitals had to compete on price to be included in the insurer's provider network before they could compete for physicians.

Hospitals became concerned that they were being moved from the center of the delivery system to its periphery.

As the entity with the largest investment in fixed assets and greatest access to capital, hospitals sought to preserve their centrality by changing their role. In addition to integrating horizontally to take advantage of economies of scale and to increase its market power in an area, hospitals attempted to become vertically integrated organizations, also referred to as Integrated Delivery Systems (IDS). An IDS encompasses the entire production function for health care; it combines the successive stages of production and distribution of medical services into one organization. For example, in a capitated environment the IDS will include services such as wellness care, acute care, as well as recovery and rehabilitation. All of the various institutional settings are included, from ambulatory care, inpatient care, outpatient care, and home health care.

A hospital can produce a particular service itself or purchase it from suppliers. Important to the hospital's decision of "make or buy" is whether there are economies of scale in the production of the service and differences in the transaction costs of these options. These transaction costs, in addition to the actual prices paid for supplies and labor, are part of the costs of producing a service. To be efficient, a firm must also minimize its transaction costs. When the transaction costs of dealing with suppliers exceeds the transaction cost of producing the service itself, all else being equal, then the firm is likely to vertically integrate the supply of that input.

A hospital's transaction costs (or the costs of controlling and coordinating the delivery of medical services) involve the collection of information about the different suppliers of each of the components of medical services, the negotiation of separate contracts

with each set of suppliers, monitoring compliance with the contract, and the hospital's ability to enforce such contracts. The necessity for frequent negotiations with suppliers, uncertainty as to the suppliers' quality, and the difficulty of monitoring a supplier's behavior increase transaction costs to the firm. (7)

When payment systems were cost based and each provider was separately reimbursed, a provider had little incentive to be concerned either with economies of scale or with transaction costs. They were not at risk for either their own or other providers' behavior.

In the new competitive environment and fixed Medicare DRG prices, the dependence of hospitals on providers in other parts of the production process particularly physicians, increased. Hospitals were placed at financial risk for their physicians' behavior and they controlled hospital referrals.

The shift to fixed DRG prices also increased the interdependency between hospitals and nursing homes. Under DRGs, hospitals have a financial incentive to discharge a patient early since they will not be reimbursed for the additional costs they incur on behalf of a patient. Many aged patients, however, cannot be immediately discharged to their home but need to be in a nursing home. Nursing homes, however, have an incentive to accept less severely ill patients since they are separately reimbursed by Medicare according to maximum prices. Given the uncertainties of having adequate facilities to discharge their patients, some hospitals purchased nursing homes. It is costly for the hospital to negotiate customized contracts with the nursing home for each of its discharged patients, who vary in their care needs and discharge dates.

The dependence of hospitals upon other providers and the difficulty of specifying contracts in great detail resulted in hospitals purchasing the separate components of the delivery and distribution system.

By coordinating care in different settings, the IDS expected to have a competitive cost advantage over less integrated delivery systems. Patients would be able to move smoothly throughout the system and through different levels of care with their medical information available to each provider and without having unnecessary duplication of services or tests.

Essential to the success of an IDS are appropriate financial incentives among the various components of the system, primary care physicians, specialists, hospital administrators, etc., capital to invest in developing an exclusive physician infrastructure, and an information system that enables coordination of patient care to occur without duplication of tests, etc.

Although a number of organizations attempted vertical integration, few, if any, were successful. Hospitals purchased physician practices only to find that physician productivity declined since physicians no longer had the same financial incentives as previously. Other hospitals invested in medical groups only to find that the medical groups did not share a common vision, or that the group's financial incentives resulted in conflict with the hospital. Hospitals were also unable to develop the necessary information systems to coordinate care within the entire delivery system. Physicians were also concerned with the governance of the IDS, believing that too much control rested with the hospital. The lack of a culture of cooperation between non-profit hospitals and affiliated physicians also limited the organization's integration.

Several larger medical groups believed their organization should be the one to integrate the delivery of medical services. The growth of very large medical groups resulted in an increase in their market power relative to that of hospitals. These medical groups decided that they could make more money by contracting with an HMO for all the patient's medical services. The medical group would receive a capitation payment from the HMO for either all of the medical services, such as 85 percent of the premium, or for just the medical portion, e.g., 40 percent of the premium, and share in the savings from reduced hospital use and cost. The medical group would then manage the production function for healthcare (produce medical services) less expensively by contracting with hospitals and other providers rather than integrating with a hospital under a common ownership and governance. Given hospitals' excess capacity, these large medical groups believed they could negotiate better hospital rates than if they had to purchase or use the hospitals within their own organization.

In a virtually integrated organization, the medical groups believed that the alignment of organizational incentives were improved in a contractual rather than in an ownership relationship.

Few medical groups were successful at integrating the delivery of medical services. These groups did not have the management expertise, the necessary capital for expansion, the information systems, or the group culture for working together. Several large medical groups sold their assets to publicly traded physician management companies in return for management expertise and capital but were still unsuccessful at fulfilling their promise. Both the physician management companies and the medical groups suffered financially.

Organizations attempting vertical or virtual integration have been unsuccessful in being able to coordinate performance among the different entities in the delivery of care, developing an acceptable structure of organizational governance, and instituting an approach for managing clinical innovation.

The different providers of medical services, e.g., hospitals and physicians, have divergent interests. What are the most effective incentives to be used so that providers will coordinate their activities? Two approaches that are used to improve performance are, first, cooperation between different providers (as occurs when all providers work for one organization) and, second, relying on financial incentives, as when different providers engage in contractual relationships. Each approach has advantages and disadvantages. Developing specific contracts to govern all aspects of a provider's performance is difficult given differences among the patient population and their severity of illness. Alternatively, relying on provider cooperation entails weaker financial incentives for providers to be productive. Alignment of financial incentives among mutually dependent provider groups is difficult to achieve.

With regard to governance structures, the for-profit model is clear in its objectives and results in quicker response to poor management. However, for-profit companies have a shorter time horizon in calculating their investment return; they may also have less of a commitment to their communities since a subsidiary may be closed or merged with another organization depending upon its profitability. Conversely, non-profit organizations are less accountable for their performance and slower to react to market changes.

Important to the future success of any organization is their ability to innovate. Do vertically integrated systems have a greater commitment to maintaining their large investment in fixed assets and their current provider network than in developing innovations that threaten their existing stakeholders? Do virtually integrated systems have greater financial incentives to innovate than systems that rely on cooperative relationships? Which type of organization and which incentives offer the greatest encouragement to undertake risk? The rewards of risk and innovation in a large organization are diffused throughout that organization, while failure resulting from risk is more apt to be concentrated among several persons.

Organizational change is constantly occurring as the competitive market evolves. While it is difficult to anticipate new types of organizations, virtual organizations (based on contractual relationships) appear to offer more promise in solving the problems of an acceptable governance structure, performance incentives, and incentives for innovation.

HOSPITAL CONDUCT AND BEHAVIOR

To understand and to be able to evaluate the performance of the hospital industry, it is first important to examine three aspects of this sector: the determinants of the industry's structure, payment systems and their effect on hospitals' incentives, and the objectives of hospital decision-makers. The industry's market structure, based on economies of scale and legal restraints on entry, is typically an important factor determining the number of competitors in a market, the type of competition among firms, as well as the performance of that industry.

In addition to market structure, hospital objectives and the payment incentives facing hospitals affect the type of competition among hospitals (and their consequent performance). Most hospitals are non-profit organizations, thus it is important to determine whether their market behavior is likely to differ from for-profit hospitals.

In a competitive system, the assumption that firms will attempt to maximize their profits makes it possible to predict what a firm's supply response will be to changes in demand and/or changes in its input prices. With entry into the industry permitted, firms would be expected to minimize their costs, and their prices will reflect the costs of production; there would be no internal cross-subsidization of patients or of users of different services. If prices are higher than production costs, new firms will enter the market and sell the service at a lower price. Because of the assumption of profit maximization and entry, prices would (in the long run) be expected to equal costs (which includes a normal profit); the different mix of services provided would reflect what people are willing to pay for those services, which in turn would reflect their full costs. Competing firms would attempt to minimize their costs, and investment decisions would be based on profitability (i.e., demand and cost conditions).

Hospitals are predominantly non-profit organizations, which means restrictions are placed on how surpluses are distributed. For-profit firms can distribute surpluses (earnings) to shareholders, non-profit firms cannot. This technical distinction between firms of different ownership types is less important than any potential behavioral distinctions.

The non-profit form of organization raises several questions: Why are hospitals non-profit? For-profit firms dominate most markets with few, if any, firms organized as not-for-profit organizations. In contrast, non-profit firms have traditionally dominated healthcare markets. What does this difference in ownership imply for the behavior and performance of the hospital industry? Does it, as some persons have alleged, result in lower costs of production since the hospital does not have to earn a profit and pay dividends? Or are the objectives of the non-profit hospital decision-makers such that non-profit hospitals have poorer performance? Further, important for anti-trust issues is whether non-profits act in the community's interest and therefore should not be subject to the same merger guidelines as for-profit hospitals. A model of the non-profit hospital is needed to explain its past and current behavior.

Why Non-Profit Firms Exist

The Public Interest Explanation: There are generally two alternative hypotheses to explain why non-profit hospitals exist. The first may be termed the "Public Interest" view; the hospital's Board of Trustees operate the non-profit hospital to primarily benefit the community. According to this view, non-profits are likely to develop for those services considered to be "collective goods," such as charity care. For-profit firms would not serve the healthcare market when there was insufficient demand to generate a profit. Yet, the importance of health and the desire of individuals to support healthcare allowed non-profit firms to exist, supported by charitable donations.

Undoubtedly, hospitals as charitable institutions are part of the explanation, particularly in the years before insurance coverage and when hospitals primarily served the poor. Further, it was difficult for state governments to monitor how well subsidies to the poor were provided. By subsidizing the non-profit hospital (and nursing homes), the hospital is trusted to provide those services desired by the government. Three types of subsidies are received by the non-profit hospital to enable them to provide charity care. Donations are tax deductible; the hospital is exempt from property taxes; and it is exempt from corporate income taxes.

The co-existence of for-profit firms suggests another public interest explanation. Based on imperfections in the healthcare sector, coupled with the importance of healthcare to consumers, Arrow suggested that non-profit hospitals were a response to consumers' inability to judge the quality of medical services (8). In markets where there is a lack of information (informational asymmetries), such as medical care, consumers might believe that a greater degree of trust can be placed in the non-profit form of organization. Consumers in healthcare markets cannot easily verify the quality of the services that they purchase, and if they purchase services with inferior quality, it is often difficult and costly to obtain a suitable remedy after the fact. As a result, they must place considerable trust in the firm or organization providing the service. Non-profit ownership is taken as a

signal of quality because such firms presumably desire to produce high-quality services and have less of an incentive to skimp on quality and save money to increase profits.

Consequently, non-profit firms are more likely to exist in industries where the quality of the product is very important and difficult to measure and monitor. If information about quality becomes more widespread, one would expect the prevalence of non-profit firms to diminish because consumers can observe quality more directly (9).

If the predominance of non-profit hospitals was based on patient trust, then why does the non-profit form of organization not also apply to physicians? After all, patients have little information on their medical condition and it is the physician—not the hospital—who decides upon the medical treatment.

A Physician Control Model of Hospitals: A more cynical view of the non-profit form of organization is based on economic self interest, namely, the physician-control model. Physicians favor subsidies to their inputs of production when they are concerned with the total price of care paid by or on behalf of the patient. Inputs in a for-profit hospital have to be paid their market price. However, when hospitals are non-profit, the hospital can become the recipient of philanthropic contributions (which are tax deductible), accept volunteers (who provide services at no charge), and receive substantial government subsidies, such as the Hill-Burton program. The effect of these various subsidies is to cause hospital costs to be lower than they would be otherwise. The advantages to physicians of non-profit hospitals are several. For-profit hospitals would have to pay property, sales, and corporate income taxes as well as dividends to their shareholders, thereby leaving less of the total price available to the physician (10). Further, physicians did not have to invest their own capital to own and control the hospital—the community donated it.

Another advantage to the physician is that the non-profit hospital can only use surplus funds internally. Using a criterion other than profitability, such as prestige (which would also be consistent with the goals of the trustees and managers), would be used for the investment of their funds. The institution would be more willing to invest in duplicative services and facilities, which would be more advantageous to the staff physicians than if it were accountable to stockholders.

Physician control also enabled physicians to enforce a cartel arrangement. In the past, medical societies have been viewed as being similar to a physicians' cartel. The individual producer in a cartel always has an incentive to increase output since the costs of doing so are less than the cartel's profit-maximizing price. Unless the cartel can prevent its members from expanding their output, the monopoly price will fall. Since there are so many physicians, it is relatively costly to monitor the output of individual physicians in their offices (although the cartel can limit the use of inputs contributing to increased production, i.e., which personnel can undertake different tasks). It was far easier to limit the number of hospital beds per physician, which also acted as a constraint on the physician's productivity. By controlling the number of hospital beds, the medical society was able to limit competition among physicians for patients. Limiting the number of hospital beds, however, makes them a scarce resource. If physicians were to bid for these scarce inputs, it would transfer income from the physician to the hospital. To retain these monopoly profits for themselves, the physicians in control of the hospital used a form of non-price rationing, either seniority or some other standard, to distribute the scarce hospital privileges among themselves (11).

Physician control over the hospital prevents the hospital from hiring physicians and jointly producing hospital and medical services. If it were able to do so, then the hospital would receive the difference between the average costs of production and the total price charged. Medical societies ensured that hospitals would not be able to compete with physicians by having many states enact legislation prohibiting the corporate practice of medicine; only physicians could practice medicine, not organizations operated by nonphysicians. If a patient required hospitalization, they had to have a physician on the staff of that hospital.

(The physician-control model would be less applicable to university teaching hospitals where decision-making is shared among different constituencies, such as the clinical departments, medical school, and the university.)

Theories of Hospital Behavior

Three different models of non-profit hospital behavior are analyzed and their predictions compared to actual hospital performance. The first is the Public Interest model, which assumes that the non-profit hospital acts as though it were a for-profit hospital but uses the "profits" to benefit the community it serves. The second and third models of hospital behavior are based on economic self-interest; in the second model (Utility Maximizing model) the main beneficiaries are the hospital managers and employees, while in the third (Physician-Control model), it is the medical staff. Each model of hospital behavior is examined with respect to how the hospital determines its prices, output, and investment policies. Several aspects of hospital behavior are similar in each of these models.

A Profit-Maximizing Model of Hospital Behavior

This first model of hospital behavior assumes that the non-profit hospital acts as a profit-maximizing hospital and returns the "profits" to the community.

Hospitals are assumed to have a downward sloping demand curve; each hospital has a somewhat differentiated product in that not all of its physicians have staff appointments at the other hospitals, its mix of services may differ, as does its location and reputation. To maximize profits, the hospital would select that price on the demand curve where its marginal cost curve intersects the marginal revenue curve; this is shown in Figure 11-3. The profit-maximizing price and output would be P_1 and Q_1, respectively, and the amount of profit would be the difference between P_1 and the average cost curve at that price multiplied by Q_1.

Further, since the hospital is a multi-product firm with different payers, it can increase its profits by price discriminating according to the price elasticity of demand for each class of patient and type of service. (The ability of the hospital to practice price

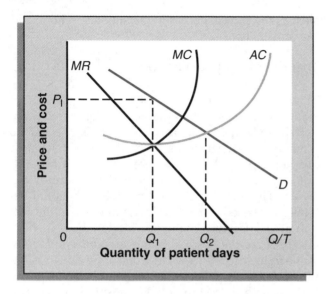

Figure 11-3. Price and output policies of a profit-making hospital.

discrimination implies that the hospital has market power.) The hospital's room rate is more price elastic than is the demand for ancillary services because, once in the hospital, the patient cannot substitute other providers' ancillary services. Thus the demand for ancillary services is believed to be less price elastic. To maximize its profits, the hospital will charge higher prices (relative to costs) for those services and that class of patients whose demands are less price elastic.

The Profit-Maximizing model of hospital behavior predicts that hospitals will increase their prices if demand either increases or becomes less price elastic, or if the prices of their inputs (i.e., the hospital's marginal cost curve) increase. Hospitals are also expected to minimize their costs of operation, otherwise they forego profits. Further, hospitals will invest on the basis of which investments offer the highest rate of return. Examples of the types of investments hospitals could undertake would be cost-saving technology and expanding or adding new facilities and services. New facilities and services could be profitable in their

own right or could serve to attract a greater number of physicians to the hospital's staff, thereby indirectly increasing the demand for the hospital's beds. According to this model, the hospital would determine its prices as would a profit maximizer, minimize its costs (since higher costs represent foregone profits), and invest only in projects that offer a profitable return.

With free market entry and price-sensitive purchasers, prices in excess of average costs and above-normal profits could not persist in the long run. The performance of the industry would be similar to that of a monopolistically competitive industry; along with price competition and competition for physicians, hospitals would attempt to differentiate themselves from other hospitals. The prices of their services and classes of patients would, in the long run, reflect their respective average costs.

A non-profit hospital acting as a profit maximizer would use its profits and contributions from the community to achieve the community's desires, such as engaging in altruistic activities, such as charity care to the poor.

A non-profit hospital is not required to pay taxes nor dividends to its stockholders, thereby providing the non-profit form of ownership with a cost advantage over the for-profit hospital. If both types of hospitals behaved similarly and were equally efficient, then the non-profit hospital would be able to drive for-profit competitors out of the market.

How well does a model of the non-profit hospital as a profit-maximizing firm reflect past hospital behavior? There is evidence that non-profit hospitals priced according to their price elasticity of demand (12). Prices have been much greater than marginal costs for those services believed to be less price elastic (ancillary services), but closer to marginal costs for those services believed to be more price elastic (room rates and delivery room). Obstetric care has lower price-cost ratios since obstetric patients have the time to compare prices among hospitals.

After the introduction of Medicare in 1966, the aged represented about 40 percent of hospital patient days, and the federal government paid hospitals their costs for providing services to the aged. Because hospitals did not have cost accounting systems in place, the payment method was the "ratio of charges to charges to cost." The hospital's charges to Medicare patients as a portion of its charges to all patients was the ratio of the hospital's total costs that would be reimbursed by the government. As the proportion of Medicare charges increased, so did the portion of the hospital's costs that would be paid for by the government. Anecdotal evidence indicated that many hospitals increased their charges for those services that were used predominately by the aged, such as bed rails. The effect of these policies was to increase the portion of the hospital's total costs that was reimbursed by Medicare. Medicare patients were only responsible for a deductible when they were admitted to the hospital; the patient had little incentive to choose a less costly hospital or to be concerned with the cost of their hospital stay.

Also during this period, private hospital insurance by the non-aged increased. As shown previously in Table 3-2, out-of-pocket payments by patients for hospital care decreased so that patients were, on average, responsible for less than 10 percent of their hospital expenditures. Patient sensitivity to hospital charges diminished. Other third-party payers of hospital care (such as Blue Cross) also paid hospitals according to their costs. The effect of extensive government and private insurance payment lessened patient sensitivity to the costs of their care and enabled hospitals to engage in non-price competition, resulting in very rapid increases in hospital expenditures.

The assumption that non-profit hospitals (in general) minimized their costs and returned their profits to the community in the form of additional care to the poor is not supported by the data. The amount of charity care, bad debt care, and percent of Medicaid patients served was similar to for-profit hospitals (13). Under cost-based payment prior to the mid 1980s, non-profit hospitals invested in facilities and services that were expected to result in substantial losses; cross subsidies were provided to certain facilities and services to offset their losses rather than closing them. These money-losing facilities and services were not the sole source of such services in the community, but were instead duplicative of others.

An additional problem with this model of the hospital is that it excludes any important role for the physician. According to this model, the hospital competes for physicians who then refer their patients to the hospital. The physicians' role is a passive one, to increase demand for the hospital. The model assumes that the hospital will attempt to keep adding physicians to its staff, whereas in the past the medical staff tightly controlled staff appointments and sought to limit rather than expand physician staff appointments.

Utility Maximizing Models of Hospital Behavior

The next set of models incorporates some of the observed inconsistencies of the previous model. This model suggests that the beneficiary of the non-profit form of ownership is not the community but the decision-makers, namely the managers and trustees of non-profit hospitals. One version of this model assumes that the managers themselves benefit (in terms of higher salaries) by being the administrator of the largest full-service hospital in the area.

According to this model, hospitals act as if they wanted to maximize their output or revenues. In the short run, hospitals attempt to maximize their profits and then invest those profits either in additional capacity, cost-saving technology, or facilities and services that result in the *largest increases in their output.* Hospitals still have an incentive to minimize their costs since to do otherwise is to forego revenue, which could be used to increase output. With reference to Figure 11-3, an output maximizer would increase output to Q_2, which would represent the point on the demand curve where average cost equals price. This does not mean that for every service or class of patients price equals average cost, but it does in the aggregate. For different services the hospital would set profit maximizing prices and use the profits to cross-subsidize other, money losing services.

A more sophisticated version of this model assumes that the decision-makers have a utility function that includes some measure of the quality of the institution as well as its size (14). Greater prestige is associated with being an administrator or trustee of a large prestigious hospital. Prior to the 1980s, hospital quality data was not collected, and results of surveys performed by the Joint Commission on Accreditation of Hospitals was not publicly available, thus a hospital's reputation was often indicated by the range of facilities and services offered.

Under this "quality-quantity" behavioral model, the hospital will still seek to maximize its profits in the short run through its pricing strategy, but it will then attempt to invest that profit either in increased quantity—increased capacity, cost-saving technology, or facilities and services that result in an increase in quantity of patients—or in prestige/quality investments. Because quantity and quality are to some extent substitutable for one another in the utility function, the decision-makers will have to make a trade-off according to the marginal increase in utility resulting from increased quality or from increased quantity.

The effect of adding quality to the decision-maker's objective is to cause an increase in hospital costs, as shown in Figure 11-4. Assume that the hospital is operating on average-cost curve AC_1. Since it cannot keep any profits, its long-run price and output will be P_1 and Q_1, respectively. If the hospital invests in increased quality, the average cost curve rises to AC_2, but the increased quality also results in an increase in the hospital's demand, shifting its demand to D_2. The increase in demand may occur as a result of attracting additional physicians to the hospital.

After some point, increased expenditures for quality will result in small or negligible increases in demand (competing non-profit hospitals will attempt to match these additional investments in quality); at this point, the additional cost of increased quality may exceed the additional revenue resulting from the small increments in demand. Additions to quality beyond that point continue to raise the average cost curve to AC_3 but do not result in further shifts in demand. Since funds that are used to increase quality could be used to increase quantity by adding to capacity, the decision-maker has to determine the relative weights to be placed on the quantity-quality trade-off.

The consequences for economic efficiency of a utility model of a hospital attempting to maximize both quantity and quality is that the price of hospital care

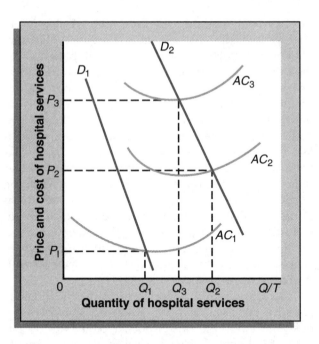

Figure 11-4. The effect on hospital costs of increases in hospital quality.

will be higher than if quality were not continually increased. Continued increases in quality without increased demand will shift the average cost curve higher, possibly decreasing quantity and raising price. Further, hospitals will be producing a higher quality product (greater unused facilities and services) than consumers might be willing to pay for. Such a behavioral model would be more typical of the cost-based payment period before managed care competition became prevalent and hospitals did not have to compete on price to be included in the insurer's provider network.

In a market characterized by entry and price competition, consumers (through their choice of health plans) would select that combination of price and quality that corresponded to what they were willing to pay rather than to the quality-quantity preferences of the hospital administrator. In a price-competitive market, quality would increase in response to consumer demands for quality.

How consistent was the quantity-quality model with observed behavior in the period before managed care? This model still implies a profit-maximizing pricing strategy and cost-minimizing behavior since the foregone revenues could be used to increase quality or quantity. However, it does explain why hospitals made unprofitable investments and maintained unprofitable services, as long as these services added prestige to the institution. This model also suggests that hospitals invested in new technology as soon as it became available, not necessarily because of its effect on demand, but because of its effect on the perceived image of the hospital.

Hospitals having a quantity-quality objective would be expected to oppose the entry of for-profit hospitals. For-profit hospitals, which do not have a prestige objective, would not have to cross-subsidize money-losing prestige services. Thus for-profits would compete with non-profits by lowering the price of the "profitable" services in comparison with the prices charged by the non-profits. Non-profits claimed that for-profit hospitals "skimmed the cream" by not offering such money-losing services.

Extensive cross subsidization of expensive, money-losing services were often duplicative, *resulted in lower quality outcomes*, and should not have been offered by multiple hospitals. An example of duplication of prestigious investments was the number of hospitals with open heart surgery facilities. Luft, et al., found that for complicated types of surgery, the greater the volume of surgery performed, the lower the surgical mortality rates (after controlling for other factors that might affect mortality, such as the patient's age, sex, and health status.) (15).

One of the drawbacks to the quantity-quality model is an expectation of cost-minimizing behavior. This can be corrected by including a "slack" variable in the manager's utility function. Hospital administrators are assumed to also be interested in working in a pleasant environment, as defined by such amenities as additional administrative personnel and higher wages for employees so as to minimize conflict. This broader utility function of the hospital administrator predicts that hospitals would still price to maximize profits, and then spend those profits to achieve some combination of quantity, quality, and slack.

With the inclusion of slack in the manager's utility function, prices will be even higher than under the previous models. Under these circumstances, hospitals would compete with one another, but the competition would be to see which hospitals could become the most prestigious while providing the administrative staff with a pleasant working environment. There would be a great deal of duplication within the industry, as well as excess capacity, high costs, and rapidly rising prices to finance the described behavior. This type of non-price competition was referred to as a "medical arms race."

These utility-maximizing models of hospital behavior explain much of the observed data in the period *before* the early 1980s, prior to Medicare DRGs and managed care competition. However, they attribute a passive role to physicians. The decision-makers in the foregoing models are the hospital administrators and trustees, but in reality physicians had a great deal of control over the hospital, its pricing policies, and investment behavior.

Physician-Control Model of Hospital Behavior

This model assumes that the medical staff effectively controls the hospital, and that hospital decisions reflect the medical staff's objectives. Physicians, not the community nor the administrative staff, were the major beneficiaries of the non-profit form of hospital organization.

The physician is the manager of the patient's illness, with responsibility for deciding upon the components to be used in providing treatment. Under this model, the physician combines the treatment inputs in such a manner so as to increase his or her own income and/or productivity. The relevant price to the consumer (e.g., under indemnity insurance in the period before Medicare and health plan physician fee schedules) is the total amount of out-of-pocket expenditure for a treatment, not the individual price of specific inputs, such as hospital care. The physician is able to retain more of the total price, the less the patient has to pay for any one component, such as hospital care.

When the total price of medical care is the relevant price to the payer, physician pricing and behavior can be illustrated with reference to the previous Figure 11-3. The profit-maximizing price of the treatment is that point on the demand curve above the intersection of marginal revenue and marginal cost. The amount of profit is the difference between price and average cost. The higher (lower) the cost of other inputs, the less (more) profit available to the physician. For example, if two inputs are used in providing a medical treatment—hospital and physician services—then the average cost curve represents the cost of hospital care. The difference between the price charged the patient (P_1) and the amount that goes to pay the hospital (AC at Q_1) is available to the physician.

The physician acts as a contractor, retaining the amount left over after all the other inputs have been paid. In this situation, the physician has an incentive to minimize the cost of providing the treatment since higher input costs represent foregone revenue to the physician. (This situation is also similar to when medical groups are capitated and have a risk-sharing bonus for reduced hospital use. The physician's incentive is to similarly minimize total treatment cost.)

Such profit-maximizing behavior on the part of the physician is not necessarily inconsistent with the physician's acting in the patient's economic interest as well. If hospital care is free to the patient (because of the pre-1980s Blue Cross hospital service benefit policy) while the patient must pay the full price for use of other components, it was in both the patient's and the physician's interest to hospitalize the patient.

With increased demands for medical services, physicians would be expected to favor increases in their hospital's capacity in order to increase their productivity, such as by increasing the number of interns and residents who provide physician services for which the physician can charge the patient; additional facilities and services, such as an excess of operating rooms and obstetric facilities so the physician does not have to wait or be inconvenienced; and facilities and services that are available in their hospital so that the physician does not have to refer a patient to another hospital and physician, thereby risking the loss of the patient and their fee. Physicians who do not have appointments at other hospitals would favor investment by their hospital even though it may be duplicative for the community because it increases

their productivity and income. (See Appendix 1: Using A Physician Control Model To Increase Physician Productivity.)

Physicians would also prefer some hospital slack if it enables them to economize on their own time.

Physician control over hospital investment policies results in economic inefficiency. It is a more costly approach for producing additional output (increased demands for medical care). The price to the physician for these other inputs is zero, particularly if some third-party payer or the government pays them in full.

Before the mid 1960s when hospital insurance was not as extensive as it is today, the physician was more concerned with the hospital's costs since the greater the patient's financial burden for hospital care, the lower would be the payment available to the physician. In large hospitals, however, the effect on any one physician's income of inefficient behavior on the part of the hospital would be small. Only in smaller hospitals, with correspondingly fewer physicians, would physicians be expected to be concerned with the efficiency of the hospital's operation.

As insurance coverage for hospital care became more widespread and as hospital payment was cost based, physicians were able to increase their charges to the patient and were unconcerned with the hospital's inefficiency and rapidly increasing costs.

The physician-control model also explains hospital pricing behavior. Prior to the widespread availability of hospital insurance, physicians preferred that the hospital assign relatively low prices to services that were complementary to the physician's services; for example, the surgeons wanted hospital charges for the operating room priced at or below cost. Similarly, obstetricians preferred the same type of pricing policy for the hospital's delivery room. As the out-of-pocket price for hospital care declined, physicians favored hospital profit-maximizing pricing policies (as long as they did not conflict with their own pricing strategies) since such prices would result in greater hospital profits which could then be invested internally according to physician preferences.

Physicians also wanted their hospital to have an outpatient department and for the hospital to provide health screening services, both of which might appear to be competitive with physicians. However, the outpatient department was a convenient way of avoiding the financial risk of caring for low-income patients, and physicians were relieved of providing emergency services. Physicians were thereby able to allocate more of their time to higher-income patients and/or for leisure. Similarly, when the hospital provided free screening services (a form of marketing), the physician's time is freed for acute services, which offer a higher return per unit of time. Patients with health problems are referred to physicians on the hospital's staff, thereby increasing demand for those physicians.

Physicians also had an economic interest in the size of their medical staff. The Pauly-Redisch physician-control model posits that physician incomes would be higher under a closed rather than an open staff model of the hospital. Under a closed staff model, physicians would be willing to add additional members to the staff as long as each additional physician increased the incomes of other physicians on the staff. (As long as the marginal revenue product (MRP) of additional physicians is greater than average revenue product (ARP), which is equal to average income, additional physicians would be added.) An open staff model would have a greater number of staff physicians, and the average income of staff members would be less than under a closed staff. Physicians would have an incentive to join the staff as long as staff members' incomes were higher in that hospital than elsewhere. Thus each physician specialty, e.g., surgeons, is interested in limiting hospital privileges; too many surgeons would decrease the average surgeon's income. (If other inputs increase, for example hospital beds or residents, then this would cause an increase in the MRP and ARP curves of the medical staff.)

To sum up the physician-control model, before the mid 1960s when hospital insurance was not widespread and major medical insurance was more prevalent, physicians would have been expected to minimize the cost of all the medical inputs used in providing a medical treatment. Patients were concerned about their total out-of-pocket price for medical services, and physicians received the difference between the cost of the inputs and the total price of medical care charged to the patient. As hospital coverage became more extensive and hospitals were reimbursed for their costs, physicians no longer had to be concerned with the cost of hospital care. Physician payment was separated from payment for hospital services, and physicians were neither financially responsible nor accountable for their decisions. There were no constraints on how the physician used the hospital or influenced its investment decisions. (During the 1970s, state health planning efforts intended to reduce duplication of hospital facilities failed because they were contrary to both the physicians' and the hospital's interests.)

Effect of Price Competition on Hospital Behavioral Models

Differences in hospital objectives and the degree of competitiveness in the marketplace are key factors that affect the behavior of firms. Historically, cost-based hospital payment systems enabled non-profit hospitals to achieve objectives not otherwise possible in a price-competitive market. Profit-maximizing behavior with the profits returned to the community, utility-maximizing behavior benefiting hospital management and employees, and a physician-control model benefiting the medical staff are alternative models to explain the non-profit hospital's pricing, output, and investment policies. Several models predict similar behavior, such as profit-maximizing pricing on certain services, hospital inefficiency (higher wages and a greater number of employees), and duplication of expensive facilities and services.

The ability of non-profit hospitals to achieve their non-profit objectives changed once hospital payment systems changed (see Appendix 2: Cost Shifting).

In late 1983, the federal government began to phase in a new method of hospital payment called Diagnostic Related Groupings (DRGs). The hospital was reimbursed for each Medicare admission according to a fixed price. Also in the mid 1980s, as employers and unions became more concerned with their medical costs particularly with the rising costs of hospital care, pressure was placed on insurers to reduce the rise in health insurance premiums. Managed care competition began and hospitals had to compete on price to be included in an insurer's provider network.

Price competition among hospitals to be included in an insurer's provider network and fixed DRG prices per admission changed non-profit hospitals' behavior. To survive in the new price-competitive environment, non-profit and for-profit hospitals began to behave similarly; the difference between non-profit and for-profit hospitals narrowed. Many non-profits no longer had the funds to achieve their non-profit goals.

Empirical Evidence on Differences Between Non-Profit and For-Profit Hospitals

The for-profit form of ownership in healthcare presents the concern that to make a profit, the firm or hospital will sacrifice the consumer's interest to that of the stockholder. Will the for-profit firm raise prices more than a non-profit firm? Will the for-profit firm inadequately pay its employees to ensure dividends to its stockholders? Will the for-profit firm provide lower quality services, reduce access to care, and have lower customer satisfaction than a non-profit firm? More generally, would for-profit hospitals behave any differently than private non-profit hospitals in a price-competitive market?

A number of studies have been conducted on the differences between for-profit and non-profit hospitals (16). These studies have attempted to determine whether for-profits are more efficient than non-profits, whether for-profits charge higher prices, whether non-profits provide higher quality of care, and whether non-profits provide more charity care.

Comparative studies are difficult since there are numerous measurement problems with regard to adjusting for differences in the hospital's output, namely its case mix of patients, as well as being able to adequately measure differences in patient severity of illness, quality of care, and amenities. Also affecting the comparison are the different time periods examined. Prior to the mid 1980s, non-profit hospitals were reimbursed according to their costs; since that time, their financial incentives changed.

Ownership Status and Efficiency: The evidence on whether non-profit hospitals are less efficient (more costly) is mixed. One cannot conclude that there are significant differences in efficiency between profit

and non-profit hospitals. One study using a matched sample of hospitals found that there was no significant difference in their costs per admission adjusted for case mix, but for-profit hospitals generally charged higher prices for their ancillary services than did non-profits. One explanation for the higher mark-up prices by for-profits is that they have entered markets where the population is growing rapidly (e.g., the South and Southwest). Expanding markets typically have less price competition. Thus the association of higher prices with for-profit hospitals may have more to do with the characteristics of the markets in which they compete than with their form of ownership.

Ownership Status and Profit-Maximization: Hospital mergers that reduce competition are likely to result in higher prices at both the merging hospitals as well as their competitors. Will merging non-profit hospitals that gain market power behave any differently than merging for-profit hospitals? Proponents of non-profit mergers claim that prices will be reduced because of scale economies. The federal government lost several anti-trust cases brought against merging non-profit hospitals because the judge believed that non-profit hospitals would not exploit their market power by raising prices.

Several studies analyzing non-profit hospitals' pricing behavior as a result of mergers that lessen competition have concluded that such mergers lead to higher, not lower, prices. This finding suggests that non-profit hospitals, similar to for-profit hospitals, price according to the competitiveness of the market. Empirical evidence is consistent with economic theory that competition among hospitals leads to lower prices (markups over cost). Both types of hospitals will use market power gained from mergers that lessen competition to increase their prices (17). For anti-trust analysis, therefore, ownership differences should not be considered a mitigating factor in hospital mergers that lessen competition.

Ownership Status and Quality of Care: With respect to the effect of ownership on quality of care, studies have again been inconclusive. Three types of quality measures have been used: structure (the inputs used in treatment), process (how care is provided), and outcomes. Studies using structural measures such as hospital accreditation and percent of hospitals with cardiac and intensive care units find no differences by ownership.

Keeler, et al., reviewed 14,000 medical records for five diseases and compared several process measures of quality, namely that specific diagnostic and therapeutic treatments were competently provided, to the difference between the actual mortality rate and the expected mortality rate based on the patient's characteristics. The authors concluded that overall quality of care in for-profit and non-profit hospitals were similar (18).

Using survival, functional status, cognitive status, and probability of living in a nursing home as outcome measures, Sloan, et al., examined elderly patients hospitalized for hip fracture, stroke, coronary heart disease, and congestive heart failure by hospital ownership. The authors found that there were no significant differences between for-profit and non-profit (non-teaching) hospitals according to the above outcome measures. Major teaching hospitals, however, did perform better on several outcome measures (19).

Ownership Status and Uncompensated Care: There is very little difference in the provision of uncompensated care between non-profit (non-teaching) and for-profit hospitals. (Uncompensated care consists of charity care [care for which the hospital did not expect compensation] and bad debts [care for which the hospital did expect to be compensated at time of service].) In 1999, uncompensated care costs as a percent of total hospital costs were, on average, 4.7 percent for non-profit (non-governmental) hospitals and 4.2 percent for for-profits (20). The amount of uncompensated care varies greatly among the non-profits themselves. When comparisons are made between non-profit and for-profit hospitals located in the same area, it was found that they care for a similar number of uninsured patients. Large non-profit teaching hospitals located in urban areas amidst low-income populations provide most of the charity care. For-profits are typically not located in areas with low-income populations (21).

Competitive pressures make it difficult for non-profit hospitals to cross-subsidize patients or to behave differently from for-profit hospitals. Increased competition to be included in an insurer's provider network increases a hospital's price elasticity of demand resulting in a lower price, hence lower profitability. Studies have indicated that in highly price-competitive hospitals markets (relative to less-competitive markets), uncompensated care by non-profits has sharply decreased (22).

As non-profit hospitals merge and compete on price, their tax-exempt status is being questioned. Some communities believe that their non-profits are providing little, if anything, to the community in return for their tax-exempt status. To retain their favored tax-exempt status, several states have established standards as to the amount of charity care non-profit hospitals have to provide. Similar legislation is being considered at the federal level. (Also driving the re-examination of hospitals' non-profit status by states is the billions of new tax dollars that states and communities could receive if the tax exemption rules were changed.)

Summary of Differences by Ownership Status: On average, there does not appear to be significant differences between for-profit and private (non-governmental) non-profit hospitals in their efficiency, prices charged, quality of care, and the amount of uncompensated care provided. Major teaching hospitals, however, generally provide higher quality of care and a greater amount of uncompensated care. It is important to note that the percent of hospitals that are for-profit has remained constant (about 20 percent) for the last 25 years. This is an indication that neither form of ownership has a dominant economic advantage over the other. Market competitiveness is likely to be a more important determinant of performance than ownership status.

HOSPITAL PERFORMANCE

Non-Price Competition and Hospital Performance

The major determinant of hospital performance after the enactment of Medicare in 1965 was not the structure of the industry, but the methods used to pay hospitals. Medicare paid hospitals according to their costs for treating Medicare patients and private health insurers, who paid hospitals either their costs or charges, were merely a passive intermediary between the employer and provider; insurers simply passed higher hospital costs to employers in the form of higher premiums. Government and privately insured patients, the aged, the poor under Medicaid, and insured families, were not price sensitive because of their extensive hospital insurance.

Employers had little incentive to be concerned with rising hospital costs and insurance premiums because, not being subject to much import competition, they could pass on higher labor costs through increased product prices. Further, purchasers of hospital care had little information on which to judge hospitals according to their prices and quality. And many state laws precluded insurers from establishing provider networks based on negotiated discounts.

As budget constraints were removed from hospitals, the responsibility for hospital performance was placed on the hospital's decision-makers; their decisions were based on what objectives they hoped to achieve.

The physician played a decisive role during this period. As the patient's agent, the physician selected the hospital to which the patient was admitted. Hospitals competed for physicians by offering them greater bed availability, the latest in technology, and increased staffing. The consequence was higher costs and duplication of expensive technology and facilities. Under a hospital cost-based payment system, physicians could serve the patient and hospital as well as themselves without making any conflicting choices.

The type of competition that occurred during this period was *non-price competition* (23). To compete for patients, hospitals had to compete amongst themselves for physicians. Non-price competition manifested itself in several ways. Hospitals in more competitive markets (a greater number of hospitals) maintained more excess capacity than hospitals in less competitive (more concentrated) markets. Physicians were thus assured that by affiliating with a particular hospital their patients were likely to have a bed when one was needed. Greater amenities were provided to patients as well as to physicians (offices next to the hospital at below market rents). To increase the productivity of physicians on their medical staff, hospitals provided them with more support staff such as interns and residents and a higher proportion of registered nurses in their nursing units. Hospitals also purchased the latest in medical technology and added facilities and services. Physicians did not have to refer their patients (and possibly lose them) to other institutions. High-tech services also provided a means for the hospital to indicate to prospective patients that it was a high-quality institution.

Non-price competition led to rapidly rising hospital costs. Using data from the period 1972 and 1982, Robinson and Luft found that in *more competitive markets*, hospital costs were higher, they offered more services, and average length of stay was longer (24). More competitive hospitals were also reluctant to engage in cost containment activities for fear of losing their physician referrals.

The finding of higher costs in more competitive (less concentrated) hospital markets was contrary to the expectations of traditional economic theory, namely that in more competitive industries firms become more efficient. (What was lacking, however, were the incentives for hospitals to compete on price.)

As shown in Figure 11-5A, in the first few years after Medicare began (1966), hospital expenditures per capita increased at a much more rapid rate than previously. In 1971, wage and price controls were imposed on the entire economy (the Economic Stabilization Program [ESP] by the Nixon Administration. These controls were removed from the rest of the economy in 1972 and from the health industry in April 1974. Once free of price controls, per capita hospital expenditures increased sharply. For the remainder of the 1970s, hospital expenditures continued to increase rapidly.

Proponents of hospital planning argued that the way to reduce rapidly rising hospital expenditures and to eliminate "wasteful" competition it was necessary to encourage *monopolization* of the hospital industry. (Changing hospital incentives was not proposed as an alternative to government planning.)

Relying on Regulation to Improve Hospital Performance

After the passage of Medicare and Medicaid, rapidly rising hospital costs led to the imposition of regula-

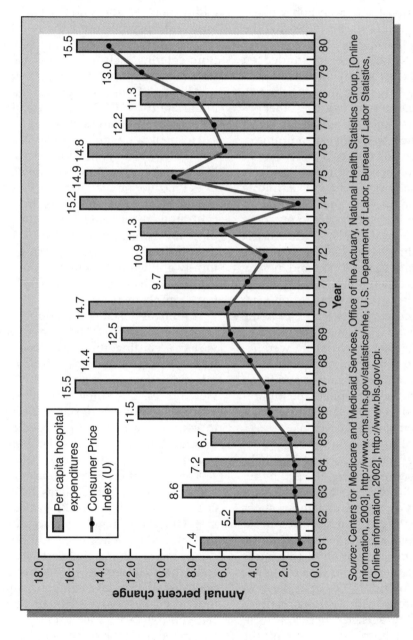

Source: Centers for Medicare and Medicaid Services, Office of the Actuary, National Health Statistics Group. [Online information, 2003], http://www.cms.hhs.gov/statistics/nhe; U.S. Department of Labor, Bureau of Labor Statistics, [Online information, 2002], http://www.bls.gov/cpi.

Figure 11-5A.   Annual percent changes in per capita hospital expenditures and consumer price index, 1960–1980.

tory controls on hospitals. As Medicare hospital expenditures rose faster than expected, the federal government had to continually increase the Medicare payroll tax and the wage base to which it applied to prevent the Medicare Trust Fund from going bankrupt. Neither raising payroll taxes nor increasing the aged's financial contribution was politically popular. State Medicaid expenditures, which are funded on average equally by the states and by the federal government, were also increasing faster than anticipated. Rather than increasing state taxes or reducing other politically popular programs such as education, states sought ways to reduce their Medicaid expenditures.

Hospital regulation appeared to be a direct way of reducing the pressures on state and federal budgets (25). In the late 1960s, many states enacted Certificate of Need (CON) legislation which required hospitals to have their capital expenditures (typically in excess of $100,000) to be approved by state planning agencies. Planning proponents claimed that CON would reduce duplication of costly facilities and services and thereby reduce the rise in hospital expenditures. As hospital expenditure increases placed greater pressure on state and federal budgets, more states enacted CON in the early 1970s; in 1974 a federal CON law was enacted.

Planning controls on hospital investment were *ineffective* in limiting the rise in hospital expenditures. Economists conducted a number of studies and failed to find a lower rate of increase in hospital expenditures that could be contributed to state planning agencies' decisions on the allocation of hospital capital.

The failure of hospital planning to more "rationally" allocate hospital capital was because hospitals, who would presumably be adversely affected by investment controls, used the regulatory process to benefit themselves. One study found that those states more likely to adopt CON legislation had lower occupancy levels (thereby favoring entry controls) and a higher degree of hospital concentration (the more highly concentrated the market, the easier it is for hospitals to collude and lobby for CON). Further, hospitals were the major group with a strong (concentrated) interest in the CON agencies' decisions; consequently, it appears that hospitals "captured" the decision-making process. Thus the actual effect of CON laws was to benefit hospitals.

The CON investment regulations were used to deny entry into the market by new competitors, such as for-profit hospitals; large urban hospitals used the regulations to prevent suburban hospitals from adding new facilities and thereby becoming competitors; and hospitals used the regulations to prevent free-standing (lower cost) outpatient surgery centers from entering their market for fear that they would take away some of the hospital's surgical cases.

Although Congress repealed the federal CON law in the late 1970s, CON is still used in an anti-competitive manner in many states.

Hospital rate regulation was also used to limit the rise in hospital expenditures. In 1971, President Nixon mandated economy-wide wage and price controls ("Economic Stabilization Program," or ESP) to limit the rising rate of inflation in the economy. These controls were removed in 1972, but they were kept in place for medical care until 1974. Research indicates that these stringent price controls, which were uniformly applied to hospitals, reduced hospital expenditure increases. Once removed, hospital expenditures rapidly increased.

A number of states also adopted hospital rate regulation in the 1970s. The form of rate controls used varied according to which payers were included, whether the program was voluntary, and whether the rate regulation used a hospital-by-hospital budget review process or a single formula was used across all hospitals. A number of states enacted rate regulation to control the rise in their Medicaid expenditures. Several states, such as Maryland, included all payers under the rate regulation.

The motivation for the rate regulation, hence its success, varied. Those states facing severe budget crises (such as New York) instituted stringent and mandatory rate regulation according to a formula that applied to all hospitals. Although these states reduced the rise in hospital costs, over time there were concerns that service quality was being reduced. States relying on less stringent approaches (such as individual hospital budget reviews) and applying rate controls to just Medicaid patients were not effective in reducing the rise in hospital costs.

In 1983, to limit its growing budgetary commitment under Medicare, the Reagan administration began to phase in (over a 5-year period) price controls on hospitals. Medicare paid hospitals fixed prices per admission according to Diagnostic Related Groupings (DRGs). (This payment system is also referred to the Prospective Payment System, or PPS). Although PPS only applied to Medicare patients, it had an important effect on hospital costs since Medicare patients represent about 40 percent of hospital patient days. The DRG system worked to limit hospital costs in two ways: first, faced with a fixed price per Medicare admission, hospitals had an incentive to reduce the costs of caring for Medicare patients and to discharge them sooner; hospital occupancy rates declined. Second, Congress limited the rate of increase in DRG prices by an annual update percentage.

Hospital rate regulation, whether implemented by the federal or state governments, can be effective in reducing the rate of increase in hospital expenditures. Mandatory rate regulation applied to all hospitals according to a formula, such as used by New York State, Medicare PPS, and the Economic Stabilization Program, reduced the rate of increase in hospital expenses. These regulatory programs, however, do not achieve their savings by simply making hospitals more efficient. Stringent rate controls are based on an average of hospital costs (such as DRG prices) and an annual percent increase, which is the same for all hospitals. Thus some hospitals receive windfall gains while others losses, unrelated to their efficiency.

Further, it is not possible for a regulatory system to mimic a competitive market. Regulations provide incentives to "game" the system, such as "upcoding," which is classifying patients into a higher DRG category to receive a higher level of payment. Also, politics surrounding the federal budget influences the government's decision on the annual percent increase in DRG prices. Similar to other regulated industries (such as price controls on housing in New York), price regulation has undesirable consequences. Stringent regulated prices eventually lead to decreased access, reductions in service quality, and a lower rate of innovation.

Hospital Performance Under Managed Care

In the 1980s, hospital performance began to change. This change was brought about by a change in pur-

chaser demands for lower hospital costs, excess hospital capacity, and the U.S. Supreme Court ruling in 1982, which upheld the applicability of the anti-trust laws to the health field.

Large employers and their unions, threatened by increased import competition, pressured their insurers to limit rising medical expenses. To compete on the basis of their premiums for large employers, insurers had to lower the cost of their benefits; they instituted utilization review, changed their benefits to include lower-cost substitutes to hospitals, and instituted increased patient cost sharing.

The competitive environment facing hospitals began to change. Hospital occupancy fell as a result of Medicare's fixed price system and private insurer's utilization management. HMOs and PPOs formed provider networks based on the provider's price, the provider's reputation, and its location. Health plans were able to influence the patient's choice of provider by channeling patients to the insurer's network providers. Before hospitals were able to compete for physicians, they first had to compete on price to be included in the insurer's network. Regardless of hospital decision-makers' previous objectives, hospitals had to minimize their costs if they were to be able to compete on price.

The movement toward shifting inpatient services to an outpatient setting also adversely affected hospitals. Currently, more surgeries are performed in outpatient facilities than in hospitals. The increase in hospital outpatient services occurred for four reasons. Third-party payers tried to decrease the use of the most costly component of care—the hospital—by expanding insurance coverage to include the outpatient setting. In addition, insurers instituted utilization review mechanisms to ensure that surgical procedures that could be performed in less expensive outpatient surgery centers would not be performed in the hospital. Third, when medical groups and hospitals were paid on a capitation basis, it was more profitable (less costly) to treat patients in an outpatient setting. And lastly, advances in medical technology made it possible to perform more procedures in an outpatient facility.

The change to price competition among hospitals was not uniform throughout the country. In some areas, such as in California, competition developed much more rapidly than in other areas. In 1982, California legalized selective contracting which meant that third-party payers could negotiate discounted prices with a group of hospitals while excluding other hospitals from participating in the contract. Enrollment in PPOs in California grew rapidly. HMO growth in California, which was historically high because of Kaiser, also rapidly increased. Many studies, therefore, used California hospital data to determine the effect of the new competitive environment.

Hospital demand curves became more price elastic as hospitals competed on price to be included in an insurer's provider network. Empirical estimates of average hospital price elasticities of demand (as high as –5.67) shown in Table 11-3 indicate that other community hospitals are very good substitutes; a hospital increasing its price will lose significant market share.

The effect of price competition on California hospitals produced dramatic results. In a study of California hospitals, Melnick, et al., were able to examine actual prices paid to hospitals by California Blue Cross. It was thus possible to determine the effect of differences in hospital market structure on actual prices paid by a large purchaser. This data shows that Blue Cross was able to receive greater discounts from hospitals located in more competitive markets; further, these discounts were larger the greater was Blue Cross' leverage within the hospital (as measured by Blue Cross' percent of that hospital's total revenue). Conversely, the greater the hospital's leverage over Blue Cross (as measured by the hospital's market share in Blue Cross' network), the higher the price charged to Blue Cross by that hospital (26).

As managed care spread to the rest of the United States, Melnick et al., using data for the period 1989 to 1994, attempted to determine the answers to two questions: first, did areas with high managed care penetration result in lower rates of increase in hospital costs and, second, did hospital costs increase less rapidly in more competitive compared to less competitive markets (27)?

Using each hospital's HHI index as the measure of competition, the authors found results shown in Table 11-4. This table shows the percent increase in hospital costs according to whether the hospital is in a high- or low-competition market, and also whether the managed care penetration is high or low.

An increase in managed care penetration reduces the rise in hospital costs. The reduction, however, is much greater for hospitals in more competitive markets. Further, holding the degree of managed care penetration constant, hospitals in more competitive markets had lower rates of increase than hospitals in less competitive markets. The largest reduction occurs for competitive hospitals in high managed care markets.

A recent study examined the effect of the number of competitors in a market on hospital prices and profitability. The authors analyzed the number of hospitals providing coronary artery bypass graft surgery (CABG) in a market with HMO penetration. With only two to three CABG providers competing for HMO patients, the profitability of CABG services declines to zero. Thus it takes very few competitors in a market with a large purchaser willing to shift volume for competition to reduce prices (28).

The above findings are important for anti-trust policy that seeks to prevent hospital mergers that lessen competition. Those who advocate permitting hospital mergers that tend to monopolize the market emphasize the early studies that indicate that more competitive hospital markets lead to greater duplica-

Table 11-3. Price Elasticities of Demand for Individual Hospital Services

Study	Dependent Variable	Elasticity
M. Gaynor and W. Vogt (2003)	hospital services	–5.67 (California hospitals)
R. Feldman and B. Dowd (1986)		–1.12

Sources: R. Feldman and B. Dowd, "Is There a Competitive Market for Hospital Services?" *Journal of Health Economics,* September 1986, 5(3), pp. 277–292; M. Gaynor and W. B. Vogt, "Competition Among Hospitals," *NBER working paper #9471,* January 2003, http://www.nber.org/paper/w9471 (accessed on May 14, 2003).

Table 11-4. Hospital Cost Growth in the U.S. by Level of Managed Care Penetration and Hospital Market Competitiveness, 1989–1994

Level of Managed Care Penetration	Level of Hospital Competition		% Difference
	Low	High	
Low	65	56	16(a)
High	52	39	33(a)
% Difference	25(a)	44(a)	67(b)

Source: Table is based on the authors' simulation of the results presented in Bamezai, A., Zwanziger, J., Melnick, G. A., and Mann, J. "Price Competition and Hospital Cost Growth in the United States (1989–1994)," *Health Economics,* 8(3), May 1999: 233–243.

(a) % Difference = [(High - Low)/Low]

(b) [Low/Low (65) – High/High (39)] / [High/High (39)]

tion and higher costs. The above studies, based on data from the mid 1980s to the present, demonstrating that hospital costs and prices are lower in more competitive markets provide definitive evidence that hospital mergers that lessen competition would result in higher hospital prices.

If the number of competing hospitals declined (their concentration increased), the remaining hospitals would have fewer substitutes, greater market power to increase price, and would be less responsive to purchaser demands for quality. Enforcement of the anti-trust laws is necessary to prevent mergers that increase hospital market power.

Decreased inpatient utilization and intense price competition had an adverse affect on hospitals. As in any industry facing a declining demand and/or reimbursement, a number of hospitals closed or merged with stronger institutions. Hospitals that are smaller, offer less specialized services, are located in inner cities or rural areas, and serve a greater portion of Medicaid patients were at greater risk of closure.

Increased market power was an important reason for hospital consolidation. Some merger proponents claim that fewer hospitals will result in efficiencies which will be passed on by non-profit hospitals in the form of lower prices. Opponents of this view claim that scale economies are relatively small and that non-

profit hospital boards do not have objectives that are necessarily in the community's interest; they may behave no differently in their pricing strategies than for-profit hospitals. Further, unless the anti-trust laws are vigorously applied to mergers that tend to lessen competition, hospital prices will increase more rapidly as hospitals gain increased market power.

The beneficial effects on hospital performance of increased price competition (which started in the mid 1980s) have been documented in a number of studies discussed earlier. An indication of the slower rate of increase in hospital expenses is shown in Figure 11-5B. The annual percent increase in hospital expenditures per capita over the period 1980 to 2000 declined relative to the previous period as a result of Medicare's PPS system, managed care, and hospital price competition. By the early 1990s, managed care and price competition had become prevalent throughout the U.S., and hospital cost increases were dramatically reduced. These slower rates of increase in expenses have occurred even though there have been continual increases in technology (see Table 11-2), an older patient population, a sicker patient mix, and treatment for illnesses for which little could have been previously provided.

The differences between Figures 11-5A and 11-5B demonstrate the changes that managed care and price competition brought about in the healthcare industry.

The Effect of Competition on Hospital Quality

Critics of price competition are concerned that in a price-competitive market, hospitals will be forced to reduce their quality of care to be able to compete on price. As profit margins decline, hospitals will be unable to adequately staff their critical care units, recruit the most qualified surgeons, and invest in the latest technology. Only in less competitive, more concentrated markets will hospitals be able to raise their prices and have the necessary funds to invest in higher quality. Consequently, these critics claim price competitive markets in healthcare will reduce patient quality.

Proponents of competition counter that in a price-competitive market, hospitals will compete not only on price but also on other attributes such as quality of

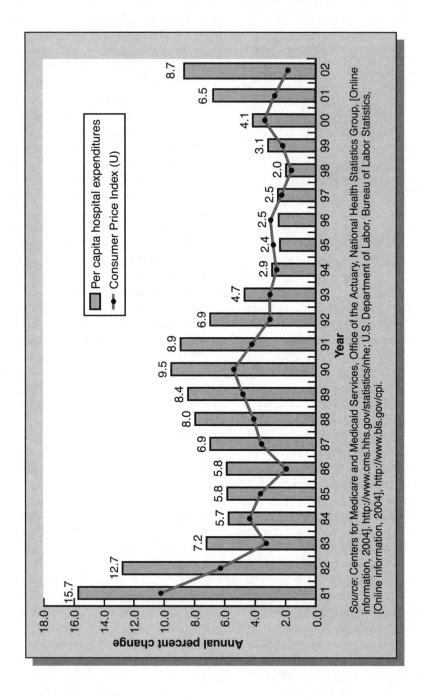

Source: Centers for Medicare and Medicaid Services, Office of the Actuary, National Health Statistics Group, [Online information, 2004]. http://www.cms.hhs.gov/statistics/nhe; U.S. Department of Labor, Bureau of Labor Statistics, [Online information, 2004], http://www.bls.gov/cpi.

Figure 11-5B.   Annual percent changes in per capita hospital expenditures and consumer price index, 1981–2002.

care. Patients (perhaps through their choice of physician and/or employer) choose health plans in part based on the quality of its provider network. Health plans compete on their premiums as well as their provider network, which would include those hospitals having good reputations and that perform a high volume of complex procedures. Competitive markets should therefore result in increased quality.

The research literature on the effect of hospital competition and HMO penetration rates on hospital quality is limited. However, several studies indicate that increased HMO penetration rates and hospital competition are associated with increased hospital quality. For example, HMO patients are more likely to be admitted to higher quality hospitals for bypass surgery than privately insured fee-for-service patients.

Outcome studies have used as quality measures risk-adjusted (for patient characteristics) hospital mortality rates for heart disease, e.g., coronary artery bypass graft (CABG). The lower the risk-adjusted mortality rate, the higher the quality. CABG surgery is often used in these studies because it is a high volume procedure performed in many community hospitals as well as in academic medical centers. CABG is also a procedure where there is a strong relationship between the volume of such surgeries and outcome.

Escarce, et al., examined the quality of hospitals used by HMO and non-HMO insured patients for CABG surgery during the period 1992 to 1994 in California and Florida. It is hypothesized that HMOs have an incentive to use high-quality hospitals when employers are interested in quality as well as premiums. When the health plan purchaser is not interested in quality or quality cannot be measured, then the HMO has an incentive to select the lowest priced hospitals. The authors found that HMO patients in California used higher quality hospitals than privately insured non-HMO patients. In Florida, there was no difference between HMO and non-HMO insured patients. The authors suggest that the difference in findings between the two states is because California was a mature managed care market with large HMOs who were able to use their market power compared to Florida. In Florida, the authors also found that Medicare HMO patients were less likely to use high-quality hospitals than Medicare non-HMO

patients. Florida Medicare HMO patients were believed to have less information on quality, they were more dependent on their physician's hospital affiliation, and there was no large buyer (like an employer) to demand quality data from the HMO (29).

The Current Market for Hospitals and A Look Ahead

The relative balance of market power between hospitals and health plans has changed in the last several years. During the 1980s and 1990s, many hospitals were independent, they had excess capacity, health plans shifted patients to those hospitals willing to provide sharply discounted prices, and hospitals competed on price to be included in an insurer's provider network. Hospital profitability declined and they were a distressed industry. Over time hospitals closed, others merged, excess capacity declined, and health plans broadened their provider networks to meet consumer demands for greater access to more providers.

The decline in excess capacity and in the number of hospital competitors in a market increased hospitals' bargaining power. With increased market power, hospitals increased their prices to health plans, and hospital profitability rose. Federal anti-trust agencies are closely examining hospital mergers for their possible anti-competitive effects.

The economic outlook for hospitals has improved, and an increasingly aged population will demand more hospital care. However, uncertainties exist that could adversely affect their profitability. Medicare, an important payer of inpatient care for the aged, faces a large budget deficit as the baby boomers begin to retire in 2011. To the extent that Medicare reduces the rate of increase in hospital payments to limit its future deficits, hospital profitability will decline. At the same time, hospital input costs are increasing more rapidly. A severe nursing "shortage" (see the chapter on The Market for Registered Nurses) will require hospitals to increase nurse wages. Also, hospitals will have to hire more nurses if legislation, similar to that enacted in California, on minimum nurse staffing ratios is enacted by other states. Technological advances will continue to increase hospital costs as well.

Lastly, several physician specialties are establishing specialty hospitals, such as cardiology, oncology, and orthopedic hospitals that directly compete with their own hospital. These physicians retain their staff appointments at the community hospital but direct some patients to their own hospital. To the extent that physicians are able to move the most profitable services to their specialty hospital, the community hospital's profitability will decline. How hospitals respond to competition from their own specialists will be an important issue in coming years. (As a result of hospital lobbying, the recently enacted Medicare Prescription Drug Act placed a moratorium on new competing physician-owned specialty hospitals.)

SUMMARY

In the period before managed care, given the type of payment systems, hospitals had little concern with efficiency, hospital expenditures rose rapidly, there was unnecessary duplication of costly facilities and services, and, because many hospitals performed few complex procedures, the quality *outcomes* of these procedures was lower than if the volume were greater at each hospital. (Quality was perceived in terms of process or structural measures, such as the latest technology, rather than by outcomes of medical services.)

The structure of the hospital industry has been undergoing dramatic changes since the mid 1980s. The applicability of the anti-trust laws, purchaser incentives to reduce the cost of hospital care, excess hospital capacity, and increasing physician-to-population ratios changed the form of hospital competition. There was a shift from non-price to price competition. In the period before 1983, hospitals competed largely on the basis of non-price factors such as technology, bed availability, services, and amenities. Studies based on data from this earlier period concluded that hospital competition led to higher rather than lower costs. While hospitals still compete on non-price factors, they now also compete on price. Large health insurers negotiate prices with high-quality regional health centers for specialized services, such as for transplants. These regional centers are also likely to have better treatment outcomes than local institutions that perform few such complex procedures.

As a means of increasing referrals to their institution, hospitals attempted to develop stronger relationships with their medical staffs and physician groups. Many hospitals purchased physicians' practices and lost large sums on these ventures as physicians no longer had the same productivity incentives as they did previously. Hospitals are still searching for ways to work together with physicians in a price competitive environment.

In addition to price competition, hospital systems will have to compete on quality, outcomes, and patient satisfaction. Employers and insurers are developing sophisticated data systems that will enable them to determine the clinical outcomes for specific services within a hospital. In the years ahead, purchasers will have data on prices and clinical outcomes upon which to base their decisions. A competitive market whereby competition is based on prices, outcomes, and satisfaction should lead to improved market performance.

As the hospital market becomes more price competitive, there is a concern over who will serve the uninsured. Certain non-profit teaching institutions located in low-income areas provided a great deal of charity care. This care was paid for through a system of cross subsidies that is being eliminated through price competition and lower Medicare payments. Competitive markets cannot be expected to finance care for the uninsured; thus the issue of payment for the uninsured is becoming more visible and must be addressed by government.

APPENDIX 1: USING A PHYSICIAN CONTROL MODEL TO INCREASE PHYSICIAN PRODUCTIVITY

The profit-maximizing model of the physician explains the American Medical Association's political positions on a number of issues. When the demand for medical care increased, it was in physicians' economic interest that it was met by an increase in physicians' productivity which would increase physicians' incomes, rather than by an increase in the number of physicians. For example, with reference to Figure 11-6, physician and hospital services are two inputs in a production function. With an increase in the demand for medical care, the increased output, represented by the highest isoquant, can be produced with different quantities of either physician or hospital services. At the initial amount of medical care being produced, isoquant Q_{MC1}, the combination of physician and hospital care is Q_{MD0} and Q_{H1}, respectively. As the quantity of medical care to be provided increases to isoquant Q_{MC4}, the number of physicians and the quantity of hospital care can be increased in the same proportions as previously. It will, however, be in the economic interest of physicians if their number remains the same while the quantity of hospital care is increased. With the same number of physicians, Q_{H4} of hospital care will be required. Since the quantity of medical care produced is greater even though the number of physicians has remained unchanged, their marginal productivity has increased; correspondingly, the marginal productivity of the hospital has fallen. The higher the physician's productivity, the greater their income.

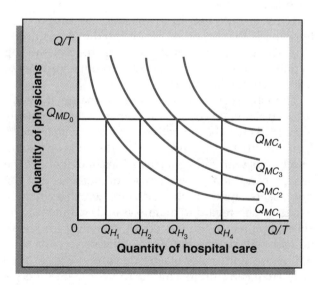

Figure 11-6. A production function for medical care.

(Increasing output by expanding one input while keeping the quantity of the other input constant is the concept of the law of variable proportions. The marginal productivity of the variable input—in this case the hospital—will eventually decline, while that of the fixed input—physicians—will increase.)

APPENDIX 2: COST SHIFTING

Large employers have expressed concern over the pricing behavior of non-profit hospitals referred to as "cost shifting," which is the practice of raising prices to privately insured patients because Medicare, Medicaid, or the uninsured do not pay their full charges. Many employers believe that hospitals increase their charges to privately insured patients to make up shortfalls from the government; consequently, private insurers, hence employers and employees, subsidize those who do not pay their "fair" share. The 1990 price-to-cost ratios of Medicare (about 0.9), Medicaid (about 0.8), and private payers (about 1.3) are considered to be evidence of cost shifting.

Cost shifting would be an indication of market power; the hospital is able to increase its prices to certain classes of patients without losing a sufficient number of those patients to make the price increase profitable. To determine whether cost shifting occurs, it is necessary to understand a hospital's pricing objectives. Different objectives result in different pricing strategies.

If a hospital prices so as to maximize its profits, then the hospital will set a profit-maximizing price to each payer class. Assuming there are two types of patients, privately insured and Medicare patients, then the hospital will have two sets of prices, the fixed DRG price per admission for Medicare patients and a price for the privately insured. The hospital is a price taker in the Medicare market and a price setter in the privately insured market.

In the private market, the hospital will set price at that point on its demand curve where marginal revenue (MR) equals marginal cost (MC). As shown in Figure 11-7, this profit-maximizing price will be P_1. (This price would change only if the hospital's

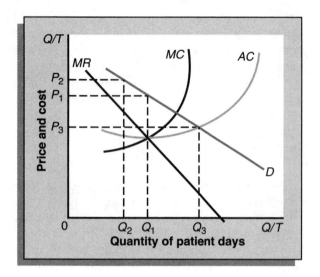

Figure 11-7. Hospital cost shifting.

How likely is it that hospitals did not profit maximize so as to have more than the profit-maximizing number of private patients? As discussed previously, hospitals have certain objectives. If physicians were the dominant group in control of the hospital, they would prefer that any additional hospital revenues be used to increase their productivity and income. Increased numbers of hospital personnel, interns and residents, new equipment, or even lower charges for hospital services that are complementary to their own are examples of the opportunity costs of charging "too low" a price to private patients.

Even using a different behavioral model of the hospital, there is an opportunity cost of foregoing additional profit. Managers could be given higher salaries and more assistants, hospital staff could be paid higher wages, additional personnel could be hired, the physical facilities could be enhanced, or a greater amount of charity could be provided. Given the different ways in which the foregone profit could be used—namely, to charge private patients less or to forego ways of achieving the hospital decision-makers' objectives—it is more likely that the profit would be used by the hospital decision-makers than for a group (e.g., private-pay patients or insurance companies) that is not as politically important to the hospital.

There is little empirical evidence to support the hypothesis that hospitals are engaged in cost shifting (30). The few examples supporting the cost-shifting hypothesis are from the period before the mid 1980s, prior to price competition.

The observation that hospitals charge different prices (relative to cost) to different classes of patients is more likely to be indicative of *price discrimination*. A firm's ability to price discriminate depends on having purchasers with different elasticities of demand. (The second condition for price discrimination is that the purchasers cannot resell the service, which is unlikely to occur with regard to diagnosis and treatment.) The class of patients with less elastic demands for hospital care will pay higher prices relative to costs than will those with more elastic demands (e.g., a large HMO that can shift its volume to a competitor hospital). For example, with reference to Figure 13-2, the two demand curves have different elasticities of de-

variable costs (MC) change or if the elasticity of the demand curve changes, thereby changing the MR curve. Changes in fixed costs would not change the profit-maximizing price.) If for some reason Medicare pays the hospital less, the MC and MR curves in the private market will not change. Consequently, the profit-maximizing price in the private market should not change.

If the hospital decided to increase the price to private patients to P_2 from P_1, then the hospital would be worse off, they would be foregoing profit they could have earned, the difference between MR and MC. Thus it is unlikely that the hospital would increase price if they were already at the profit-maximizing price.

Only if the hospital is *not* profit maximizing could the hospital increase its price and make additional profits. If the hospital were a utility-maximizer (charging less than the profit-maximizing price so as to increase its number of patients), then the hospital's price would be at P_3; increasing price to P_1 would increase profits. For cost shifting to occur, the hospital's objective must have been to have a larger number of private patients rather than to maximize profits.

mand. The group of patients represented by D_1 is less price elastic, hence has a higher price to cost ratio, than those represented by D_2.

Price discrimination also occurs between the prices paid by privately insured and Medicare patients. The federal government, as a large purchaser of hospital care for Medicare patients, uses its market power and establishes a single hospital price for all Medicare patients. As shown in Figure 10-6, the hospital faces a horizontal demand curve for its Medicare patients. Assuming that private insurers do not have as much market power as the government, the hospital faces a downward-sloping demand curve by private (non-Medicare) patients. If the hospital sets its prices so as to maximize its profits, it will establish a price for private patients that will be higher than the fixed Medicare price; the private price will be at that point on the demand curve where the marginal revenues from both types of patients are equal. If the Medicare price were decreased, the profit-maximizing strategy for the hospital would be to *decrease*, not increase, the price to its private patients (assuming no change in the marginal costs of treating its private patients).

The above analysis is contrary to what many believe happens when the government reduces its payments to hospitals. The hospital may want to increase its price to private patients when it receives less from government. However, if the hospital is pricing to maximize its profits, then increasing its price beyond that point will reduce its profits. Only if the hospital's costs of serving private patients increase (e.g., inflation or a sicker mix of private patients) will the hospital raise its prices. As these costs increase and the price to private patients increase, it may be thought to be the result of low Medicare payment; however, these increased prices would have occurred anyway. The hospital may say that it will raise prices to private patients if the government pays hospitals less; however, this may be more of an attempt by hospitals to scare private payers into lobbying with them against government reductions in Medicare prices.

The market for hospital services has become very price competitive. Hospital demand curves became more price elastic as private insurers formed PPOs and chose network hospitals according to their prices. Only those hospitals possessing market power are

able to "cost shift," assuming that they are not currently pricing to maximize their profits. With increased price competition, hospital demand curves become more price elastic, and prices will reflect the cost of providing those services. Faced with competition from other hospitals it will not be possible for a hospital to raise its prices when the government reduces its payments.

REVIEW QUESTIONS

1. What effect do economies of scale have on the market structure of an industry?

2. How are the following terms important for determining whether a hospital merger will be challenged on anti-trust grounds: Herfindal Index, failing hospital doctrine, economies of scale, entry barriers, and geographic and product market definition?

3. Contrast the use of government-determined areas, such as Counties and Metropolitan Statistical Areas (MSAs) with patient origin studies as a means of determining the geographic market of a hospital for use in hospital anti-trust cases.

4. Two models of hospital behavior are the profit-maximizing and utility- or prestige-maximizing models. Describe each model and then contrast their predictions in the period before and after managed care competition.

5. What are the advantages to physicians of hospitals being organized as non-profit institutions?

6. In a "Physician-Control" model of hospital behavior, explain how the physician's incentive to minimize the cost of producing a treatment has changed in the period before and after the introduction of managed care.

7. The move from cost-based payment for hospital services to payment based on DRGs was expected to change hospital behavior. Discuss what you would have expected to observe as the payment method changed.

8. What are the similarities and differences between DRG prices and hospital prices determined in a price-competitive market?

9. What is "cost-shifting"? Explain why an increase in a hospital's fixed costs or an increase in the number of uninsured cared for by the hospital will not change the hospital's profit-maximizing price. Similarly, why would a change in a hospital's variable costs change the hospital's profit-maximizing price?

10. Why are hospitals able to charge different purchasers different prices for the same medical services?

11. How does cost shifting differ from price discrimination?

12. Hospitals have always competed for patients. Contrast the effects of such competition (in terms of cost per admission, length of stay, services offered, and introduction of new technology) in the period of cost-based payment and after the introduction of managed care.

13. Within an economic framework, discuss the changing economic outlook for hospitals.

REFERENCES

1. Harold S. Luft, et al., "Does Quality Influence Choice of Hospital?," *Journal of the American Medical Association*, 263(21), June 6, 1990, 2899–2906.

2. See the *Journal of Health Economics*, 8(4), February 1990 issue for several articles, editorials, and comments and rejoinders on the subject of hospital geographic markets. The Spring 1988 issue of *Law and Contemporary Problems*, edited by James F. Blumstein and Frank A. Sloan, 51(2), is a special issue devoted to anti-trust issues in healthcare; included are several excellent articles on definitions of relevant hospital markets for anti-trust analyses. For a discussion and analysis of hospital merger cases, together with a review of empirical evidence on the effect of hospital mergers on price, see Martin Gaynor and W. Vogt, "Antitrust and Competition in Health Care Markets," in *Handbook of Health Economics*, vol. 1B, eds. A. J. Culyer and J. P. Newhouse, (New York: North-Holland Press, 2000), 1405–1487.

3. There have been a large number of hospital cost studies. See for example, T. G. Cowing, A. G. Holtmann, and S. Powers, "Hospital Cost Analysis: A Survey and Evaluation of Recent Studies," in R. Scheffler and L. Rossiter, eds., *Advances in Health Economics and Health Services*, Vol. 4 JAI Press, (Greenwich, Conn.: 1983); Thomas Grannemann, Randall Brown, and Mark Pauly, "Estimating Hospital Costs: A Multiple Output Analysis," *Journal of Health Economics*, 5(2) June 1986, 107–127; and Martin Gaynor and Gerard Anderson, "Uncertain Demand, the Structure of Hospital Costs, and the Cost of Empty Hospital Beds," *Journal of Health Economics*, 14(3) August 1995, 291–317.

4. Mark V. Pauly, "Medical Staff Characteristics and Hospital Costs," *Journal of Human Resources*, 13, Supplement, 1978, 77–111 and Gail A. Jensen and Michael A. Morrisey, "Medical Staff Specialty Mix and Hospital Production," *Journal of Health Economics*, 5(3), September 1986: 253–276.

5. Carson Bays, "The Determinants of Hospital Size: A Survivor Analysis," *Applied Economics*, 18(4), April 1986, 359–377.

6. D. Bellandi, Kirchheimer B., and Saphir, A. "Profitability a matter of ownership status. For-profit systems see earnings rise, while not-for-profits lag." *Modern Healthcare*, 30(24), June 12, 2000, 24–26, 30–40, 42–49.

7. For an excellent discussion of hospital integration, complete with full references, see James C. Robinson, "Physician-Hospital Integration and the Economic Theory of the Firm," *Medical Care Research and Review*, 54(1), March 1997, 3–24.

8. Kenneth J. Arrow, "Uncertainty and the Welfare Economics of Medical Care," *American Economic Review*, 53(5), December 1963, 941–973.

9. For a review of different hypotheses for the existence of non-profit hospitals, see Frank A. Sloan, "Not-For-Profit Ownership and Hospital Behavior," in *Handbook of Health Economics*, vol. 1B, eds. A. J. Culyer and J. P. Newhouse, (New York: North-Holland Press, 2000), 1141–1174.

10. Tax exemption, by itself, is hypothesized to provide a significant reason for non-profit organization. The value of tax exemption varies from state to state since states vary in their property, sales, and corporate income taxes. Henry B. Hansmann, "The Effect of Tax Exemption and Other Factors on the Market Share of Non-Profit Versus For-Profit Firms," *National Tax Journal*, 40(1) March 1987, 71–82.

11. For a more complete discussion of the hospital control mechanism used by physicians, see Mark V. Pauly and M. Redisch, "The Not-for-Profit Hospital as a Physicians' Cooperative," *American Economic Review*, 63(1) March 1973, 87–99; Mark V. Pauly, "Non-Profit

Firms in Medical Markets," *American Economic Review,* Papers and Proceedings, 77(2), May 1987: 257–262; S. Shalit, "A Doctor-Hospital Cartel Theory," *Journal of Business,* 50(1), January 1977, 1–20.

12. Patricia M. Danzon, "Hospital 'Profits': The Effects of Reimbursement Policies," *Journal of Health Economics,* 1(1), May 1982: 29–52.

13. Frank A. Sloan, "Property Rights in the Hospital Industry," in H. E. Frech, ed., *Health Care in America,* (Pacific Research Institute for Public Policy: San Francisco, Ca.), 1988, 103–141.

14. For an example of this model, see Joseph P. Newhouse, "Toward a Theory of Non-Profit Institutions: An Economic Model of a Hospital," *American Economic Review,* 60(1), March 1970, 64–74.

15. Harold Luft, John Bunker, and Alain Enthoven, "Should Operations Be Regionalized," *New England Journal of Medicine,* 301(25), December 20, 1979, 1364–1369. See also Robert Hughes, Sandra Hunt, and Harold Luft, "Effects of Surgeon Volume and Hospital Volume on Quality of Care in Hospitals," *Medical Care,* 25(6), June 1987, 489–503.

16. David M. Cutler, ed., *The Changing Hospital Industry: Comparing Not-For-Profit and For-Profit Institutions,* (Chicago: University of Chicago Press) 2000. Also see Frank Sloan, "Not-For-Profit Ownership and Behavior," *op. cit.*

17. Emmett Keeler, G. Melnick, and J. Zwanziger, "The Changing Effects of Competition on Non-Profit and For-Profit Pricing Behavior," *Journal of Health Economics,* 18(1), January 1999, 69–86, and David Dranove and R. Ludwick, "Competition and Pricing by Nonprofit Hospitals: A Reassessment of Lynk's Analysis," *Journal of Health Economics,* 18(1), January 1999, 87–98.

18. Emmett B. Keeler, et al., "Hospital Characteristics and Quality of Care," *Journal of the American Medical Association,* 268(13), 1992, 1709–1714.

19. Frank A. Sloan, et al., "Does Where You Are Admitted Make A Difference? An Analysis of Medicare Data," in Alan Garber, ed., NBER *Frontiers in Health Policy Research,* v.2, (MIT Press: Cambridge, Mass.) December 1999, pp. 1–27.

20. Medicare Payment Advisory Commission, Report to the Congress: Medicare Payment Policy (March 2001) table B-14, [online information] http://www.medpac.gov/publications/congressional_reports/Mar01%20App%20B.pdf accessed on Oct. 18, 2002.

21. For a review of studies in this area, see Richard G. Frank and D. Salkever, "Non-Profit Organizations in the Health Sector," *Journal of Economic Perspectives,* 8(4) Fall 1994, 129–144.

22. Jonathan Gruber, "The Effect of Competitive Pressures on Charity: Hospital Responses to Price Shopping in California," *Journal of Health Economics,* 13(2), July 1994, 183–212.

23. James C. Robinson, "Hospital Quality Competition and the Economics of Imperfect Information," *The Milbank Quarterly,* 66(3), 1988, 465–481, and James C. Robinson and H. Luft, "The Impact of Hospital Market Structure on Patient Volume, Average Length of Stay, and the Cost of Care," *Journal of Health Economics,* 4(4), December 1985, 333–356.

24. James C. Robinson and H. Luft, "Competition and the Cost of Hospital Care 1972–1982," *Journal of the American Medical Association,* 257(23), June 19, 1987, 3241–3245.

25. For a review of the literature on hospital regulation, see David S. Salkever, "Regulation of Prices and Investment in Hospitals in the U.S.," in *Handbook of Health Economics,* vol. 1B, eds. A. J. Culyer and J. P. Newhouse, (New York: North-Holland Press, 2000), 1489–1535.

26. Glenn Melnick, J. Zwanziger, A. Bamezai, and R. Patterson, "The Effect of Market Structure and Bargaining Position on Hospital Prices," *Journal of Health Economics,* 11(3), October 1992, 217–233.

27. Anil Bamezi, Zwanziger, J., Melnick, G., and Mann, J., "Price Competition and Hospital Cost Growth in the United States (1989–1994)," *Health Economics,* 8(3), May 1999, 233–243.

28. Michael Chernew, G. Gowrisankaran, and A. Fendrick, "Payer Type and the Returns to Bypass Surgery: Evidence From Hospital Entry Behavior," *Journal of Health Economics,* 21(3), May 2002, 451–474.

29. Jose Escarce, et al., "Health Maintenance Organizations and Hospital Quality For Coronary Artery Bypass Surgery," *Medical Care Research and Review,* 56(3), September 1999, 340–362, Michael Chernew, D. Scanlon, and R. Hayward, "Insurance Type and Choice of Hospital For Coronary Artery Bypass Graft Surgery," *Health Services Research,* 33(3), August 1998, 447–466, and Daniel Kessler and M. McClellan, "Is Hospital Competition Socially Wasteful?" *Quarterly Journal of Economics,* 115(2), 2000, 577–615.

30. For a comprehensive discussion of cost shifting, see Michael Morrisey, *Cost Shifting in Health Care: Separating Evidence from Rhetoric,* (Washington, D.C.: American Enterprise Institute Press) 1994.

CHAPTER
~ 12 ~

The Pharmaceutical Industry

KEY TERMS AND CONCEPTS

- Patented versus generic drugs
- Therapeutic class
- "Me-too" drugs
- Drug formularies
- FDA safety and efficacy standards
- Hatch-Waxman Act
- Tiered co-payments
- Re-importation

Learning Objectives

Upon completing this chapter, the reader should be able to:

- Explain the contribution of innovative new drugs as a contributor to rising drug expenditures.
- Understand the lengthy drug approval process.
- Describe how prices for both innovative and "me-too" drugs are determined.
- Explain why drug price discounts are not based on purchaser volume but ability to shift drug purchases.
- Describe drug companies' response to managed care's use of formularies.
- Discuss the effect of imposing price controls on existing innovative drugs versus those drugs not yet discovered.
- Understand why re-importation laws will not reduce U.S. drug prices to those prevailing overseas.

INTRODUCTION

Innovative new drugs have improved the quality and length of life for many millions of people. New drugs have also reduced the cost of medical care, substituting medicines for more costly surgeries and long hospital stays. At time of discovery, however, the effects of new drugs are not fully known. Powerful drugs that have the potential for curing cancer may also have harmful side effects. Some drugs may cause illness or even death to some, which would outweigh any possible beneficial effects to others. New drugs offer a trade-off: improvements in the quality and length of life versus possible serious adverse consequences.

Along with their beneficial effects, however, the expense of new drugs has become a financial burden to many. Although prescription drug expenditures represent a smaller percentage of total health expenditures (10 percent) than hospital or physician services (31 percent and 22 percent, respectively), the sharp increase in drug expenditures has become a cause for concern in both the public and private sectors. Rapidly increasing drug expenditures are an increasing burden to state Medicaid programs and a major contributing factor to higher private insurance premiums. Further, patients pay a higher percent out of pocket for drugs than they do for other major health expenditures. It is therefore not surprising that patients are more likely to complain about paying $50 for a prescription drug than for a $20,000 hospital stay that is covered by insurance.

Reasons for the Rapid Increase in Pharmaceutical Expenditures

Drug expenditures had been increasing at double-digit rates since the early 1980s. This rate of increase slowed in the early 1990s and then once again began to increase sharply in the latter part of the 1990s, more rapidly than other medical expenditures. For example, from 1999 to 2000, total prescription drug expenditures rose 17.3 percent, reaching $122 billion. Government researchers forecast that drug expenditures will continue to increase rapidly for the rest of this decade. If Congress adds a prescription drug benefit to the Medicare program, spending on drugs will increase even more rapidly.

Increased Prices and Utilization of Drugs: Annual percentage increases in prescription drug expenditures and drug prices since 1980 are shown in Figure 12-1 (page 298). What is different about the most recent increase in drug expenditures is that price increases (as measured by the Bureau of Labor Statistics) do not appear to be as important a contributing factor to expenditure increases as they were in the period before the mid 1990s.

Instead, increased use of drugs has been an important contributor to increased drug expenditures. As shown in Figure 12-2 (page 299), the total number of prescriptions filled increased during the last decade, reaching 3.1 billion. On a per capita basis, the average number of prescriptions increased sharply, from 7.3 in 1992 to 10.6 in 2002.

The increase in the number of aged and increased insurance coverage for prescription drugs are two important reasons for the large rise in number of prescriptions. Although population growth is about 1 percent per year, the aged population has been increasing more rapidly, and the aged have the highest use rate of prescription drugs. While those between the ages 35 and 44 use 2.9 prescriptions each per year, those between the ages 55 and 64 receive about 6.5 prescriptions each. Between the ages 65 and 74, the number of prescriptions increases to more than 9 per person, and those 75 years of age and older receive more than 11 prescriptions each. See Figure 12-3 (page 300).

As the aged, the greatest users (and beneficiaries) of prescription drugs, become an increasing proportion of the population, the volume of prescriptions should continue to increase. Starting in 2011, the first of the baby boom generation begins to reach 65 years of age. The increasing number of aged and the greater number of prescriptions per aged should result in rapidly increasing drug expenditures.

The second reason for the increase in number of prescriptions per capita has been growth in insurance coverage for prescription drugs. The percentage of the population with some form of third-party pay-

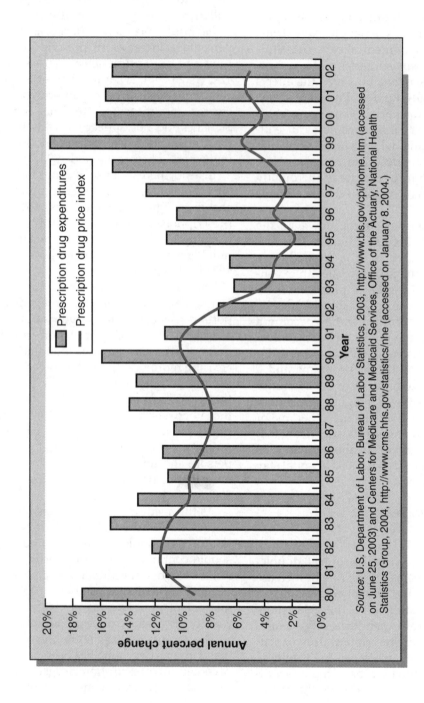

Figure 12-1. Annual percent changes in the Prescription Drug Price Index and Prescription Drug Expenditures, 1980–2002.

Source: U.S. Department of Labor, Bureau of Labor Statistics, 2003, http://www.bls.gov/cpi/home.htm (accessed on June 25, 2003) and Centers for Medicare and Medicaid Services, Office of the Actuary, National Health Statistics Group, 2004, http://www.cms.hhs.gov/statistics/nhe (accessed on January 8. 2004.)

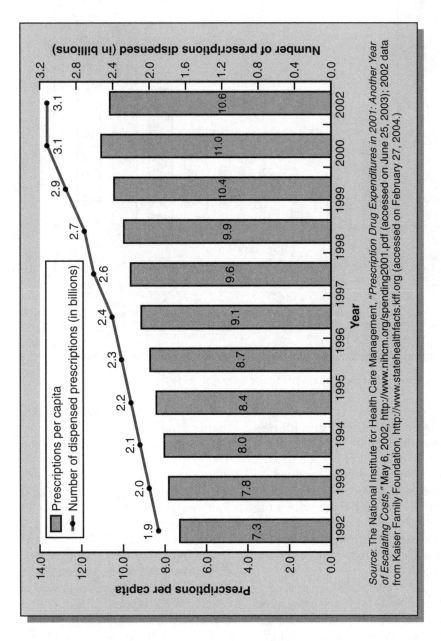

Source: The National Institute for Health Care Management, "*Prescription Drug Expenditures in 2001: Another Year of Escalating Costs*," May 6, 2002, http://www.nihcm.org/spending2001.pdf (accessed on June 25, 2003); 2002 data from Kaiser Family Foundation, http://www.statehealthfacts.kff.org (accessed on February 27, 2004.)

Figure 12-2.   Total prescriptions dispensed and prescriptions per capita, 1992–2002.

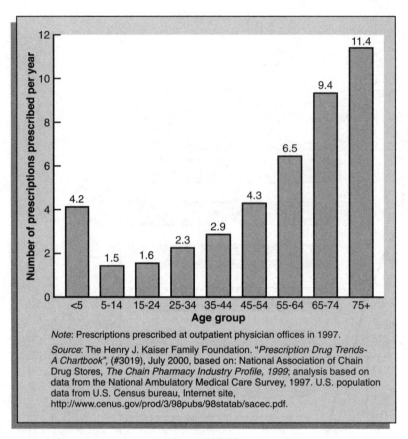

Figure 12-3. Average number of prescriptions prescribed, by age, 1997

ment for prescription drugs has been increasing over time. Conversely, out-of-pocket expenditures for prescription drugs have been falling. In 1970, 82 percent of drug expenditures were paid out of pocket. In each of the following 10 years this percentage declined, to 69 percent in 1980, 59 percent in 1990, and down to 30 percent in 2002. Providing a drug benefit where the patient's co-payment may be $5 per prescription represents a large price decrease, and drug plans offered by managed care insurers led to large increases in the use of prescription drugs.

As shown in Figure 12-4, the largest share of spending on drugs is paid for by private health insurance and health plans, which increased from 24 percent in 1990 to 48 percent in 2002. Government payment for drugs, primarily by Medicaid and Medicare HMOs, increased from 16 percent to 22 percent over that same period. (Medicare does not include a drug benefit.)

Innovative Drugs: Increased use of drugs and higher drug prices do not, by themselves, explain the rapid rise in drug expenditures since the mid-1990s. The 1990s saw a large increase in the number of innovative new drugs that cost more and have preventive and curative effects that result in greater use. These innovative new drugs can treat illnesses that were previously untreatable and have substituted for more costly, invasive medical treatments. This has led to lower overall treatment costs. Some of these new drugs also have fewer adverse side effects. Many new "lifestyle" drugs improve quality of life, e.g., Viagra, relief from allergies (Claritin) and stomach upsets (Prilosec), anti-depressants, and pain relievers. For example, there are new pain relievers to treat severe arthritis but they cost $150 a month, nearly 20 times more than previous pain relievers. A new biotech drug, Enbrel, to treat rheumatoid arthritis can cost

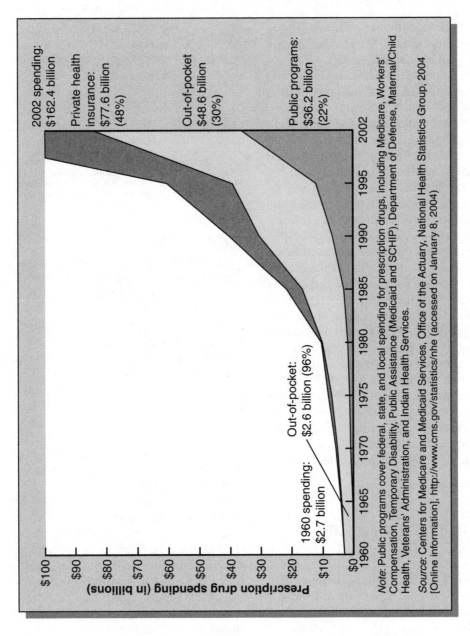

Figure 12-4. Share of prescription drug spending, by source of funds, selected years, 1960–2002.

$1,500 a month. While drugs such as penicillin would be prescribed for a brief period to cure an infection, some modern drugs, including lifestyle drugs, can be taken for decades.

The prospect of better health and a higher quality of life has led to increases in both the number of prescriptions and the price of new drugs.

For a better understanding of the increase in drug expenditures, one must account for the contribution of new drugs. Table 12-1, based on a study examining the period 1993 to 1998, categorizes the increase in prescription drug expenditures into price and utilization increases. Overall utilization of prescription drugs accounted for about one-third (7.3 percent per year) of the expenditure increase, while price increases accounted for the remaining two-thirds of the increase (12.8 percent per year) in drug expenditures. However, when the expenditure increase over this time period was classified by new drugs (introduced after 1992) versus old drugs, two-thirds of the expenditure increase (13.1 percent per year) was due to new drugs (8.4 percent per year increase in prices and 4.7 percent per year increased use). Older drugs accounted for only one-third of total expenditure increase over this period (4.4 percent per year increase in price and 2.6 percent per year increase in use).

The implication of these findings is that *the replacement of old drugs by new drugs is the most important reason for rising drug expenditures.* Prescription drug expenditures are likely to continue their rapid rise driven by new drug discoveries and greater use of drugs, particularly among an increasingly older population.

THE STRUCTURE OF THE PHARMACEUTICAL INDUSTRY

A brief description is provided of the different types of drugs provided by the pharmaceutical industry since substitutes and competition occur among drugs within a specific therapeutic class and not among all drugs (1).

Table 12-1. Percentage Contribution of Changes in Price and Utilization to 1993–1998 Increase in Prescription Drug Spending

	Average Annual Percent Increase in Price Effect	Average Annual Percent Increase in Utilization Effect	Total Average Annual Percent Increase
New drugs (1992 and later)	8.4%	4.6%	13.0%
Older drugs	4.4%	2.6%	7.0%
Total	12.8%	7.2%	20.0%

Source: Data based on National Institute for Health Care Management Research and Educational Foundation, *Factors Affecting the Growth of Prescription Drug Expenditures,* July 1999. Internet site: http://www.nihcm.org/FinalText3.pdf [accessed on December 18, 2001].

Types of Drugs:

There are two general types of drugs, those that require a physician's prescription and those that can be purchased without a prescription. (Certain prescription drugs may eventually be sold over the counter without a prescription, as has recently occurred with Claritin when the government regulatory agency, the Food and Drug Administration [FDA], believes that experience with use of the drug has demonstrated that there is minimal risk to the patient and that the physician's advice regarding the drug's use is no longer required.) The analysis of the pharmaceutical industry is concerned with prescription drugs.

There are two types of prescription drugs: drugs that receive a patent on their chemical formulation, and generic drugs which are a copy of a patented drug. Patented drugs are approved by the FDA for particular usage after an extensive testing process and are sold under a brand name. Generic drugs have the same active ingredients as the original patented drug and are judged by the FDA to be comparable in terms of strength, quality, and therapeutic effectiveness. (The generic drug must demonstrate bio-equivalence of ±20 percent of the original drug.) Generic drugs are generally sold under their chemical name after the patent on a brand-name drug has expired.

A drug patent, however, does not necessarily provide a firm with a complete monopoly on a particular therapeutic market. Within a therapeutic market, there may be a single patented brand-name drug for treating an illness, or there may be several patented brand-name drugs. Multiple patented drugs can be therapeutically similar, but each has received a patent based on a different chemical formulation. A "me-too" drug uses the same therapeutic mechanism as a breakthrough drug and therefore competes directly with it. When there is a single breakthrough (innovator) drug with no close substitutes, the firm producing that drug will have a great deal of monopoly power. In many therapeutic markets, however, over time there are multiple patented drugs providing each firm with some monopoly power but less than if there were no close substitutes.

The Role of the Physician:

There are both demand- and supply-side characteristics of the pharmaceutical industry that distinguish it from other industries.

A crucial factor that determines the demand for prescription drugs is the role of the physician as the patient's agent in prescribing medications. When treating a patient, physicians do not have perfect information on the most appropriate drug to prescribe, the possible substitute drugs that are available, their side effects, and their relative costs. As a result, pharmaceutical companies devote a great deal of effort in marketing their drugs to physicians. Physicians are also unaffected by the cost of the drugs they prescribe, as may be the patient whose costs are covered by prescription drug insurance.

The lack of physician knowledge on prescription drugs, as well as their lack of a financial incentive to be concerned with the cost of drugs, combined with insurance to cover the patient's costs, have affected the structure of this industry. These demand-side characteristics, together with the life-saving and quality-of-life benefits of innovative drugs, made patients insensitive to drug prices.

Economies of Scale, Mergers, and Biotechnology Firms

The pharmaceutical industry is comprised of two types of drug manufacturers: those that engage in research and development and also market brand-name drugs and, second, generic manufacturers.[1] Public concerns about the performance of the industry have been directed at firms that develop and produce branded drugs.

As measured by the degree of market concentration, pharmaceutical manufacturers appear to be a relatively competitive industry. Concentration, which is measured by the combined market share of the top four firms, is only about 22 percent. However, when therapeutic categories are used, the degree of market concentration is much higher. In some cases it is 100 percent since there may be only one drug in that therapeutic category. Thus the competitiveness of the pharmaceutical industry depends upon the definition of the market.

More highly concentrated markets are typically less price competitive. As the degree of market concentration increases, there are fewer substitutes available to a particular drug, and firms generally have greater market power, that is, the ability to raise price without losing sales. Thus the manufacturer of the first breakthrough drug in a therapeutic category has a great deal of market power. As other companies eventually patent drugs that use the same mechanism to treat that illness, additional branded drugs in that therapeutic category ("me-too" drugs) become available as substitutes, and price competition increases.

---

1. With regard to the distribution channel for prescription drugs, manufacturers produce the drugs and, for the most part, sell them to wholesalers, who then sell them to pharmacies where they are purchased by patients. Pharmacies can be chain drug stores, such as Longs Drug stores; mass merchandisers, such as Wal-Mart; food store pharmacies, such as Safeway; mail order or retail pharmacies, and, more recently, Internet pharmacy websites. Over time, the number of independent retail pharmacies has been declining. Wholesalers and retail pharmacies are competitive industries.

Once patent protection expires, generic versions are introduced, and a great deal of price competition occurs. Generics are priced much below the branded drug and quickly increase their share of the market. For example, in 1997, the patent on Zantac expired and the generic version captured 90 percent of the market served by Zantac within 2 years. Currently, about one-half of all prescription drugs dispensed are off-patent generic drugs. At each of these stages, purchasers are able to buy the prescription drug at a lower price.

During the last decade, a large number of mergers have occurred among pharmaceutical companies. These mergers have been of two types. The first were vertical mergers, whereby the firm diversifies into another product line. The growth of managed care led to the development of Pharmacy Benefit Managers (PBMs), which are firms that provide administrative services and process outpatient prescription drug claims for health insurers' prescription drug plans.[2] The growing importance of PBMs led several large drug manufacturers to spend many billions of dollars to buy PBMs in the early 1990s. (Merck paid $6.6 billion for Medco in 1993.) These drug firms believed that by buying PBMs they could gain greater control over the market for their drugs; the PBMs would presumably substitute their drugs over those of their competitors, thereby increasing their market share and drug sales. PBMs, however, were unable to merely include their owner's drugs to the exclusion of others since their credibility in serving health plans would be adversely affected. (It does not appear that the drug firms' PBM strategy was worthwhile. Drug companies that did not buy PBMs were also able to in-crease their drug sales, and companies that bought PBMs are now selling them.)

The growth of managed care turned out to be a benefit rather than a threat to drug manufacturers. As more people enrolled in managed care, they received prescription drug coverage, use of prescription drugs increased, and sales at all drug firms sharply increased.

The second type of merger that has been occurring is horizontal, where one drug manufacturer purchases another. The reason for horizontal mergers is twofold: First, there is the expectation that by becoming larger, economies of scale will increase efficiency and decrease costs. Merging two companies can result in decreased administrative costs and increased efficiency of the two company's sales forces, which is critical to the success of any drug firm. There are also large economies in conducting research and developing new drugs. Consolidating research units can eliminate competing efforts.

The second reason for horizontal mergers is to take advantage of economies in marketing and to improve the combined drug firm's market power. Few mergers have been between firms with drugs in the same therapeutic category. Instead, the types of drugs offered by the combined drug firms are in different therapeutic categories, thereby enabling the firm to market a broader range of prescription drugs across many therapeutic categories to large purchasers.

Large drug firms have also purchased smaller biotechnology companies. Small firms have their capital invested in the particular drug that is going through the research and development (R & D) and approval process. The longer the delay in being able to market their drug, the greater is their capital requirement. These small firms face large risks and huge investment costs before their products can be marketed. The process of discovery, clinical trials, and drug approval is lengthy and costs hundreds of millions of dollars. Larger firms are able to bear these costs and have the expertise to navigate the drug-approval process. There is also greater risk pooling when many different drugs are in the discovery and development phase since only a few of the many drugs developed will be successful. Only a large firm can afford to undertake these large research efforts.

---

2. To control growth in prescription drug expenditures, PBMs will also contract with a network of pharmacies, negotiate pharmacy payments, negotiate with drug manufacturers for drug discounts and rebates, develop a drug formulary listing preferred drugs for treating an illness, encourage use of generic drugs instead of high-priced brand-name drugs, operate a mail-order pharmacy, and analyze and monitor patient-compliance programs. Some PBMs have been very aggressive in switching physicians' prescriptions. They may call up the physician and tell them that a less expensive drug is available for the same medical condition and suggest switching to a drug for which the PBM receives a large price discount or rebate.

To minimize their chance of running out of money, small drug firms with a promising new drug will merge/partner with larger firms that have greater capital resources and experience with the drug-approval process.

The longer and more costly the FDA's research and approval process, the greater is the burden on small drug firms.

Thus, while the drug industry is characterized by several large firms, these firms typically do not have a monopoly over any particular therapeutic market. Generally, several firms compete within a therapeutic class. And once a patent expires, there is quick entry by generic firms, making the market more competitive and leading to much lower prices.

The Patent Process: A Barrier to Entry

To understand the structure, hence conduct, and performance of the pharmaceutical industry, it is necessary to understand the role of patent protection and the high cost of developing new drugs. The following is a history of the regulatory process and the requirement that the federal Food and Drug Administration (FDA) approve any new drug before it can be marketed in the U.S.

The Pure Food and Drug Act of 1906 was the federal government's first major effort at regulating the pharmaceutical industry. The supporters of this act were primarily concerned with the quality of food rather than with drugs. Pure food acts had been submitted to Congress at least 10 years before one was finally passed. Media publicity on the ingredients of food and drugs generated popular support for legislative action. A great deal of publicity was generated by newspapers, magazine articles, and Upton Sinclair's *The Jungle*, with its graphic descriptions of what was being included in the foods the public was eating. The result was public outrage, to which Congress responded by passing the 1906 Pure Food and Drug Act.

The American Medical Association led the political fight to include drugs as part of the Pure Food and Drug Act. The AMA had been opposed to "patent" medicines, which contained secret ingredients, favoring instead "ethical" drugs, which were advertised to physicians and whose ingredients were not kept secret. The act required drug companies to provide accurate labeling information, including whether the drug was addictive. (A number of medicines contained alcohol, opium, heroin, and cocaine, which were legal at that time.) The drug-related portion of the act was quite limited and was modeled by the public's concern with the contents of food.

In the 1930s, the modern drug era began with the development of sulfa drugs. As drugs were introduced, a tragedy provided the impetus for new legislation. A company seeking to make a liquid form of Elixir Sulfanilamide for children dissolved it in ethylene glycol (antifreeze). The company was unaware of the toxic effects. As a result, more than 100 children died before the drug was recalled. Responding to the public outcry, Congress passed the Food, Drug, and Cosmetic Act in 1938. The 1938 law, which created the Food and Drug Administration, was intended to protect the public from unsafe, potentially harmful drugs. A company had to seek approval from the FDA before it could market a new drug. *It was left up to the drug company* to determine the necessary amount and type of pre-market testing to prove to the government that the drug was safe for its intended use.

A 1950 amendment to the 1938 Act authorized the FDA to distinguish prescription from non-prescription drugs by stating that some types of drugs could be sold only by prescription since they could be harmful to the individual if bought on their own.

In 1959, Senator Estes Kefauver held hearings on the drug industry. (He was running for the Democratic nomination for President at that time.) Critics of the industry were concerned that drug prices were too high, that drug companies undertook unnecessary and wasteful advertising expenditures, and that the drug industry earned excessive profits.

In the late 1950s, a new drug was introduced in Europe to treat morning sickness for pregnant women. Following the introduction of thalidomide in Europe, an FDA staff member expressed doubts about the safety of the drug because of reported side effects and delayed its approval in the U.S. As reports began to appear in Europe that deformed babies were born to mothers who had taken the drug during pregnancy, media attention shifted Congress' concern over high drug prices, wasteful expenditures, and excessive profits to concern with public safety. Congress responded to the public's fears over drug safety and passed the 1962 Amendments to the Food, Drug, and Cosmetic Act.

The 1962 Drug Amendments:

The 1962 Amendments resulted in a major change in the regulation of pharmaceuticals (2). Drug companies were now required to prove the safety of their new drug and also its efficacy (beyond a "placebo" effect) for the indications claimed for it in treating a particular disease or condition. (Effectiveness must be determined by a controlled study where some patients are given the new drug and others are given a placebo, an inactive substance such as a salt or sugar pill. Once the FDA approves a new drug for marketing, the drug is approved only for specific claims. If the drug company wants to broaden those claims, it must file a new application with the FDA and provide evidence to support the new uses of that drug. Physicians may, however, prescribe a drug for a use for which the FDA has not approved the drug.)

The steps that a drug company must take to meet the FDA's safety and efficacy standards are both costly and time consuming. The FDA specifies the type of pre-marketing tests that are required. Before undertaking clinical trials using humans, animal trials are used to determine whether the drug is sufficiently safe and promising to justify human trials. Based on this evidence, the FDA will approve clinical trials using humans. There are three different stages of clinical trials, and each stage uses a greater number of subjects so that more dangerous drugs are identified before they can affect larger numbers of patients. Stage 1 introduces the drug to a small number of healthy individuals, and stage 2 uses a small number of diseased persons. The third stage using a large number of patients, half of whom take a placebo, is designed to demonstrate efficacy as well as additional evidence of safety. Clinical trials take on average 6 years to complete. Once completed, the drug firm must receive FDA approval, which can take an additional several years (3). Once approved by the FDA,

the new drug must be manufactured according to specified standards.

After the 1962 Amendments were enacted, generic and patented drugs were treated the same. Both had to meet the same stringent FDA requirements as a new drug seeking a patent. Generic drugs had to independently prove the safety and efficacy of their product in order to receive FDA approval. Because generic drugs had to undertake the same research as the patented drug, the cost and time for developing generic drugs increased. Once a new drug received its patent and was approved by the FDA, the drug had no competition and the price could be kept high for a longer period of time. Consumers continued to face high prices for prescription drugs whose patents had expired because of the FDA requirements that delayed the entry of generic substitutes.

The 1984 Hatch-Waxman Act:

The 1984 Drug Price Competition and Patent Term Restoration (Hatch-Waxman) Act simplified and streamlined the process for FDA approval of generic drugs in exchange for granting patent extensions to innovative drugs. Generic drugs no longer had to replicate many of the clinical trials performed by the original manufacturer to prove safety and efficacy. Instead, the generic drug manufacturer was only required to demonstrate that the generic drug was "bioequivalent" to the already approved patented drug, which was much less costly than proving safety and efficacy. (Bioequivalence means that the active ingredient is absorbed at the same rate and to the same extent for the generic drug as for the patented drug.) The effect of this Act was to reduce the delay between patent expiration and generic entry from more than 3 years to less than 3 months. Generic drugs are now quickly available at prices greatly reduced from those of branded drugs whose patents expired. The market share of the generic substitute rapidly increased after patent expiration. Previously, only 35 percent of top-selling drugs whose patents expired had generic copies; currently almost all do.

Although the 1984 Act made generic drug entry easier and less costly once the patent expired, the Act also extended the patent life of branded drugs to compensate for patent life lost during the long FDA-approval process. (Effective patent life is the time a new drug is approved by the FDA to the end of the patent.) The Act permitted drugs that contain a new chemical entity to qualify for a patent life extension. These patent extensions postpone generic entry by an average of about 2.8 years. The 1984 Act was a compromise between the generic drug manufacturers who wanted easier entry and the drug manufacturers who wanted a longer patent life (4).

State legislation in the 1970s and 1980s also enabled generic drugs to rapidly increase their market share once the drug patent expired. Through the early 1970s, it was illegal in many states for a pharmacist to dispense a generic drug when a prescription specified a brand-name drug. By 1984, all states had enacted drug substitution legislation that permitted a pharmacist to substitute a generic drug even when a brand-name drug was specified, as long as the physician had not indicated otherwise on the prescription.

More Rapid FDA Approval Process:

During the 1980s and 1990s, AIDs activists were very critical of the FDA's approval process. AIDs patients were dying from the disease and wanted promising new drugs to be immediately available. It would be too late for many if these drugs were delayed for years because of research protocols required by the FDA. To provide half of terminally ill AIDs patients with a placebo was believed to be immoral; they would be denied a possible life-saving drug. Terminally ill AIDs patients were willing to bear the risk of taking drugs that might prove to be unsafe or have adverse side effects.

AIDs activists applied pressure on Congress and on the FDA for an accelerated approval process. As a result, new laws and regulations were enacted between 1987 and 1992 that enabled seriously ill patients to have access to experimental drugs. These types of drugs were provided with a "fast-track" approval process. Also, drugs in the clinical trial stages for other diseases that were serious or life threatening and that were shown to have meaningful therapeutic

benefit compared to existing treatments were given an expedited review. In return for the early approval of these new drugs, the drug firm had to periodically notify the FDA about any adverse reactions to the drug that were not detected during the clinical trial periods. In 1992, Congress enacted the Prescription Drug User Fee Act (renewable every five years), which authorized the FDA to collect fees from drug manufacturers seeking a drug approval. The revenues from these fees were to be used to increase the number of FDA staff reviewing drug approvals. As a result, there was a speedup in the approval process and an increase in the number of new drugs approved compared to previous years (5).

Both the fast-tracking approval process and the funds from user fees reduced FDA approval time for new drugs.

Patent protection, which gives a drug manufacturer market power, is essential for protecting R & D investments. Once a new drug is discovered, it is relatively easy to reproduce. Without the period of market exclusivity that patents provide, drug manufacturers could not recover their R & D investments.

It is the patented brand-name drugs that have few competitors within a therapeutic class and whose patents have not yet expired that are the focus of public policy.

CONDUCT

The Pricing Practices of U.S. Pharmaceutical Companies

Drug manufacturers sell their drugs to different purchasers (intermediaries), who in turn sell them to patients. Retail (independent and chain) pharmacies sell about 48 percent of all prescription drugs; mail-order pharmacies, 12 percent; food stores and mass merchandisers, 16 percent; and healthcare organizations, such as HMOs, hospitals, long-term care facilities, and clinics, 24 percent. (HMO and insurance company patients rely on mail-order and retail pharmacies that are in their insurer's network to pick up their drugs.) See Figure 12-5.

The drug manufacturer sells the same prescription drug to different purchasers at different prices. HMOs pay less for their drugs than independent retail pharmacies, even though the latter sell a much greater volume of drugs. Similarly, patients without any prescription drug coverage (often the poor and sick) pay more for the same drug at a retail pharmacy than those who are part of a managed care plan.

There are two aspects of the pricing practices of pharmaceutical companies that have been criticized as being unfair and have led to proposals for government intervention: First, there is a very high price mark-up for prescription drugs and, second, different purchasers are charged different prices for the same drug.

Pricing in Relation to Cost: A new prescription drug is priced many times higher than its actual cost of production. This high mark-up of price over marginal cost has generated a great deal of criticism. If the drug were priced closer to its production cost, it would be less of a financial burden on those with low incomes, those without prescription drug coverage, and state Medicaid budgets.

Drug manufacturers often claim that their drug prices are determined by the high cost of developing those drugs. High R & D costs, however, are *not* the reason for high or rising drug prices. Large fixed or "sunk" costs are costs that have already been incurred; hence they are not relevant for setting a drug's price. It is true that fixed costs must eventually be recovered, otherwise the drug company will lose money. However, a new drug that was no different than drugs already on the market could not sell for more than these competitive drugs, regardless of how much it cost to develop that drug.

Pricing Innovative Drugs: Pharmaceutical manufacturers are strategic in how they mark up the price of their drugs (price-to-marginal cost ratio) and negotiate price discounts. *A drug's price mark-up is determined*

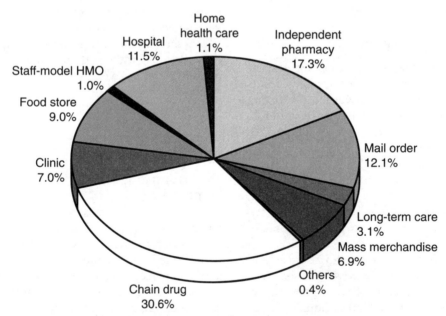

Source: Pharmaceutical Research and Manufacturers of America, PhRMA Annual Survey, 2001. [Online information], http:phrma.org/publications/profile01/chapter4.pdf; based on data from IMS Health, 2001.

Figure 12-5. Prescription sales by outlet, U.S. market, 2000.

by the purchaser's price elasticity of demand. New drugs are priced according to their therapeutic value and the availability of good substitutes. When a new drug for which there is no close substitute comes on the market and it is clearly therapeutically superior to existing drugs, it will have a high price mark-up. Sometimes a drug is priced according to some concept of value, that is, comparing the drug's price to the surgical procedure that it replaces. Approving an existing drug for a new use also increases its value since it provides greater therapeutic effects for that new use than existing drugs; the drug company is thus able to increase its price.

The greater the price mark-up over costs, the more innovative the drug and the fewer the close substitutes to it.[3]

As shown in Figure 12-6, the profit-maximizing price is determined by a firm's marginal cost curve and the elasticity of its demand curve. (The marginal cost curves are assumed to be equal.) A new drug that cost more to develop would have higher average fixed costs, indicated in Figure 12-6 by a higher average total cost curve (ATC). However, if that new drug is less innovative (a more price elastic demand curve) than a drug that cost less to develop (lower ATC) but whose demand curve is less price elastic, then the drug that cost more to develop will have a lower profit-maximizing price than the more innovative drug.

Innovative drugs command higher price mark-ups than imitative drugs. The price of a new drug is determined by a purchaser's willingness to pay for its greater therapeutic benefits. A new breakthrough drug that is the first to treat a disease is priced much higher than any other drug in its therapeutic class (over three times the price) because there are no good substitutes. New drugs with modest therapeutic gains are priced about two times the average for available drug substitutes. New drugs with little or no gain over existing drugs are priced at about the same level as existing substitutes (6). Once the patent has expired on a branded drug, generic drugs are priced at about 30 to 70 percent of the branded drug before its patent expired. As more generic versions become available, the prices of generic drugs fall.

---

3. Assuming that the marginal cost (MC) of a breakthrough drug is $10 and its price elasticity of demand is –1.1, then the price mark-up will be 10 times its marginal cost.

$$\text{Price} = \text{MC}/(1+1/-\text{Pe}) = \$10/(1+1/-1.1) = \$10/(1-0.9)$$
$$= \$10/0.1 = \$100, \text{ or } 10 \text{ times MC.}$$

A more price elastic demand curve, –1.3, would result in a smaller mark-up over marginal cost.

$$\text{Price} = \$10/(1+1/-1.3) = \$10/(1-0.77) = \$10/0.23 = \$43.$$

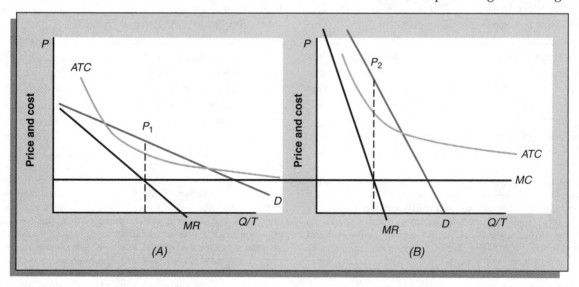

Figure 12-6. Drug price profit maximization when fixed cost and demand elasticities differ.

New, higher-priced drugs will fail commercially if their therapeutic benefits are similar to existing drugs. As managed care organizations evaluate drugs for inclusion in their formulary based on therapeutic benefits and price, *differences in drug prices will reflect differences in therapeutic benefits.* Knowledgeable purchasers evaluating a higher-priced new drug would pay a higher price only if its therapeutic benefits were greater than the older drug.

A new drug that is similar to an existing drug (a "me-too" drug), regardless of its R & D costs, cannot be priced much higher than the existing drug because purchasers will switch to a good substitute (the existing drug) at a lower price.

Although drug companies have been criticized for producing "me-too" types of drugs, the availability of "me-too" drugs contributes to price competition by creating substitutes to the innovative drug. Once "me-too" drugs enter the market originally served by an innovative drug, demand curves become more price elastic, hence prices decline, and purchasers will have greater choice regarding the drug's duration, severity of its side effects, and convenience of administering the drug.

Interestingly, when generic versions enter the market after the patent on a branded drug has expired, the branded drug loses market share to the generic drug but *the price of the branded product actually increases.* The reason is that the price-sensitive customers switch to the generic drug, and those who do not switch are not price-sensitive. Thus the seller of the branded drug is able to raise its price. (Although the demand for the branded drug shifts to the left, it becomes less price elastic.) Some physicians (and consumers) have strong preferences for the branded drug and do not want to substitute the generic version; they are willing to pay more for the security of the brand-name drug.[4] The

drug manufacturer has determined it is more profitable to serve a smaller market at a higher price than reduce the price of the branded drug to compete with generic versions.

Pricing According to Differences in Demand: Drug manufacturers price their drugs differently when they sell to different purchasers. When price differences for the same drug cannot be entirely explained by cost differences, then according to economic theory, the reason for price differences must be related to differences in the purchaser's price sensitivity or price elasticity of demand. Purchasers who are not price sensitive will be charged higher prices than those who are. A purchaser who is willing to buy less or switch to other drugs when the price is increased is more price-sensitive than one who will not.

The higher price charged to one purchaser is not meant to make up for the lower price charged to another purchaser. Instead, the reason for different prices is that the seller can simply make more money by practicing price discrimination, that is, charging according to each purchaser's willingness to pay (7).

It is the ability to shift market share rather than just the volume purchased that drives discounts. Not all large-volume purchasers receive price discounts. Retail pharmacies in total sell a large volume of drugs, but they do not receive the same price discounts as do managed care plans. When an HMO negotiates with a drug company on one of several competing brand-name drugs within a therapeutic class, the HMO's willingness to place the drug on its formulary, while excluding a competitor's drugs, can result in substantial discounts for the HMO.[5] Similarly, pharmacy benefit managers (PBMs) who, on behalf of health plans,

---

4. The Bureau of Labor Statistics' drug price index overstates drug price increases when a generic equivalent of a branded drug comes on the market. The lower-priced generic drug rapidly expands its market share at the expense of the branded drug. As the branded drug loses market share to the generic drug, its price is increased to the remaining patients who are less price sensitive and are reluctant to use the generic version of the drug. The BLS picks up the price increase of the branded drug, but does not measure the price decline experienced by the large proportion of consumers who switch to the generic version.

5. As HMOs and health plans seek volume discounts from drug companies, they are willing to limit their subscribers' choice of drugs in return for negotiating lower drug prices. Drug formulary committees focus on drugs where there are therapeutic substitutes and evaluate different drugs according to their therapeutic value and their price; higher-priced drugs are used only when justified by greater therapeutic benefits. Restrictions are then placed on their physicians' prescribing behavior. These organizations also use computer technology to conduct drug utilization review; each physician's prescription is instantly checked against the formulary, and data is gathered on the performance of each physician as well as on the health plan's use of specific drugs.

manage their drug benefits for drugs sold through retail pharmacies can promote brand name substitution and thereby receive large discounts.

Retail pharmacies pay the highest prices for their prescription drugs because they must carry all branded drugs. Also, the pharmacy cannot promote substitution between branded drugs because the physician may be prescribing according to a health plan's formulary. Since the pharmacy cannot shift volume, there is no need for the drug manufacturer to give them a price discount.[6]

Price discrimination promotes price competition between drug manufacturers for more price-sensitive purchasers resulting in lower prices for purchasers and consumers. Unless a drug manufacturer gave discounts to more price-sensitive purchasers, they would lose sales to other drug companies that are willing to provide such discounts. (To price discriminate, a seller must prevent low-price buyers from reselling the product to those who are charged more. A 1987 federal law prevented resale of prescription drugs on the basis of preserving the safety and integrity of those drugs.)

In addition to being a profit-maximizing strategy for pharmaceutical companies, price discrimination also increases sales of the product. If price discrimination were prohibited and a single pricing system

for a drug was mandated, price-sensitive customers would be less willing to pay higher prices, and use of the drug would decline.

Thus the pricing strategy of pharmaceutical companies is based on two principles. First, the more innovative the drug, such as when a close substitute drug is not available, the higher will be the price mark-up. Second, the greater the price sensitivity of the purchaser, such as an HMO willing to shift its drug purchases to a competitor's drug, the lower the price. These pricing strategies are designed to maximize drug firm profits.

Drug Companies' Marketing Response To Managed Care Plans: Decision-making with respect to pharmaceuticals has changed. Previously, physicians decided the patient's prescription drug. As a result, drug manufacturers spent a great deal of money marketing directly to physicians. With the growth of managed care and their use of closed formularies, drug companies began to develop new marketing strategies. As the purchasing decision over prescription drugs shifted from the individual physician to the committee overseeing the organization's formulary, sending sales representatives to individual physicians caring for an HMO's patients was less useful than marketing to the HMO itself. Drug companies have had to demonstrate that their drugs were not only therapeutically superior to competitive drugs, but that they were also "cost-effective," namely, that the additional benefits of their drug were worth a higher price.

Physicians continue to be important in prescribing drugs to their patients, but PBMs and health plans determine which brand-name drugs the physician is able to prescribe and the prices paid for those drugs.

To counteract the closed formularies, drug manufacturers started direct-to-consumer TV and newspaper advertising to generate consumer pressure to demand certain drugs from their physician (8). Direct-to-consumer advertising, which increased from about $600 million in 1997 (the first year it was permitted by the FDA) to $2.5 billion by 2000, has proved very effective in increasing sales of advertised prescription drugs. Previously, physicians almost never wrote prescriptions for drugs requested by patients because most patients did not know enough to demand drugs by name or therapeutic class. As more

---

6. In 1993, an anti-trust suit was filed by 31,000 retail pharmacies against 24 pharmaceutical manufacturers claiming that the drug companies conspired to charge HMOs, PBMs, and hospitals lower prices while denying price discounts to retail pharmacies. Most of the drug companies settled by paying a relatively small average amount per retail pharmacy and said they would give the same discounts to retail pharmacies if they could demonstrate that they were able to shift market share of their drugs. Five drug companies refused to settle. The retail pharmacies had to prove that price discrimination harmed competition and that the discounts were not a competitive response to another drug firm's lower prices. At the trial in 1998, the judge dismissed the lawsuit, which was upheld on appeal.

The drug companies claimed that price discounts to retail pharmacies would not increase the drug company's market share. Retail pharmacies had to carry a wide selection of drugs because they merely filled orders of prescribing physicians. The greater the ability of the buyer to switch market share from one drug manufacturer to a competitor's drug, the greater was the discount. The drug companies claimed that retail pharmacies were unable to switch volume from one drug company to another; therefore there was no reason to give them a discount.

medical information has become available to patients, they have begun demanding more input into the therapeutic decisions that affect their lives.

Drug companies claim that ads are meant to inform patients and to stimulate discussions between patients and physicians. Critics claim that the ads do not inform patients about who is most likely to benefit from that drug, possible side effects, or other treatment options.

Drug costs have become health plans' fastest growing expense. In response to rising costs, health plans have given patients incentives to use less expensive drugs. A three-tiered co-payment system is used: patients pay a small co-payment for generic drugs, a higher co-payment for prescription drugs on the insurer's formulary (where the manufacturer gives a large discount), and a much higher co-payment for branded drugs not on the health plan's formulary. (Recently, insurers, to further lower their drug costs, have been successful in having the FDA declare that certain prescription drugs can be sold over the counter without a prescription. Once this occurs, the insurer is no longer liable for the cost of that drug since over-the-counter drugs are not covered under the insurer's prescription drug plan.)

Anti-Competitive Behavior by Drug Manufacturers to Delay Entry of Generics: Once generic drugs enter the market, profitability of the branded drug quickly falls. It is therefore in the interest of the drug firm to delay generic entry as long as possible. Certain practices have led the Federal Trade Commission (FTC) to investigate anticompetitive behavior in the drug industry. For example, drug companies that hold patents on brand-name drugs have been accused of making special deals with generic drug manufacturers (such as paying them) to keep the low-priced generic drug off the market, thereby not competing with the branded drug. Another tactic used by drug companies to delay the entry of generic drugs is to sue the generic manufacturer for patent infringement by filing false secondary patents on new uses of the branded drug, thereby allowing the branded drugs months more of lucrative, exclusive sales. Drug companies have also sought to extend the patent life of their drug by making minor changes to the drug, thereby delaying entry of the generic copy. Congress

and the FDA are examining whether changes to the 1984 Hatch-Waxman Act are required to allow generic drugs to enter the market more quickly.

Lower Overseas Prices for Prescription Drugs: An Example of Price Discrimination

There are numerous anecdotes of people traveling to Canada or Mexico to buy a prescription drug at a much lower price than it can be purchased from a retail pharmacy in this country. In addition to anecdotal evidence, there have been several studies showing that branded prescription drugs are more expensive in the U.S. than in other countries. The Government Accounting Office concluded that U.S. prices were 32 percent higher than in Canada and 60 percent higher than in the U.K. Another study found that senior citizens in Maine pay an average retail price of $116.01 for Prilosec, while consumers in Canada and Mexico pay $53.05 and $29.46, respectively (9). See Figure 12-7.[7]

---

7. Typically, cross-national studies compare the retail prices of selected prescription drugs in the U.S. that are bought by cash-paying patients to the retail prices of those same drugs in another country. These comparisons greatly *overstate* U.S. drug prices since it is assumed that all purchasers of the prescription drug in the U.S. pay the same retail price. Although the retail prices of certain prescription drugs may be lower overseas than in the U.S., only a small percentage of the U.S. population pays retail prices for drugs. The majority of the U.S. population has some form of third-party payment for drugs, and these large purchasers buy their drugs at discounted prices. Further, patients with drug insurance pay a co-payment that is a small fraction of the price the organizations pay for the drug.

Cross-national studies have also excluded generic drugs (which are priced 40 to 80 percent lower than branded drugs), and U.S. purchasers rely much more on generic drugs than do patients in other countries. (Generics accounted for 46 percent of prescriptions in the U.S. in 1998 while use of generics in countries with strict drug price regulation, such as France and Italy, is very small.) Thus a comparison based solely on branded drugs overstates the cost of a prescription for U.S. patients.

Rather than assuming a single U.S. retail price, it would be more appropriate to compare prices paid, on average, for all those purchasing drugs in the U.S. (including both branded and generic drugs) to the prices paid by overseas patients. For a detailed discussion of cross-national comparisons, including limitations, see Patricia M. Danzon and Li-Wei Chao, "Cross-national price differences for pharmaceuticals: How large and why?," *Journal of Health Economics,* March 2000, 19(2): 159–195.

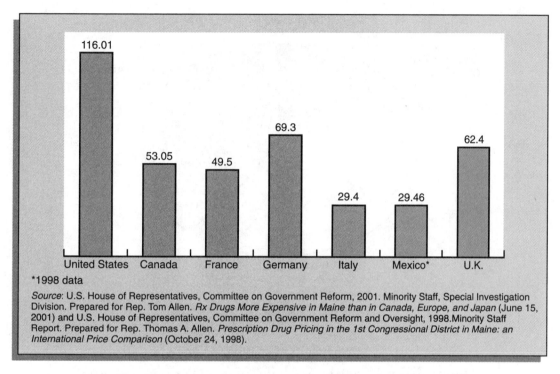

Figure 12-7.   Prices for PRILOSEC, United States, Canada, France, Germany, Italy, Mexico, and U.K., 2001.

Why would a manufacturer of a patented prescription drug be willing to sell the same drug at greatly reduced prices overseas?

The costs involved in developing and bringing to market an innovative new drug are very high. R & D for a prescription drug can cost as much as $700 million. Experimental trials must be conducted, and FDA approval is required. It may take 7 to 10 years to develop a new drug and receive FDA approval. R & D expenses and costs involved in receiving FDA approval are termed fixed costs. These development costs are the same regardless of how much of the patented new drug is produced and sold.

The actual costs of producing the new drug (variable costs), once its chemical entities have been determined through the R & D process and it has received FDA approval, are relatively small. Thus patented drugs are characterized by very large fixed costs and relatively small variable costs.

Although the drug manufacturer would like to receive the highest possible price for a new drug, the manufacturer would be willing to accept any price that exceeds its variable costs. A price in excess of variable costs makes a contribution to covering those large fixed costs and to profit. The manufacturer is better off receiving $5 even if it costs $4 to produce that drug. The $1 profit from some purchasers is better than nothing.

The drug manufacturer would like to add new users (sell the drug in different countries) since the variable costs of producing the drug are so low. But the drug manufacturer is not willing to add new users if it has to reduce the price and revenues it earns in its higher-priced markets. The single largest market for new innovative drugs is in the U.S., which accounts for 42 percent of the world pharmaceutical market. (See Figure 12-8.) People in the U.S. are, on average, wealthier than those in other countries, and they want

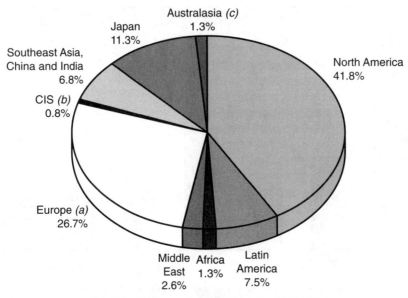

Australasia *(c)*
1.3%

Japan
11.3%

Southeast Asia,
China and India
6.8%

CIS *(b)*
0.8%

North America
41.8%

Europe *(a)*
26.7%

Middle
East
2.6%

Africa
1.3%

Latin
America
7.5%

Total World Pharmaceutical Market = $406 billion

(a) Europe includes Eastern Europe
(b) CIS - Commonwealth of Independent States (former Soviet Union)
(c) Australasia includes Australia, New Zealand, and Melanasia.

Source: IMS Health, 2003 [Online information], http://www.ims-global.com/insight/report.htm
(accessed on June 25, 2003.)

Figure 12-8. World pharmaceutical market, 2002.

access to innovative drugs as soon as possible. Therefore, they are less sensitive to high drug prices (about two-thirds of the U.S. population have insurance to pay for prescription drugs). It is not surprising that the drug manufacturer would charge higher prices when consumers are less price sensitive.

In countries that regulate drug prices, the same manufacturer is willing to sell that same drug at a lower price as long as the regulated price exceeds the manufacturer's variable cost.

An important condition for price discrimination, however, is that purchasers in the lower-priced countries cannot resell the drug in the higher-priced markets. If resale were possible, then a differential pricing system could not persist. As long as the manufacturer is able to prevent resale of the same drug from the low-priced to the high-priced country, then this sys-

tem of differential pricing allows markets to be served that would otherwise be neglected. Price discrimination results in the greatest number of people gaining access to that drug. The manufacturer is willing to reduce its price to countries that regulate drugs and to poor countries that cannot afford to pay much for drugs, not because the manufacturer has a social conscience, but because any sales at a price that exceeds the drug's variable cost contributes to profits.

PERFORMANCE

The performance of the pharmaceutical industry is affected both by the industry's behavior as well as government regulations directly or indirectly affecting the price and availability of new drugs.

Measurement of Industry Profitability

Published data on pharmaceutical industry profitability show that rates of return are much higher than other industries. Critics of the industry claim that these higher rates of return on equity (or assets) over long periods of time are evidence of monopoly power and that the industry should be subject to greater regulation, namely, policies to lower prices, require cross-licensing of patents, and a shorter patent life of new drugs. If implemented, each of these policies would decrease profitability. If, however, drug firm profitability has not been excessive, policies to decrease profitability in this industry would cause the rate of return to be below that earned in other industries; with a lower return on investment, there would be a consequent decline in research and development, hence drug innovation would fall.

Economists who have examined the method by which rates of return are calculated for the pharmaceutical industry have concluded that published profit data significantly *overstate* the true rate of profit earned by drug companies. When corrections are made to the published data, drug company rates of return are approximately comparable to those earned in other industries. (Although drug firms might have temporary monopoly power, it is eroded over time.)

To understand why economists believe drug industry rates of return are not excessive, it is necessary to examine how profits are calculated.

Accountants calculate profitability (R_{acc}) by subtracting all expenses (E) from sales revenue (S) and divide this by the firm's capital or the stockholders' equity (C).

$$R_{acc} = \frac{(S - E)}{C}$$

Net income ($S - E$) is the income remaining after all expenses and taxes have been paid. This accountant's definition of profitability is the method used to compare profitability between different industries. According to the definition above, advertising, research and development, and promotional expenses are all treated as current expenses; they are deducted from sales revenue in the year they are incurred.

Economists have argued that these expenditures are more than current expenses. They are, in fact, intangible capital since their effect continues beyond the year in which they are incurred. For example, research and development expenditures might not yield any benefit in the current year; but if a successful drug is developed, benefits will accrue in future years. It takes a number of years before a successful drug is finally marketed. The testing process to receive FDA approval alone takes many years. These expenditures are incurred so as to receive future benefits. A similar case can be made for advertising and other promotional expenditures, such as detail personnel; these expenditures increase revenues over long periods of time, their effects are longer lasting than for the year in which they were made. The average life of a new drug, including its R & D time may be 20 to 30 years.

The foregoing types of expenditures have an economic life greater than one year since they provide future benefits. They are a form of intangible capital of the firm and should therefore be depreciated rather than expensed all at once. The current years R & D do not yield revenues in the current year, but they represent an asset and should therefore be added to the asset base.

In accordance with conservative accounting principles, such expenditures are expensed since there is uncertainty as to future benefits they may provide and over how many years such future revenues may accrue. Therefore the most conservative approach is to assume that there are no benefits in future periods from these expenditures.

The economists' definition of profitability (R_{econ}) would treat these expenditures as intangible assets (A), thus a portion of these assets would be depreciated (D) each year (i.e., treated as an expense). The remainder (that is, the undepreciated portion of the asset) would then be added to the firm's capital or assets. Thus the economists' definition of profitability would be stated as follows:

$$R_{econ} = \frac{(S - E - D)}{C + (A - D)}$$

The effect of this change in the treatment of advertising, research and development, and promotional expenditures is to cause net income to be greater than it would otherwise be since only a part of the expenditure is deducted from sales revenue. However, the capital base of the firm is increased by the amount of the undepreciated asset. Under the accountants' definition of profitability (R_{acc}) the capital base is smaller than under the economists' definition of profitability (R_{econ}); the economist includes the undepreciated asset as part of capital while the accountant does not. Therefore the accountants' definition will show a higher rate of profitability than would the economists.'

Using data from a large pharmaceutical firm, Clarkson determined that the average accounting rate of return on book equity over the period 1980 to 1993 was 27.5 percent. After correcting accounting income for the expensing of investment outlays and recalculating the firm's equity for the omission of intangible assets (expenditures on R & D and promotion), the return on equity declined to 14.3 percent (10).

Accounting definitions of profitability are used by all industries. The pharmaceutical industry, however, is more affected by this definition of profit than any other industry. Expenditures for intangible capital, research and development, advertising, and other promotional expenditures are greater in the drug industry than for any other industry. It is still possible that after similarly correcting rates of return for other industries, drug firms would still have a higher rate of return. Thus another reason for increased returns in the drug industry is the greater risks in returns. In competitive markets, the rate of return would move toward the opportunity cost of capital adjusted for risk. Industries with less predictable returns on their investment require a greater risk premium to attract investors; the drug industry is considered to have higher risk returns than industries that explore for natural resources, such as oil companies.

Published data on drug industry profits, based on the accounting rate of return, showing continued high rates of profitability, have been one of the reasons for proposals to change the structure of the industry. It would be unfortunate, not only for the drug firms, but for consumers of drugs as well, if public policies to reduce industry profitability were based on misleading profitability data.

Prices, Expenditures, and Industry Profitability

The pharmaceutical industry is characterized by high price mark-ups (over production costs) on branded drugs, rapidly rising drug expenditures, large expenditures on marketing, relative high profitability, and research and development investments that are among the highest of all industries.

The pharmaceutical market has become more price competitive over time. Although drug companies continue to spend large sums to market their branded drugs to physicians and to patients (direct-to-consumer advertising), legislation to speed the entry of generics and the rise of managed care have changed competition in the drug industry. Managed care companies and PBMs are informed purchasers. Thus, to market to these organizations and to have their branded drug included in their drug formularies, drug manufacturers have to demonstrate that their drugs are cost-effective. The rapid introduction of lower-priced generic substitutes when patents on branded drugs expire has resulted in generics quickly increasing their market share, thereby increasing the drug's availability and reducing the purchaser's financial burden.

Of continuing concern about the industry's performance are the high price mark-ups and rapidly rising drug expenditures.

Patent protection provides branded drugs with monopoly power. However, unless a new drug was an improvement over existing drugs, the new drug could not be priced higher than existing drugs. The willingness of managed care organizations to pay a high price (relative to cost) for a new drug is an indication that the new drug represents a significant improvement over alternative treatment methods. Under managed care, *high drug prices reflect greater drug benefits.*

Rising drug expenditures should be viewed with favor. Higher prices for new drugs likely indicate new and improved drugs. And with a greater number of prescriptions per person, particularly for the aged, chronic diseases can be better managed, there is less need for expensive surgery, patients can live longer, and their quality of life can be improved.

It is important to the performance of the drug industry that there are informed purchasers who are able to evaluate the cost-effectiveness of new drugs, as well as financial incentives (patent protection) to develop new drugs that patients (or purchasers on their behalf) are willing to buy. It is also important that, once the patent on a branded drug has expired, generics are able to quickly enter the market.

Profitability of pharmaceutical firms over time has generally been higher than any other industry. Although profits are high, so are the risks since the cost of developing a new drug and bringing it to market have been estimated to be at least $300 million and as high as $800 million. Drug development is a very risky business; only a small percentage of drugs make it through all the clinical phases and become financially viable.

The high rates of profit earned by drug manufacturers to finance R & D result from the few breakthrough drugs that are discovered. Even those that are marketed may not be financially successful; about three out of ten drugs that are marketed make a profit, and about 10 percent of all drugs that are marketed provide 55 percent of the industry's profits. Figure 12-9 describes the percentage of drugs whose profits exceed average R & D costs. As can be seen, the distribution of profits is very skewed. Very few drugs offer a profitable return, but for the 10 percent of drugs that are considered to be "blockbuster" drugs, the profits are substantial. Thus, a drug company needs a few "winners," especially "blockbusters," to repay the costs on the majority of drugs that do not even repay their R & D investments.

High price mark-ups on branded drugs, large expenditures on drug marketing, and high profitability have led some industry critics to advocate price controls on branded drugs. These regulatory policies (discussed below), if enacted, will affect drug manufacturers' financial incentives and, consequently, the development of new innovative drugs.

The pharmaceutical industry's performance should not be evaluated solely in terms of its market

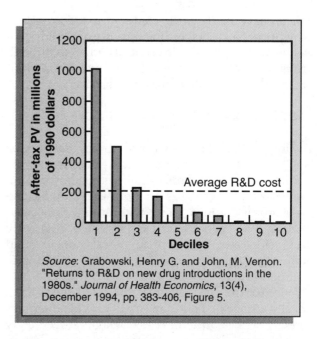

Figure 12-9.   Decile distribution of present values of post-launch returns for the sample of 1980–84 NCEs.

power, high price mark-ups, ability to engage in price discrimination, and profitability (all of which are indicative of market power). Instead, this industry's performance is more appropriately judged according to the rate of discovery of innovative new drugs and whether price competition is able to occur within therapeutic classes by substitute branded drugs and by generics after the patent has expired.

Government Regulation Affecting Industry Performance

Essential to this industry's performance are its financial incentives to invest in research and development. The industry's incentives have been greatly affected by government policies regarding the safety and efficacy requirements (hence development time and cost) before the FDA approves a new drug. Government policies have also been directed at measures to reduce drug prices (such as speeding up entry of generics), as well as proposals for price controls on breakthrough drugs which, if enacted, will have a major impact on the industry's incentives for drug discovery.

Price Controls on Prescription Drugs

The implication of cross-national studies that find the U.S. has higher prescription drug prices is that the U.S. should institute a price-control system, similar to countries that have lower drug prices. By publicizing these study findings, along with examples of aged persons who cannot afford to pay these high retail drug prices, advocates of price controls hope to build political support for imposing controls on U.S. prescription drugs.

Price controls on new breakthrough drugs are politically attractive. Politicians try to provide their constituents with short-term visible benefits at seemingly no cost. Since the costs of research and development have already been incurred, the only cost of producing an existing drug is its relatively small variable costs. As long as the regulated drug price is greater than the drug's variable costs, the firm will continue selling the drug. Profits from that drug will be lower, but the drug firm will make more money by continuing to sell the drug (even at the regulated price) than by not selling it.

Price controls would not decrease access to innovative drugs *currently* on the market or even to those that are in the drug approval process. *There would seemingly be no adverse effect of imposing price controls.* Patients who cannot afford expensive drugs would benefit, as would states with rapidly increasing Medicaid expenditures. Both patients and state Medicaid programs are likely to favor legislation to reduce drug prices. The only apparent loser would be drug companies.

The real concern with price controls is not their effects on current drugs, but on R & D for future drugs. Price controls reduce profitability of new, innovative drugs. With lower expected profits, drug companies would be less willing to risk hundreds of millions of dollars on R & D. Most new drugs (about 70 to 80 per-

cent) are not therapeutic breakthroughs and do not recoup their R & D investment. Although their price may exceed their variable costs, the drugs do not generate sufficient profit to cover their R & D costs; thus the drug company loses money on these drugs. The small percentage of drugs that are considered "blockbuster" drugs have high price mark-ups over their variable costs and generate most of the profit. The drugs that would be targeted by price controls would be these breakthrough drugs whose price is relatively high.

With fewer breakthrough drugs, treating disease will be more costly; these drugs might make surgical intervention unnecessary and can even prevent a disease from occurring. It is through R & D and the development of new drugs that the total cost of medical treatment is lowered. With price controls, R & D investments would decline. For example, if Medicare provided a new prescription drug benefit to the elderly and relied on price controls to reduce government expenditures, drug companies would reallocate their R & D away from diseases affecting the elderly (where price controls limit profits) toward diseases affecting other population groups where profits are not limited.

Price controls on drugs will not necessarily reduce drug expenditures. Drug expenditures represent a *higher* portion of total medical expenditures in countries that regulate drug prices than in the U.S. See Figure 12-10. Drug prices in price-controlled countries are quite low (generally for older molecules), and neither patients nor their physicians have an incentive to use fewer drugs. For example, to reduce drug expenditures, the German government in recent years imposed financial penalties on physicians to limit their prescribing too many drugs. The U.S. spends a smaller portion on drugs (12.4 percent) than Germany (14.3 percent), France (21.0 percent), or Canada (16.2 percent).

Examples of Price Controls on Prescription Drugs

The federal government requires drug manufacturers to sell their drugs to the government at the "best"

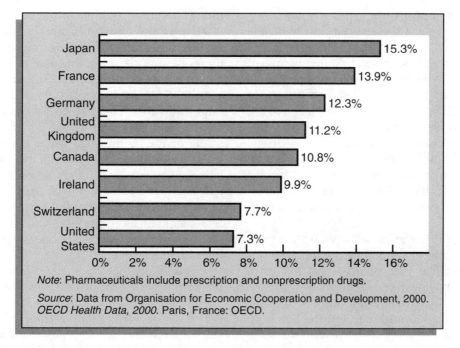

Figure 12-10. Pharmaceutical expenditures as a percentage of total health expenditures, selected countries, 2001.

price. In the 1980s, as a result of price competition among drug companies to have their drugs selected for inclusion in the drug formularies of HMOs and Group Purchasing Organizations (GPOs), drug manufacturers had been giving large price discounts to certain HMOs and GPOs. In 1990, the federal government, in an attempt to reduce Medicaid expenditures, enacted a law that required drug manufacturers to give state Medicaid programs the same discounts they gave to their best customers. Consequently, drug companies gave smaller discounts to these HMOs and GPOs. A study by the Congressional Budget Office (CBO) found that the best (lowest) price discount given to HMOs and GPOs declined from 24 percent and 28 percent in 1991 to 14 percent and 15 percent, respectively, which was the minimum amount required by the government, by 1994 (11).

The CBO concluded that drug companies were much less willing to give steep discounts to large purchasers when they had to give the same discounts to Medicaid. Drug prices and expenditures increased for many private buyers.

To reduce the cost of drugs in their state Medicaid programs, several states are attempting to receive greater price discounts than the minimum mandated by the federal government. Maine, for example, enacted a law in May 2000 that authorizes the state to negotiate deep price discounts with drug manufacturers for the 325,000 state residents without prescription drug coverage. If the drug manufacturer does not agree to offer a discount for a specific drug, Maine could require prior authorization before the drug could be dispensed in the Medicaid program (thereby sharply limiting its use).

Maine does not appear to be willing to shift volume to only one drug in a therapeutic class, which is the way HMOs and GPOs negotiated price discounts for their drug formularies. Instead, Maine wants all prescription drugs to be discounted. Drug companies that have branded drugs with no close substitutes are less likely to be willing to give deep discounts and are therefore likely to be excluded from the state's formulary in favor of less expensive, less effective drugs. In Medicaid programs that have excluded expensive innovative drugs from their formulary, the lack of access to these drugs has led to an increase in hospitalizations, the costs of which exceeded any savings in drug costs (12).

Re-Importation of Prescription Drugs: One regulatory approach to reducing U.S. retail prices for prescription drugs is to allow U.S. pharmacists and drug wholesalers to buy lower-priced supplies of FDA-approved medicines in Canada and other nations for resale in the U.S. Drugs re-imported into the U.S. from Canada would likely be less expensive than the same drugs sold in the U.S. because of Canadian price controls on those drugs. The presumed effect of this policy would be to reduce the U.S. retail price of drugs to prices comparable in other countries from which they are re-imported.

A federal law permitting licensed pharmacists and drug distributors to re-import prescription drugs was enacted in October 2000. This law overturned a 1988 law that permitted only pharmaceutical manufacturers to re-import prescription drugs, based on the concern that drugs were being improperly stored and repackaged overseas. Although re-importation was vigorously opposed by the pharmaceutical industry, senators and congressional candidates from both political parties running for re-election during Fall 2000 voted for the bill, which was then signed into law by President Clinton. Legislators running for re-election believed that voting for re-importation would be viewed by the public as being in favor of helping the aged with their prescription drug costs.

The re-importation law required the Secretary of Health and Human Services to certify that the re-imported drugs would be safe and save consumers money before it could be implemented. In December 2000, after the election, Donna Shalala, Secretary of Health and Human Services, refused to implement the new law, claiming that it was unworkable and would not lower drug costs (13). At the time of the debate, the FDA said that it could oversee the drug re-importation system, but only at considerable cost. Unless funding was provided ($93 million a year), the safety of the re-imported drugs could not be monitored. The full funding was not included in the legislation. Further, the Administration believed that the bill had several fatal flaws that would deter re-importation, namely, that the drug companies would retaliate against re-importers and would not provide the re-importers with the necessary package labeling inserts.

It is unlikely that a U.S. manufacturer of a branded prescription drug would increase its sales to a country that then resells that drug in the U.S. It would be very easy for a drug manufacturer to monitor its drug sales to each country to determine whether sales of a particular drug have suddenly increased. (If the drug importer in a country resells the country's limited supply of that drug back to the U.S., then patients in that country are harmed by not having access to that drug.) Thus to be able to re-import drugs into the U.S., U.S. pharmacists and wholesalers would have to buy those chemical entities from a foreign producer of those drugs.

When a drug is manufactured in the U.S., the manufacturer must adhere to strict FDA guidelines to ensure that the drug is produced with certain quality standards. If the drug were to be manufactured in another country without extensive monitoring of the re-imported drug by the FDA, there is no guarantee that the drug meets the same quality standards. The concern over drug safety resulted in eleven former FDA commissioners opposing the re-importation bill.

Thousands of illegal shipments of prescription drugs have been entering the U.S. each month through the postal service. This growth in overseas sales to U.S. patients has dramatically increased because of the Internet. The sheer volume of such overseas drug shipments has overwhelmed the FDA and custom officials in their ability to verify the safety of the imported drugs. Finally, on June 7, 2001, the FDA proposed stopping overseas drug products mailed from overseas to individuals unless they met certain strict conditions. The FDA claims that these drug products may be counterfeit or even dangerous and that the volume is so large that they no longer have the ability to inspect them.

Re-importation is unlikely to be effective in reducing U.S. prescription drug prices for several reasons. First, U.S. drug manufacturers will be unwilling to sell large quantities of their drugs at greatly reduced prices to other countries so that these countries can then sell the same drugs back to U.S. pharmacists at lower prices. Price discrimination can no longer be profitable if high-priced and low-priced markets cannot be kept separate. Second, if foreign drug manufacturers are permitted to produce the same drug that is patented by the U.S. drug manufacturer and sell that drug to customers in the U.S., then those foreign producers would be violating U.S. patent laws, and the imports would be prohibited. Lastly, the FDA has decided to restrict overseas mail order sales to U.S. patients for safety reasons.

A Single Price For Prescription Drugs Across Countries: Another approach favored by proponents of price controls is having the U.S. government require that the retail price of prescription drugs sold in the U.S. be no different than the price at which those same drugs are sold in other countries, such as Canada and Mexico.

Proponents of this approach assume that the uniform price will be the lower of the different prices for that same drug. Assume that a prescription drug, ABC, sells for $10 in the U.S. and for $5 in Canada. Further assume that the U.S. enacts a law stating that the manufacturer of drug ABC must charge the same price, regardless of the country in which the drug is sold. Would the price of drug ABC be reduced to $5 and U.S. consumers receive a $5 benefit? The answer is "No."

The manufacturer of drug ABC would have to determine which single price would result in the greatest amount of profit. Since the U.S. is the largest single market for innovative branded drugs and its consumers are less price sensitive, greatly reducing the drug's price in the U.S. market would not result in

a large increase in the number of users of that drug. Consequently, a large decrease in price (without a corresponding large increase in volume) would cause a large decrease in revenue. Given the large profits earned in the U.S. (the price mark-up over variable cost in the U.S. multiplied by the large number of users), it is likely that the uniform price of the drug will be closer to the U.S. price than the lower prices paid in other countries. The drug company will lose less money if it raises the prices in other countries by a greater amount than it lowers the U.S. price.

Keeping the uniform price closer to the U.S. price for that drug means that the new uniform price of the drug will be increased in other countries. Raising the price in these countries is likely to cause a decrease in use. These countries typically have limited government budgets for healthcare, and a large increase in the price of drugs is likely to cause the government to restrict their use. Overseas patients who need that drug will be worse off. Whereas formerly they (or the government on their behalf) paid $5, they would now have to pay a higher price. Some patients would no longer have access to the drug. If close substitute drugs are available, they will buy these other drugs (assuming the price of these other drugs has not also been similarly increased). If close substitutes are not available on innovative drugs, then patients/government will have to spend more of their income on this drug.

If patients cannot afford to buy the drug or their government restricts its use because of its higher price, there will be adverse health consequences. Requiring a uniform pricing policy in the U.S. and in other countries is likely to lead to a small reduction in the U.S. price of that drug and an increase in the drug's overseas price so that it is equal to the new U.S. price. This policy would inflict a tragic loss on patients in other countries who would have to go without innovative drugs.

Government Regulation of the Safety and Efficacy of New Drugs

The FDA attempts to achieve a balance between the concerns of drug safety and the prospective benefits of pharmaceutical innovation. Ensuring that a new drug does not harm anyone delays the introduction of a beneficial drug that may save many lives. Regulatory delay increases the time and cost of bringing a new drug to market. Thus excessive caution or expediency incurs risks. This delay may result in the deaths of thousands of people whose lives could have been saved had the new drug been approved much earlier. Similarly, introducing potential breakthrough drugs immediately may cause the deaths of many since the full effects of the new drug are not completely understood.

How should this trade-off in lives be evaluated? Is each type of life—those potentially saved from early introduction of a new drug (statistical lives) versus those who might die from early approval (visible deaths)—valued equally?[8]

---

8. (Statistical deaths are calculated as follows: Assume that a new drug is introduced in Europe and that there is a two-year lag before that same drug receives FDA approval to be marketed in the U.S. Further assume that the new drug is more effective than the drug currently on the market treating that same disease, such that it is able to decrease mortality from 5 percent to 1 percent. Suppose that 100,000 persons each year are affected by that illness. The number of lives that would have been saved by earlier FDA approval is 8,000. The percent difference in mortality rate [0.05–0.01 = 0.04], multiplied by the 2-year lag when the drug could have been on the market [0.04 x 2 = 0.08], multiplied by the number of people at risk each year [0.08 multiplied by 100,000] equals 8,000 statistical deaths due to the two-year delay.)

Those who die because a drug that could save their lives has not yet received FDA approval (even though it may be available in Europe) are not as visible or identifiable as those who die because they used a new drug. Yet, statistical deaths due to drug lag (particularly the early beta blockers to prevent heart attacks) number in the tens of thousands and have greatly outweighed the number of victims of all drug tragedies prior to the 1962 Amendments (including those deaths caused by Elixir Sulfanilamide in the 1930s).

The FDA's incentives are clearly to minimize the loss of identifiable lives at the expense of a greater loss of statistical lives. The political pressure on FDA staff to justify their decision will cause them to be overly cautious in approving new drugs until they can be sure there will be minimal loss of life.

The two main criticisms of FDA regulation are the long delays before new drugs are approved once their data is submitted to the FDA (currently about 18 months) and the increasing research and development cost imposed on drug companies for bringing a new drug to market.

Increased Cost of Drug Development: Stringent FDA guidelines and long approval times have greatly increased the cost of developing new drugs. After the enactment of the 1962 Drug Amendments requiring more stringent clinical testing requirements and use of the efficacy as well as the safety criteria for FDA approval, the cost and time for bringing a new drug to market increased sharply. The median time that it takes for a new drug to go from the start of clinical testing to receiving FDA approval has increased from 4.7 years on average during the 1960s (after the 1962 Drug Amendments) to about 12 years (2001).

A recent study estimated that the average (pre-approval) cost of developing a new drug was $802 million (14). An important reason for the rapidly increasing cost of drug development is the cost of human trials. The typical clinical trial involves 4,000 people currently, compared with 1,300 in the 1980s.

Included in the cost of drug development are actual expenditures, as well as the opportunity cost of the interest foregone on these investment costs. For example, only $403 million of the estimated $802 million are actual out-of-pocket costs. The rest is the estimated cost of capital, or the amount that investing the money at an 11 percent rate of return would have earned over time. This opportunity cost of capital is significant since there are long time lags between investment expenditures and revenues generated by the new drug.

These investment costs include expenditures on many drugs that never make it to market (failures). Of every 5,000 potential new drugs tested in animals, only five are likely to reach human clinical trials, and of those five only one will eventually be marketed.

Also important to a drug firm's profitability is that the longer it takes to achieve the FDA's stringent research guidelines and receive FDA approval, the shorter is the remaining patent life on the drug and the period to make profits.

Since profit is the motivating factor behind drug companies' willingness to assume risk and invest large amounts in R & D, the larger the R & D cost, the lower the potential profit.

The U.S. Drug Lag: One measure of the FDA's performance is how long it takes to approve a drug here compared to other countries. After the 1962 Drug Amendments were enacted, a long time lag developed between when drugs were available for use in other countries and when they could be used in the U.S. For example, drugs proven effective for the treatment of heart disease and hypertension were used in Great Britain as early as 1965, but it was 1976 before they were fully approved for use in the United States.

Criticism of the FDA's slow approval process has come from two groups: drug firms that would like to start earning revenues sooner and organized patient groups, such as those with AIDs, that want quicker access to possible life-saving drugs.

Early studies looking at data through the 1970s concluded that there was a drug lag. Researchers compared drugs approved in the United Kingdom (U.K.) and the U.S. and concluded that drugs approved in the U.S. lagged behind those approved in the U.K. by about 2 years. However, in more recent years it appears that the U.S. drug lag has disappeared.

Orphan Drugs: As R & D costs and drug approval time have increased, it became unprofitable for drug companies to undertake long and costly clinical trials to develop "orphan" drugs, i.e., drugs that benefit small population groups. The potential revenue for a new drug may be small because few people are affected with a particular disease or a small percentage of those afflicted do not respond to the standard treatment. With rising R & D costs, it is not profitable for drug companies to target these small therapeutic markets. Market size (potential revenue) is an important determinant of drug development. Congress enacted the Orphan Drug Act in 1984 to provide drug companies with a financial incentive (tax incentives and/or exclusive marketing rights) to develop drugs

providing therapeutic benefits affecting fewer than 200,000 patients.

Similar to the orphan drug issue is the concern that drug development is targeted toward people living in wealthy countries. Only 5 percent of global R & D is directed at health problems unique to developing nations, even though 90 percent of the global disease burden is in the developing world. Private sector R & D is determined by prospective demand conditions. For example, malaria is a parasitic disease having a global incidence of 200 to 300 million cases annually. There are approximately 856,000 deaths each year due to malaria, and the majority of these deaths are children under 5 years of age living in sub-Saharan Africa. Drug development aimed at health problems confronting people in poor countries will need to be subsidized from government sources, as are orphan drugs.

Public policy with respect to the drug industry must deal with the following trade-off. To increase R & D investments, drug manufacturers must earn high profits on innovative drugs that provide significant increases in therapeutic value. However, the variable cost of producing these drugs is but a small fraction of their selling price. If prices on these breakthrough drugs were made more affordable through price controls (closer to their production costs) so as not to be a large burden on those with low incomes, the high profits that provide the incentive to invest in R & D would disappear. Lower drug prices that benefit today's patients mean fewer innovative drugs in the future.

SUMMARY

Prescription drug expenditures will continue to increase, both because of increased use of drugs (particularly among the increasing number of aged) and the introduction of newer, higher-priced drugs. A new Medicare prescription drug benefit will be an additional stimulus to sharply increasing drug expenditures. Prices of new drugs have a very high mark-up in relation to their cost of production. To those without drug coverage and to large purchasers of drugs, such as HMOs and state Medicaid agencies, these facts are a cause for concern.

However, the public should view rising drug expenditures and even high price mark-ups favorably. New drugs reduce non-pharmaceutical medical costs. For example, new antidepressants have reduced the need for costly psychotherapy, and beta blockers and blood pressure drugs have reduced the costs of cardiovascular-related hospital admissions and surgeries. Further, when new drugs replace older drugs, purchasers value the greater therapeutic benefits of the newer drugs more and are willing to pay higher prices for their increased value. Consumers are clearly better off. A recent study concluded that the replacement of older by newer drugs results in reductions in mortality, lower morbidity, as indicated by fewer days lost from work, and reduced total treatment costs, particularly for inpatient care. The use of new drugs results in large hospital savings because of reductions in lengths of stay and in the number of hospital admissions. The total reduction in non-drug medical expenses is about four times the increase in the costs of drugs (15).

Rising drug prices are often an indication that new drugs are more effective than existing drugs (or alternative treatments). (When new drugs are of higher quality, i.e., provide greater benefits, than the drugs they replace, then the "quality-adjusted" price of these drugs may well be lower than the price of older drugs. Thus counting the higher prices of new drugs as mere price increases is misleading.) The replacement of older drugs by newer drugs is the most important reason for the increase in drug expenditures.

Drug manufacturers charge different prices to different buyers for the same drug (price discrimination) so as to give price discounts to those purchasers willing to shift their drug purchases; those who are less price sensitive are charged higher prices.

The cost-containment strategies of health plans and PBMs have caused drug firms to emphasize the cost-effectiveness of their drugs and to compete on price to have their drugs included in insurers' formularies. Drug firms have also started direct-to-consumer advertising to develop consumer pressure to demand the drug from their physician. To limit the effect of such tactics, health plans have instituted three-tiered co-payment systems that give consumers incentives to use drugs on the health plan's formulary.

The pharmaceutical market is becoming more competitive with the growth of managed care companies and changes in regulations permitting earlier approval of generic substitutes (16).

The rationale for FDA regulation of drugs is presumably to provide a remedy for the lack of information that exists among both physicians and consumers when buying drugs. Lack of information on a drug's safety could cause serious harm to patients. Given this serious information problem, what should be the role of the FDA? Should the FDA continue to be the sole decision-maker on the availability of new drugs? Or should the FDA play a more passive role by merely providing information on the safety and efficacy of new drugs and then leaving it up to the physician and/or patient to decide whether to use a new drug?

There is a trade-off between ensuring safety and efficacy of new drugs with consequent higher development costs and longer approval times versus having a greater number of innovative drugs more quickly available that might save many lives, but with a greater possible risk to the patient.

The "costs" of delay vary depending upon the seriousness of the illness. Even for the same disease, two patients will differ on the two types of risks they are willing to accept. Under the current system, the FDA is determining the level of risk acceptable to society while some patients would be willing to go below that level. Who should make this decision?

Various proposals have been made to speed up the FDA's review process for drug approval, such as having the FDA also rely on evidence gathered from other countries that have high approval standards, dropping the proof of efficacy requirement, and also having the FDA rely on less evidence of a drug's safety for those drugs that are life saving where no alternative therapy is available.

Speeding up the FDA's approval process will require greater post-marketing surveillance of drug interactions and safety; physicians are alerted to watch for harmful side-effects. Evidence of the effects of a new drug may not be known for several years. The long pre-approval process continues to miss dangerous drugs. Only after a drug has been on the market and is used by large numbers of people can its safety and efficacy be truly evaluated.

In addition to speeding up the FDA's approval process and expanding post-market surveillance of new drugs, there is a concern with the time and cost required to bring a new drug to market.

High R & D costs (just like longer times for approval that shorten patent life) decrease the profitability of an investment in new drugs. Decreased profitability leading to a lower investment results in fewer new drugs being discovered. As the costs of drug discovery are increased, drug companies are less likely to develop drugs that have small market potential.

An additional consequence of the high cost and long time requirements to introduce a new drug is that with fewer new drugs being introduced, drug prices are higher than if there were more competition.

Economics is concerned with trade-offs. Choosing one policy, namely increased drug safety and efficacy, has a "cost," namely fewer new drugs will be developed. There will be a greater number of statistical deaths, the drug industry will become more consolidated, and drug prices will be higher since there are fewer new drugs to compete with existing drugs. Thus merely favoring increased drug safety and efficacy is not a simple choice without consequences. The issue is how to strike an appropriate balance between these choices.

Any public policy should consider its effect on R & D expenditures. The incentive for drug manufacturers to invest large sums in R & D and develop breakthrough drugs is based on the prospect of earning large profits. Once a drug has been discovered and approved by the FDA for marketing, the actual cost of producing that drug is very low. Therefore, it is not surprising that countries can regulate the price of drugs and still have access to U.S. drugs. However, if the U.S. were to regulate its drug prices as do other countries or permit re-importation by foreign drug producers, then R & D investment would decline, as would the supply of innovative drugs.

An alternative approach to solving the concern over high drug prices and rising expenditures through price controls is a policy that subsidizes the purchase of drugs for those with low incomes and/or catastrophic drug expenditures. Their health plan or a pharmacy benefit manager will then negotiate lower drug prices from the drug manufacturer, substitute generic drugs when appropriate, and manage the drug benefit to reduce the total cost of drug therapy. Those with low incomes will have access to needed drugs, and competition will reduce prescription drug prices.

In coming years there is likely to be enormous scientific progress. The mapping of the human genome and advances in molecular biology are expected to lead to drug solutions for many diseases. It is also likely that drug prices and expenditures will be higher to reflect the increased willingness of people to pay for these new discoveries. It would be unfortunate if the desire to reduce the cost of drugs through price controls decreased the availability of breakthrough drugs. Given the trade-off between regulation to reduce the cost of drugs or having innovative drugs to cure disease, reduce mortality, and reduce the cost of medical treatment, it is likely society would choose the full benefits that scientific discovery can offer.

REVIEW QUESTIONS

1. Which factors have contributed most to the sharp increase in drug expenditures?
2. Are rising drug expenditures necessarily bad?
3. Is the high price of drugs determined by the high cost of developing a new drug?
4. Why do drug manufacturers charge different purchasers different prices for the same prescription drug?
5. What methods have managed care plans used to limit their enrollees' drug costs?

6. How have the 1962 Drug Amendments affected the profitability of new drugs?
7. What is the consequence of the FDA providing the public with greater assurance that a new drug is safe?
8. What are "orphan" drugs and why are drug firms less likely to develop such drugs today?
9. Why would a policy of re-importation of prescription drugs be ineffective?
10. Why are price controls on prescription drugs politically attractive?

REFERENCES

1. For excellent discussions of the pharmaceutical industry, see F.M. Scherer, "The Pharmaceutical Industry" in *Handbook of Health Economics*, Vol. 1, ed. A. J. Culyer and J. P. Newhouse, (Elsevier Science: New York), 2000 and Stuart O. Schweitzer, *Pharmaceutical Economics and Policy*, (Oxford University Press: New York), 1997.
2. For a history of the 1962 FDA Amendments, see Richard Harris, *The Real Voice*, (New York: Macmillan Company, 1964). Also see, Peter Temin, *Taking Your Medicine: Drug Regulation in the United States*, (Cambridge, MA: Harvard University Press, 1980).
3. Once a new drug is approved by the FDA as being safe and efficacious for its intended use, the new drug must also pass the health plan's review process, which determines whether the drug is also cost-effective. Unless the drug can also pass this review, the new drug may not be added to the health plan's drug formulary.
4. Olson describes why, after several years of failure, the 1984 drug legislation was ultimately enacted. His analysis includes the proposals of different interest groups and turnover in key Senate committees, as well as a change in the majority party. Mark K. Olson, "Political Influence and Regulatory Policy: The 1984 Drug Legislation," *Economic Inquiry*, 32(3), July 1994.
5. In 1994 new federal legislation (the Uruguay Round Agreements Act) changed the patent life of prescription drugs (and all types of inventions) from 17 years from the date a patent is granted to 20 years from the date the application is filed. It takes 2 to 3 years from the time an application is filed until a patent is granted. The average period of time that a new drug can be marketed under patent protection has risen from about 9 years to about 11.5 years.
6. J. L. Lu and W. Comanor, "Strategic Pricing of New Pharmaceuticals," *Review of Economics and Statistics*, 80(1), February 1998, 108–118.
7. Richard G. Frank, "Prescription Drug Prices: Why Do Some Pay More Than Others Do?," *Health Affairs*, 20(2), March/April 2001, 115–128.
8. Ronald J. Vogel, Sulabha Ramachandran, and Woodie Zachry, "A 3 Stage Model for Assessing the Probable Economic Effects of Direct To Consumer Advertising of Pharmaceuticals," *Clinical Therapeutics*, January 2003, 25(1) 309–329.
9. U.S. General Accounting Office, *Prescription Drugs: Companies typically charge more in the United States than in Canada*, 1992, GAO/HRD 92-110. U.S. General Accounting Office, *Prescription Drugs: Companies typically charge more in the United States than in the United Kingdom*, 1994, GAO/HEHS 94-29. Also see U.S. House of Representatives, Committee on Government Reform and Oversight, 1998. Minority Staff Report. Prepared for Rep. Thomas A. Allen. *Prescription Drug Pricing in the 1st Congressional District in Maine: An International Price Comparison*, (October 24, 1998).
10. Kenneth W. Clarkson, "The Effects of Research and Promotion on Rates of Return," in Robert B. Helms, ed., *Competitive Strategies in the Pharmaceutical Industry*, (American Enterprise Institute Press: Washington, D.C.) 1996, pp. 238–268.
11. Congressional Budget Office, *How the Medicaid Rebate on Prescription Drugs Affects Pricing in the Pharmaceutical Industry*, (U.S. Government Printing Office: Washington, D.C.) 1996.
12. Stephan Soumerai, et al., "Effects of Medicaid Drug-Payment Limits on Admissions to Hospitals and Nursing Homes," *New England Journal of Medicine*, 325 (15), October 10, 1991, 1072–1077.
13. "Shalala Halts Bid To Lower Drug Costs," *The Washington Post*, December 27, 2000, p. A1.
14. Joseph A. DiMasi, Ronald Hansen, and Henry Grabowski, "The Price of Innovation: New Estimates of Drug Development Costs," *Journal of Health Economics*, 22(2), March 2003, 151–185.
15. Frank R. Lichtenberg, "The Benefits and Costs of Newer Drugs: Evidence from the 1996 Medical Expenditure Panel Survey," NBER Working Paper No. 8147,

(National Bureau of Economic Research: Cambridge, Mass.), March 2001.

16. Congressional Budget Office, *How Increased Competition from Generic Drugs Has Affected Prices and Returns in the Pharmaceutical Industry*, (U.S. Government printing Office: Washington, D.C.) July 1998.

CHAPTER

13

Health Manpower Shortages and Surpluses: Definitions, Measurement, and Policies

KEY TERMS AND CONCEPTS

- Applicant/acceptance ratio
- Derived demand
- Physician/population ratio
- Definition of a health manpower surplus
- Economic definition of a shortage
- Normative judgment of a shortage
- Professional determination of shortages and surpluses
- Rate of return to a professional education
- Static and dynamic shortages

Learning Objectives

Upon completing this chapter, the reader should be able to:

- Explain the differences between an economic and non-economic definition of a shortage.
- Distinguish between a dynamic and a static shortage.
- Define an economic definition of a health manpower surplus.
- Critique the use of health manpower ratios for measuring a shortage and/or a surplus.
- Explain, based on empirical evidence, whether there has been a surplus or shortage of physicians.
- Evaluate alternative proposed public policies for alleviating health manpower shortages or surpluses.

HEALTH MANPOWER MARKET PERFORMANCE

Within the context of the overall market for medical care, the various categories of health manpower comprise separate sub-markets. The health manpower professions are thus an *input* to the provision of medical services. In Chapter 3 it was shown that the overall market for medical care consists of a set of institutional markets, a set of health manpower markets, and a set of markets in which the demand and supply of health manpower education occurs. With a change in the demand for medical care, perhaps resulting from an increase in the population with insurance coverage, there will be increases in demand for the institutional settings in which medical care is provided and, subsequently, an increase in demand by the different institutional settings for inputs used in the production of their services.

The demand for the different health manpower professions is, therefore, a *derived* demand, derived from the demand for medical and institutional services. These demands by the various institutions for different types of health manpower, together with the existing stock of trained health manpower, will determine the wages, the number of persons employed, and their participation rate (the percent of the available stock of each health manpower profession that is employed). The health education institutions determine the long-run supply or stock of health manpower in each profession. (Immigration laws that affect entry by foreign trained health professionals also affect the long-run supply.)

How well the different health manpower and education markets perform has an effect not only on the wages and number of health professionals, but also on the price and quantity of medical and institutional services. Since the various sub-markets are interrelated and feed into the market for medical services, the efficiency with which the health manpower market performs will affect prices and outputs in each of the other markets; the more efficient a market is, the greater will be its output. Thus an important reason for examining the separate health manpower markets for different categories of health professionals is to determine how well each market performs. If the markets are determined not to perform well, alternative approaches for improving their performance will be examined, giving due consideration to the reasons for inadequate performance.

The market for health professional *education* will also be examined to determine whether it is performing efficiently—that is, whether the quantity of health professional education has been "optimal" over different time periods and whether health education is being produced efficiently. The market for health professional education is important not only because it determines the long-run supply of health manpower, but also because it has been the recipient of a great deal of federal and state funding. Examples of federal and state health manpower legislation will be analyzed to determine both its purpose and how effective it has been in achieving its stated goals.

In addition to analyzing the efficiency, performance, and public policies of the separate health manpower and health professional education markets, alternative approaches for forecasting health manpower "requirements" will be examined. Historically, the physician and registered nurse markets have changed from one of "shortages" to "surplus" and back to a "shortage." These definitions will be analyzed since, together with the approaches used for forecasting shortages and surpluses, they have served as the basis for much of the federal and state legislation dealing with health manpower.

DEFINITIONS OF A HEALTH MANPOWER SHORTAGE

For many years, public policy was concerned with reducing health manpower shortages. Various estimates were made as to the magnitude of these shortages, and legislation was enacted to decrease these shortages. Throughout the 1990s there was concern of a growing surplus of physicians, and policies were proposed to reverse this trend. Currently there is a belief that there is a shortage of registered nurses, and policies are being debated to rectify this shortage. Essential to fully understanding the debate over shortages and surpluses, and consequently appropriate public policy, is their definition.

The economic definition of a shortage or a surplus is different than how it is defined by non-economists. Further, a continuing disequilibrium in a market indicates that the market is not performing efficiently. Policies to improve market performance should therefore be based on the reasons for its inadequate performance. Thus unless there is agreement on what constitutes a shortage and surplus, proposals for subsequent government intervention to improve market performance may be misguided.

This section therefore starts with a discussion of different definitions of shortage. Surpluses are discussed next. For each type of market disequilibrium, various approaches used to measure shortages and surpluses are discussed together with appropriate policy prescriptions.

Normative Judgment of a Shortage

There are several *non-economic* definitions of health manpower shortages. An example is the statement that the demand for physicians "ought" to be greater. It has also been said that the "need" for physicians is greater than the demand, or that the price of physician services is "too high" thereby preventing people from consuming all the physician services they need. A normative judgment of a shortage means that there is a shortage of effective demand relative to what it should be. The non-economic definitions of a shortage are based either upon a value judgment of how much care people should receive, or upon a professional determination of how much physician care is appropriate in the population.

Such normative judgments of shortage are based upon a determination of "need" in the population, or upon some professional estimate of health manpower requirements. For example, physician/population ratios in high-income states are contrasted with physician/population ratios in low-income states. The differences in the ratio are believed to indicate the "need" for physicians in low-income states, which is the number of physicians "required" to achieve a physician/population ratio equal to that of the high-income states. (The ratio technique is discussed in more detail below.)

The classic example of the use of professional determination to determine the number of physicians "needed" was the 1930s study by Lee and Jones (1). Lee and Jones based their estimate of the number of physicians required on estimates of the incidence of morbidity and on the number of physician hours required to provide both preventive and therapeutic services to the population. The policy proposals resulting from normative definitions of a shortage of health manpower are generally the same: increase the number of trained professionals through increased federal funding.

In Figure 13-1 it is assumed that the initial situation is represented by the supply and demand diagrams S_1 and D_1, resulting in the quantity of physician services Q_1. The number of physician services for the population, based on either need or professional determination, is determined to be Q_2. The usual policy prescription to achieve an increase in physician services is to shift the supply of physicians to S_2, thereby increasing physician services to Q_2. The same increase in quantity, Q_2, of physician services can also be achieved by shifting the demand schedule to D_2. This

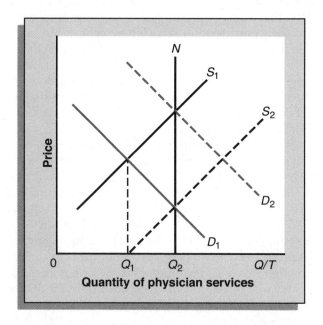

Figure 13-1. Alternative policy prescriptions based upon a normative shortage of health manpower.

would not require a shift in supply or in the number of physicians. (A shift in demand can be achieved through a demand subsidy, such as insurance coverage for physician services.)

Thus the normative judgment of a shortage of physician services, Q_1–Q_2, can be alleviated either by increasing the number of physicians (shifting S_1 to S_2) or by subsidizing the demand for physician services (shifting D_1 to D_2) along a given supply curve. A movement along a given supply curve represents increased production by existing physicians; physicians either work longer hours and/or they use more auxiliary personnel.

Which policy alternative—the demand or the supply shift—is preferable depends upon the cost of each proposal, the population groups receiving the benefits, and the length of time required to achieve the increase in services consumed. Normative judgments of a manpower shortage can be alleviated in various ways; however, these judgments of a shortage say nothing about how well the market for health professionals is functioning. The market for physicians may be functioning efficiently, although some persons may believe there "should" be more physicians; conversely, the number of physicians may be less than would be produced in an efficiently functioning market. The basic policy prescription using a normative definition of a shortage, however, is always for federal funding to achieve an increase in the number of physicians.

If the market is not performing efficiently, there might be alternative ways of achieving an increase in the number of physicians or physician services *without* resorting to federal funding. Perhaps some legal barriers might be changed to permit an increase in the physician supply. To determine how well the market for health professionals is functioning, we must establish the economic definitions of a shortage and examine how such shortages may occur. Possible policy prescriptions for correcting these shortages will be an outgrowth of their analysis.

Economic Definitions of Shortages in Health Manpower

In a competitive market, market equilibrium occurs when the value placed on a good or service by its de-

manders (marginal benefit) equals the cost of the resources used in its production (marginal cost). When the value placed on that good or service exceeds its cost of production, too little of that good is produced, creating a shortage.[1] In freely operating markets, shortages can exist in the short run but not in the long run.

There are two ways of analyzing how an economic shortage can occur with respect to health manpower. First, the quantity demanded of a particular health profession (i.e., hospitals' demands for registered nurses) can exceed the quantity supplied at a given market price (wage). For this to occur, the wage would have to be below the equilibrium wage.

The second way in which a shortage can occur is when the income of a health profession (relative to other occupations) exceeds the additional costs of entering that profession. In this example, the income of a health profession such as physicians reflects the value of the services that the profession produces. The costs of entering the profession include the out-of-pocket costs of training for that profession, as well as the value of the entrants' time, that is, their opportunity costs. (Since the time streams at which the income is earned and the costs incurred differ, an appropriate discount rate must be used in equating the two. It is also assumed that all other differences between occupations, such as variability in incomes, mortality risk, etc., are equal.)

The latter situation may be illustrated by use of Figure 13-2. D_1 is the demand by firms for a particular health manpower occupation. SL represents the long-run supply curve and is the number of persons willing to enter that occupation at different wage rates. S_1 is the current number of persons in that health profession. (S_1 could be more elastic since the supply of work effort from the current stock of trained professionals depends upon the responsiveness of their hours worked and their participation rate to different wage rates.) With a supply equal to S_1, the wage will be W_1. If the market were operating freely, the wage would fall to W_0 as the supply of labor to that occupation increases. If the health manpower profession in question were able to establish

---

1. This situation also occurs when a monopolist establishes a price for its service greater than the marginal cost of producing that service.

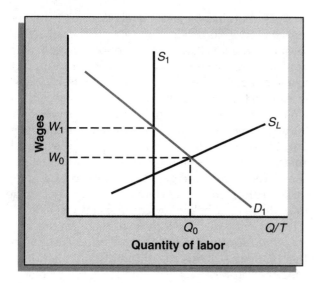

Figure 13-2. A shortage created by restriction of supply.

entry barriers, S_1 would not shift to the right along S_L, and the resulting wage would be W_1. Wage W_1 represents the value placed on that labor input by its demanders, and it exceeds the cost of inducing additions to the supply of that health profession.

Each of these two types of shortage—the first example, where the wage is held below the equilibrium level, and the case just considered where the wage exceeds the wage at which persons are willing to enter that occupation—is caused by market power on either the demand or supply side of the health manpower market. When the wage is prevented from rising to its equilibrium level, the demanders of labor are exercising monopoly power; in the latter case, the suppliers of labor services are the monopolists. In both of these types of shortage situations, the shortage would disappear with an increase in supply. Supply would increase in the first case if the price of the service were allowed to rise, and in the second case if more persons were allowed to enter the profession.

These discussions of economic shortage indicate what information should be examined to determine whether or not an economic shortage exists or has occurred. Since each of these approaches will be used with regard to different health professions (i.e., physicians and registered nurses), these approaches are discussed in more detail.

When quantity demanded exceeds quantity supplied at a given market price as in Figure 13-3, the price will rise (to P_2), and there will be no excess demand. All who are willing to pay price P_2 will be able to purchase as much as they want of the commodity they are seeking. (There may be persons who cannot afford to buy as much of the commodity as others believe they should purchase at the new, higher price; however, such a normative judgment can still be handled using a market mechanism by providing subsidies directly to such persons.) An economic shortage would occur in the situation above if, with an increase in demand from D_1 to D_2, the price of the service were prevented from rising to its new equilibrium point P_2. With an increase in demand and a price of P_1, the demand would be for Q_3 units of service. However, at a price of P_1, the supply of that service would be Q_1. The shortage would be the excess of demand over supply at the prevailing price, of Q_3–Q_1.

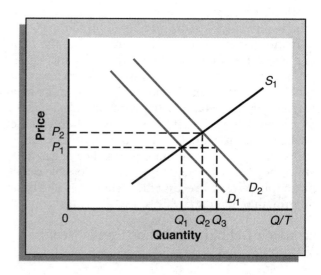

Figure 13-3. An economic shortage.

There are two types of economic shortage: a temporary (dynamic) shortage or a static (long-run) shortage. Both types of economic shortage are believed to have existed at one time or another in the health professions.

Dynamic Shortage

A dynamic or temporary shortage occurs when, as in Figure 13-3, there is an increase in demand but the new price has not yet reached its new equilibrium point of P_2. Demand will exceed supply at the old price of P_1. Not everyone who is willing to pay P_1 will receive as much as he or she wants. In the long run, however, this form of temporary or dynamic shortage will work itself out; the price will rise to the equilibrium level and there will no longer be a shortage. If demand continues to increase, it will take longer to achieve the equilibrium situation. There will be continued claims of a shortage while the price is rising, although supply will also be increasing.

Increases in quantity supplied, as well as rising prices, distinguish a dynamic shortage from a static shortage.

How long will a dynamic shortage persist? Arrow and Capron state, "the amount of shortage will tend to disappear faster the greater the reaction speed and also the greater the elasticity of supply (or demand)" (2). The reaction speed is the time it takes for price to reach its equilibrium level given the excess of demand over supply. It will take time for firms to realize that there is a shortage at the old price and that they must raise wages to attract more personnel. Firms must also decide how many more persons they want in the event that they have to pay higher wage rates. It also takes time for employees to react to these higher salaries. If demand and supply are relatively elastic, it will take smaller price increases to bring about a new equilibrium situation. Thus, in a dynamic situation where demands are increasing, temporary shortages can exist. The magnitude of the dynamic shortage will depend upon how fast demand is increasing, the reaction speed of increased prices to the excess demand, and the elasticities of supply and demand.

The policy prescriptions for a dynamic shortage differ from those prescribed for a shortage based on a "normative" judgment or for a static shortage. Increasing information to both demanders and suppliers in a market where dynamic shortages exist will make the equilibrium situation occur more quickly. Career information given to prospective applicants in professions where demand is increasing, and similar information given to prospective employers regarding the higher wages they will have to pay for such personnel, will bring about a quicker adjustment process. Massive supply subsidies to finance additional applicants entering those professions for which demands are increasing cannot be justified on grounds of economic efficiency. Such subsidies would have to be justified on the basis of other reasons, such as a normative shortage.

Static Economic Shortages

A static or long-run shortage occurs because supply does not increase; market equilibrium is therefore not achieved. In the typical case of a static shortage, prices are controlled and prevented from rising to their equilibrium level. If prices are not able to rise, the suppliers cannot pay higher prices to attract personnel away from other occupations. Similarly, a given health professional will not increase the amount of time that he or she is willing to work if the wage rate per hour does not increase; at some point the person will prefer leisure to more work. Thus suppliers will not increase the services they offer unless the prices paid for their services rise. The available supply in such situations is rationed by other methods: there may be long waiting lines to see a physician, and only those willing to wait (those with low time costs) will see the physician; there may be a decrease in quality (i.e., physicians may spend less time with each patient); physicians may also refuse to see new patients.

It is possible that either a static shortage or a market equilibrium situation could exist in the physician *services* market, while in the market for physician *manpower* either equilibrium or a static shortage could exist. It is important to keep the analysis of these two markets—the services and manpower markets—separate. For example, in Figure 13-4, the left-hand diagram represents the market for physician services,

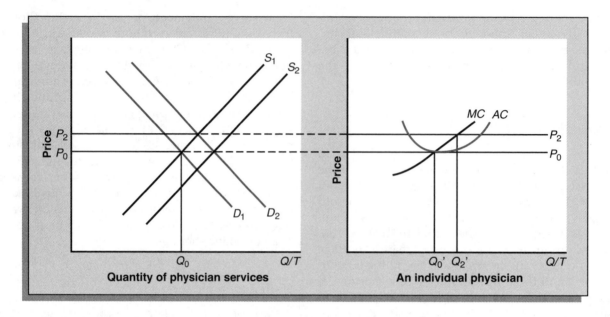

Figure 13-4. The market for physician services and for an individual physician firm.

while the right-hand diagram represents a typical firm (i.e., a physician in solo or group practice) within the overall market for physician services. Starting from an equilibrium situation in both markets, with price equal to P_0 and quantity of physician services equal to Q_0, the physician as a firm faces a price of P_0 and produces a quantity of services given by Q_0', which is the intersection of the physician firm's marginal cost curve (MC) and the market price P_0. (For simplicity, we are assuming a competitive market in both the production and demand for physician services.) The physician firm is in equilibrium (physicians will neither leave the industry nor enter it) since they are earning a normal rate of return with no excess profits, as shown by the position of the physician firm's average cost curve (AC) and the market price P_0.

Given the foregoing initial equilibrium position in both the services and manpower markets, let us assume that there is an increase in demand for physician services, possibly as a result of increased income in the population. The demand for physician services will increase from D_1 to D_2. Given the same number of physicians, physicians will either work longer

hours or increase their productivity by hiring auxiliary personnel. This increased output is shown by a movement up the industry's supply curve (S_1), which is the sum of the physician firms' marginal cost curves. The market price will rise to P_2, and each physician will be making excess profits (the distance from P_2 to the firm's average cost curve at output level Q_2'). The increase in price and output in the market for physician services is the short-run reaction to the increase in demand for physician services.

In this situation, there is no shortage in the physicians' services market. If there is an increase in the number of physicians (i.e., firms) in the long run in the manpower market because of excess profits, the industry supply curve will shift to the right (shown by S_2), and each physician firm will be producing at the point where the new price equals average cost and marginal cost. The increase in the number of physicians in the long run will also bring about an equilibrium situation in the manpower market, and no shortage will exist in either market.

If, however, with an increase in the demand for physician services the price is *prevented* from rising, a static shortage will occur in the services market. Equilibrium could still exist in the physician manpower market since there will not be an excess of profits (or losses). Alternatively, if the price is allowed to reach its equilibrium level in the services market but new physicians are not permitted to enter the manpower market, a shortage situation will exist in the physician manpower market. Physicians will be earning excess profits, and we would observe little, if any, addition to the number of physicians.

A static shortage in the number of physicians will be represented by high rates of returns (excess profits) to physicians and little or no entry into the physician market.

The policy implications for a static shortage situation are to allow the price to rise if the shortage is in the services market. If the shortage is in the physician manpower market, then easing the entry barriers will result in an increase in the number of physicians. With an increase in the number of physicians, excess profits per physician will fall until profits are "normal," and there will no longer be an economic shortage of physicians.

If a static shortage exists because of barriers to entry, providing subsidies to the new entrants will not resolve the static shortage. The entry barriers are not eliminated by such subsidies. Subsidizing the limited number of new entrants will merely increase their return in a profession whose members are already receiving excess profits.

The Definitions of a Surplus of Health Manpower

The above discussion defined a shortage in the physician manpower market as occurring when the physician earned an above-normal rate of return, or excess profits, on their investment in a medical education. A surplus of physicians would exist when the opposite occurs, that is, when physicians are earning a below-normal rate of return. (This would be characterized on the previous graph by the price being below the average-cost curve.)

A surplus situation can occur if one or both of the following situations occur. First, as a result of government regulation, the price of physician services is not permitted to rise as rapidly as the costs of providing physician services. Over time, the relative rate of return to becoming a physician falls below a normal rate of return. The second way in which a surplus could occur is through a change in market conditions. The growth in managed care, together with HMOs limiting their enrollees' access to specialists, decreased the demand for specialists. As a result, specialist fees and incomes declined. Exacerbating this situation was that the supply of specialists continued to increase faster than increases in demand for their services.

Similar to the definition of shortages, surpluses are often defined in non-economic terms. Typical approaches are to estimate the number of specialists, of various types, that are "needed." For example, how many specialists would be needed if, e.g., the population were half enrolled in HMOs and the other half in FFS, with their differing use of specialists. These needs or "requirements" for specialists are then compared to the number of specialists available. The difference is the surplus of specialists.

Surpluses are resolved more easily than static shortages (although there is a great deal of financial hardship to those in the surplus profession). As prospective applicants perceive a lowering in their rate of return to a medical education, fewer will apply to medical school; there will be a shift away from those specialties in greater surplus; some physicians may decide to retire earlier, while others move into management positions. Over time, the number of new entrants into the profession will be less than those exiting, and the smaller increase in the physician supply will bring about a new equilibrium situation.

In a surplus situation as described above, the physician *services* market is in equilibrium (although fees are lower than physicians would prefer), and in the manpower market physicians are earning a lower rate of return than other professions. The professional societies seek legislative remedies (higher prices for their services, e.g., higher Medicare physician fees, Any Willing Provider laws, and decreased entry into the profession) to mitigate the financial hardship on their members.

Income redistribution occurs in surplus and shortage situations. When there is a surplus of physicians, incomes of practicing physicians decline while purchasers of physician services pay lower prices and have greater access to care. The fortunes of physicians and patients are reversed in a shortage situation.

THE MEASUREMENT OF HEALTH MANPOWER SHORTAGES AND SURPLUSES

In defining and distinguishing between normative, dynamic, and static shortages, it is clear that the latter two are different types of economic shortages, and that the normative shortage is based upon either a professional determination or a value judgment of how many professionals of a particular type of manpower are needed. Similarly, there are economic and non-economic definitions of a physician surplus. The alternative policy prescriptions for the different types of shortages and surpluses were also indicated. In this section, the methods by which each of these types of shortages and surpluses have been measured is discussed. The measurement of a shortage and/or surplus is important since it enables us to distinguish between the different types of shortages and/or surpluses.

Professional Determination

Non-economic shortages have traditionally been measured in one of two ways: The first is professional determination. The earliest approach, used by Lee and Jones, calculated the number of physicians required in the population based upon an estimate of the number of physician hours needed (as determined by professional judgment) to provide medical care to the population. The authors developed a table of annual expectancy rates for diseases and injuries; they then asked leading physicians to determine the number of services required to diagnose and treat a given illness; the number of physician hours required to provide care for each illness category was then estimated; finally, assuming a 40-hour workweek per physician, the authors translated these hours into a requirement for 165,000 physicians, or a proposed physician/population ratio of 135 per 100,000 population. The difference between the then-current num-

ber of physicians (which was lower) and the number of physicians arrived at by the foregoing method was the "shortage" of physicians.

One of the problems with using such an approach for estimating shortages and for proposing government subsidies to increase the number of needed physicians is that the additional physicians do not necessarily go where they are most needed. Further, those persons most in need of physician services may not be able to pay for them even if they are made available.

The same approach has also been used to estimate a physician surplus. Concern by medical associations and educational institutions about a possible surplus of physicians led to the 1980 Graduate Medical Education National Advisory Committee (GEMENAC) report to the Secretary of Health and Human Services on the future supply and requirements for physicians (3). The approach used by the GEMENAC committee was similar to the methodology used by Lee and Jones in the 1930s.

Estimates of future supplies of physicians were generated based on estimates of current numbers of medical school graduates, foreign medical graduates, residents, and deaths and retirements. No attempt was made to relate entry into medicine, into different specialties, or entry by foreign medical graduates to economic factors or to any other causal factors. Instead, it was implicitly assumed that such factors would not change over the period studied. Nor did this approach consider changes in physician productivity that might be occurring. It was a mechanical approach to generating future estimates of physicians and their specialty distribution.

The estimates of physician requirements were developed by combining data on current utilization and the "need" for physicians. Within each physician specialty, physicians were asked how many physicians were needed in that specialty. Again, such an approach does not explicitly consider patient preferences for care or economic factors such as changes in insurance coverage, factors which in the past have been important determinants of physician utilization.

The "desired balance" between physician supply and requirements in 1990 did not consider any equilibrating mechanisms such as changes in physician prices or hours worked. The GEMENAC report forecast a "surplus" of 70,000 physicians by 1990.

At any given time, there is an equilibrium price resulting from the interaction of the demand for and supply of physicians. If the number of physicians exceeds the professionally determined estimate and if such a "surplus" of physicians were to be eliminated (a shift to the left in the supply of physicians), the consequence would be an increase in price and a decrease in quantity. If the price were a government-determined price and did not rise as the "surplus" is eliminated, then an *economic shortage* would occur (demand would exceed supply at the fixed price). The above methodology for estimating a surplus is silent on this issue either because the profession is unaware that this will occur or, more likely, they are aware of it and that is the reason for favoring an elimination of the surplus.

The Ratio Technique

The second and most popular approach to determining health manpower shortages and surpluses has been the ratio technique. When used to estimate a shortage, this method generally uses the existing physician/population ratio (or other health manpower/population ratio) and compares it with the physician/population ratio that is likely to occur in some future period. To calculate the future ratio, the proponents of this approach estimate the future population and then calculate the likely number of additional graduates to the stock of physicians, less the expected number of deaths and retirements. The difference between the existing physician/population ratio and the future physician/population ratio is the extent of the shortage (or surplus).

Until the late 1970s, studies using this approach consistently found the future ratio to be lower than the current ratio, meaning that an increased number of physicians were needed if the future ratio was to be at least equal to the current ratio. The policy proposal that was always prescribed based upon the finding that increased numbers of physicians needed was that federal subsidies should be provided to health professional educational institutions to produce more graduates.

There were variations in the use of the ratio technique for determining the number of needed physicians. For example, the highest regional or statewide physician/population ratio observed might be used as the ratio to be achieved for the entire country in some future period.

The ratio technique has served as the basis for much of the health manpower legislation in this country. It has been used for physicians, dentists, and registered nurses. Other health professional educational organizations also made use of this approach in their requests for federal subsidies. Since this approach has had such an important legislative role and has resulted in many billions of dollars of subsidies both by the federal and state governments, it deserves a critical evaluation.

One way of thinking of the physician/population ratio is that it is the outcome of an equilibrium situation. At any point in time there is a demand for physicians and a supply of physicians; the intersection of the demand and supply curves results in physician incomes and in a physician/population ratio. Attempts to change the physician/population ratio generally ignore the fact that this ratio is the result of demand and other supply factors. Any significant change simply in the number of physicians will cause changes in the demands for other inputs (substitutes for and complements to physicians), as well as in the demands for physicians themselves, which would mean a movement along the physician demand curve.

Three basic problems are associated with the use of the ratio technique for forecasting manpower requirements. The first problem is that the method does not consider any changes that may occur in the demand for physician (or other health manpower) services. If demand were to increase, then even maintaining an existing ratio is likely to result in an *increase* in the price of physician services (i.e., the shift in demand is greater than the change in the physician/population ratio). Demand changes could occur because of changes in financing care, such as Medicare, Medicaid, and tax-free employer-paid health insurance. Other demand factors include the aging of the population, changes in lifestyle factors that decrease the demand for medical services, and the increased use of other treatment inputs, such as pharmaceuticals.

Since the ratio technique basically ignores the demand side, differences between the future ratio of physicians to population and the ratio that would be demanded will be resolved through changes in the *price* of physician services. Some persons will be even less likely to buy physician services if the price of those services were to increase.

Thus, maintaining a given ratio says nothing about whether the future price of physician services will be the same; it may be higher or lower, but it is highly unlikely that it will be the same. Since the future price is likely to be different, what is the real purpose of maintaining a given ratio? If, under a projected "shortage" scenario, the objective were to provide more services to certain population groups or to the entire population, it would be important to lower the price of the service so as to increase consumption. The ratio technique and its basic policy prescription of changing the number of physicians does not even consider price or alternative ways to affect consumption of services.

The second problem with the use of the ratio technique is that it does not consider productivity changes that are likely to occur or that are possible to achieve. The ratio of farmers to the population has fallen drastically in the last 100 years (from a ratio of 60 farmers to every 100 persons in 1860 to 3.5 per 100 persons today), yet few people would maintain that there is a shortage of farmers or that it would be desirable to retain the previous farmer/population ratio. Because of enormous increases in farm productivity, it takes fewer farmers today to produce more food than their predecessors did.

Although productivity gains in medical care appear to be more limited than what has occurred in agriculture, it is possible to achieve an increase in physician services without increasing the number of physicians. Technology and lesser-trained personnel can be used to relieve physicians of many of the tasks they perform; delegation of tasks would permit an increase in the number of physician visits. If increased productivity were considered, a smaller physician/population ratio would be needed in the future. To alleviate a projected "shortage," increasing productivity is an alternative approach for achieving

an increase in the quantity of physician services. Policies to increase productivity require smaller subsidies than do policies to increase the number of physicians.

(An indication of the real intent underlying the use of physician/population ratios is that the subsidies should be provided to the medical schools, who would not be the recipients if the less costly approach of increasing physician productivity were used.)

The third problem with the use of the ratio technique is that no indication of the importance of the shortage of physicians is provided. For example, an earlier Bane Report estimated that to maintain a specific physician/population ratio 15 years hence, an additional 11,000 physicians would be needed. These projections assumed that without federal support for medical education there would be 319,000 physicians with a resulting shortage of 11,000 physicians (4). How much is it worth (in terms of governmental subsidies) to reduce this shortage to 7,000 physicians or to no shortage whatsoever? It is difficult, if not impossible, to use the ratio technique to compare the additional cost of decreasing the estimated shortage of physicians with their marginal contribution to medical care, to increased health, or lower physician fees.

There are a number of other difficulties inherent in using the ratio technique that can cause variations in its estimates. It is necessary to exclude non-patient care physicians from the physician/population ratio, to correct for the age distribution of physicians (since it may affect productivity), to adjust for the percentage of female physicians (who see fewer patients), to correct for the expected number of foreign medical graduates, to estimate the percentage of the population in HMOs (which use fewer physicians per 1,000 enrollees), to account for changes in the institutional settings where care is provided (hospitals use a greater mix of certain manpower than do ambulatory care settings or care in the home), and to develop an accurate forecast of the population in a future period.

However, the three conceptual problems inherent in this approach—no consideration given to demand or productivity changes and no understanding of the importance of the shortage estimate—are more difficult shortcomings to correct.

The Rate-of-Return Approach

In an equilibrium situation, physicians earn normal profits. With an increase (decrease) in demand in the physician services market, physicians would, in the short run, experience higher (lower) prices leading to above (below) normal profits, and in the long run (assuming no barriers to entry), the change in the number of physicians would cause physician profits to return to normal.

This analogy of the physician as a firm is useful because it helps to delineate what we expect to observe. Normal, above, or below normal profits mean that the rate of return to a medical education is either normal, high, or low relative to equivalent investments. Although not all, nor even perhaps most, physicians seek a medical education because of its value as a remunerative investment, enough persons do so that if one profession becomes more lucrative than another, some persons will change their occupation. This just means that as some professions and occupations become relatively more rewarding financially, some potential applicants who are relatively indifferent between one occupation or another will switch their preferences to the more rewarding profession. This switching between occupations and professions will, on average, equalize returns among different occupations. (Because there are always large variations in skills and abilities, returns *within* an occupation or profession will vary. In the long run, however, the average return should be similar among different occupations.)

When viewing medical education as an investment, the rate of return is calculated by estimating the costs of that investment and the expected higher financial returns achievable as a result of that investment. The profitability of a medical education can then be compared with alternative investments, educational and otherwise. The costs of purchasing a medical education are the direct outlays, such as tuition, laboratory, and book fees, and the foregone income had the student gone to work immediately upon graduating from college. These opportunity costs of the medical student's time are the more significant costs of securing a professional education. The financial return of an investment in a medical education is the higher income that a physician earns compared with the income of not having gone for a medical education. Since these higher incomes occur in the future, they are worth less than if they occurred immediately; the financial returns between being a physician as compared to not having gone on for a medical education must be discounted to the present. The comparison between these higher returns and the costs required to receive them is the rate of return to a medical education.

In similar fashion, the rate of return to a medical education can be compared to an investment in a legal education, a dental education, a PhD degree, or an MBA. (More precisely, the internal rate of return is that discount rate which, when applied to the future earnings stream, will make its present value equal to the cost of entry into that profession, i.e., the present value of the expected outlay or cost stream.)

A normal rate of return might be similar to the rate of return on a college education or on the return the individual could have received had he or she invested a sum of money comparable to what was spent on a medical education. It is necessary to compare the rate of return on a medical education with an alternative rate of return to be able to determine whether or not physicians are receiving a normal return.

Returning to our analogy of the physician as a firm, if physicians were receiving "excess" profits, this would be translated into a high relative rate of return to a medical education.[2] If rates of return to medicine

2. An economist's rate of return calculation differs from that of an accountant in that economists include opportunity costs while accountants do not. By excluding foregone earnings, accountants overstate the profitability of a medical career; accountants similarly overstate the profitability of any business where the owner invests their own capital and/or their own time. For example, accountants calculate net income by subtracting all (explicit) expenses from the firm's revenue. (Dividing the resulting net income by the firm's invested capital (or stockholder's equity) is the rate of return earned by the firm.) Assume that after subtracting explicit expenses from the firm's revenue, $50,000 remains; an accounting definition of profit would conclude that the firm is generating positive net income. However, assume that the owner could have invested their $1 million elsewhere and earned risk-free 5 percent on their capital and, similarly, could have earned $100,000 a year working for another firm. Based on the same data, an economist would conclude that the firm is not profitable; failure to include opportunity costs, often not easily observable, overstates the firm's profitability.

are higher than those received in other occupations, there will be a greater number of applicants to medical schools. As the number of physicians increase over time, the rate of return to a medical career will become comparable to other occupations or investments.

With regard to shortages, to distinguish between a dynamic and a static shortage, it is necessary to examine the rate of return to a medical education relative to some standard or to another profession, and also whether there is an increase in the number of physicians. A dynamic shortage would be characterized by a high relative rate of return in the short run, increases in the number of physicians, and eventually normal rates of return. A static shortage would also be characterized by a high relative rate of return, but it would persist since there would be little or no entry into the profession to drive these rates of return down. If rates of return remained relatively high and there was a large increase in the supply of physicians, this would be indicative of a persistent dynamic shortage.

The key difference between the dynamic and static shortage is whether additions to the stock of physicians occurs over time. A dynamic shortage will eventually resolve itself; a static shortage requires intervention since entry into the profession is prevented from occurring.

Similarly, a surplus of physicians would be indicated by a rate of return that is *below* that of a college graduate. As prospective medical students become more aware of the lower expected rate of return to becoming a physician, fewer students will seek a medical education. With a smaller influx of new physicians, the rate of return will eventually rise so that it once again becomes "normal." How long it takes for a surplus to be reduced depends upon growth in demand for physician services, the age distribution of physicians and how rapidly physicians decide to retire, the opportunity for physicians to move into managerial (or other) positions, how responsive prospective medical students are to the lower rate of return, and the size of the inflow of foreign trained physicians. It is unlikely that a large surplus could be reduced quickly since many physicians do not have the skills or opportunities to earn an income comparable to what they receive, even when it is at a below-normal rate of return. (Since the costs of becoming a physician have already been incurred, the relevant comparison is between the income

they would continue to earn as a physician relative to that of another occupation, plus any training costs for that new occupation.)

The main indicators of the performance of the physician market, as well as other health manpower markets, are data on relative rates of return and changes to the stock of physicians (or other health manpower). Changes in the use of various manpower categories, such as increases and decreases in the use of substitutes, are indicative of changes in the relative wages of such inputs rather than being indicative of a shortage or surplus of physicians. For example, if both incomes and costs of becoming a physician increased, the relative rate of return between occupations could still be similar but because there is a change in relative wages, substitution would occur. Thus the main method whereby different types of shortages are distinguished is in the use of relative rates of return and entry into the profession.[3]

EMPIRICAL ESTIMATES OF SHORTAGES AND SURPLUSES

Several studies have estimated the rate of return to a medical education. The earliest such study, undertaken in the early 1930s, was Friedman and Kuznets who found that physicians earned, on average, 32 percent per year more than dentists (5). This higher income for physicians was, in part, offset by the 17 percent higher cost of becoming a physician. Friedman

---

3. Another approach suggested for measuring whether or not a shortage exists is to examine changes in relative incomes. If one profession's income rises more rapidly than another profession's, a relative shortage is said to exist. (See, for example, Elton Rayack, "The Supply of Physicians' Services," *Industrial and Labor Relations Review*, January 1964.) The problem with this approach is that it does not consider differences in the relative costs of entering different professions. If training times have increased or if there is a decrease in the number of working years, we would expect higher relative incomes for this profession in order for the relative rates of return to be similar. Another problem in using the relative income approach is that the base year for making comparisons among professions is quite important. Depending upon which base year is used, the relative income approach can show a shortage or a surplus of the manpower in a particular profession. Finally, the relative income approach cannot distinguish between relative shortages in all professions and a shortage situation in only one profession.

and Kuznets attributed part of the increased income of physicians to greater entry barriers into the profession. The greater return to physicians represented a relative shortage of physicians; that is, their marginal value as represented by their incomes exceeded the costs of producing additional physicians.

A subsequent study by Hansen found that by 1939 there was a slight *surplus* of physicians and dentists (their rates of return were below those of college graduates). However, by 1949, physicians and dentists had a 16 percent greater rate of return than did college graduates, indicating a shortage. By 1956, the shortage had decreased slightly: physician rates of return were only 10 percent greater than for college graduates; the comparable figure for dentists was 4 percent. This data is shown in Table 13-l, which is reproduced from Hansen's work.[4]

Several additional studies have estimated the internal rate of return to a medical education; these results are presented in Table 13-2 (6). The rates of return are shown for all physicians and separately for general practitioners. The "all physicians" estimate includes general practitioners as well as the various physician specialties. The rates of return to all physicians over the period 1955 to 1985 were sufficiently high to make medicine a financially attractive profession. Between 1974 and 1985, there was a slight decline in the return to a medical education.

---

4. There is a difference in the method used by Hansen and the other studies. Hansen's income and cost streams begin at the first year of undergraduate college, and his foregone earnings are based on those of a high school graduate. The other studies are based on the forgone earnings of a college graduate, and the income and cost streams begin at the first year of medical school.

Table 13-2. Internal Rates of Return, All Physicians and General Practitioners, 1955–1997

Year	All Physicians		General Practitioners
1997		21.8(a)	18.4(a)
1990		24.7(a)	16.6(a)
1985	16.0(b)		4.1(c)
1980	—	14.0(d)	16.7(d)
1976	17.5(e)	13.3(d)	16.4(d)
1974	16.7(d)		
1970	22.0(f)	14.7(d)	16.8(d)
1965	17.5(g)		21.4(h)
1962	16.6(g)		—
1959	14.7(g)		23.7(h)
1955	13.5(g)		29.1(h)

Sources:

(a) Personal correspondence with William B. Weeks, Assistant Professor of Psychiatry and of Community and Family Medicine, Dartmouth Medical School, November 2002.

(b) William Marder, Phillip Kletke, Anne Silberger, and Richard Wilke, *Physician Supply and Utilization by Specialty: Trends and Projections*, (Chicago, IL: American Medical Association, 1988), p. 79.

(c) William D. Marder and Richard J. Wilke, "The Value of Physician Time: Comparisons Across Specialists," in H. E. Frech, editor, *Regulating Doctors Fees*, (Washington, D.C.: American Enterprise Institute, 1991).

(d) Phillip Burstein and Jerry Cromwell, "Relative Incomes and Rates of Return for U.S. Physicians," *Journal of Health Economics*, March 1985, 4(1), pp. 63–78.

(e) Stephen Dresch, "Marginal Wage Rates, Hours of Work, and Returns to Physicians Training and Specialization," in Nancy Greenspan, editor, *Health Care Financing, Conference Proceedings: Issues in Physician Reimbursement*, (Washington, D.C.: Department of Health and Human Services, 1981), pp. 199–200.

(f) Roger Feldman and Richard M. Schefler, "The Supply of Medical School Applicants and the Rate of Return of Training," *Quarterly Review of Economics and Business*, Spring 1978, 18(1), pp. 91–98, table 1.

(g) Frank Sloan, *Economic Models of Physician Supply*, unpublished doctoral dissertation, Harvard University, 1968, p. 164.

(h) Frank Sloan, "Lifetime Earnings and the Physicians Choice of Specialty," *Industrial and Labor Relations Review*, October 1970, 24(1), pp. 47–56.

Table 13-1. Internal Rates of Return to Male College Graduates, Physicians, Dentists, and Ratios of Internal Rates of Return of Physicians and Dentists to Male College Graduates, United States, 1939, 1949, and 1956

	1939		1949		1956	
	Rates	Ratios	Rates	Ratios	Rates	Ratios
Male college graduates	13.7	1.00	11.5	1.00	11.6	1.00
Physicians	13.5	.98	13.4	1.16	12.8	1.10
Dentists	12.3	.90	13.4	1.16	12.0	1.04

Source: W. Lee Hansen, "Shortages and Investment in Health Manpower," in *The Economics of Health and Medical Care* (Ann Arbor, MI: University of Michigan, 1964), p. 86.

The rate of return to different specialties varies greatly according to Marder, et al., and Dresch, who find that in 1985 some specialties, such as anesthesiology and surgical sub-specialties, earned 40 and 35 percent returns, while for pediatrics it was only 1.3 percent. Rates of return were typically higher for hospital-based specialties than for those in primary care. Dresch compared the rates of return to medicine with other professions and found that the rates of return varied greatly depending upon which occupation was compared to medicine. For example, the rate of return to a medical education was over 100 percent greater than that of a college professor. Recent calculations by Weeks indicate that physicians continue to earn, on average, above-normal rates of return, although these returns have declined between 1990 and 1997.

What can we conclude based on the above rate of return data? In the pre-World War II period there appeared to be a slight surplus of physicians and dentists. The rate of return to a medical and dental education was lower than for comparable investments. After World War II, however, the rate of return to a medical and dental education increased. The rates of return during this period were sufficiently high to indicate a shortage situation. With increasing rates of return, increased demands for a medical education would be expected. If the stock of physicians were expanding rapidly, then it would appear that a dynamic shortage existed. If, however, the rates of return remained high (and in fact increased) and there were few or no additions to the stock of physicians, then one would have to conclude that a static shortage situation existed, and that barriers prevented an adjustment process from occurring.

To determine whether a dynamic or a static shortage of physicians existed throughout the post-World War II period, one must examine data on changes in the stock of physicians during these periods, as presented in Table 13-3.

In 1950 there were 209,000 active physicians in the United States. By 1965, the number of active physicians reached 278,000, which is a rate of increase of about 2.2 percent per year. When the increase in the number of physicians is adjusted for increases in the population, the physician/population ratio remained virtually unchanged between 1950 and 1963 (140 physicians per 100,000 population and 142 per 100,000, respectively). After 1963, the total number of active physicians began to increase at a slightly more rapid rate, averaging between 1.5 and 3.0 percent per year until 1975 when the annual increase was 3.5 percent. The physician/population ratio also began to show a gradual annual increase during this same period, reaching 173 physicians per 100,000 in 1975.

Part of the increase in physicians over this period was a result of increases in foreign medical graduates (FMGs). The Immigration Act of 1965 permitted large numbers of foreign medical graduates (FMGs) to enter the US.[5] As a result, there was a rapid rise in FMGs

---

5. Before the 1965 Act, immigration quotas were based on national origin (which limited Asian migration). The Act eliminated quotas based on national origin and instead established a more flexible system of hemispheric quotas. (Migration from Asia represented the largest portion of the increased migration.) In addition, two new immigration categories, professional members with exceptional ability and workers in short supply (as determined by the Secretary of Labor), favored foreign trained physicians.

There are two main classifications of FMGs: those that have permanent immigrant status and those that have exchange visitor status. Exchange visitor FMGs are supposed to return to their own countries after they have received graduate medical training. In 1971, the requirement that persons with exchange visitor status had to spend two years overseas before being able to permanently immigrate to the U.S. was eliminated. This law further eased the migration of FMGs to the U.S. The annual increase in exchange visitor FMGs exceeded the number of FMGs permanently immigrating up until the mid 1970s. Exchange visitor FMGs were an important component of total FMGs, and they were becoming a significant portion of all physicians.

In 1976, Congress changed the immigration laws affecting FMGs. Newly entering FMGs were now required to pass more rigorous medical exams, as well as exams in written and oral English. The legislation also restricted the number of FMGs who can remain indefinitely by requiring exchange visitor FMGs to return to their own countries after two years of U.S. graduate medical education. This legislation had its greatest impact on newly entering FMGs with exchange visitor status; their numbers decreased from 2,563 in 1976 to 544 in 1982. The number of newly entering permanent immigrants also declined. As a percentage of total new licensees, FMGs decreased from 36.0 percent in 1976 to 17.9 percent by 1985. In 1984, a more rigorous certification exam was introduced which also reduced the number of FMGs being admitted to U.S. residency programs.

In 1991, the immigration laws were once again liberalized and the demand by teaching hospitals for residents resulted in a large increase in the number of foreign-born FMGs entering U.S. residency positions, from 2201 in 1988 to 5891 in 1994. U.S. Department of Health and Human Services, Division of Health Professions Analysis, *Report to the President and Congress on the Status of Health Professions Personnel in the United States,* (1981 and 1986), (Washington, D.C.: U.S. Government Printing Office, 1981), pp. III-20, III-143; (1986): III-36, III-38. John K. Iglehart, *op. cit.*

Table 13-3. Number of Physicians and Physician/Population Ratios, United States, 1950–2001

Year	Active Physicians	Annual Percent Change	Physicians Per 100,000 Population	Annual Percent Change	Foreign-Trained Physicians	Foreign-Trained Physicians as a Percentage of All Active Physicians	Physician/ Population Ratios Excluding Foreign-Trained Physicians (Physicians per 100,000 Population)
1950	208,997		140				
1955	228,553	1.9	142	0.3			
1960	247,257	1.6	140	−0.3	15,154	6.1	131
1963	261,728	1.8	142	0.5	30.925	11.8	125
1965	277,575	3.0	146	1.4	38,380	13.8	126
1967	294,072	3.0	152	2.1	45,816	15.6	128
1969	302,966	1.5	154	0.7	53,552	17.7	127
1970	311,203	2.7	156	1.3	54,418	17.5	129
1975	366,425	3.5	173	2.2	76,784	21.0	137
1980	435,545	3.8	195	2.5	91,826	21.1	154
1985	511,090	3.5	219	2.5	112,660	22.0	171
1990	572,660	2.4	234	1.4	122,823	21.4	184
1995	646,022	2.6	247	1.1	153,792	23.8	188
2000	737,504	2.8	273	2.1	177,681	24.1	207
2001	794,895	7.8	285	4.4	186,013	23.4	218

Sources: U.S. Department of Health, Education, and Welfare, National Center for Health Services, *Health Resources Statistics, Health Manpower and Health Facilities, 1970,* Public Health Service Publication 1509 (Rockville, MD., Public Health Service, 1971), pp. 133, Table 81; *Physician Characteristics and Distribution in the United States, 1981, and 2003–2004 eds.,* Division of Survey and Data Resources, (Chicago: American Medical Association, 1982, 2003); U.S. Department of Health and Human Services, Bureau of Health Professions, *A Report to the President and Congress on the Status of Health Professions Personnel in the United States,* (Washington, D.C.: U.S. Department of Commerce), various editions: 1970, 91st ed., p. 40, Table 48; 1985, 105th ed., p. 49, Table 72; 1995, 115th ed., p. 67, Table 82; 2001, 121st ed., p. 54, and 2002, 122nd ed., p. 8.

between 1966 and 1976. During this period, approximately one-third of the permanent increase in physician supply was attributed to the inflow of FMGs. In 1960, 6.1 percent of the total number of active physicians were FMGs; by 1975, FMGs comprised 21 percent of active physicians. By the early 1970s, the number of FMGs entering the United States exceeded the number of U.S. medical graduates (USMGs). When the physician-to-population ratio is adjusted for the number of FMGs, the ratio of U.S.-trained physicians changed very little between 1960 and 1975 (131 and 137, respectively).

Not all active physicians are involved in patient care. When the growth in the number of physicians is adjusted to determine those in patient care activities and the number of FMGs is excluded, the physician/population ratio for U.S. physicians engaged in patient care actually *declined* between 1960 and 1975, from 115 to 111 per 100,000 population.

The large increase in the supply of foreign-trained physicians benefited consumers while eventually leading to a decline in physicians' earnings (7). This effect is illustrated in Figure 13-5 (page 344). The initial demand curve facing physicians is shown as D_1. The initial supply curve, S_1, is relatively inelastic over a short period because of the time it takes for medical schools to produce new medical graduates. (For simplicity, increases in physician productivity and hours of work are assumed to be constant.) In 1966, Medicare and Medicaid had increased the demand for physician services by both the aged and the poor. The demand for physician services in the private sector also increased as employers provided their employees with more comprehensive health insurance. This increased

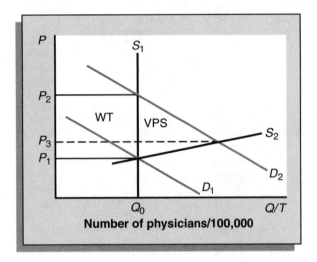

Figure 13-5. An increase in foreign medical graduates on physician earnings and consumer benefit.

demand is shown by D_2. With the increased demand and the inelastic supply, price would have increased to P_2.

However, as a result of the 1965 law which increased the number of FMGs, the new short-run supply of physicians includes the rapid increase in FMGs and is very elastic, S_2. The new price, P_3, is the intersection of the increased demand and S_2.

The benefit to consumers is the rectangular area or wealth transfer (WT) shown by $(P_2-P_3)Q_0$ and the remainder (VPS) is the value to consumers of the additional units of physician services. Svorny estimated the size of WT for the period 1966 to 1972 using different assumptions of demand elasticity. The size of WT was estimated to be 1 percent of total physician expenditures in 1966, increasing to 12 percent by 1972.

Svorny further estimates that physician earnings would have been 11 percent higher by 1971 had there not been any change in the 1965 immigration law.

It is not surprising, given these large wealth transfers from physicians to consumers as a result of the 1965 law, that the immigration laws affecting FMGs were changed in 1976.

Demand for physicians had been increasing during the period from 1950 to 1965, as indicated by the relatively high rates of return to a medical education. Large increases in the number of physicians would therefore be expected. However, rather than increasing, U.S. physicians involved in patient care as a ratio to the population actually decreased during this 15-year period; the absolute increase in the number of U.S.-trained physicians was very small.

The small increase in the number of physicians was not a result of a lack of applicants to medical schools. As shown in Table 13-4, the applicants/acceptances ratio during this period was continually greater than 1.

In fact, the applicant/acceptance ratio appears to track changes in physician rates of return fairly well. The high rates of return in the late 1940s (Table 13-1) show a correspondingly high applicant/acceptance ratio. As rates of return declined during the 1950s (Tables 13-1 and 13-2), the applicant/acceptance ratio similarly declined. With the rise in the rate of return during the 1960s and 1970s, the applicant/acceptance

Table 13-4. Ratio of Applicants to Acceptances, 1947–1948 to 2002–2003

Year	Applicants/Acceptance Ratio
1947–1948	2.9
1950–1951	3.1
1955–1956	1.9
1960–1961	1.7
1965–1966	2.1
1970–1971	2.2
1975–1976	2.8
1980–1981	2.1
1985–1986	1.9
1990–1991	1.7
1995–1996	2.7
2000–2001	2.1
2002–2003	1.9

Source: American Medical Association, "Medical Education in the United States, 1971–1972," *Journal of the American Medical Association,* 222 (8), November 20, 1972: p. 979, table 12; "Undergraduate Medical Education," *Journal of the American Medical Association,* 256 (12), September 26, 1986: p. 1561, table 5, copyright 1971, 1986, American Medical Association; B. Barzansky and S. I. Etzel, "Educational Programs in U.S. Medical Schools, 2002–2003," *Journal of the American Medical Association,* 290 (9), September 3, 2003: p. 1193, table 3.

ratio also increased. The decline in the rate of return in 1985 was matched by falling applicant/acceptance ratios throughout the 1980s.

In 1965, Congress passed the Health Professions Educational Assistance Act in response to claims of a "shortage" of physicians and other health manpower. As a result of this legislation, which provided generous subsidies to health professional educational institutions, medical schools were required to increase their enrollments to qualify for federal funds. The effect of this legislation began to be felt by the late 1960s when the number of U.S.-trained physicians began to increase at a more rapid rate.

By 1980, the total number of physicians per 100,000 population reached 195, and by 2001 it rose to 285. Even when adjusted for the increase in FMGs, the physician/population ratio is greater than it has been for many years. The expansion in medical school spaces resulting from the previous manpower legislation continues to have an effect.

Even with the increase in the physician-to-population ratio, the ratio of applicants to acceptances, which had been declining since 1975 (when it was 2.8) to 1.7 by 1990, increased to 2.7 in 1995, and since then declined to 1.9 in 2002. The rising applicant/acceptance ratio during the 1990s to a high of 2.7 was surprising to those who claimed there was a surplus of physicians during this period.

What can we conclude from the data on rates of return, physician-to-population ratios, and the ratio of applicants to acceptances to medical schools? During the entire post-World War II period, rates of return to medicine were high and rising. Based on these higher returns, greater entry by U.S.-trained physicians would have been expected. However, it appears that there was very little entry into the profession by U.S.-trained physicians. Although a large number of students demanded a medical education as indicated by the applicant/acceptance ratio, very few additional physicians were produced. Even after the introduction of federal legislation that led to increases in the production of physicians, there was still an excess demand for a medical education. The only possible conclusion, based on the minimal increase in the number of U.S.-trained physicians until the mid 1970s and the

continued high rates of return, is that a static shortage situation existed.

(The mechanisms used by the medical profession to create and maintain a static shortage of physicians for so many years are discussed in the next chapter.)

IS THERE A PHYSICIAN SURPLUS?

During the late 1970s, the medical profession and medical school educators became increasingly concerned that the rapid rise in the physician/population ratio was causing a physician "surplus." Further, the growth of managed care during the 1980s, with its reliance on primary care physicians and decreased demand for specialists, led to the belief that there would also be a serious surplus of specialists. Medical societies, representing the economic interests of their members, were concerned with the effect of the increased supply on physicians' incomes. Medical schools became concerned about their own survival if there was a decreased demand for a medical education. For the first time since the early 1960s, the decline in the applicant/acceptance ratio in 1985 to below 2 lent credence to the medical schools' fears. Several dental schools closed when their applicant pool decreased.

The Graduate Medical Education Advisory Committee (GMENAC) was established in 1976 to provide forecasts and recommendations to the country on the number of physicians needed to serve the population. In 1980, GMENAC, relying primarily on the ratio technique, forecast a surplus of 70,000 physicians by 1990 (approximately 15 percent more than "needed") and 145,000 (or a 30 percent surplus) by the year 2000. GMENAC issued additional reports during the 1990s reiterating its concern with the impending physician surplus. Based on these forecasts of a large physician surplus, GMENAC recommended placing limits on the number of new U.S. medical graduates and reductions on the number of international medical graduates (IMGs) entering the U.S.

In 1986, Congress created the Commission on Graduate Medical Education (COGME) and charged it with the mission of analyzing trends in physician supply, specialty distribution, and financing graduate medical education (in addition to several other tasks). Based on their estimates of a growing surplus of physicians, particularly specialists, COGME issued a series of reports in the 1990s that included the following proposals. First, that the number of residency positions should be reduced to 110 percent (or less) of the number of U.S. medical school graduates (rather than the current 140 percent). This policy would reduce the supply of new physicians by decreasing the number of residencies for foreign trained physicians by 7,000 a year. Second, 50 percent of the residency positions should be for training generalists, thereby correcting the specialist imbalance. COGME proposed that teaching institutions that did not comply with these guidelines should be denied federal funding.

In 1995, the PEW Commission issued its report of the physician surplus, recommending reductions in medical school spaces by 20 to 25 percent by the year 2005 and reductions in the number of residency positions to 110 percent of the number of U.S. graduates (8).

In addition to these Commissions, academic researchers also forecast a large physician surplus. In one of the more detailed approaches using the ratio technique to derive an estimate of the physician surplus, Weiner, in a 1994 article, forecasted a huge overall surplus of 165,000 physicians, or 30 percent of the total number of patient care physicians by the year 2000 (9).

Weiner's approach to estimating the "need" (or "requirements") for physicians and the available supply was to use data based on ten large HMOs to determine the ratio of physicians to HMO members; he found a wide range of physician staffing within those HMOs, from 97 to 163 physicians per 100,000 members. He also examined the non-physician staffing patterns, the use of nurse practitioners and physician assistants per 100,000 HMO members. The range was also quite wide, from 0 to 37 per 100,000 members. Estimates were also calculated of the ratio of primary care physicians and specialists.

Weiner made a series of adjustments to HMO staffing patterns since the HMOs surveyed were less likely to serve the aged, those on Medicaid, and the uninsured. The purpose of these adjustments was to increase HMO staffing levels if HMOs were to enroll a more diverse population with higher care needs as HMOs expanded to include a greater percentage of the population. Adjustments were also made for out-of-plan use by HMO enrollees. Several scenarios were used which varied the percentage of the population that would be enrolled in different financing and delivery systems, e.g., HMOs, managed, and unmanaged fee-for-service. Different staffing patterns were also estimated for the fee-for-service sector.

Projections to the year 2000 were then derived for the likely number of physicians by specialty. The difference between the need forecast and the number of physicians available was the likely surplus.

Although the above study was more detailed than previous ratio techniques and attempted to include many relevant factors in making a forecast of physician requirements, its forecasts are affected by the same problems inherent in all ratio studies. For example, no consideration was given to the effect of financial incentives on demands for care, physician productivity, or PCP/specialty mix. Choice of health plan and use of services are affected by enrollee co-premiums and co-payments, employee price sensitivity, in addition to employee preferences and incomes. Unless these factors are accurately accounted for (which is difficult to do) forecasts of the percentage of the population in HMOs, with HMO staffing patterns, will be inaccurate.

Further, if the supply of physicians exceeds demand, physician fees will decline. Yet the effect of lower fees on an increased quantity demanded of physician services was ignored, as were the effects of lower fees on physician behavior, such as the decision to choose a medical career, specialty choice, and practice behavior. Changes in Medicare policy will greatly affect the elderly's behavior and choice of health plan, similar to the way changes in financial incentives have affected employees' choice of plan and use of services.

According to Weiner's estimates, the need for PCPs was roughly in balance with future supply estimates, but the number of specialists was likely to be about 60 percent greater than those needed. However, specialists and primary care physicians cannot be analyzed separately. If a surplus of specialists occurred, more medical graduates would decide to become primary care physicians which would cause a decrease in incomes of primary care physicians, as well as leading to fewer applicants to medical school.

The use of the ratio technique simply assumes trends in supply and demand for physicians will continue and will be unaffected by changes in health plan premiums, physician fees, increases in physician productivity, the growth and use of non-physician practitioners, or by changes in physicians' incomes.

Contrary to the above study's findings, as well as estimates of a huge physician surplus by the various Commissions, Schwartz, et al., believed the medical profession's fear of a surplus was overstated (10). They contended that a surplus would be characterized by declining physician incomes. However, during the late 1980s, real physician incomes increased which is indicative of demand increasing faster than physician supply. Schwartz, et al., claim that one important way in which their study differs from those predicting a surplus is that they include estimates of increased per capita demands for medical care based on past trends that they believed would continue.

Schwartz, et al., calculated the likely future supply of physicians, taking care to project only those engaged in patient care, changes in the supply of residents' services, and the fewer working hours of female physicians. With respect to the demand for physicians, the authors projected the proportion of the population that will be enrolled in HMOs, the effect on demand of the aging of the population, as well as a per capita growth in demand based on prior periods. Based on these demand and supply projections, the authors concluded that it was unlikely that there would be a surplus, and based on certain assumptions with regard to medical advances, there could even be a *shortage* of physicians.

Even if there was a slight surplus, the authors believed that it would largely remedy itself; physicians would become more involved in long term care, move into administrative positions, as well as move to underserved areas.

If a physician surplus were to occur, the relative rate of return to a medical career would fall below that of a college graduate (or comparable group of college graduates), fewer medical graduates would take specialty residencies, and there would be a de-

clining ratio of medical school applicants to acceptances, similar to the situation that existed in the 1930s, as shown in Table 13-1. Until these indications occur, there would not appear to be a surplus.

Throughout the 1990s, incomes of all specialists declined, which is consistent with anecdotal evidence during that time of falling specialist incomes, particularly in certain geographic areas. Incomes for general practitioners and internal medicine physicians, however, increased. Income data for specialists and non-specialists, presented in the chapter on "The Market For Physician Services," is consistent with the findings on rates of return shown in Table 13-2. Overall, however, this economic data do not indicate a physician surplus.

Even though physician incomes may have fallen and reduced the rate of return of prospective medical students, the rate of return to a medical career is still sufficiently high and is not indicative of a surplus. Data on the applicant/acceptance ratio, although declining, continue to indicate that there is an excess demand for a medical education, also not indicative of a surplus. Recently, anecdotal evidence is more indicative of a growing shortage; it is becoming more difficult for both privately and governmentally (Medicare) insured patients to find access to a physician.

Given the uncertainties regarding a physician surplus, particularly among specialists, what should be appropriate public policy, if any? Should reliance be placed on the market or on government intervention to adjust any imbalance between supply and demand?

PROPOSED POLICIES TO CORRECT IMBALANCES BETWEEN THE DEMAND AND SUPPLY OF PHYSICIANS

The forecasts of an impending surplus of physicians by GMENAC, COGME, PEW and others led to a number of proposals for reducing both the overall number of projected physicians and the number of specialists. GMENAC, for example, proposed that an agency (such as GMENAC) should determine both the number and size of residency programs for each specialty. Another proposal was to phase out residency opportunities for non-USFMGs. Reducing residency positions for USFMGs, while more controversial, was also proposed. The Association of American Medical Schools proposed that medical school enrollments be reduced as a means of reducing future supply. It was further proposed that the federal government provide "decapitation" grants to medical schools to offset the decline in medical school tuition as a result of having fewer students.

Defining the Optimal Number of Physicians

GMENAC had already been proven inaccurate in its 1990 and 2000 year forecasts of huge physician surpluses. Physician incomes in 1990 (and 2000) did not suffer the drastic decline that would have been indicated by such large surplus projections; nor has the excess demand by students for a medical career disappeared or the number of applicants fallen so low as to raise concerns about the quality of new medical students. Factors that contributed to the inaccuracy of the GMENAC forecast were: the percentage of physicians employed in HMOs was lower than forecasted; females as a percentage of total physicians were underestimated, thereby overestimating (according to GMENAC) overall physician productivity (female physicians were estimated to have a 78 percent lifetime productivity of male physicians); GMENAC was also inaccurate with regard to its specialty requirements (e.g., the number of cesarean deliveries has been much greater than anticipated); GMENAC did not foresee the spread of AIDS and the consequent increased demands for medical care, or the growth in transplants.

Despite the inaccuracies of their forecasts, GEMENAC, COGME, and the Pew Commission continued to recommend limiting increases in the supply of physicians by reducing the number of medical school graduates, restricting residency opportunities for FMGs, and changing the specialty distribution of physicians by increasing the percentage of primary care physicians.

How "appropriate" are the various proposals for reducing the estimated physician surplus? In other words, are the proposals likely to achieve the optimal number of physicians? Optimal is defined as when the marginal benefit of additional physicians equals their marginal cost. (This would occur when there is a normal rate of return to a medical education. Similarly, the optimal specialty mix occurs when the marginal benefit/marginal cost ratio of an additional specialist [of each type] equals the marginal benefit/marginal cost ratio of an additional primary care physician. This would occur when specialists and generalists earn equal rates of return but unequal incomes [marginal benefit] since training times [marginal cost] differ.) The optimal number of physicians is discussed more completely in the chapter on "The Market for Medical Education."

Would a regulatory policy, such as proposed by COGME, be more effective in achieving the optimal number (and specialty mix) than a market-oriented approach?

Any policy that attempts to manipulate the number of physicians involves deciding what incomes physicians (as well as specialists) should earn. When COGME claims that there is a surplus of physicians, COGME is stating that physician incomes are or will be "too low." COGME has not explicitly discussed what physicians should earn. Would the criteria be the same as that of an economist, namely a normal rate of return? Policies to determine physician and specialist incomes would be a very politically charged issue. Therefore it is unlikely that it would be resolved strictly according to economic criteria. Within any profession there is a wide range of incomes based on skills, work effort, personality, etc. Would COGME attempt to influence physician incomes or would it also try and reduce the range of physician incomes? And if so, how? And what would happen if physicians were to increase their productivity and earn more than COGME believed appropriate?

Even if an appropriate level of income could be determined for each physician specialty, it is very difficult for a quasi-regulatory body, such as COGME, to correctly estimate changing demand conditions, productivity changes, and the effect of managed care competition to be able to maintain physician incomes at a given level. COGME would have to continuously monitor these market conditions in order to make appropriate adjustments to the number of medical students and their choice of specialty. Further, given the long training times to become a physician and a specialist, COGME would have to anticipate these market changes many years into the future to correctly change the number of new medical students and their specialties.

If the supply of physicians were to be determined by an agency such as COGME, then an error in forecasting has much greater consequences in terms of the total number of physicians than if individuals forecast incorrectly. COGME's errors will result in much greater changes in the number of physicians than prospective students who differ on the outlook for physician incomes.

No other profession is subject to legislation establishing quotas or income levels to correct what that profession perceives as a surplus. The members of most professions probably favor less entry into their profession, hence less competition and higher incomes.

Physician Specialty Distribution

Specialists have exceeded the number of primary care physicians (PCPs) for many years. As shown in Figure 13-6 (page 350), in 1965 there were 13 percent more specialists than PCPs. By 1970, specialists exceeded the number of PCPs by 52 percent, reaching a high of 56 percent by 1990, and then declining to 38 percent by 2001.

The reasons why more physicians have chosen a specialty career vary; however, economic incentives, such as relative earnings and medical school indebtedness, are an important part of that decision (11).

Proponents of changing the specialty distribution and reducing the supply of physicians by limiting the number of IMGs want to use Medicare medical education subsidies to achieve this goal.

Medicare is the largest explicit source of funding for graduate medical education residencies (12). Since its inception, Medicare (Part A) has paid teaching hospitals a direct medical education subsidy based on the number of residents in that hospital. The basis for this subsidy was the belief that the education of residents, which increases the quality of that institution, increases the hospital's cost. The number of residents and the medical education subsidy has risen sharply over time; there are approximately 100,000 residents (26 percent are IMGs), and the cost to Medicare is in excess of $7 billion per year, or $70,000 per resident

annually, with several hospitals (in 1995) receiving more than $240,000.

As part of the Balanced Budget Act of 1997, to save money, Medicare limited the number of residencies it would support at the hospital's 1996 level. These payments per resident to teaching hospitals increased their demand for residents. Since these hospitals could not recruit enough U.S. medical graduates to fill all their residency positions, they recruited foreign-trained physicians. Thus Medicare policy provided an incentive to teaching hospitals to indirectly increase the supply of physicians. Further, Medicare policy provides an incentive for residents to be trained in hospitals (as specialists) and outpatient clinics rather than in primary care or managed care settings, since Medicare only supports training in the former settings.

The attempt to reduce Medicare education subsidies and/or the number of residencies has resulted in economic and, consequently, political conflict between both the AMA and medical schools (and those interested in reducing Medicare expenditures) against teaching hospitals, who do not want to lose the financial support. About one-half of all FMG residencies are in four states, New York, New Jersey, Pennsylvania, and Illinois. Thus the political battle has been geographic rather than according to political party (13). Unless the teaching hospitals are somehow compensated for the loss of Medicare support, legislators from their states are unlikely to support reductions in residencies for FMGs.

Several economists have questioned the use of any Medicare funds to pay teaching hospitals for their residents' medical educational costs. Newhouse and Wilensky claim that according to economic theory it is the resident—not the hospital—that bears the cost of educational training (14). Graduate (as well as undergraduate) medical education is an example of "general" training whereby the resident can use the skills they acquire at other places than in the hospital where they are being trained. (Specific training means that the skills can only be used at the specific institution where the person works.) Because a resident with general training can use those skills elsewhere, the cost of that training is borne by the resident.

Medical residents (as well as others receiving general training) produce services that have some value

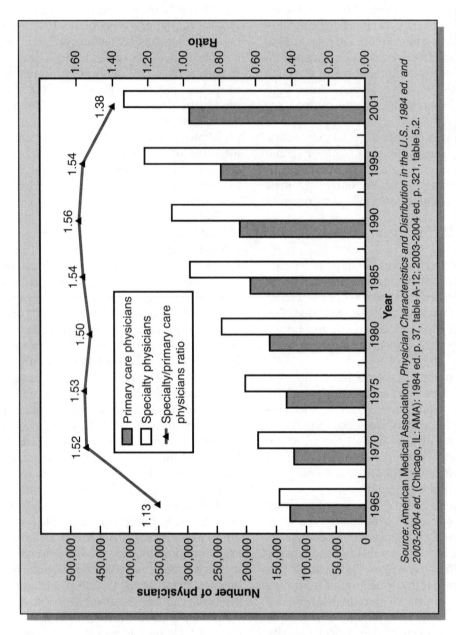

Figure 13-6. Number of Primary Care and Specialty Physicians and Specialty to Primary Care Physicians Ratio, United States, selected years, 1965–2001.

Source: American Medical Association, *Physician Characteristics and Distribution in the U.S., 1984 ed. and 2003-2004 ed.* (Chicago, IL: AMA): 1984 ed. p. 37, table A-12; 2003-2004 ed. p. 321, table 5.2.

as part of their training. When the value of those services exceeds the costs of training that resident, then it would be worthwhile to pay the resident the difference. When the costs of training exceed the value of services provided, then the student would be expected to pay the difference. The more senior the resident, the greater the value of their services, hence the greater their wage. In a competitive market for trainees with demanders of trainees having equal reputations, hospitals will be unable to attract the number of trainees they want if they do not pay a competitive wage (when the value of services exceed the costs of training).

Based on the above discussion of general versus specific training and who pays the costs of general training, teaching hospitals do not bear the educational costs of their residents, residents do. Therefore, it does not seem appropriate that Medicare should continue graduate medical education subsidies to teaching hospitals. Although there is no justification for medical education subsidies, there may, however, be other reasons for subsidizing teaching hospitals, such as their care for the uninsured and their research programs.

Determining the Optimal Number and Specialty Distribution of Physicians: Reliance on Markets or Government Planning?

Previous forecasts of society's needs for physicians have been grossly inaccurate. Had government enacted the policies recommended by those who forecast a physician surplus, physician fees and incomes would be sharply higher and there would be serious concerns today over access to care. Government policies have contributed to dissatisfaction with the current size and specialty distribution of physicians. Medicare's graduate medical education subsidies provided teaching hospitals with a financial incentive to expand their residency positions and to recruit IMGs when there were too few U.S. graduates to fill those positions. Health manpower policy overshot its mark in subsidizing the number of physicians now claimed to be in surplus. Future policy may be too restrictive with respect to new graduates.

Government is unable to quickly adapt its policies to changing market situations. Policy makers need to collect data on what is occurring, formulate proposals, and then negotiate proposed policies with those organizations (and their legislators) having an interest in the outcome, such as medical societies that are more concerned with physician incomes than an optimal number of physicians, and teaching hospitals that profit from medical education subsidies for their residents.

Professional determinations of a surplus (based on "need" for physicians) have been unable to correctly anticipate future trends. Given the "cost" of inaccurate manpower planning, namely, higher physician fees and reduced patient access to care, it would be unwise to rely on a regulatory approach for determining the optimal number and specialty mix of physicians (15).

Forecasts 15 to 20 years ahead are unlikely to be accurate given the changes occurring in medical knowledge and in the financing and delivery of medical services. However, unlike government, markets are able to adjust quickly to changes in demand and supply. Relying on market forces for defining and then correcting physician shortages and surpluses will bring about a more rapid response to imbalances in the demand and supply of physicians.

Employee price sensitivity and the lower premiums charged by HMOs increased their demand for HMOs. As more of the insured population moved into managed care, HMOs, with their greater reliance on primary care physicians, reduced the demand for specialists. Specialists' fees and incomes declined. This information was quickly transmitted to medical students who adapted by changing their career choices; fewer medical students chose specialty residencies, and the percentage of medical graduates choosing primary care increased. As managed care organizations relaxed their restrictions on use of specialists, the demand for specialists (and their incomes) increased. These changing market trends have again resulted in an increase in the demand for specialty residencies.

Allowing market forces (using prices of services and physician incomes as signals) to determine the number of physicians and the specialty mix will bring the supply and demand for physicians and specialists into closer balance. It is difficult to conceive of government responding as quickly to changes in market conditions as medical school graduates with information on their career prospects.

Permitting prospective applicants to decide whether or not they wish to enter medicine and, similarly, allowing the specialty decision to be made by residents places the burden as well as the benefits of that decision on the individuals rather than on a regulatory agency. Improved information would enable these individuals to make more informed choices. Individual decision making, based on professional and economic incentives, results in a rapid self-adjusting mechanism to changes in the marketplace. These adjustments are quicker and more accurate than an agency whose constituency (medical schools, the medical profession, and teaching hospitals) has its own economic objectives.

SUMMARY

A great deal of public policy has been directed toward the health manpower sector. Previously, public policy was concerned with perceived shortages of various types of health manpower. More recently there has been a concern over a possible surplus of physicians. Whether a shortage or surplus exists depends on how they are defined. Non-economic definitions often relied on the use of the ratio technique, that is, whether the physician/population ratio differs from a specified ratio. Problems with the ratio technique include its failure to consider changes in demand and productivity and an inability to indicate the importance of an estimated shortage or surplus, such as the changes in prices that would occur if the shortage or surplus were not eliminated.

Economic definitions of shortages and surpluses rely on the rate-of-return approach, namely, the rate of return to an investment in a medical education relative to that of a college graduate. Excess rates of return indicate an economic shortage, while below normal returns are indicative of a surplus. Static, as compared to temporary, shortages are characterized by increased demand and rising prices but limited entry into the profession. Entry barriers prevent the elimination of a static shortage.

Concern over a possible surplus of physicians arose because of the increase in the physician/population ratio and the movement to managed care. The various approaches used to define a surplus provided differing conclusions as to whether a surplus existed. While the physician/population ratio has greatly increased, there is still an excess demand for a medical education, the applicant-to-acceptances ratio to medical schools is about 2:1.

Proponents of reducing a possible physician surplus have proposed limiting the number of medical school graduates and the number of residencies. If implemented, these policies would increase the prices of physician services and physician incomes, while decreasing access to care.

Having too many or too few physicians has costs and benefits to different groups. Using regulation to determine future supplies is likely to result in too few physicians because current physicians want to have high rates of return, and medical schools want excess demand for their spaces. The representatives of these constituencies will dominate the regulatory body as they have with GMENAC, COGME, other commissions, and as they have in the past in determining the number of medical school spaces. Too few physicians imposes a cost on society; fewer physicians means that the prices of their services are higher, access to care by those with low incomes is reduced, fewer physicians would locate in underserved areas, and fewer physicians would be available to work in innovative organizational settings.

Unlike regulatory policy, relying on the market does not have to consider the political interests of those who may be adversely affected by changing market conditions. Often the economic interests of those affected will motivate the profession to seek legislative remedies that result in market inefficiencies.

Consumers bear the cost of too few physicians, whereas physicians bear the cost of too many. Thus whether greater caution should be placed on eliminating a surplus or a shortage depends upon one's economic perspective.

The next two chapters describe how the economic interests of the medical profession and medical educators have determined previous health manpower policies. The mechanisms used by the medical profession to create and maintain a static shortage up until the late 1970s is discussed next.

REVIEW QUESTIONS

1. What is the difference between an economic and non-economic definition of a shortage? What are the consequences if public policy were based on a non-economic definition of a shortage?
2. Distinguish between the different economic definitions of shortage (e.g., dynamic versus static shortages), and describe the data you would need to differentiate between these different definitions. What might be appropriate public policies for each type of shortage?
3. What are the problems of using health manpower ratios to project health manpower "requirements?"
4. Through the 1960s, there was a shortage of physicians. A proposal to remedy this problem was to provide subsidies to prospective physicians (tuition, interest-free loans, etc.). Comment on the effect this proposal would have had on reducing the shortage of physicians. Be explicit regarding your assumptions.
5. "Trying to prove that there is a shortage of doctors by comparing their incomes to the incomes of lawyers only results in proving that there is a surplus of lawyers."
   a. How do you evaluate this statement?
   b. What does the relative income approach tell you about the supply of physicians?
6. Assume that a particular physician specialty association decides to limit the number of residencies in that specialty. Using diagrams, what would be the expected effect on that specialty and on other physician specialties? Should the physician specialty association be concerned about Federal Trade Commission scrutiny?
7. What are the various indications of a surplus of physicians? What would be the appropriate public policy to reduce such a surplus, if any?
8. Evaluate both regulatory and market approaches for determining the optimal number (and specialty distribution) of physicians.

REFERENCES

1. R. I. Lee and L. W. Jones, *The Fundamentals of Good Medical Care*, (Chicago: University of Chicago Press, 1933).
2. Kenneth J. Arrow and William M. Capron, "Dynamic Shortages and Price Rises: The Scientist-Engineer Case," *Quarterly Journal of Economics*, 73(2), May 1959: 299, 292–308.
3. *Summary Report of the Graduate Medical Education National Advisory Committee to the Secretary, Department of Health and Human Services*, Vol. I, DHHS Publication (HRA) 81-651, 1980: 48–56. Volume II contains a more complete description of the Modeling, Research, and Data Technical Panel.
4. *Physicians for a Growing America*, Report of the Surgeon General's Consultant Group on Medical Education, Public Health Service, U.S. Department of Health, Education, and Welfare (Washington, D.C.: U.S. Government Printing Office, 1959).
5. Milton Friedman and Simon Kuznets, *Income From Independent Practice*, (New York: National Bureau of Economic Research, 1954).
6. The rates of return shown in Table 13-2 are unadjusted for the number of hours worked by physicians. There has been substantial debate about whether the internal rates of return, unadjusted for hours worked, adequately reflect the true internal rates of return to a medical education. Lindsay claims that because of his or her training, a physician will receive a relatively high market wage. This high wage will induce the physician to substitute work for leisure; consequently, the physician will work more hours than someone with a lower market wage. Lindsay believes that there should be an adjustment for the number of hours worked before the income and cost streams are calculated. When Lindsay adjusts Sloan's data for hours worked (he assumes a 60-hour week for physicians and a 40- to 45-hour week for the alternative occupation), the internal rate of return is reduced.

Sloan's response is twofold: first, he claims that Lindsay overestimated the number of hours that physicians work; second, Sloan claims that being a physician provides intangible benefits, such as increased status in society, which compensate the physician for any additional hours worked. For this reason, Sloan argues, it is not necessary to take into consideration these extra hours when calculating the income and cost streams.

For a more detailed discussion of the Sloan and Lindsay debate see: Cotton M. Lindsay, "Real Returns to Medical Education," *Journal of Human Resources*, 8(3), Summer 1973: 331–348; "More Real Returns to Medical Education," *Journal of Human Resources*, 11(1), Winter 1976: 127–130; and Frank A. Sloan, "Real Returns to Medical Education, A Comment," *Journal of Human Resources*, 11(1), Winter 1976: 118–126.

7. This discussion is based on an article by Shirley Svorny, "Consumer Gains From Physician Immigration To the U.S.: 1966–1971," *Applied Economics*, 23(2), February 1991, 331–337.

8. The Third Report of the Pew Health Professions Commission. *Critical Challenges: Revitalizing the Health Professions for the Twenty-First Century*, (San Francisco: Center For the Health Professions, University of California), 1995.

9. Jonathan P. Weiner, "Forecasting the Effects of Health Reform on U.S. Physician Workforce Requirement: Evidence from HMO Staffing Patterns," *Journal of the American Medical Association*, 272(3), July 20, 1994, pp. 222–230.

10. William B. Schwartz, Frank A. Sloan, and Daniel Mendelson, "Why There Will Be Little Or No Physician Surplus Between Now And the Year 2000," *The New England Journal of Medicine*, 318(14), April 7, 1988, 892–897. Also see William B. Schwartz and Daniel Mendelson, "No Evidence of an Emerging Physician Surplus," *Journal of the American Medical Association*, 263(4), January 20, 1990, 557–560.

11. Niccie L. Mckay, "The Economic Determinants of Specialty Choice By Medical Residents," *Journal of Health Economics*, 9(3), November 1990, 335–357.

12. *Medicare Payment Policy: Report to the Congress*, (Medicare Payment Advisory Commission: Washington, D.C.) March 2001, describes Medicare's payment policy for graduate medical education (Chapter 10) and changes in the number of residents by specialty between 1993–1999 (Table C-1).

13. John K. Iglehart, "The Quandary Over Graduates of Foreign Medical Schools in the United States," *The New England Journal of Medicine*, 334(25), June 20, 1996, 1679–1683.

14. Joseph P. Newhouse and Gail R. Wilensky, "Paying For Graduate Medical Education: The Debate Goes On," *Health Affairs*, 20(2), March/April 2001, 136–147. The authors also discuss empirical research on the relationship between number of residents per bed and cost per case.

15. The use of regulation for determining the size and specialty distribution of physicians is proposed by Kevin Grumbach, "Fighting Hand To Hand Over Physician Workforce Policy," *Health Affairs*, September/October 2002, 21(5), 13–27. For an opposing analysis see Uwe Reinhardt, "Dreaming The American Dream: Once More Around On Physician Workforce Policy," *Health Affairs*, September/October 2002, 21(5), 28–32, and Uwe E. Reinhardt, "Planning the Nation's Health Workforce: Let the Market In," *Inquiry*, 31(3), Fall 1994, 250–263.

C H A P T E R
14

The Market for
Physician Manpower

KEY TERMS AND CONCEPTS

- The Flexner Report
- Periodic re-examination
- Task licensure
- Charity hypothesis of physician pricing
- Physician market entry barriers
- Physicians as price-discriminating monopolists
- Process versus outcome quality measures

Learning Objectives

Upon completing this chapter, the reader should be able to:

- Discuss the various entry barriers for becoming a physician.
- Contrast the physician income versus the consumer protection hypotheses for the existence of entry barriers in medicine.
- Understand, diagrammatically, how physicians have acted as price discriminating monopolists.

ENTRY RESTRICTIONS: QUALITY ASSURANCE OR MONOPOLY POWER?

To better understand the development of the physician market, it is useful to examine how a shortage situation could have existed for so many years. The concern for consumer protection and quality of care was, presumably, the basis for the various restrictions that were developed to ensure that physicians were well trained. Also to be discussed is whether these measures improved consumer protection or whether they had the opposite effect.

In the previous chapter, a dynamic shortage was differentiated from a static shortage according to whether or not there was entry into the market. Persistently high rates of return, it was suggested, could continue only if there were barriers to entry. Based on the small growth in the number of physicians until the mid-1970s, the continual excess of applicant acceptances to medical schools, the rapid growth in foreign medical graduates, and the increasing number of U.S. students studying medicine overseas, it was concluded that entry barriers must have existed to prevent an equilibrium situation from occurring in the market for physician manpower.

CONSUMER PROTECTION OR MONOPOLY POWER? ENTRY RESTRICTIONS IN MEDICINE

Three entry barriers to the physician's market have been suggested: licensure, graduation from an approved medical school, and continual increases in training, such as the movement to a three-year residency program. There is, however, an alternative hypothesis to explain why barriers in medicine exist: rather than serving to increase the economic returns to physicians, the barriers increase the quality and competence of practicing physicians. It is rationalized that these entry barriers enhance the public interest in a variety of ways. Consumers have very little information on the quality and competence of physicians. Gathering this information is costly, and the consumer may be irreparably injured if the physician is incompetent; licensure provides the consumer with protection by reducing the uncertainty as to the provider's training. Occupational licensure has also

been rationalized on grounds of "neighborhood effects"—an incompetent physician may harm persons other than the patient being treated if, for example, the physician was to cause an epidemic. Licensure is thus a means of protecting others from bearing the costs of incompetent practitioners; that is, the social costs exceed the private costs (1).

Given these alternative hypotheses to explain the reasons for entry barriers to becoming a physician (namely, to increase physician incomes or to provide consumer protection from incompetent practitioners), which is the more accurate justification? If the barriers are reduced because they are believed to provide physicians with monopoly incomes, will the public lose its protection from incompetent providers? Similarly, if such entry restrictions are maintained in the belief that they reduce consumer uncertainty and protect society from incompetent providers, but if in fact such barriers are meant to provide physicians with monopoly incomes, is the public really protected from incompetent practitioners? Could the public be better protected using other approaches and at a lower cost?

To determine which hypothesis best describes the reasons for entry restrictions in medicine, one must determine how consistent each of these hypotheses is with regard to the assurance of quality or the achievement of monopoly power. If the restrictions are for consumer protection, the medical profession should also be expected to favor other measures that have the effect of improving quality and/or offering consumers protection from incompetent practitioners. If, on the other hand, the entry restrictions were meant to provide physicians with a monopoly and to increase their incomes, the profession would only favor those quality measures that are in the economic interests of physicians; the profession would be expected to oppose quality measures that would adversely affect physicians' incomes.

BARRIERS TO ENTRY IN MEDICINE

The first step in controlling entry into a profession is to establish a licensure requirement. Each state has the authority to license occupations under the power granted to it to protect the public's health. A license to practice medicine, therefore, can be granted only by a state. Beginning in the mid 1800s when the American Medical Association (AMA) was formed and extending until 1900, the medical profession sought and received licensure in each state (2). The states, in turn, delegated this licensure authority to medical licensing boards which have the authority to determine the requirements for licensure. These state licensing boards also have the authority to set the conditions for suspending or revoking a license once it has been granted. The conditions for licensure and for maintaining a license can be placed on the quality of care that the physician provides, and/or they can be used to impose restrictions on who can practice thereby limiting the number of persons entering the profession. The membership of the medical licensing boards in each state consisted of physicians who were either nominated by or were representatives of the state and county medical associations. It was in this manner that county and state medical associations influenced the conditions for licensure in each state.

The earliest requirement for licensure was an examination. Examination by itself, however, is a weak barrier to entry. A person may try to pass the examination many times, and the number of people taking the examination is not limited (3). A more effective barrier is one that raises the cost to those wishing to take the examination. Not everyone would be willing to bear this cost, particularly if there was uncertainty as to whether they would pass the licensure exam.

The second barrier to entry into the medical profession, therefore, was the imposition of an educational requirement and a limit on the number of institutions that could provide such an education. This stage began in 1904 with the AMA's founding of its Council on Medical Education. This group had the task of upgrading the quality of medical education offered by existing medical schools. Of the 160 medical schools in 1906, the Council on Medical Education found only 82 offering a fully acceptable medical education (4). To achieve greater recognition of its findings, the Council on Medical Education induced the Carnegie Commission to survey the existing medical schools and publish a report. The resulting report, popularly known as the Flexner Report, recommended the closing of many medical schools and an upgrading of the educational standards in the other schools. "Flexner forcefully argued that the country was suffering from an overproduction of doctors, and that it was in the public interest to have fewer doctors who were better trained" (5).

The result of the Flexner Report was that state medical licensing boards instituted an additional requirement for state licensure: before taking an examination for licensure, an applicant had to be a graduate of an approved medical school. The approval of medical schools was conducted by the AMA's own Council on Medical Education. In the years that followed, as expected, the number of medical schools decreased, from 162 in 1906, to 85 in 1920, to 76 in 1930, to 69 in 1944. The number of physicians per 100,000 similarly declined. The graduates of those medical schools that were closed continued to practice. No attempts were made to rectify any supposed inadequacies in their educational backgrounds.

Whenever standards are raised, grandfather clauses protect the right of existing practitioners, regardless of their abilities.

The AMA now had control over entry into the profession in two ways: first, through its Council on Medical Education, the AMA was able to limit the number of approved medical schools and hence the number of applicants for licensure exams; second, entrants into the profession then had to pass state licensure exams and any other prerequisites promulgated by the individual state medical licensing boards. Thus the AMA, through its Council on Medical Education, was able to determine the "appropriate" number of physicians in the United States.

The third method used by the medical profession to restrict entry, which is also meant to increase the competence of the new physician, is to lengthen the training time required for the student to become a practicing physician. Increased educational requirements increase the investment cost of becoming a physician, thereby decreasing the rate of return to entering physicians. Before entering medical school, a student has to have 4 years of undergraduate education. Medical school is 4 years, and the time spent in internship and residency programs continually increase; medical school graduates usually take a minimum 3-year residency. For students desiring to enter certain specialties, more than 3 years is required. The effect of continually increasing the training required before entering a profession is to raise the costs to the entering student. Not only are tuition costs higher the longer the requirements for undergraduate and medical school education, but more important, the income forgone because of the additional years of training is very large. These increased costs reduce the rate of return to prospective physicians.

The emphasis in terms of quality is always on the training of entering physicians and not on those currently practicing in the profession. It is in the economic interests of current practitioners that the costs of entering the profession continually increase; since the training of those currently practicing occurred in the past at a lower cost, they would receive higher prices and higher incomes in the form of economic rent (6).

Until the anti-trust laws were ruled to be applicable to healthcare in the early 1980s, more highly trained physicians were prohibited by the medical profession from advertising their additional training and more recent knowledge. Thus they could not receive a higher price for their services than physicians without this additional training. To prevent new physicians from receiving higher returns than existing physicians who had less training, it was necessary for the medical profession to maintain the fiction that all physicians were of uniform quality. To enforce this impression among patients, the medical profession discouraged any intra-professional criticism and, until recently, prohibited the advertisement of differences in training or any other quality differentials among physicians.

Whether or not a person was permitted to perform certain medical tasks depended upon whether or not they were a physician. A physician was provided with an unlimited scope of practice; it did not matter whether the physician had specialized training. Anesthesiologists, for example, can be physicians who are board certified in anesthesiology, they can be physicians with additional training but who are not board certified, or they can be physicians without any additional training in anesthesia. Merely being licensed was sufficient to allow physicians to undertake tasks performed by other physicians who have had additional training.

This third barrier to entry, which has taken the form of continual increases in the training costs for entering physicians, suggests that measures to increase the quality of physician services were independent of demands by consumers for increased quality and instead were related to the income considerations of the medical profession.

In addition to entry barriers, it was necessary for physicians to control productivity increases amongst themselves if they were to receive monopoly profits. Otherwise, it would be possible for some physicians to greatly increase their output, with a corresponding loss of business to other physicians, and consequently, a decrease in their rate of return. Productivity increases were (and, in some cases, still are) limited in two ways. First, only licensed physicians are allowed to perform certain tasks thereby severely limiting the ability of physicians to increase their output by delegating tasks to other personnel.

Second, when new types of health personnel, such as physicians' assistants, were trained to undertake certain tasks, previously the sole prerogative of the physician, state boards of medical examiners retained the authority to certify their use on an individual physician-by-physician basis. In this manner, a particular physician would not be able to hire a large number of such personnel and greatly increase his or her output. The medical licensing boards' control over physicians' assistants can be used to approve their use in situations where demand for physician services has increased, or in areas where physicians are not available, such as in rural areas. Their employment can be limited in those places where physicians' practices, from the standpoint of the physicians, are underutilized.

The above barriers to entry and increased training costs, which have been used successfully by the medical profession to restrict both entry into the profession and productivity, have been adopted by other health professions as well. The American Dental Association (ADA), after successfully achieving state licensure of dentists, had a study conducted on dental education, which resulted in the Gies Report in the early 1920s. As a result of this report, applicants for state dental examinations had to be graduated from approved dental schools, with the accreditation being conducted by the ADA's own Council on Dental Education. The number of dental schools declined as standards, mandated by the ADA and carried out by its Council, were increased. The length of the training time to become a dentist also increased. In more recent years, as the number of dentists have increased, the ADA has called for new dentists to have an additional year of training in a hospital.

The price of physician services and physicians' incomes will rise in response to fewer physicians, the extent to which it will rise depends upon the elasticities of the demand and supply of physician services. Barriers to entry in the physician market are consistent with a monopoly model that would confer higher incomes on physicians.

ENTRY BARRIERS AND CONSUMER PROTECTION

Next is an examination of an alternative hypothesis, namely, these barriers are a means of protecting the consumer from incompetent providers. For this hypothesis to be an accurate description of the justification for such restrictions, the medical profession, through its representatives in county, state, and national organizations, should favor all policies, not just entry barriers, to protect the consumer from incompetent practitioners. If the AMA only favors those quality measures that favorably affect its members' incomes while opposing those that adversely affect its members' incomes, then it should be concluded that the real motivation for such measures is to enhance the monopoly power of its members.

If the AMA were in favor of protecting consumers from incompetent physicians, one measure the AMA would be expected to favor would be re-examination and re-licensure of physicians. One justification given for increased training requirements for new physicians is that there has been an explosion of medical knowledge. Some physicians received their medical education 30 to 40 years ago; re-examination and re-licensure would ensure that existing physicians have kept up with this increase in knowledge. Re-examination for re-licensure is required in other areas, such as for renewal of driver licenses and for commercial airline pilots.

There can be little justification for favoring increased training for new physicians but not for existing physicians if quality and consumer protection is of concern to the medical profession. Yet the AMA is opposed to re-examination and/or re-licensure. If re-examination and re-licensure were required, then unless the passing level were set so low that everyone always passed, either a large number of physicians would fail the re-examination and be unable to practice, or different levels of licensure would be established to recognize what exists in practice. Namely, not all physicians are equally competent to perform certain tasks.

(For physicians to be board certified, they must pass additional examinations. However, a physician does not need to be board certified to perform various tasks. A primary care physician in California recently received a great deal of publicity when he started to perform liposuction, and several of his liposuction patients died.)

Not all physicians should be permitted to undertake all tasks even though they are licensed. With the realization that licensure should exist by tasks or by levels would come the recognition that it is possible to prepare for different levels by using different educational requirements. It should be possible to have lower training requirements for some tasks; as the complexity of the task to be performed increased, so would the training requirements. One would expect, therefore, that the number of entrants would be greater the lower the training requirements.

If different levels of licensure were to exist, barriers to entry would be lowered and the incomes of practicing physicians would be decreased. Since such an approach to increasing quality among physicians would decrease the monopoly power of physicians, the AMA would be expected to oppose re-examination and licensure by task.

The emphasis on quality control in medicine is on the "process" of becoming a physician and not on the care that is provided ("outcome") once a person has become a physician. Controlling quality and competency of physicians through process measures (which require an undergraduate education, 4 years of education in an approved medical school, a minimum of 3 years in residency) is consistent with constructing barriers to entry and raising training costs, thereby lowering the entering physician's rate of return. Once the physician has met all these requirements, there is no monitoring of the care that he or she provides.

Physicians may be well trained when they begin practicing, but this does not mean that they will be ethical. A number of studies have documented the amount of "unnecessary" surgery performed under fee-for-service payment; other studies showed that a significant portion of all surgery was undertaken by unethical or unqualified practitioners.

Virtually no quality control programs were instituted by the medical profession that were directed toward practicing physicians. It was for precisely this reason that in the 1970s Congress enacted the professional standards review organizations (PSROs) legislation in an attempt to develop peer review mechanisms to monitor the quality of care provided by physicians. The AMA opposed this legislation. If the medical profession were concerned primarily with quality rather than with monopoly power, the profession would place at least some emphasis on the quality of care provided by practicing physicians.

Requiring citizenship for physician licensure as a number of states once did (it is now unconstitutional) is another example of the use of entry barriers to achieve monopoly power instead of promoting quality. If a prospective physician has met all the educational and licensure requirements, a citizenship requirement can only be viewed as a means of preventing entry into the profession by foreign-trained physicians. Although the quality of foreign-trained physicians varies, examinations and other procedures, such as monitoring of care, would be a more direct and accurate measure of quality than whether or not the person is a U.S. citizen.

Similar to citizenship is the requirement by some professional associations (e.g., state dental associa-

tions) of residency in a state before a person is permitted to practice. A year's residency is imposed on dentists who wish to locate in Hawaii. Such a requirement, which forces the practitioner to be without income for a year, decreases the attractiveness to dentists in other states of moving to that particular location. Such a barrier to entry is unrelated to quality since it does not differentiate among the educational or performance backgrounds of the persons wishing to locate there. It is solely a device to enhance the monopoly power of the practicing professionals in that location.

It would appear, therefore, that the concern of the medical profession (as well as of other health professions) with quality is selective. Quality measures that might adversely affect the incomes of their members, such as re-examination and re-licensure, are opposed, as are any measures that attempt to monitor the quality of care delivered. The hypothesis that quality measures are instituted to raise the rate of return to practicing physicians appears to be consistent with the positions on quality taken by the medical profession.

It has been claimed that the selective approach to quality favored by the medical profession may actually have served to lower the quality of care available to the U.S. population (7). Once entry into a profession is restricted, the prices of those services are higher than they would be otherwise, and there is an increase in the growth and use of substitutes for that profession. Patients begin searching for lower-priced substitutes, such as faith healers. Patients also substitute self-diagnosis and treatment for the physician's services. Some of these alternatives may be of lower quality than if the restrictions on medicine were lower. Fewer, more highly trained physicians mean that a smaller percentage of the population will have access to medical care. When only physicians are permitted to perform certain tasks, even though other trained personnel might be equally capable of performing them, this will again mean that a smaller percentage of the population will have access to such services.

A relevant measure of the quality of care in society should not be confined to the care received only by those persons receiving physician services; it should incorporate the size of the population that does not receive any (or many fewer) physician services or that uses poorer substitutes.[1]

The current system of medical licensure, with its attendant requirements and emphasis on entry into the profession, imposes certain "costs" on society. The presumed successes of such a system of licensure in protecting consumers against unethical and incompetent practitioners are uncertain. What is desirable is the least costly system for alleviating consumer uncertainty and for meeting society's demand for protection.

Groups other than organized medicine are currently pursuing the measurement and monitoring of quality of care. Under pressure from large employers and business coalitions, HMOs, medical groups, and hospitals are being forced to collect and publish data on medical outcomes. Physicians are being profiled on the quality of care they provide, and provider groups (such as medical groups) have their own quality assurance programs. Information on patient satisfaction, outcomes, and quality of care is being made available by business coalitions to assist their employees in choosing a health plan and their provider groups.

State medical licensing boards and medical societies have remained passive and reactive with respect to monitoring the quality of care practiced by physicians.

THE PHYSICIAN AS A PRICE-DISCRIMINATING MONOPOLIST

The establishment of barriers to entry and limits on physician productivity under FFS provided physicians with a greater rate of return than if such restraints had not existed. However, a monopolist can

earn still greater returns if they were to become a price-discriminating monopolist. Profit-maximizing monopolists charge the same price to all of their consumers; that price and the resulting output would be determined by the intersection of their marginal revenue and marginal cost curves. This situation is shown in Figure 14-1. The profit-maximizing price and output would be P_0 and Q_0, respectively. The amount of "profit" in this situation is the shaded area between marginal revenue (MR) and marginal cost (MC). (The firm's profit is also the difference between price and average total cost per unit. But since in the diagram fixed cost and average total cost are not shown, the contribution to profit from each additional unit is the difference between the marginal cost and marginal revenue from each additional unit sold.)

When a monopolist is able to become a price-discriminating monopolist (e.g., first degree), thereby able to charge each patient a separate price for the same service, the monopolist's demand curve also becomes the marginal revenue curve. The profit per unit is the difference between the price along each point on the demand curve and the marginal cost curve at that price. To sell more services, the monopolist does not have to lower its price to all of its patients, just to

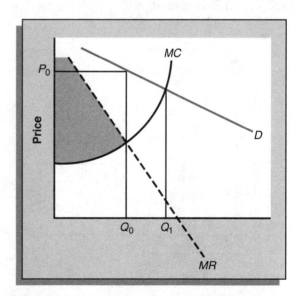

Figure 14-1. Determination of price and output by a profit-making monopolist.

---

1. Milton Friedman has claimed that quality has been adversely affected because there was less experimentation in treatment, which tends to reduce the rate of growth in medical knowledge since a person desiring to experiment in treatment must be a member of the medical profession. The profession also encouraged conformity in medical practice and discouraged malpractice suits against physicians by discouraging physicians from testifying against one another. This action also limited the consumer's protection against unethical and incompetent practitioners. The possibility of high malpractice awards would discourage incompetent practitioners from practicing, thereby providing protection to future patients.

those patients willing to pay a lower price. When the demand curve becomes the marginal revenue curve, then with the same marginal cost curve the monopolist's profit will have increased: instead of being just the shaded area, the profit now includes the entire area between the demand and marginal cost curve. The price-discriminating monopolist's output is also larger (Q_1) since he or she will produce to the point where the marginal cost curve intersects the demand curve, which is equivalent to the marginal revenue curve.

No single price is charged to everyone; the price-discriminating monopolist tries to charge each patient a different price. Because the profit can be greater if the monopolist can charge different prices to different purchasers for essentially the same service, we would expect monopolists to try and become price-discriminating monopolists.

Two conditions must be met if price discrimination is to be successfully applied in any market. The first is that the different purchasers of the service must have different elasticities of demand for the same service. Unless the elasticities of demand are different, the profit-maximizing price will be the same for each purchaser. The second condition is that it is necessary to separate the different markets in which the service is

sold so that the purchaser paying a lower price for the service cannot resell it in the higher-priced market. If such markets are not kept separate, prices will eventually become the same for all purchasers. Figure 14-2 is an illustration of price discrimination where the price elasticities differ between two purchasers or markets. Assuming a constant and similar marginal cost curve for serving each market, the profit-maximizing price would be higher in the market with a less price elastic demand curve, P_1, and lower when the demand curve is more price elastic, P_2.

Since price discrimination results in greater profits than would occur from setting the same price for each purchaser, it was hypothesized that physicians would attempt to maximize their "profits" by becoming price-discriminating monopolists. The necessary conditions for price discrimination are rather easily met in the physician sector. Patients paying lower prices for a physician's services cannot resell those services, thereby keeping the markets separate. The elasticities of demand for physician services differ since persons with higher incomes are willing to pay more than are persons with lower incomes for the same services.

Prior to widespread health insurance for physician services, physicians would price discriminate according to their patient's income; for example, a surgeon

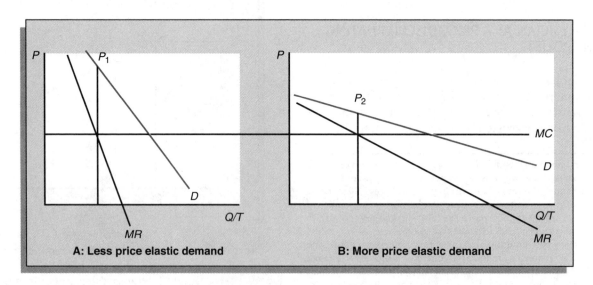

Figure 14-2. Determination of prices and outputs by a price-discriminating monopolist.

would charge high-income patients a higher price for the same surgery than a lower income patient. As insurance coverage among the population began to increase, the price-discriminating model would predict that physicians would still try to maintain their ability to price discriminate.

An alternative model used to explain physician pricing behavior postulates that differences in prices charged to different patients for the same service were because the physician was acting as a charitable agency. By charging higher prices to those who can afford to pay more, the physician is able to provide services to lower income patients who could not afford to pay as much. The physician thus acted as a charitable agency in determining who received care and how much each was charged. The medical profession used the charity hypothesis to rationalize price discrimination. According to the charity hypothesis, however, as insurance coverage (both private and public) became more widespread among those with low incomes, there should no longer have been a need for the physician to price discriminate. There was less of a need for the physician to charge higher prices to those with higher incomes.

When public and private insurance coverage for physician services was examined, however, it was observed that physicians still practiced price discrimination. Until the 1980s, physicians had the option of accepting assignment under Medicare. Physicians could do so on a case-by-case basis. When the physician accepted assignment, he or she agreed to accept the Medicare fee schedule. For patients who had a greater ability to pay, the physician could decide not to be a participating physician. The patient would then pay the physician's higher fee and apply to Medicare for partial reimbursement. The physician received a higher fee from the patient while the patient paid a greater amount out of pocket than if the physician accepted assignment. (An illustration of this form of price discrimination was shown in Figure 10-6.)

The same method of price discrimination occurred among privately insured patients, such as those with Blue Shield coverage. The physician could choose to become a participating physician or to bill the higher income patient directly.

To distinguish further between the two hypotheses and to test whether physicians acted as price-discriminating monopolists, it is instructive to examine the past behavior of county and state medical societies. In this way it can be determined whether the societies' actions and political positions have consistently been directed toward maintaining a situation that enabled individual physicians to price discriminate.

Unless a cartel-like organization such as a medical society were able to enforce sanctions against price cutters, price discrimination could not have survived in what would otherwise be a price-competitive market. Even though entry barriers existed, there was still such a large number of physicians that the market could have been price competitive. If one physician charged a higher price for a given surgical procedure, for example, other physicians could have been able to increase their market share by offering to sell the procedure at a lower price; price discrimination cannot exist in a price-competitive market. Higher income patients, when charged higher prices, would seek out lower-priced, equally qualified physicians. Prices for medical services would become similar to patients with different incomes. Differences in prices for medical services would be related only to differences in the costs of providing those services, not to differences in the patient's price elasticity of demand.

To understand how price discrimination could have existed in what would otherwise have been a competitive industry, it is necessary to examine the sanctions that could have been applied to physicians if they attempted to compete on price.

In his classic article entitled "Price Discrimination in Medicine," Kessel claimed that control over physician pricing behavior was related to the physician's need for hospital privileges and the prerequisite requirement of membership in the county medical society (8).

Internship and residency programs were once offered only in hospitals approved by the AMA. Physicians wanted the hospitals they were associated with to be approved for such programs since interns and residents increase the physician's productivity, hence income. The availability of interns and residents in a hospital enables a physician to see more patients and/or to have more leisure time. Interns and residents are thus demanded by physicians. The hospital pays the salaries of interns and residents while the physician receives the benefits of the services of a resident; the resident cares for the physicians' patients in the hospital. The Mundt resolution, which was declared unconstitutional in the mid-1960s, required that for the hospital to be approved for intern and residency training, the entire attending medical staff in the hospital be members of the county medical society.

Membership in the county medical society thus became important to physicians if they wanted hospital privileges, a necessity for almost all specialties of medicine. Membership in the county society was also a prerequisite if a physician wanted to take an examination to qualify for a specialty board. If a physician engaged in any form of competitive behavior that was branded "unethical," the county medical society, which determined its own rules for membership, could deny membership in the society, thereby denying that physician hospital privileges and access to specialty certification.

Those physicians who potentially offered the greatest threat to the existence of price discrimination were new physicians entering the community. To establish a market, new firms must advertise their availability, competence, and specialty, and also offer lower prices to attract consumers away from established firms. To prevent such competitive behavior from occurring, county medical societies gave new physicians probationary membership. If the new physician engaged in any of the above "unethical" activities to establish a practice in the community, the county medical society would revoke membership and thereby deny hospital privileges to that physician. Probationary status was granted, not just to recent graduates, but also to physicians who had been in practice for a long time in another area (and were members of another county medical society) but had recently moved into the community.

After the invalidation of the Mundt resolution, medical societies developed other sanctions for use against physicians who wished to compete on price. Some states enacted legislation proposed by the medical society while other states delegated their authority to the medical licensing board, thereby enabling the board to determine the conditions for medical licensure. Included in state laws and licensing board rules were severe penalties for advertising and fee splitting. Although the mechanism for inhibiting price competition among physicians shifted from control over hospital privileges by county medical societies to state laws that prohibited such behavior, the effect was the same. Strong sanctions and penalties were available to organized medicine (which may be viewed as a cartel) to inhibit price competition which would have eroded the physician's ability to price discriminate.

According to the above, medical societies had the ability to control price discrimination. However, is there any evidence to suggest that medical societies used the above-listed sanctions to maintain physicians' ability to price discriminate? Does the evidence indicate whether the sanctions were imposed for reasons of "quality" or whether they were consistently imposed on physicians who attempted to engage in price competition?

The AMA's position with regard to health insurance was the first evidence that Kessel examined in his test of the price discrimination hypothesis. Physicians would be expected to favor insurance coverage for physician services since it would increase their demand. Health insurance, however, can vary with regard to the way in which physicians are reimbursed. Indemnity plans reimburse the patient a certain dollar amount (or percentage) and allow the physician to charge the patient whatever he or she believes the patient can pay. Such plans are the most conducive to price discrimination by physicians. Health insurance plans that guaranteed medical services rather than dollars would be opposed by the medical profession because high-income persons can purchase the same medical service at the same price as can a person with low income. Medical service benefit plans are also price competitive with indemnity plans.

According to the charity hypothesis explanation of physician pricing, medical societies would not be expected to oppose medical service benefit plans. Thus the only conceivable reason for the medical profession's opposition to such medical service plans is that they undercut the ability of physicians to price dis-

CHAPTER 14 *The Market for Physician Manpower* • 365

criminate. Examples of such medical service plans are HMOs where the consumer pays a yearly capitation fee regardless of family income, and is then entitled to hospital and medical services when ill. It is interesting, therefore, to examine the sanctions that local medical societies have applied to prevent the development of HMOs, formerly referred to as Prepaid Health Plans.

The opposition mounted by organized medicine against early HMOs was unaffected by the location of these plans or their sponsorship. The first type of sanction, aimed at putting such plans out of business, was to deny hospital privileges to physicians associated with such plans. If the physician was already a member of the county medical society, the medical society would disband and re-establish itself without including the particular physician. New physicians entering the area with the intention of joining an HMO in the community would not be permitted to join the county medical society. Whether or not an HMO had its own hospital determined whether it was able to survive. It is for this reason that Kaiser Foundation, a well-known HMO on the West coast, operated its own hospitals; otherwise, it could not have offered hospital care to its subscribers and would not have been able to compete. County medical societies tried other tactics against the Kaiser Foundation. The State Board of Medical Examiners in California tried Dr. Garfield, the medical director of Kaiser, for unprofessional conduct and suspended his license to practice. In subsequent legal rulings the suspension was overruled; the board's action was considered arbitrary in that Dr. Garfield did not have a fair trial.

Another approach used by medical societies to inhibit the development of HMOs was to have a higher proportion of HMO physicians drafted during World War II. (The medical society played a strong role with regard to the drafting of physicians at that time.) Because they could not obtain a letter from their county medical society stating that they were members in good standing, a number of physicians serving during World War II were unable to qualify as officers in the Navy and had to serve as enlisted men. These physicians believed they were discriminated against because they were associated with HMOs. In other instances where local medical societies ousted

physicians belonging to HMOs, successful lawsuits were brought against the medical societies under the Sherman Anti-Trust Act (9).

In addition to attempting to terminate HMOs through the use of sanctions against HMO physicians, medical societies attempted to legislate them out of business. State medical societies sponsored legislation in many states (and were successful in more than 20 states) in having restrictions placed on HMOs, thereby inhibiting their growth. These restrictive statutes permitted only the medical profession to operate or to control prepaid medical plans. (Federal HMO legislation enacted in 1973 specifically preempted federally qualified HMOs from such restrictive statutes.)

Another example of the medical profession's desire to maintain physicians' ability to price discriminate is the type of medical insurance plan favored by organized medicine. Blue Shield plans were developed and controlled by state medical societies and (during the 1940s and 1950s) offered physician coverage to consumers under the following terms. For subscribers whose income was less than a certain amount, generally $7,500 a year, the participating physician would accept the Blue Shield fee as full payment for physician services. However, if the patient's income was in excess of the stated amount, the physician was permitted to bill the patient an amount in excess of the Blue Shield fee for that service.

The medical profession favored Blue Shield because physicians would be assured of payment from low-income subscribers and would still be able to price discriminate among higher-income subscribers. If physicians were charitable agencies, there would no longer be any need for them to charge higher-income patients an additional amount once the lower-income patient was able to pay the full fee for their services (using Blue Shield). During the 1970s, to be competitive with other insurance plans, Blue Shield plans either raised the income limits or dropped them entirely. As a result, a number of medical societies dropped their sponsorship of Blue Shield plans since physicians could no longer price discriminate.

Kessel provides additional evidence that the charity hypothesis is inapplicable for explaining physician pricing behavior in the following statement:

Most of the "free" care that was traditionally provided by the medical profession fell into three categories: (a) work done by neophytes, particularly in the surgical specialties, who wanted to develop their skills and therefore require practice; (b) services of experienced physicians in free clinics who wish to develop new skills or maintain existing skills so they can better serve their private, paying patients; and (c) services to maintain staff and medical appointments which are of great value financially. The advent of Medicare has reduced the availability of "charity" patients used as teaching material, and has led to readjustments in training procedures, particularly for residents (10).

The sanctions available to the medical profession for preventing price competition have changed over time. Advertising can no longer be prohibited by state practice acts. That the medical profession had been successful in inhibiting price competition is evidenced by the successful suit brought by the Federal Trade Commission (FTC) against the AMA and several medical specialty societies (decided by the U.S. Supreme Court in 1982). The FTC claimed that the AMA's "Principles of Medical Ethics," which banned advertising, price competition, and other forms of competitive practices, resulted in a situation in which

prices of physician services have been stabilized, fixed, or otherwise interfered with; competition between medical doctors in the provision of such services has been hindered, restrained, foreclosed and frustrated; and consumers have been deprived of information pertinent to the selection of a physician and of the benefits of competition (11).

The desire by organized medicine to maintain physicians' ability to price discriminate has influenced public policy on financing of medical care for many years. The AMA has always opposed any government program that required all physicians to participate according to a fixed fee schedule. The design of Medicare and Medicaid are indicative of the polit-

ical power of the AMA. Both programs permitted physicians to participate on a case-by-case basis and to be able to bill the patient a higher fee when the physician did not participate ("balance billing"). The economic power of medical societies (the threat to boycott insurers) similarly influenced the design of private health insurance plans. Initially, private health plans also permitted physicians to balance bill the patient.

Both the political and economic power of organized medicine has declined in recent years as other groups, e.g., the purchasers of health care (employers, unions, and the government) sought to lessen their financial burden and the applicability of the anti-trust laws to health care eliminated medical societies' economic power.

The medical profession has been successful in acting in the economic interest of its members. The medical profession constructed entry barriers into the profession to limit the supply of physicians. Under the guise of controlling quality of care and eliminating unqualified practitioners, the medical profession emphasized "process" measures of quality control. Quality assurance was present only at the point of entry into the profession by means of requiring attendance at an approved medical school, licensure examinations, and longer minimum times spent in postgraduate training programs; virtually no quality control measures were directed at practicing physicians.

The continually high rates of return to an investment in a medical education and the excess of applicants to acceptances in medical schools are evidence of the successful strategies of organized medicine in creating a static shortage of physicians.

With the authority delegated to medical licensing boards by the state, the medical profession was able to go beyond the establishment of a simple monopoly. The medical profession, acting as a cartel to protect the economic interests of its members, was able to establish and enforce the necessary conditions to enable physicians to practice price discrimination. The sanctions used by the medical profession against members who participated in prepaid medical plans were sufficiently severe as to retard the development of such plans for many years. The consequences to society of these actions by organized medicine were that prices of medical services were higher than they would have been otherwise, the availability of such services was less, and importantly, consumers were (and still are) not as well protected from unqualified and unethical practitioners as they have been led to believe.

PROPOSED CHANGES IN THE PHYSICIAN MANPOWER MARKET

The objective of proposing changes in the market for physicians is twofold: first, the demand for consumer protection should be achieved in the least costly manner possible, and second, the market for physicians should perform efficiently. The key to improving market performance is to deal first with the issue of consumer protection.

Entry into The Medical Profession

If a prospective physician can pass the licensing examination, it is not clear why he or she also has to have attended an approved medical school. The only logical reason for also requiring attendance at an approved medical school is that the licensing examination is not a sufficient assurance of the physician's knowledge. If this is the case, the examination process should be improved and less emphasis placed on the number of years of education required and on attendance at approved schools.

A second approach to lowering the cost of licensure, while also achieving a certain performance level of entering physicians, is to have "task" licensure. Currently, physicians are either licensed or they are not. Once licensed, they are permitted to undertake many tasks and practice the full scope of medicine, including a number of tasks for which they might not be well trained, such as in the case of the practitioner who is legally permitted to perform surgery, provide anesthesia services, as well as provide medical care to the patient.

Physicians should instead be licensed to perform specific tasks. Such task or specific-purpose licenses would recognize what exists in the real world: namely, even though physicians are licensed, the public would be better protected if they performed only those tasks which they are qualified to perform.

Task licensure would mean that all physicians would not need to take the same educational training; it might be possible to provide alternative levels of training (or train certain types of physicians) in a much shorter period. Different educational requirements would lower the costs of a medical education since both educational and opportunity costs would be reduced. If physicians wanted additional specific-purpose licenses, they could return to school and receive additional training before taking the qualifying examination for that license. (In this way a career ladder could be developed for medicine.) Under such a proposal, the training requirements to enter the medical profession would not be determined by the medical profession itself but would be related to the demand for different types of physicians and the least-cost manner of producing them.

Continuing Assurance of the Quality of Physician Services

As discussed earlier, once a physician is licensed, the medical profession undertakes virtually no quality assurance mechanisms. Several proposals to deal with the issue of unethical and unqualified physicians should be considered. First, periodic re-examination and re-licensure would require physicians to maintain their qualifications. Rather than mandating a certain number of hours of continuing education, re-examination would determine the appropriate amount and type of continuing education.[2] Re-examination would also be a more direct measure of whether or not the physician has achieved the objectives of continuing education. Periodic re-examination and re-licensure would be consistent with the earlier proposal of task or specific purpose licensure.

---

2. After speaking to a hospital's medical staff on the "Economic Outlook for Physicians," I received a letter awarding me continuing medical education credits, which my audience had also received.

(Several physician specialty boards require re-examination as a condition for re-certification, but the AMA has opposed requiring all physicians be re-evaluated for re-licensure).

If physicians were re-examined and re-licensed every few years for specific-purpose licenses, the public would have greater assurance that physicians were practicing in the fields of medicine in which they were qualified.

Even with re-examination, however, there would still be a concern about qualified but unethical physicians who perform unnecessary services and charge for services not rendered. Continual monitoring of the care provided by physicians is essential. Physicians should be assessed financial penalties which should vary according to the severity of their misbehavior. Penalties that remove or suspend the physician's license are usually considered to be so severe that they are rarely undertaken. Financial penalties would be more likely to be imposed for actions that are not sufficiently flagrant to call for removal of the physician's license but are in need of redress.

Unfortunately, the performance of state licensing boards in monitoring and disciplining physicians has been poor. Although there have been some improvements in certain states in recent years, the number of disciplinary actions against physicians varies greatly among states (see Figure 14-3). As of 2002, the number of disciplinary actions per 1,000 practicing physicians was 6.5 in Florida, 6.9 in New York, 3.9 in Pennsylvania, and 5.1 in California (12). Many states had much lower disciplinary rates. These numbers,

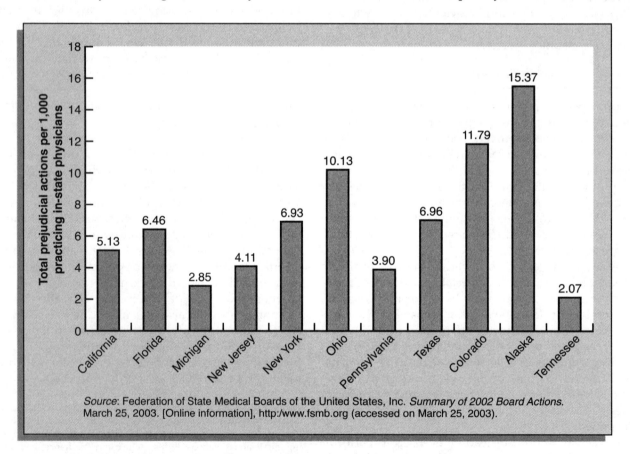

Source: Federation of State Medical Boards of the United States, Inc. *Summary of 2002 Board Actions.* March 25, 2003. [Online information], http:/www.fsmb.org (accessed on March 25, 2003).

Figure 14-3. Disciplinary actions per 1,000 practicing physicians, selected states, 2002.

although inadequate in many states, still represent a great improvement over their previous state licensing board's performance. In 1982, the disciplinary rates were 7.4 in Florida, 1.1 for New York, 0.5 in Pennsylvania, and 2.8 in California. In fourteen states the disciplinary rate was less than one per 1,000 physicians. In 1972, the disciplinary rate was only 0.74 per 1,000 physicians, which included a number of states that had not undertaken any disciplinary actions against their physicians.

There is no reason to believe that unqualified and/or unethical physicians are concentrated (at a greater rate) in some states more than in others. Instead, it is likely that variations in disciplinary rates across states and over time is more a result of the diligence with which the licensing board decides to pursue complaints against negligent physicians.

It is also unfortunate that for most states physicians who lose their license in one state can then move to another state and practice again.

It is difficult to develop appropriate incentive structures for these state regulatory agencies to act in the public interest. State medical societies are important contributors to state legislators, who would likely incur the displeasure of the medical association if they were to hold annual oversight hearings on the performance of the state licensing board. Thus other mechanisms must be relied upon to monitor physician practice behavior.

Malpractice has been the traditional approach used against unqualified and unethical physicians. The purpose of malpractice laws should be twofold: to compensate the injured party as a result of the physician's negligence and, second, to serve as a deterrence of future negligence. Damages to the injured party include economic losses (lost wages and medical bills) and "pain and suffering." Medical societies have, however, successfully lobbied many state legislatures in establishing financial limits ($250,000) on "pain and suffering."

Most instances of malpractice are not pursued. A 1990 study found that less than 2 percent of patients identified as victims of negligence filed a malpractice claim. And about 1 percent of patients injured through negligence received some compensation. Further, of those patients who did not file malpractice

claims for negligence, about 20 percent of those negligent injuries were serious, disabilities that lasted 6 months or more, including fatalities (13). Critics of the current system claim that the current system does not deter physician negligence since only 2 percent of negligence victims filed claims.

Reliance on the malpractice system alone, therefore, is insufficient to provide the public with assurance that physicians performing the service are qualified and that they act in an ethical manner. Reforms are needed to the current malpractice system to enable it to achieve its twin objectives, deterrence of future negligence and compensation to the victims of negligence (14).

The performance of the medical profession, state regulatory agencies, and the malpractice system in protecting patients against negligent physicians has been inadequate. One of the consequences of organized medicine's process approach toward quality and its sanctions for violating certain ethical standards was to prohibit the free flow of information on physician performance. Without the availability of data on physician performance, actions taken by state licensing boards, and comparative information on physicians, the public was less able to choose high-quality physicians.

It appears that reliance upon a competitive health care market might well be the most useful approach to improving physician performance and providing consumers with the necessary information to make informed choices. Informed purchasers, such as large employers and business coalitions, are beginning to pressure managed care organizations to provide performance data on the health plan itself and on the health care providers with whom they contract. As employers make this data available to their employees in choosing a health plan, employees will become better informed. Competition among health plans will be based on premiums as well as on other performance measures of the plan and on its provider network. Health plans and their provider networks are recognizing that they have a financial incentive to monitor the performance of their participating physicians.

It is important to understand the historical development of the physician manpower market. Many current policies are both the result of and reaction to previous behavior by medical associations. To understand the behavior of medical associations in the past, present, as well as in the future, it is important to understand the causal relationship between the medical association's economic interests and their political positions.

SUMMARY

The entry barriers to becoming a physician are a licensing exam, an educational requirement met by attendance at an approved medical institution, and increased training times. These "process" measures of quality control have been justified in terms of consumer protection. An alternative explanation is that these entry barriers were designed to limit physician supply and provide physicians with higher incomes.

If the medical profession were primarily concerned with consumer protection, then the profession should be expected to favor all quality measures regardless of their effects on physician incomes. Favoring only those quality measures that enhance (or do not decrease) physician incomes suggests that entry barriers are meant to increase physician incomes rather than protect the consumer from incompetent and unethical providers. In support of the latter hypothesis, it was noted that the medical profession's emphasis on quality control has been on the process of becoming a physician and not on the quality of care provided. The medical profession has not instituted any quality control measures that were directed toward practicing physicians. Quality measures that the profession should favor but does not are re-examination and re-licensure.

Charging consumers according to their willingness to pay (differing price elasticities of demand) would increase physician incomes more than if all consumers were charged the same price. The historical sanctions used by the medical profession to maintain a physician's ability to price discriminate were examined, as were organized medicine's positions on physician payment under public programs.

To enhance consumer protection, several policies, such as specific-purpose (task) licenses and periodic re-examination and re-licensure were proposed. Further, reliance on a price-competitive market in which large purchasers (such as business coalitions) require performance data from health plans and their providers appear to offer consumers more consumer protection than just relying on inadequately performing medical licensing boards.

REVIEW QUESTIONS

1. Contrast the use of entry restrictions in medicine according to both the quality and monopoly hypotheses.
2. Why does price discrimination result in greater physician incomes than a single price to everyone?
3. What are the necessary conditions for price discrimination? How well have the conditions for price discrimination been satisfied in the case of surgeons? In the case of primary care physicians?
4. What sanctions were available to county medical societies to prevent price competition?
5. What types of health insurance plans were favored by organized medicine (why)?

REFERENCES

1. A discussion of the reasons offered for licensure may be found in Thomas G. Moore, "The Purpose of Licensing," *Journal of Law and Economics*, 4, October 1961: 93–117; and Simon Rottenberg, "Economics of Occupational Licensing," *Aspects of Labor Economics*, National Bureau of Economic Research (Princeton, N.J.: Princeton University Press, 1962): 3–20. K. Leffler, "Physician Licensure: Competition and Monopoly in American Medicine," *Journal of Law and Economics*, 21(1), April 1978: 165–186 hypothesizes that the restrictions cited are in response to consumer demand. See also Lee Benham, "Licensure and Competition in Medical Markets," in H. E. Frech, ed., *Regulating Doctor's Fees*, (Washington, D.C.: American Enterprise Institute Press) 1991, 75–90.
2. Reuben Kessel, "Price Discrimination in Medicine," *Journal of Law and Economics*, 1, October 1958: 20–53.

3. Milton Friedman, *Capitalism and Freedom*, (Chicago: University of Chicago Press, 1962): 151.

4. Kessel, *op. cit.*: 27.

5. Ibid.

6. This aspect of licensing board behavior is discussed in Rottenberg, *op. cit.*

7. Friedman, *op. cit.*: 155–158.

8. Kessel, *op. cit.*: 29.

9. This example of Group Health Association in Washington, D.C., and other examples cited are from Kessel, *op. cit.*: 30–41.

10. Reuben Kessel, "The AMA and the Supply of Physicians," *Law and Contemporary Problems*, 35(2), (Chapel Hill, N.C.: Duke University Press), Spring 1970): 267–283.

11. United States of America Before Federal Trade Commission in the Matter of the American Medical Association, a corporation, The Connecticut State Medical Society, a corporation, The New Haven County Medical Association, Inc., Docket 9064, p. 3, December 1975.

12. The Federation of State Medical Boards. Annual Summary of Board Actions [Online information, 2003.] http://www.fsmb.org.

13. A. R. Localio, et al., "Relation Between Malpractice Claims and Adverse Events Due to Negligence," *New England Journal of Medicine*, 325(4), July 25, 1991, 245–51.

14. Patricia M. Danzon, "Liability for Medical Malpractice," *Journal of Economic Perspectives*, 5(3), Summer 1991, 51–69.

C H A P T E R

15

The Market for Medical Education:
Equity and Efficiency

KEY TERMS AND CONCEPTS

- Full-cost tuition
- Infra-marginal externalities
- Prestige maximization goal
- Private and external benefits
- Income Contingent Loan Repayment plans
- Opportunity costs of a medical education
- Optimal number of graduates
- Tuition as an equilibrating mechanism

Learning Objectives

Upon completing this chapter, the reader should be able to:

- Describe how a competitive market for medical education might theoretically perform.

- Describe how the current market for medical education differs from a competitive market.

- Evaluate the economic performance of the current market for medical education.

- Explain whether the existence of externalities justify medical education subsidies.

- Evaluate the equity of the current system for financing medical education.

THE PERFORMANCE OF THE MEDICAL EDUCATION SECTOR

In the previous chapter it was shown that barriers to entry into medicine have contributed to the high rate of return from becoming a physician. Perhaps the most important barrier to entry into the health professions is the requirement of having graduated from an approved educational institution. Since such educational institutions determine the number of new graduates, it is important to examine the performance of the medical education sector. Medical schools, dental schools, and other health professional education institutions are the main determinants of the number of health professionals in the United States. They have also been the recipients of large federal and state subsidies. Because of their combined role as the only approved health professional training institutions, as the determinants of the number of health professionals, and as the recipients of public funds, their performance should be examined in terms of (a) the economic efficiency with which this sector performs, and (b) whether there are any redistributive effects (the equity issue) in the manner in which this sector is financed.

THE ECONOMIC EFFICIENCY OF THE MEDICAL EDUCATION SECTOR

Every market performs certain functions; we are interested in two aspects of efficiency with respect to medical (and other health) education. First, is the industry producing an "optimal" number of health professionals? The appropriate or optimal rate of output in medical (or other health professional) education is concerned with both the number of graduates and their type (i.e., the level of training). Second, is the output (a physician or other health professional) being produced at minimum cost? Efficiency in production is judged on the basis of the extent of economies of scale in medical education (the number of schools) and whether each school is minimizing its costs.

To establish an appropriate yardstick by which the performance of the medical education sector can be evaluated, a model of a purely competitive market is used. In examining the medical education sector as if it were similar to a competitive market, we look for any divergences between a competitive market and the current system of medical education to determine the reasons (and justification) for such differences. Using the yardstick of a competitive model and any possible economic rationales for differences between the two, we will evaluate the performance of the market for medical education and, if need be, offer proposals for improving its performance.

Medical Education in a Competitive Market

Both economic and noneconomic determinants affect the demand for a medical education. The major economic determinant of an investment in a medical education is the expected rate of return. One component of the rate of return is the price, or tuition, of a medical education. If other factors, such as physician incomes and the opportunity cost of attending medical school (incomes earned by college graduates) are held constant, a change in the tuition level would be a movement along the demand curve for a medical education. Shifts (to the right) in the demand for a medical education are caused by an increase in physician incomes or a decrease in the opportunity cost of attending medical school.

Tuition, in a competitive market, equilibrates the demand and supply of a medical education. In the short run, with a given stock of medical education capacity, changes in demand for a medical education would cause a shift along a given supply curve of medical education; the tuition level would rise, and at the higher levels of tuition all those demanding a medical education would receive it. The level of tuition would serve as a rationing device, and there would be no excess demand (applicants over acceptances). The demand and the supply of medical education would jointly determine the number of enrollments and the tuition level.

The supply response in a competitive market would be as follows. In the short run, each medical school facing an increased demand for its spaces would raise its prices (tuition). The higher tuition levels would enable the schools to attract more resources, namely to hire additional faculty by raising salaries. As a response to higher tuition levels, additional medical schools will be started (entry into the industry). The long-run effect of the increased tuition would be increased medical school capacity.

Each school would not necessarily increase its capacity as demand increases; some schools might prefer to remain small and offer a "higher"-quality product than other schools, such as more inputs per student or longer training times. Tuition levels in such schools would be higher than in schools that had much larger class sizes and lower training requirements. Whether or not such differences in types of schools could exist would depend upon whether students demanded such differences in the quality of education.

Presumably, just as there are differences in tuition levels and in the perceived quality of undergraduate and graduate schools, there would be a demand for different types of medical education at different levels of tuition. In a competitive system, as in pre-Flexnerian days, the graduates of diverse educational institutions would have to pass a licensing examination. Some schools would have a much higher passing rate for their graduates than would other schools. Graduates from higher-quality medical schools would also find it easier to enter certain residency programs, achieve higher specialization, gain staff privileges at prestigious hospitals, have better liability experience, and be more sought after by certain medical groups. Presumably, the schools would advertise such differences as they would their tuition levels and other educational requirements.[1]

Not all schools under such a competitive situation would be for-profit. Some schools might be nonprofit and have objectives similar to those of medical schools today, such as prestige maximization. As long as entry was permitted into the medical education market, differences in a school's "product"—educational requirements, pass rate on licensing examina-

tions, and perceived quality of that institution—would have to justify the higher input costs, which would, in turn, be passed on to prospective students in the form of higher tuition levels. Unless students (or their parents) were willing to pay for such differences in quality, these educational institutions would either exit from the industry or, more likely, change their product to conform to what was being demanded.

The supply side of the medical education sector, then, would consist of many firms; economies of scale in medical education, such as in library and clinical facilities, are not large enough to result in only one school's being sufficiently lower in cost to preclude competition from other firms. Further, it would be expected that the schools would take advantage of any economies of scale that might exist in medical education since that would improve their competitive position.

Each school, in addition to moving to that size of operation that was of lowest per-unit cost (for the type of product it was producing), would also attempt to minimize its own costs of operation. Again, the incentives for cost minimization would come either from the school's desire to increase its revenues or from competition from other schools offering prospective students lower tuition levels. Needless to say, schools would be forced to compete among themselves for prospective students.

Thus a competitive market in medical education, with the only entry barrier into the profession being a licensing examination, would result in the following scenario. A variety of types of medical education (different training times, different input ratios of faculty to students, and so on) would be offered by different medical schools. Tuition levels would differ and reflect the minimum costs of producing different levels of "quality" of education. Medical schools would use different input ratios appropriate to the differing outputs they produce, they would seek to become economically efficient in producing their product, and medical schools would become more innovative in their teaching methods, in curriculum design, and in the institutional settings where physicians are trained, i.e., ambulatory care settings rather than in a hospital setting as has been the practice. A price com-

1. Not all professional schools are considered to be similar. Graduates from the Harvard and Stanford Business Schools are in greater demand than graduates from other business schools. The job opportunities for graduates of law school are also dissimilar. A similar quality spectrum would exist among medical schools.

petitive medical education system should result in greater efficiency in production, both for the individual school and for the system as a whole, a greater incentive for innovation, and greater responsiveness to demands for a medical education.

A competitive system in medical education, as just described, would produce an "optimal" number of medical school graduates which, according to economic criteria, would occur when the benefits of a medical education to the student equaled the costs of that education. The demand for a medical education, at a given level of tuition, would represent the perceived private benefits of that education to the student; tuition would also reflect the costs of producing that education. As the equilibrating mechanism, tuition would reflect both the costs of producing the education and the benefits received from it. The resulting number of medical school graduates would therefore be optimal, inasmuch as the costs of education would equal the benefits from it.

It may be argued that the private benefits under such a system are less than the social benefits of having a greater number of physicians in society. Under such a circumstance, the number of physicians would be too few. If there are external benefits to having a greater number of physicians (this will be discussed shortly), subsidies can be provided under a competitive system to increase the quantity of medical education demanded. The subsidies can be given directly to students which, in lowering their tuition, would increase their demand, or they can be provided to the suppliers. When given directly to the students, students would have an incentive to seek out those medical schools that will provide them with the type of education they desire at minimum cost.

The foregoing scenario describes how a competitive system for medical education would perform in achieving, at minimum cost, the optimal rate of output of medical school graduates and the different levels of quality in medical education. The crucial role of tuition in a competitive medical education market is to equilibrate demand and supply, thereby providing both the demanders and suppliers of medical education with price incentives as to the quantity demanded and the quantity supplied of medical education.

The Current Market for Medical Education

Under the current system of medical education, tuition does not serve as an equilibrating mechanism. Medical schools receive, on average, less than 6 percent of their income from tuition payment, as shown in Table 15-1. (For public medical schools, tuition is only 2.6 percent of their income while for private schools it is 3.9 percent.) Since medical schools are not very reliant on tuition as a source of revenue, it is not necessary for them to respond to changes in demand for a medical education. Further, for many medical schools, the operating funds they receive from their university are unrelated to changes in their enrollment levels.

Medical schools are able to survive and to produce the type of medical education they want because they receive large, relatively unrestricted government subsidies. (Revenues from state and local governments represent 14 percent of public medical schools' unrestricted support, down from 33.9 percent in 1979 to 1980.) The large educational subsidies received by the schools (and research grants and contracts that have also been used to subsidize educational activities) permit the schools to set tuition levels below actual costs of production.

According to several studies, tuition and fees covered less than 10 percent of the cost of education in 1972 and 15 percent in 1989 (1). (In 1989, this percentage was 27 percent for private schools and 8 percent for public schools.) When these figures were updated to 2001, tuition and fees were about 14 percent of the cost of education.[2]

---

2. A rough estimate of the costs of medical education were calculated as follows: Based on Table 15-1, total unrestricted support for medical schools in 2001 to 2002 was $39 billion, and there were about 66,000 medical students during that year. Assuming that educational costs were at least one-third of the $39 billion unrestricted budget, then the average educational cost per student was in excess of $190,000. Further, dividing the amount of revenue generated by tuition and fees (about $26,000 per student on average) by the estimated cost of education ($190,000) results in tuition and fees representing, on average, 14 percent of educational costs. The difference between the educational costs and revenues generated by tuition and fees is the size of the student subsidy. The same approach was used to calculate the costs of education and the size of the student subsidy for earlier years.

Table 15-1. Patterns of Support for General Operations of Public and Private Medical Schools, 1968–1969, 1979–1980, and 2001–2002 (Millions of Dollars)

	1968–1969		1979–1980		2001–2002	
Public Schools						
Number of medical schools reporting	47		73		75	
Total restricted support	$330	(52.0)	$1,102	(34.7)	$6,248	(24.7)
Total unrestricted support	305	(48.0)	2,076	(63.5)	19,045	(75.3)
State and local government appropriations and subsidies	171	(26.9)	1,078	(33.9)	3,539	(14.0)
Professional fee (medical service plan) income	38	(6.0)	359	(11.3)	8,291	(32.8)
Recovery of indirect cost on contracts and grants	38	(6.0)	105	(3.3)	1,511	(6.0)
Tuition and fees	16	(2.5)	89	(2.8)	655	(2.6)
Income from college services	3	(0.5)	36	(1.1)		
Endowment income	1	(0.2)	2	(0.1)	303*	(1.2)
Gifts	2	(0.3)	31	(1.1)	489	(1.9)
Hospital and clinics	—	—	191	(6.0)	3,145	(12.4)
Other income	36	(5.6)	185	(5.8)	1,114	(4.4)
Total public schools support	$635	(100.0)	$3,178	(100.0)	$25,293	(100.0)
Private Schools						
Number of medical schools reporting	44		46		50	
Total restricted support	$450	(62.8)	$1,283	(50.9)	$6,958	(25.4)
Total unrestricted support	272	(37.2)	1,240	(49.1)	20,400	(74.6)
State and local government appropriations and subsidies	17	(2.3)	82	(3.3)	182	(0.7)
Professional fee (medical service plan) income	28	(3.8)	311	(12.3)	10,667	(39.0)
Recovery of indirect cost on contracts and grants	56	(7.7)	215	(8.5)	2,115	(7.7)
Tuition and fees	36	(4.9)	219	(8.6)	1,061	(3.9)
Income from college services	19	(2.6)	23	(0.9)		
Endowment income	31	(4.2)	52	(2.1)	789*	(2.9)
Gifts	21	(2.9)	49	(1.9)	777	(2.8)
Hospital and clinics	—	—	189	(7.5)	3,414	(12.5)
Other income	64	(8.8)	100	(4.0)	1,394	(5.1)
Total public schools support	$731	(100.0)	$2,523	(100.0)	$27,358	(100.0)
Total medical schools support private and public	$1,366		$5,701		$52,651	

Sources: American Medical Association, *Journal of the American Medical Association,* 246 (25), December 25, 1981: p. 2929, Table 34; American Association of Medical Colleges, *2001–2002 Financial Tables on U.S. Medical Schools,* Online information, http://www.aamc.org/data/finance/2002tables/table2_2002.pdf (accessed on October 5, 2003).

*Endowment income for 2001–2002 includes both restricted and unrestricted.

Subsidized tuition causes demand for a medical education to be greater than it would be otherwise. This increased demand as a result of subsidized tuition, however, is not satisfied. The number of available spaces determines the number of applicants admitted by medical schools. The number of spaces, in turn, is unrelated to the demand for a medical education or to tuition levels; instead, the number is determined by the goals and objectives of the schools themselves. There is thus a continual excess demand for medical education by qualified students given the high rates of return to a career in medicine and subsidized tuition.

This excess demand is shown schematically in Figure 15-1. With an initial demand for medical education shown by the demand curve D_1 and the supply of spaces shown by S, the amount of excess demand for medical school spaces would be Q_1–Q_0 when the tuition level is T_1, which is below the equilibrium level. As physician incomes increase (or other demand shift variables change), there is an increase in the demand for a medical education to D_2. Again,

since tuition does not serve its rationing function, the excess demand for a medical education increases to Q_2–Q_0.

On what basis does the medical school ration its spaces since it does not rely on tuition to perform this function? It is hypothesized that the medical school will select students that are most compatible with the goals of the school. Because all approved medical schools are nonprofit, they must have an objective other than trying to make the most money. It is hypothesized that their objective is one of prestige maximization, which is accomplished by retaining a faculty that is interested in research, a low student-to-faculty ratio that allows more time for research, and training medical students to be teachers and researchers rather than family practitioners.

The average medical school is likely to try and emulate Johns Hopkins and Harvard medical schools with their small class sizes, low student-to-faculty ratios, and emphasis on research. To achieve these goals, medical schools and their faculties want to select students based on high academic qualifications rather than on their future work preferences, such as desiring to work in rural areas. (There is little prestige among medical schools in having the highest percentage of its graduates become primary care practitioners in a rural area.) The excess of applicants resulting from setting tuition levels below the equilibrium level allows the faculty to select those students who most closely correspond to their goals.[3]

Attaining the goal of prestige maximization requires medical schools to be free from competitive pressures. If a school has to compete, then, as we have

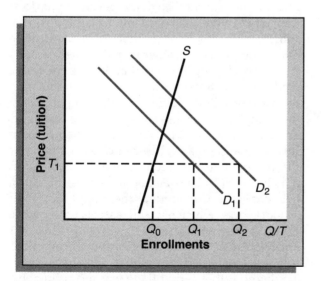

Figure 15-1.   The excess demand for a medical education.

---

3. It has been claimed that the reduction in the number of medical schools as a result of the Flexner Report and the consequent excess demand for spaces enabled medical schools to discriminate against certain population groups in society (i.e., Jews, blacks, and women). Reuben Kessel, "The AMA and the Supply of Physicians," *Law and Contemporary Problems,* Duke University, Spring 1970: 270–272. In the 1970 Carnegie Commission Report on Medical Education, *Higher Education and the Nation's Health,* they suggest that medical schools "Refrain from discrimination on the basis of race, creed, or sex and also pursue positive policies to encourage the admission of members of minority groups" (p. 69).

seen in the discussion of the competitive model, it will be forced to respond to the demands of students. Essential to freeing schools from competition are huge outside subsidies that relieve the school of reliance on tuition as a sole source of revenue.

Also important to achieving their goal are limits on entry into the medical school market by new medical schools that might have different objectives. The manner in which this restriction is achieved is through the accreditation process of new medical schools. It would be very difficult for a new medical school to start if its stated intention was to produce its graduates in a vastly shorter period, using a different curriculum and different input ratios to train its students. Because it might produce graduates at a much lower cost with the same probability of their passing the licensing examination, such a school would be a potential threat to other schools, and therefore it is in these schools' interests to prevent such a school from developing.

The Liaison Committee on Medical Education (LCME) accredits schools providing an MD degree and establishes the criteria the school must adhere to if it is to be accredited (2). For example, a minimum number of weeks of instruction and 4 calendar years for the instruction to occur are specified. An undergraduate education, usually 4 years, is required for admission to a medical school. Innovations in curriculum and changes in the length of time for becoming a physician (and to prepare for admission to a medical school) must be approved by the LCME. The LCME further states that the cost of a medical education should be supported from diverse sources: tuition, endowment, faculty earnings, government grants and appropriations, parent university, and gifts. By its concern that there not be too great a reliance on tuition, the LCME encourages the schools to pursue revenue sources and goals unrelated to educational concerns.

Medical schools must also be not-for-profit if they are to be accredited. There is no incentive for private organizations (such as HMOs) to invest capital to start a new school by demonstrating that they could produce physicians at lower cost and of equal, if not higher, than many non-profit medical schools.

It has been generally recognized for some time that medical schools are in need of reform. Since the 1960s there have been nine commissions to recommend changes to be undertaken by medical schools. A 1989 survey found medical school deans, department chairs, and faculty overwhelmingly endorsed the need for "fundamental changes" or "thorough reform" in medical education (3). However, because faculty promotion and tenure are based on research productivity and clinical expertise, they do not have incentives to reform the educational process. Instead, the faculty emphasizes the goals of their own academic specialty and department rather than the educational goals of the school.

What are the consequences of the current system for producing physicians? On the supply side of the market, the educational requirements for producing physicians are determined by the suppliers themselves without regard to demands for such an education. The product is relatively standard, and many years of education are required: 4 years of undergraduate education before admission to a 4-year medical school. The product is relatively costly to produce, and there are large variations among schools in their costs of production. There are strong indications, based on the wide variations in cost data, that the schools are not minimizing their cost of production, nor do they have any incentive to do so as long as they are the recipients of large government subsidies. It thus appears that efficiency in production is the exception rather than the rule.

It is also highly unlikely that the current system of medical education produces the appropriate number of graduates. Since tuition is only a small portion of the actual costs of education, the demand is much greater than it might be otherwise. (The price elasticity of demand for a medical education with respect to the tuition rate has been estimated to be approximately –0.4) (4). The demand for a medical education has continually exceeded the supply of medical school spaces, which have increased very slowly over time. As shown in Table 15-2, between 1946 and 1947 and 1965 and 1966, the number of medical school enrollments increased by less than 2.0 percent per year. Throughout this period there was a continual excess demand for medical school spaces.

The number of physicians produced was determined by the suppliers of education, either in conjunction with other organizations' requirements or solely in response to their own. The goals of medical schools appear to have been synonymous with the objectives of the American Medical Association. The AMA also prefers small additions to the stock of physicians. It is therefore in the AMA's interest that medical schools be nonprofit. The schools' incentive thereby changes from cost minimization to responding to increased demands for spaces to becoming prestigious.

The result of the constraint on the number of medical school spaces was twofold. First, there was a large demand by American students for a foreign medical education. Large numbers of qualified but rejected medical school applicants went overseas to study medicine and then re-entered the United States to practice. These American students were willing to pay a much higher tuition level in places such as Guadalajara, Mexico, to spend additional years in residence (thereby increasing their opportunity costs) to receive an education considered inferior to that received in U.S. medical schools. Second, as a result of increased demands for medical care during this period, the rates of return for practicing medicine became even greater in the United States than in other countries, thereby providing foreign medical graduates (FMGs) with an even greater incentive to migrate to this country. These FMGs came predominately from less-developed countries to work on hospital staffs and, in many cases, they provided the medical care for the urban poor in the United States.

The U.S. Congress responded to the demands by U.S. citizens to stem the inflow of foreign-trained physicians and enable their own children to have an opportunity for a medical education by passing the Health Professions Educational Assistance Act (HPEA) in the mid 1960s. The effect of this Act was to increase the supply of medical school spaces. It was, therefore, the perception of Congress that the medical education market was not producing an appropriate number of physicians. To achieve an increase in the supply of physicians, funds were provided for new medical schools, and existing medical schools received capitation funds on the condition that they increase their enrollments.

Although the AMA and medical schools opposed mandatory enrollment increases, medical schools

Table 15-2. U.S. Medical School Enrollment, First-Year Students and Graduates, 1946–1947 to 2002–2003

| Academic Year | Students | | | Number of Schools |
	Total	First-Year	Graduates	
1946–1947	23,900	6,564	6,389	77
1950–1951	26,189	7,177	6,135	79
1955–1956	28,639	7,686	6,845	82
1960–1961	30,288	8,298	6,994	86
1965–1966	32,835	8,759	7,574	88
1970–1971	40,487	11,348	8,974	103
1975–1976	56,244	15,351	13,561	114
1980–1981	65,497	17,204	15,667	126
1985–1986	66,604	16,929	16,125	127
1990–1991	64,986	16,803	15,499	126
1995–1996	66,906	17,024	16,029	125
2000–2001	66,295	16,813	15,901	125
2002–2003	66,677	17,120	15,704	126

Sources: American Medical Association, *JAMA,* 226 (8), November 19, 1973: p. 910; H. S. Jonas, S. I. Etzel, and B. Barzansky, "Educational Programs in U.S. Medical Schools," *JAMA,* 266 (7), August 21, 1991: p. 916; B. Barzansky, and S. I. Etzel, "Educational Programs in U.S. Medical Schools, 2000–2001," *JAMA,* 286 (9), September 5, 2001, Table 5; B. Barzansky, and S. I. Etzel, "Educational Programs in U.S. Medical Schools, 2002–2003," *JAMA,* 290 (9), September 3, 2003, Appendix 1A, Table 2, p. 1231.

were in need of additional funds. These congressional financial incentives to medical schools proved to be effective. As a result of the HPEA legislation, enrollments and graduates began to increase. In 1965 to 1966, there were 32,835 medical students in 88 medical schools. By 1980, the number of students had risen to 65,497 in 126 schools. See Table 15-2. (The consequence of this increase in medical school enrollment was a 50 percent increase in the number of physicians between 1965 and 1980.)

By the late 1970s, these large projected increases in the supply of physicians led to a concern, particularly among organized medicine and government, that "too many" physicians were being produced. As a result, the preferential immigration treatment for FMGs was removed, making it more difficult for FMGs to enter this country, and the HPEA financial assistance to medical schools began to be phased out in the early 1980s.

As shown in Table 15-2, between 1980 and 2002 the number of students in medical schools has been approximately constant each year, regardless of the demand for such an education. This limit on the number of medical school admissions is expected to continue as decisions on the number of physicians are made by the suppliers rather than the demanders of a medical education.

Efficiency, Externalities, and the Optimal Number of Physicians

The optimal quantity of output in an industry occurs when the cost of producing the last unit equals the additional benefits from consuming it. The price that people are willing to pay for that output is an indication of the marginal benefits they hope to receive from consuming it. When price is equal to marginal cost (as would occur in a competitive market), the marginal private benefits equal the marginal private costs of production, and the optimal quantity of that good or service is produced (assuming no external effects). Those persons receiving the benefits of the good or service are paying the full costs of producing it.

When the concept of marginal benefits and marginal costs is applied to the number of physicians, the optimal number of physicians is produced when the cost of producing physicians is equal to the price (tuition) of a medical education. The price that a student is willing to pay for a medical education reflects the private benefits the student hopes to receive as a result of that education. If the price that prospective students are willing to pay for a medical education is greater than the price charged for a medical education, too few physicians are being produced. More resources should flow into that industry until the cost of producing additional physicians equals the price that students are willing to pay for that education.

Under the current system of medical education, however, the costs of producing physicians are greater than they would be in a system where there were fewer artificial educational requirements, such as minimum years required both before entering and during medical school, and where there were incentives for efficiency. Thus even if tuition were equal to the full costs of a medical education, too few physicians would be produced. Since the price is greater than minimum cost, demand would be greater. And additional physicians could be produced if the producers were more efficient and tuition reflected those lower costs of production.

It has been alleged, however, that in addition to the private benefits gained by the student receiving a medical education, there are benefits to the public at large from having a greater number of physicians (5). According to this argument, basing the demand for a medical education on just the private benefits to be received by students would result in too low an estimate of the demand for a medical education. The existence of additional (external) benefits (to be received by persons other than students) when added to the private demand by students would result in a greater demand for a medical education.

As shown in Figure 15-2, MPB represents the marginal private benefits received by students from a medical education. MPC represents the marginal private costs of producing additional physicians. The intersection of these marginal private benefit and cost curves would result in Q_0 number of physicians. Q_0 physicians is believed by some persons to be a nonoptimal number, i.e., too few, because the external benefits to others from having physicians (MEB) are excluded from this calculation. If these external benefits are included, the sum of both the private and external benefits, shown by the line MTB, would intersect the MPC curve at a point to the right of Q_0 physicians; Q_1 would then be the optimal quantity of physicians.

The manner in which these external benefits would be included in the foregoing calculation would be to provide a government subsidy, the size of which would reflect the magnitude of the external benefits. To achieve the increased output, the government could provide a subsidy to the suppliers sufficient to shift the MPC curve down so that it intersects the MPB curve along the dotted line to the point where MPB and the new MPC result in output Q_1. This government subsidy could be distributed either to prospective medical students, which would lower their tuition costs and increase the quantity demanded of a medical education, or, in a competitive market, the subsidy could be provided to the medical schools, thereby lowering their cost and, consequently, tuition.

It is important to determine whether or not there are external benefits (and, if so, their magnitude) from having additional physicians. If there are sufficient external benefits, this would justify government subsidization of medical education so as to achieve an optimal number of physicians. (It would still be necessary to calculate the size of the external benefits in order to calculate the number of additional physicians that would have to be produced and the consequent size of the government subsidy.)

Before attempting to answer the question of whether external benefits exist with regard to the number of physicians, an externality should be defined. When someone undertakes an action, such as purchasing or producing a good or service in the private market, and this action has side effects on other persons or firms that are *not* taken into account by the normal operations of the price system, an externality is said to have occurred. Since the allocation decisions of others are affected by the initial private decisions that created the externality, failure to consider these secondary allocation decisions would result in either too few or too many resources in the market. There are different types of external effects, both positive and negative, as well as externalities in consumption and in production.

For public policy purposes, it is important to distinguish between technological and pecuniary externalities. The former are direct, non-market effects on others. For example, as a result of producing a product, a firm pollutes the water, thereby imposing a cost on those using the stream. Pecuniary externalities occur *within* the market, therefore it *does not affect* the market's ability to allocate resources. For example, as a result of an increase in demand by some participants in the market, the price is increased to all other participants in the market. Government intervention is required only when the externality occurs *outside* the market (technological externality) to correct what would otherwise be a misallocation of resources.

When externalities occur, the government, by calculating the extent of external costs and/or benefits and using a system of taxes and subsidies, should attempt to achieve the optimal allocation of resources. Such a process of non-market decisionmaking would involve the use of methodologies such as cost-benefit analysis.

It is not easy to determine the extent of externalities, if any, in medicine. With regard to medical research, traditional public health programs and water

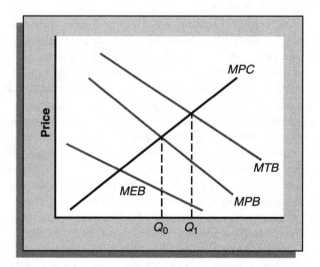

Figure 15-2. An illustration of external benefits in medical education.

fluoridation, the case for externalities seems clear. Individuals undertaking medical research do not collect from all who benefit from such knowledge. And since all those who benefit do not contribute to the production of that research, too little research would be undertaken if it were based solely on support from those who contribute. The government should, therefore, calculate the size of external benefits, levy the appropriate amount of tax on those who receive the external benefit, and subsidize the production of medical research. Only in this manner would the optimal quantity of research be undertaken.

An example of external benefits in personal medical care occurs when individuals include in their utility function greater access to medical care by those with low incomes—the non-poor benefit by knowing that the poor receive medical care when ill. Unless the government taxes the non-poor for this benefit, some non-poor would "free ride," that is, receive the benefit without contributing to assist the poor with their medical care. Government intervention in such a situation should seek to increase the consumption or availability of medical care by low-income persons. This can be more directly achieved through some form of demand-increasing program to such persons rather than by indirectly subsidizing medical schools, which may have little or no effect on increasing the availability of care to such persons.

The issue is, are there external benefits as a result of having a greater quantity of medical education or a larger number of physicians? Is it possible to specify the benefits that accrue to others—or to society as a whole—in addition to those who purchase physician services? Without government subsidies to medical education there would exist a certain stock of physicians which would be determined by the private demand and private costs of producing them. Are there external benefits to having more physicians than would be provided under the private market? (The total contribution of physicians may be large, but their marginal contribution has been estimated to be small.)

The case for public subsidies as a result of externalities in education has generally been made with regard to grade-school education: everyone in a democratic society benefits from having a better-educated

electorate. The case for public subsidies to higher education is weaker, and it is not at all clear that a case can be made for subsidies for a professional or technical education (6).

It is not enough to merely assert that there are external benefits to having a greater number of physicians and then to call for massive government support for medical schools. Not all externalities require government intervention. Even assuming that there are some external benefits of having a minimum number of physicians ("We all benefit by having physicians available in case we need them"), this would not justify government subsidies. The private market is likely to produce this minimum number. For example, externalities may be relatively small so when the MEB is added to the MPB curve, the sum of the two curves intersect at a point to the left of where MPB intersects MPC. Thus the private market will produce the optimal rate of output; it will produce more than the amount demanded by the MEB. (Visualize the MEB line in Figure 15-2 intersecting the horizontal axis to the left of Q_0, thus the optimal output is unaffected by adding MEB to MPB.) When the private market produces the optimal quantity, even though there are external benefits, it is referred to as "infra-marginal" externalities.

Since there is neither clear evidence nor strong argument that external benefits exist in medical, dental, or veterinary education, the case for public subsidies to the health professions' educational institutions on grounds of externalities should be reexamined.

There might be other grounds for providing public subsidies to the health professions, such as attracting a certain mix of students, or having medical graduates locate in an underserved area. Such subsidies are based upon societal value judgments rather than on externalities. The case for subsidies to medical education on other grounds will be discussed subsequently. These grounds include the improvement of equity in the distribution of medical care to the recipients, or the redress of possible market imperfections if medical education were to be financed through a full-cost tuition program. The equity of the current system of financing education (i.e., who receives the subsidies and who bears the cost) will also be discussed.

Some Proposals for Improving the Efficiency of the Current Market for Medical Education

An important imperfection in the current market for medical education is that there is no link between tuition and the role such a price variable should play on both the demand and the supply side of the market. When tuition acts as a price on the demand side (as would occur in a competitive market), then all who are willing to pay that price would have access to a medical education. There would be no need for thousands of Americans to pay higher costs to study medicine overseas. If medical schools were not provided with large educational subsidies, tuition would have to reflect all the costs of a medical education.

Allowing tuition to serve as a true price of medical education would encourage the suppliers to be efficient in production. If suppliers were inefficient and had to charge tuition of more than $100,000 a year (which is the educational cost per student per year in many medical schools), they would have difficulty in filling their spaces. It is highly likely that educational costs would be greatly reduced in a competitive educational market. Tuition would become a more accurate signal for determining the optimal number of physicians when supply subsidies are either eliminated or sharply reduced and entry by new suppliers of medical education are permitted. Efficiency in consumption as well as in production would then occur.

If tuition reflected all the costs of education and prospective students had to pay all these costs, low-income students might be precluded from becoming physicians. Only students from high-income families would be able to afford what would be very high tuition costs (e.g., in excess of $400,000 for 4 years of medical school). However, in a price competitive system (where quality is based on a number of examinations prior to entering the profession rather than on specific educational requirements prior to a licensure exam) full-cost tuition would be much lower than it is at present.

The cost per graduating student will be lower for two reasons. First, medical schools will have greater incentives to become more efficient and thereby reduce educational costs. Over time, the medical school has evolved into an Academic Health Center (AHC), which includes a medical school and one or more primary teaching hospitals. AHCs have increased the number of medical school faculty and residency positions in response to their funding needs, grants for undertaking research and payment for providing patient care, rather than for teaching medical students. Indicative of the AHC's response to research and patient care funding sources is that while medical school enrollment has been relatively constant over the period 1986 to 1995, full-time clinical faculty have increased by more than 50 percent along with similar increases in faculty salaries over that same period.

It is likely that if medical education costs were accurately separated from patient care and research costs, together with the faculty engaged in each activity, education costs would be much lower than they are believed to be.

Pressures to increase efficiency at the medical school and the AHC are occurring because of the increase in managed care. Managed care is reducing medical schools' clinical patient care revenues (derived from faculty practice plans and teaching hospital revenues), which account for almost one-half of the schools' budget. Managed care plans emphasize primary care while medical school faculties have been predominately specialist oriented. Medical schools have to reduce their costs and re-orient their educational objectives.

Second, educational costs will be lower because medical schools will also have an incentive to innovate in their curricula and in their teaching methods. As a result, the opportunity costs of entering the profession will be greatly reduced. Other countries, such as Great Britain, do not require a 4-year undergraduate degree before entering a 4-year medical school (7). Medical school deans acknowledge that the training times for entering the profession could be reduced by several years and the curriculum revamped. As one dean has said, "Despite the striking changes in patterns of physician education and practice, little change has occurred in the structure of the medical school curriculum since 1910." Further, there is ". . . the rigidity of the established system that is sharply demarcated by 4 years of college, 4 years of medical school, and 3 to 7 years of graduate medical education. The inflexibility of this structure has made it almost impossible to introduce new subjects into an already overcrowded medical school curriculum which, in part, reflects redundancies between college science and medical school science, as well as between clinical experience in the last 2 years of medical school and clinical experience during 3 to 7 years of graduate medical education" (8).

The opportunity costs associated with the long educational requirements to become a physician are more costly than increased tuition levels. In addition to receiving a physicians' income 3 years earlier, the student would save undergraduate tuition and fees if he or she were to enter medical school after 2 years of undergraduate education and one less year of medical school.

Previously, the Carnegie Commission Report on Medical Education recommended reducing the number of years in medical school from 4 to 3. Thus medical school tuition would be paid for only 3 years instead of 4. If a starting physician were to earn approximately $100,000 a year, each year that the educational process could be reduced saves tuition and adds to the physician's income. Tuition could be greatly increased each year to offset the benefit to the student of entering practice 1 year earlier. If, as has been recommended, the student entered medical school after 2 years of undergraduate education and medical school were reduced by one year, the rate of return to a medical education would not be adversely affected by increased tuition.

An important concern to many persons, however, is that under a system of full-cost tuition the medical profession would be comprised of only children from high-income families. To determine whether such a concern is justifiable and, if so, how to alleviate it, it is necessary to examine the "equity" of the current system of financing medical education.

EQUITY IN THE CURRENT SYSTEM OF FINANCING MEDICAL EDUCATION

In the preceding section we were concerned with the economic efficiency of the medical education market. It was determined that under the current structure of medical education, it was highly unlikely that (a) the optimal number of physicians would be produced, and (b) the production of medical education would be efficient. This section is concerned with the equity (i.e., who receives the benefits and who bears the costs) of the large governmental subsidies that support the current medical education system.

Based upon the estimate of the costs of medical education being at least $190,000 per year in 2001, as discussed above, revenues from tuition and fees represent less than 20 percent of educational costs, the average annual subsidy for 4 years of medical education in 2001 was over $500,000. The size of this subsidy (which would differ according to whether the student went to a public or private medical school) has increased over time as educational costs have increased faster than tuition payments.

These subsidies are in addition to those received during the student's 4 years of undergraduate training, since higher education is also subsidized by government funds. The subsidies received by medical students are generally larger than those received by other students in higher education and in other professional schools. The reason is that the costs of medical education are greater than the costs in other departments within the university. With such large subsidies going to each medical student, it is legitimate to question how equitably these subsidies are being distributed. Do such subsidies have desirable redistributive effects, or are they neutral with respect to their effect on incomes in society?

Income redistribution is based upon a societal value judgment that those with higher incomes should subsidize those with lower incomes. The provision of such subsidies (and the taxes to finance them) may be direct (in the form of cash grants) or indirect (in the form of grants in kind, such as lower prices for specific goods and services). Education is an in-kind subsidy to all those using it. For an in-kind subsidy to have desirable redistributive effects, low-income persons should receive a proportionately greater share of the subsidy, while the taxes to pay for it should come from those with higher incomes.

Some redistributive schemes may have perverse effects, as when a greater proportion of the cost is borne by lower-income persons and higher-income persons receive a greater proportionate share of the benefits. This occurs at times with Social Security, as when high-income aged receive benefits in excess of their contributions. A similar case occurs with high-income Medicare beneficiaries. In both cases, young low-wage employees subsidize high income beneficiaries.

In the typical market situation when a person purchases a good or service, that person receives the benefits from the purchase and pays the cost of producing it. The benefits are fully received and the costs are fully borne by the purchaser, assuming no externalities. With regard to medical education, therefore, are the sizable subsidies that go to each medical student neutral in their redistributive effects or, if not, which income groups end up subsidizing which other income groups?

An accumulation of evidence suggests that subsidies to higher education, particularly to medical education, result in a large redistribution of income; however, the costs are borne by low-income persons and are used to subsidize the highest-income groups in society. Such redistribution is inequitable. Hansen and Weisbrod's classic study that examined the financing of higher education in California and in Wisconsin determined that the size of the subsidy received by families that send their children to these state-supported schools is greater than the state taxes they pay for all state-supported services (9). On aver-

age, these families have higher incomes than families that do not send their children to such schools.

As shown in Table 15-3, which is based on the Hansen and Weisbrod study, the average income of families with children enrolled in the University of California system was $12,000 in 1964 to 1965. The average income of families with children enrolled in the California State College system was $10,000. The average for families without children in either system was $7,900. The average amount of state taxes paid by each of these families was $350, $260, and $182, respectively; the *net* subsidy to each of these family groups was +$1,350, +$1,140, and –$180. Because more children from higher-income families attended California's public higher education institutions, these families were subsidized by the remainder of the families whose income, on average, was lower.

Hansen and Weisbrod make two additional comments that are relevant to our discussion on financing medical education. First, the additional state taxes paid by the subsidized students, once they begin working and earning higher incomes as a result of their subsidized education, are less than the value of the subsidy they received (on a present-value basis). Second, a number of subsidized students never repay any of their subsidy since they leave the state. Assuming these results have persisted over time (more recent data is unavailable) and that the evidence in other states is similar to California and

Table 15-3. Average Family Incomes, Average Higher Education Subsidies Received, and Average State Taxes Paid by Families, by Type of California Higher Education Institution, 1964–1965

	Families without Children Enrolled in California Higher Education	Families with Children Enrolled in California Public Higher Education	
		University of California	California State College
Average family income	$7,900	$12,000	$10,000
Average higher education subsidy per year	0	1,700	1,400
Average State taxes paid	182	350	260
Net subsidy	–180	+1,350	+1,140

Source: Based on data in Table IV-12, p. 76, in W. Lee Hansen and Burton A. Weisbrod, *Benefits, Costs and Finance of Public Higher Education,* (Chicago, IL: Markham Publishing Co., 1969).

Wisconsin, then it is clear that prospective medical students (and others) receive substantial subsidies before they even enter medical school.

How are the subsidies in medical education distributed with regard to family income? Table 15-4 presents a comparison of family incomes for medical students with family incomes in the rest of the population for the period 1974 to 1975. Based on data from this table, it is obvious that the family incomes of medical students were higher than those of all U.S. families. Three times as many families of medical students had incomes of $25,000 or more than there were in the population at large. Similarly, twice as many families in the population had incomes less than $15,000 than did the families of medical students. The estimated median income of families of medical students was almost twice as great as the median family income in the general population.

The large subsidies to medical students, therefore, were going to students whose family incomes were much higher than those in the rest of the population. It was also highly unlikely that state taxes paid by the families of medical students were, on the average, greater than the subsidies received. The redistributive

effects of the subsidy method of financing medical education appears to be similar to the earlier examples of higher education in California and Wisconsin.

The redistributive effects of the medical school subsidies shown in Table 15-4 are actually an improvement over what they were in the past. In 1967, 20 percent of the medical students came from families with incomes greater than $25,000 a year, incomes that compared with only 2 percent of the families in the general population, a ratio of 10:1. Similarly, 42 percent of the families of medical students had incomes greater then $15,000, whereas only 12 percent of the families in the population had comparable incomes (10).

Data on family incomes of medical students published since 1974 to 1975 are surprisingly misleading. According to a 1978 publication, the highest income level used was "$20,000 or more," which characterized 46 percent of all medical student families (11). Since inflation has been causing incomes to rise generally, a larger portion of the population also ends up in that highest-income category. Thus there is only a 50 percent difference in the proportion of families in that highest-income category. Had higher income cat-

Table 15-4. Family Income of Medical Students, All U.S. Families, by Control of Medical School, 2001

Family Income	Private Schools	Public Schools	All Medical Schools	All U.S. Families
Total	100.0%	100.0%	100.0%	100.0%
Less than $10,000	1.2	1.1	1.1	5.3
$10,000–$19,999	3.2	3.0	3.1	9.7
$20,000–$29,999	3.8	4.5	4.2	11.7
$30,000–$39,999	5.4	5.6	5.5	11.5
$40,000–$49,999	5.8	6.6	6.3	10.2
$50,000–$74,999	16.9	19.5	18.4	20.8
$75,000–$99,999	12.9	15.7	14.6	13.1
$100,000–$249,000	39.1	35.5	36.9	15.9
$250,000 or more	11.7	8.5	9.7	1.7

Sources: 1. Data on 'Family Income of Medical Students' from Association of American Medical Colleges, MCAT, http://www.aamc,org, personal correspondence, January 16, 2003.

2. Data on 'All U.S. Families' from Bureau of Labor Statistics and Bureau of the Census, Current Population Survey, Mach 2002, [online information, 2003] http://ferret.bls.census.gov/macro/032002/faminc/new01_001.htm (accessed on January 16, 2003).

Note: Author calculations are for family income of students who reported their income (percent of students who did not report their family income is: 8.3% for private schools, 7.9% for public schools and 8.2% for all schools).

egories been used, the disparities in incomes would become much more obvious. A 1987 study tried to determine whether family incomes of prospective medical students relative to the population have been changing. After attempting to control for the problem of income categories with the highest income category being $50,000 and greater, the author concluded: "It appears that the incomes of families of students taking the MCAT (Medical College Admissions Test) have neither increased nor decreased to any substantial degree relative to the rest of the population over the period 1977 to 1983" (12).

Although it is undoubtedly true that some medical students came from families with low incomes, the major portion of the subsidy going to medical students goes to those with high family incomes. What is also interesting is that medical schools have shown favoritism when it comes to admitting children of physicians (13).

Another factor bearing on the inequity of the current system of financing medical education is that once medical students graduate, they enter the top 10 percent of the income distribution in society. It would seem unnecessary to subsidize medical students through their undergraduate and medical education to enable them to enter the highest income distribution, but on top of that, the students who are being selected to receive the subsidy come from the highest-income families in the first place.

In light of the foregoing discussion, the proposals of the Carnegie Commission Report on Medical Education (1970), suggesting federal subsidies to medical students and medical schools to result in a uniform level of tuition for all schools of $1,000, would worsen rather than improve the performance of the current system of medical education. At such low tuition levels, the excess demand for medical education would become greater than before. Since schools would all charge the same tuition levels, there would be no competition among schools on costs to the students and this would favor the most costly, prestigious schools: if the price is the same, why not go to the "best" school? Such a system would also provide no incentives for schools to be concerned with their costs because they would receive sufficient

subsidies to enable each school to charge only $1,000 tuition per year. A more desirable proposal could not have been developed by the deans of the most prestigious, high-cost medical schools themselves.

Are there any justifiable reasons for continuing a method of financing medical education that has the effect of worsening rather than improving the income distribution? Three rationalizations are offered for continuing the present subsidy system. The first states that if it is a societal value judgment to have physicians locate in rural and underserved areas, it is necessary to subsidize medical education (14). Similarly, if a change in the mix of physicians is desired, subsidies to medical schools are necessary. Further, some persons believe that since medical students leave the state that provided them with a subsidy, to prevent the state that is acquiring them from benefiting, that state should also subsidize its medical students.

The common fallacy in each of the above arguments is the failure to recognize that subsidies can be provided on a selective basis. For example, only those physicians locating in a rural area would be subsidized by not having to repay all or part of their educational costs. Why should all physicians be subsidized, especially since most of them locate in high-income, urban areas? Similarly, since only a portion of medical students is classified as minority students, why should the remaining medical students receive subsidies as well? If the purpose of state subsidies is to have its medical students remain in the state, then only those remaining in the state should be subsidized. By charging all students full-cost tuition, those medical students leaving the state would have paid their debt by having paid their full educational costs. Those remaining in the state could have, over time, all or part of their costs forgiven. This same argument could be applied to all persons, including lawyers, accountants, and teachers, who receive subsidized training and then leave the state to practice elsewhere.

A state should explicitly state the reasons for which it wants to provide a subsidy. The proposed subsidy would then generate discussion as to whether that is a value judgment with which others agree. Once a policy goal has been agreed upon, that objective could be achieved much less expensively by providing the subsidies directly to persons fulfilling society's needs rather than by providing a generous subsidy to all medical students. Similarly, if the subsidies went only to those participating in a particular agreed-upon program, more funds would be available to meet that objective.

A more sophisticated argument favoring subsidies to all students is that the sums of money required to pay for a medical education are so large that very few persons would be able to afford it. Banks would be unwilling to provide loans for tuition and living expenses with no collateral. Further, persons from low-income families have a higher rate of time preference (i.e., income today has a much higher value to the poor than income in the future). As a result, the poor will be less likely than those with higher incomes to invest in their own human capital (i.e., higher education). Also, undertaking an investment involves some risk that it will not pay off. Medical education is expensive, and future physician incomes may not be as attractive. If physicians have large debts to pay off, so some persons would say, they may select only the most lucrative forms of practice instead of serving certain population groups or perhaps undertaking research.

If all medical students were to be charged full-cost tuition, then such a policy would have to be accompanied by loan programs. A type of loan program that has been advocated by a number of persons is an "income contingent loan repayment plan" (ICLRP). The way in which an ICLRP would work is as follows. Students could take out a loan during the period they are in medical school to cover both tuition and living expenses. Once they have graduated and have started to earn an income, they would annually repay a fixed percent of their adjusted gross income. The fixed percent that would be assessed would depend upon how much the student borrowed (15).

By relating the ICLRP to the income of the physician, the program would not distort the preferences of physicians as to the population they serve or the type of practice they enter. A loan repayment plan similar to the one described would also minimize the risk to the student as to the size of the loan that would have

to be repaid.[4] Physicians' incomes have, in any case, been consistently high during the last 50 years. As investments go, an investment in a medical education would carry minimal risk and would be fairly predictable, as attested to by the continual excess demands for spaces and the willingness of large number of students to pay higher costs to receive such an education overseas.

What would happen to the demand for a medical education if medical students were charged the full cost of their education (and medical schools are no longer provided with education subsidies)? Would there be a large decrease in the number of medical school applicants? Assuming that full-cost tuition had been previously implemented, the results would have been as follows: The rate of return to a medical education was estimated to be between 15 and 22 percent in 1970 and between 14 and 17 percent in 1980; for many medical specialties, it was higher than that. It was estimated that the rate of return in 1976 would have declined to 13.5 percent with full cost tuition (16). Even at this lower rate of return, an investment in a medical education would still have been very worthwhile in that there would still have been an excess rate of return to medicine. There have been no recent studies to indicate the effect on the rate of return of implementing full-cost tuition today.

In any case, if full-cost tuition were combined with a reduction in both the length of the undergraduate

---

4. A problem with previous student loan programs was that former students nullified their debts by declaring bankruptcy. In 1977, however, "a new federal law went into effect that binds graduates to their student loan obligations even if they declare bankruptcy," *New York Times*, November 26, 1977: p. 25. A revolving medical student loan fund has been set up by Congress with the amount of funds available to medical students based upon the repayment of previous loans. A General Accounting Office study found, however, that medical schools were ineffective in collecting loans from their graduates. "Doctors Lagging on School Loans: Senate Panel Staff Finds Many Higher-Income Physicians Fail to Make Payments," *New York Times*, December 7, 1981: p. 13. For a report on federal loan programs to medical students, see John K. Iglehart, "Federal Support of Health Manpower Education," *New England Journal of Medicine*, 314(5), January 30, 1986: 324–328.

program and 1 year of the medical school, as discussed earlier, it should be possible to offset the increased tuition by the lower opportunity costs and the higher income as a result of entering practice 3 years earlier. There should be no diminution in the number of practicing physicians.

Medical schools would be forced to compete with one another for students if full-cost tuition were implemented. Once students have to pay a substantial cost of their education, they will become increasingly concerned with the school they select. Even if subsidies for medical education were provided to some students, the schools would have to compete for them. Medical schools would have to compete on the basis of their tuition since it would affect the size of a student's ICLRP and on their quality. It is likely that under such circumstances the schools will reexamine the number of years of undergraduate and medical education required.

Medical, dental, and other educational institutions much prefer that any subsidies go directly to the school rather than to the student. By subsidizing the school, the student has to go to that school if they are to receive subsidized education. It is for this same reason that schools prefer to distribute loans and scholarships rather than have the government or some other central agency distribute them. When the school distributes the funds, students can receive them only if they attend the institution distributing them. When students receive these funds directly and can then choose the school they wish to attend, the different schools are forced to compete for students.

SUMMARY

The economic efficiency of the medical education market was examined by contrasting its performance to that of a hypothetically competitive market. A competitive market in medical education would be more likely to produce an optimal number of physicians and at lower cost than does the current system of medical education.

One important difference between a competitive market and the current system is the role of tuition as both an equilibrating mechanism and as a source of revenue. The low levels of tuition as a result of large subsidies received by public medical schools and accreditation criteria regarding sources of revenue mean that medical schools do not have to compete on price. Further, since tuition is a small percentage of a medical school's source of revenue, medical schools have not been concerned with the costs of educating physicians.

Barriers to entry into the medical education market are a second reason for the current market's poor performance. The accreditation criteria inhibit the entry of innovative schools that would also reduce the time required to train a new physician.

The consequences of the poor market performance of the current system of medical education are that there is a continual excess demand for a medical education, there is limited curriculum innovation, educational costs are higher than if medical schools had to compete on price, and the time required to receive a medical degree is several years longer than necessary.

The equity of the present system of financing medical education was examined next. It was shown that medical students are subsidized through undergraduate education and medical school and then enter the top 10 percent of the income distribution in society. These same medical students often come from the highest-income groups to start with. There is also no equity-based argument why medical students should receive greater subsidies than students in law or those studying for a Ph.D degree. Proposals to improve the equity of the current system were suggested, such as having those students who benefit from an investment in a medical education bear the full cost of such an education. Specific value judgments of society, such as having physicians locate in certain areas, should be subsidized directly instead of rewarding all medical students regardless of whether they participate in the particular programs. A method to implement the concept of full-cost tuition, namely, income-contingent loan repayment plans, was suggested.

Eliminating medical school subsidies would also provide medical schools with the incentive to increase their efficiency and to innovate in teaching and curriculum if they are to survive. Once medical schools have to compete for students (bearing the full cost of their education), the length of the educational process would be reduced, students would be trained for the types of practice they enter (and what the managed care market demands), and the schools will have to develop quantifiable measures of the quality of their educational process.

REVIEW QUESTIONS

1. Describe the economic factors that affect the demand for a medical education. How is each of these factors likely to change in the coming years?
2. Evaluate the performance of the current market for medical education in terms of the number of qualified students admitted and the cost (medical education cost and foregone student income) of becoming a physician.
3. What would you hypothesize the consequences would be if medical education were to become a more competitive industry, like business and law schools?
4. What are the reasons for and against subsidizing all medical students seeking a medical education? How would you evaluate these reasons according to the criteria of economic efficiency and equity?
5. Currently, the public is protected from incompetent and unethical physicians by requiring graduation from an approved medical school, passing a one-time licensing exam, and continuing education. What are alternative, lower-cost approaches for achieving these objectives?
6. Evaluate in terms of both equity and economic efficiency: The Carnegie Commission Report on Medical Education (1970) recommends federal subsidies to medical schools and students in order to achieve a uniform level of tuition of $1,000 at all schools. (The subsidy would go to the schools.)
7. Medicare has been very generous in paying teaching hospitals for their residents. What would be the hypothesized effect on the demand for residents if Medicare reduces these payments?

REFERENCES

1. Institute of Medicine, National Academy of Sciences, *Costs of Education in the Health Professions,* Report of a Study, Parts I and II (Washington, D.C.: National Academy of Sciences, 1974). Paul Jolly, et al., "U.S. Medical School Finances," *Journal of the American Medical Association,* 264(7), August 15 1990, 813–820.
2. *Liaison Committee on Medical Education, Functions and Structure of a Medical School,* (Washington, D.C.: Association of American Medical Colleges and the American Medical Association), 1991.
3. C. Enarson and F. Burg, "An Overview of Reform Initiatives in Medical Education: 1906 Through 1992," *Journal of the American Medical Association,* 268(9), September 2 1992, 1141–1143.
4. Thomas Hall and Cotton Lindsay, "Medical Schools: Producers of What Sellers to Whom," *Journal of Law and Economics,* 23(1), April 1980, 55–80.
5. Rashi Fein and Gerald Weber, *Financing Medical Education,* A General Report Prepared for the Carnegie Commission on Higher Education and the Commonwealth Fund, (New York: McGraw-Hill, 1971): 131–132.
6. See Theodore W. Schultz, "Optimal Investment in College Instruction: Equity and Efficiency," *Journal of Political Economy Special Issue:* "Investment in Education: The Equity-Efficiency Quandry," 80(3), Part II (May–June 1972).
7. For some suggestions on how educational and opportunity costs might be reduced under a different system for providing medical education, see Reuben Kessel, "The AMA and the Supply of Physicians," *Law and Contemporary Problems,* Health Care Part I, School of Law, Duke University, Spring 1970: 276–278.
8. Robert H. Ebert and Eli Ginzberg, "The Reform of Medical Education," *Health Affairs,* 7(2) Supplement 1988, 5-38, quotes are on pages 15 and 19. Dr. Ebert was formerly Dean, Harvard Medical School.
9. W. Lee Hansen and Burton A. Weisbrod, *Benefits, Costs and Finance of Public Higher Education,* (Chicago: Markham Publishing, 1969): 76.
10. U.S. Department of Health, Education, and Welfare, *How Medical Students Finance Their Education,* (Washington, D.C.: U.S. Government Printing Office, 1970): 8–9.

11. W. F. Dube, *Descriptive Study of Enrolled Medical Students, 1976–1977*, final report from the Division of Student Studies, Association of American Medical Colleges for the Bureau of Health Manpower, Department of Health, Education, and Welfare, (Washington, D.C.: U.S. Government Printing Office, February 1978): 55.

12. Paul Jolly, "Family Income of Students Taking the Medical College Admissions Test," unpublished paper. (Washington, D.C.: Association of American Medical Colleges, February 17, 1987).

13. Bernard Lentz and David Laband, "Why So Many Children of Doctors Become Doctors," *The Journal of Human Resources*, 24(3), Summer 1989: 396–413.

14. An important reason why early loan forgiveness programs for physicians locating in rural and underserved areas were ineffective was that it was relatively inexpensive given the heavily subsidized cost of education for students to buy their way out of their contracted obligations.

15. The idea of an ICLRP is not new. It was proposed over 30 years ago as a means of financing higher education. Yale and Duke Universities have experimented with such plans. A good theoretical discussion of the ICLRP is presented in Marc Nerlove, "Some Problems in the Use of Income-Contingent Loans for the Finance of Higher Education," *Journal of Political Economy*, 83, February 1975: 157–183. The author also discusses the Yale Plan. A proposal to use such a plan for medical students has been proposed by Bernard Nelson, Richard Bird, and Gilbert Rogers, "An Analysis of the Educational Opportunity Bank for Medical Student Financing," *Journal of Medical Education*, August 1972. A computer simulation of such repayment plans to indicate their feasibility is performed in William C. Weiler, "Loans for Medical Students: The Issues of Manageability," *Journal of Medical Education*, June 1976. In 1986, Congress approved an ICLRP as a pilot project for ten universities.

16. Stephen P. Dresch, "Marginal Wage Rates, Hours of Work, and Returns to Physician Training and Specialization," in Nancy Greenspan, ed., *Health Care Financing Conference Proceedings: Issues in Physicians Reimbursement*, (Washington, D.C.: Department of Health and Human Services, 1981): 199.

CHAPTER
~ 16 ~

The Market for
Registered Nurses

KEY TERMS AND CONCEPTS

- Hospital collusion
- Nurse participation rates
- Vacancy rates
- Comparable worth-based wages
- Derived demand for RNs
- Determinants of a firm's demand for employees
- Dynamic and static shortages
- Federal nurse education subsidies
- Monopsony in hospital markets
- Wage disparity theories

Learning Objectives

Upon completing this chapter, the reader should be able to:

- Distinguish between a static and a dynamic shortage of nurses.
- Understand why a static shortage of registered nurses occurred in the period before Medicare.
- Explain the reasons for recurrent shortages of registered nurses.
- Evaluate federal policies for increasing the supply of registered nurses.
- Evaluate the concept of comparable worth as a method for establishing nurses' wages.
- Discuss alternative strategies for increasing nurses' wages.

A FRAMEWORK FOR UNDERSTANDING THE PERFORMANCE OF THE MARKET FOR REGISTERED NURSES

The market for registered nurses has been characterized by recurrent shortages. During each of the shortage periods there have been calls for government intervention and for subsidies to increase the supply of RNs. Economists have been concerned with the reasons for these recurrent shortages, whether they are the result of market imperfections, and whether government intervention is required to improve market performance. Because of the concern that market imperfections have caused recurrent nurse shortages, an historical approach is used to review the market for nurses and the appropriateness of government intervention.

To understand the various claims of a nurse shortage, the different types of market imperfections, and the subsequent massive federal support for nursing education, it is useful to first examine how a competitive labor market for nurses would perform. Government intervention to increase the supply of nurses would not be justified if the RN market were functioning similar to a competitive market. Other reasons would have to be examined to explain the demand for federal subsidies to nursing education.

If, on the other hand, it is found that the market for registered nurses has not been performing efficiently, certain policy prescriptions might be called for. Depending upon the particular reasons for its poor performance, federal subsidies might be one policy alternative; other forms of government intervention might also be appropriate. Only after examining the performance of the market for nurses can it be determined whether any justification for federal subsidies to nursing education exist. Also, by examining the effect of the federal subsidies we might gain some insight as to their intended as opposed to their stated purpose.

To understand the changing demand for RNs over time, it is necessary to understand the factors that both directly and indirectly affect the demand for RNs.

The Demand For RNs

The demand for RNs is a derived demand; it is derived from the demand for the institutional settings where RNs are employed. As the demand for medical services increase as a result of the growth in private and government insurance, the aging of the population, medical advances, and so on, the demand for those institutions, such as hospitals, outpatient clinics, skilled nursing homes, and home health care where patients are treated will increase. These institutions in turn have a demand for inputs used in providing care to those patients, such as capital for buildings and equipment, as well as labor inputs, particularly nursing personnel, RNs, licensed practical nurses (LPNs), and aides.

The demand for these inputs is determined by the initial demand for each of these provider organizations, that is, the admission rate per 100,000 population and the price paid for an admission. Hospitals (which provide more intensive care for a patient than, for example, nursing homes) will use a different combination of inputs than will the nursing home. As more severely ill patients are cared for and more sophisticated technology is used in these settings, the demand for RNs relative to LPNs will increase.

The institution's demand for inputs is also affected by the relative productivity of each type of input and their relative wage. For example, as the wages of RNs increase relative to LPNs, then, other factors held constant, the organization will begin to substitute LPNs for RNs (although not one for one since the RN is more productive than the LPN). Similarly, as RNs are able to perform more complex tasks (increase their productivity relative to LPNs), the organization will substitute away from LPNs to using more RNs.

The demand for an RN education is similarly derived from the institution's demand for RNs. As the number of RNs demanded and their wage increase, the rate of return to becoming an RN increases relative to other occupations. The result will be an increase in the demand for an RN education. Non-economic factors also affect the demand for an RN education. For example, fewer discriminatory barriers enabling increased opportunities for women in medicine and business will decrease the demand for an RN education, as would changing demographics, such as a smaller age cohort graduating from high school.

The factors affecting the demand for RNs have changed over time, which have caused changes in RN wages and employment.

A Competitive RN Labor Market

An efficiently performing market for nurses should perform as shown in Figure 16-1. Starting from an initial equilibrium point with the demand for registered nurses (RNs) represented by D_1 and supply by S_1, the equilibrium wage would be W_1 and the number of RNs employed Q_1. The assumption that the demand for RNs has been increasing over time would be represented by a shift in demand to D_2. With a greater demand for RNs, wages would be expected to increase to W_2 and the quantity of RNs employed to increase to Q_2. The increase in RNs employed (along S_1) would come from an increase in the nurse "participation rate," which is the percent of the existing stock of RNs that are employed, as well as an increase in hours worked by currently employed RNs.[1]

Thus the short-run effects of an increase in demand on the market for nurses is an increase in their wage from W_1 to W_2, and an increase in the nurse participation rate (and hours worked) from Q_1 to Q_2.

The long-run effect of the increase in demand from D_1 to D_2 is an increase in the stock of nurses, which is shown in Figure 16-1 by a shift to the right in the supply curve, to S_2. The new supply curve represents a greater number of trained nurses; as the wage of RNs is increased from W_1 to W_2, nursing becomes a relatively more attractive profession when compared with, for example, teaching. Assuming that all the factors that affect the demand for a nurse's and a teacher's ed-

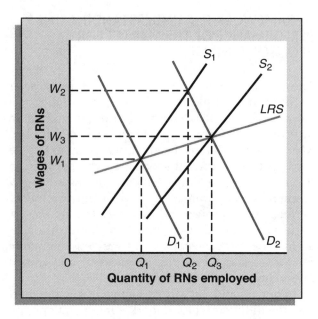

Figure 16-1. The market for registered nurses.

ucation do not change except for an increase in nurses' relative wages, some prospective teachers may instead decide to seek a nursing education. Changes in relative wages between professions do not have the same effect on all prospective students. Those who are "at the margin," i.e., perhaps prefer each profession equally, are likely to be the ones who switch careers with a change in relative incomes.

Both S_1 and S_2 are short-run supply curves for nurses; each represents the supply of nurses (hours and participation rates) for a given stock of nurses. The long-run supply curve for nurses is shown by LRS, which represents the number of persons that will become nurses over time in response to higher wages. As supply increases from S_1 to S_2, the wage rate will fall from W_2 to W_3. (Wages may not fall in absolute terms but decline relative to comparable professions as wages in other professions increase more rapidly.)

An efficiently performing RN market would, in the short run, have the following outcomes following an increase in demand:

---

1. For the majority of trained nurses who are women, a number of factors influence whether or not she will seek employment. Her wage is only one such factor. Whether she has young children and her husband's income are additional factors. However, if nurses' wages increase and all other factors remain unchanged, some inactive nurses will decide to become active.

- an increase in RN wages;

- an increase in the rate of return to being an RN, both in absolute terms and relative to other occupations;

- an increase in the RN participation rate, leading to an increase in the number of RNs employed; and

- an increase in the use of substitutes. As RN wages increase, RNs become more expensive relative to other types of nurses. Employers will substitute away from using RNs to greater use of other nursing personnel whose wages have not increased as rapidly.

Competitive markets, however, do not adjust immediately to an increase in demand. As observed in Figure 16-1, with an increase in demand from D_1 to D_2, wages would rise, the number of employed nurses would increase—in the short run through an increase in their participation rate, and in the long run through an increase in the number of persons becoming nurses (a shift to the right in the supply curve). Until the market reaches equilibrium, however, a dynamic shortage might occur. As their demand for RNs increase, the major employers of nurses may not know how much they have to increase nurses' wages to bring about an increase in their employment; similarly, it takes time for working nurses to learn which hospitals are paying higher wages and for inactive nurses both to learn of the increase in wages and to decide to become active again.

A dynamic shortage for RNs is illustrated in Figure 16-2. With the increase in demand from D_1 to D_2, the demand for RNs will initially be Q_2, which is at the old wage W_1 on the new demand curve D_2. Thus, in a dynamic shortage, until information becomes available to nurse employers that they have to raise wages to hire more nurses and to nurses that they could receive higher wages if they were to become active, there will be a shortage of magnitude Q_1–Q_2. A shortage will be indicated by an increase in nurse vacancies which are budgeted but unfilled positions. As RN wages increase and eventually reach W_2, the shortage will decrease, meaning that those employers who are

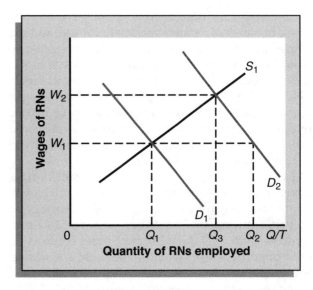

Figure 16-2. A dynamic shortage in the market for registered nurses.

willing to pay the higher price will be able to employ more nurses.

The existence of a dynamic shortage is a temporary phenomenon and will disappear over time. Unless demand for RNs continues to increase faster than the supply of RNs, equilibrium will eventually occur.

Empirical evidence of a dynamic shortage would be nurse vacancies (generally greater than 5 percent), rising (relative) nurse wages, increased RN employment, an increase in RN participation rates, and greater use of substitutes. Federal subsidies to increase the supply of nurses to resolve a dynamic shortage have no economic justification.

A static shortage in which nurses' wages are prevented from reaching equilibrium is the result of interference with a competitive market. A static shortage is illustrated in Figure 16-2. With an increase in demand from D_1 to D_2, the quantity of nurses demanded at the old wage would be Q_2. If the wage is below the equilibrium level and is prevented from rising, the shortage, Q_1–Q_2, will not disappear. In distinguishing between a static and a dynamic shortage, vacancy rates for nurses would be observed in both cases, however in a static shortage RN wages and participation rates will not increase. In both cases we would expect substitution away from the use of RNs to occur because it is more difficult to employ as many RNs as employers would like, in one case because nurses' wages have gone up and they have become relatively more expensive to employ (dynamic shortage), in the other because employers cannot hire all the nurses they would like at the old wage.

Depending upon the reason for a static shortage, government intervention is required. At times government action may have caused the shortage, as occurred during the imposition of wage and price controls from 1971 to 1974. Had these controls not been imposed, wages would have risen, and a shortage would not have occurred. The shortage ended when wage and price controls were eliminated. If the

shortage was caused by hospitals' anti-competitive behavior, then enforcement of the anti-trust laws would be appropriate. Again, federal subsidies to reduce a static shortage would not be justified. It would be more efficient (less costly) to merely eliminate the market imperfection that prevents wages from rising.

Having specified the measures of performance for determining which of the foregoing market descriptions best characterized the market for nurses, we now turn to an examination of the data.

THE PERFORMANCE OF THE MARKET FOR REGISTERED NURSES

Nurses are predominantly employed in hospitals. As shown in Figure 16-3, of the 2,201,813 registered

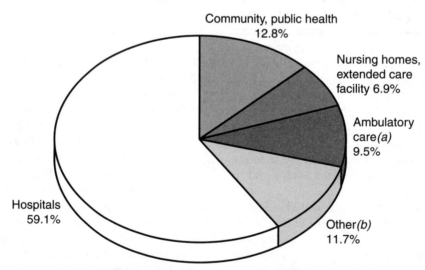

Total number of active registered nurses = 2,201,813

(a) 'Ambulatory care' includes physician or nurse solo or group practices and HMOs.
(b) 'Other' includes nursing education, student health service, occupational health, planning or licensing agency, and insurance companies.

Source: U.S. Department of Health and Human Services, Health Resources and Services Administration, Bureau of Health Professions, Division of Nursing. *The Registered Nurse Population, March 2000. Findings from the National Sample Survey of Registered Nurses*. September 2001: table 13.

Figure 16-3. Distribution of active registered nurses by place of employment, 2000.

nurses employed in 2000, 59 percent were working in hospitals. The remaining places of employment and their respective percentages were: nursing homes (6.9 percent), community or public health (12.8 percent), ambulatory care (9.5 percent), and other (11.7 percent). Thus what happens in the hospital sector has the largest effect on the employment of registered nurses.

The Market for Nurses Before Medicare and Medicaid

The demand for hospital care (hence the derived demand for RNs) has been changing over time, as described in the chapter on hospitals. Admissions and patient days in short-term general and other special hospitals (which have approximately 80 percent of all hospital admissions) had been increasing (until the early 1980s) as a result of an aging population, rising incomes and health insurance coverage, and Medicare and Medicaid, which started in 1966 and lowered the cost of hospital care to the aged and the poor. Advances in medical knowledge changed the nature of the hospital from a place that provided chronic care to an institution that provides acute care. Also, medical technology increased demands for RNs per patient day—for example, in intensive care units. Thus there was an increase in use of medical care, more of this care was provided in hospitals, and the demand for RNs increased also because of greater use of RNs in nurse staffing. An increase in the responsibilities delegated to RNs for tasks formerly performed by physicians in hospitals further increased their demand.

As a result of the above forces increasing RN demand, use of general duty nurses per patient (in nonfederal hospitals) between 1949 and 1966 increased by 65 percent (1).[2] A dynamic shortage would have been

Table 16-1. Vacancy Rates in Hospitals for General-Duty Nurses

Year	Vacancy Rate	Year	Vacancy Rate
1953	14.6	1967	18.1
1954	13.0	1968	15.0
1956	16.8	1969	11.2
1958	13.0	1971	9.3
1962	23.0		

Sources: Reprinted by permission of the publisher, from Donald E. Yett, *An Economic Analysis of the Nurse Shortage*, (Lexington, MA: Lexington Books, D.C. Health Co., 1975); copyright 1975, D.C. Health Co., p. 138, Table 3-13.

expected to occur with such a large increase in demand for RNs. Increased nurse vacancy rates, nurses' salaries, participation rates, and substitution toward the use of non-RN nurses would have been expected. As shown in Table 16-1, nurse vacancy rates were high during the 1950s, reaching a peak of 23 percent in 1962.

Other indicators of a dynamic nursing shortage, however, provide inconsistent results. Although nurses' wages rose similar to other comparable professions over a longer time period, between 1946 and 1966 nurses' salaries increased less rapidly than other professions. After 1966, nurses' salaries increased more rapidly, with hospital RN wages increasing faster than all RN wages over the longer period.

According to Table 16-2, between 1946 and 1966 the ratio of "All RN" salaries to those of teachers was approximately equal in 1946 at 1.03, for hospital RNs it was 0.95. The comparable ratios of "All RNs and Hospital RNs" to "Female Professional, Technical, and Kindred Workers" were 1.05 and 0.97 respectively. Throughout the remainder of the 1940s, 1950s, and early 1960s, RN wages declined relative to these other occupational groups. These ratios declined to a low around 1963 where, for example, Hospital RN salaries were only 0.73 of Teachers' salaries. The same decline occurred for RNs relative to other occupations in which women were predominantly employed.

After Medicare and Medicaid were enacted, RN salaries increased faster than those of Teachers or other female occupations. By 1972, RN wages, particularly Hospital RNs, once again exceeded those of other female occupations, rising to 1.10 and 1.08 for

---

2. A demand function for RNs in short-term hospitals was estimated by Donald E. Yett, et al., and it was determined that the effect of a 1 percent increase in patient days would result in a 0.86 percent increase in RNs in hospitals of 200 or more beds. The effect of a 1 percent increase in RN wages would lead to a –1.75 percent decrease in number of RNs employed, and the cross-elasticity of demand for RNs with respect to the wages of aides was 1.43. D. Yett, L. Drabek, L. Kimball, and M. Intriligator, A Forecasting and Policy Simulation Model of the Health Care Sector, (Lexington, Mass.: Lexington Books, 1979), p. 95.

Table 16-2. Ratio of all Registered Nurses' and Hospital General-Duty Registered Nurses' Salaries to Those of Teachers and Female Professional, Technical, and Kindred Workers

Year	Female Professional, Technical, and Kindred Workers		Teachers	
	All RNs	Hospital RNs	All RNs	Hospital RNs
1946	1.05	0.97	1.03	0.95
1948	1.00	0.95	0.92	0.87
1951	0.97	0.92	0.86	0.82
1954	0.89	0.82	0.82	0.76
1957	0.91	0.85	0.79	0.74
1961	0.86	0.79	0.77	0.70
1963	0.90	0.87	0.75	0.73
1966	0.93	0.87	0.79	0.73
1969	1.02	0.95	0.87	0.81
1972	1.10	1.08	0.97	0.96
1975	1.08	1.08	0.96	0.96

Source: Donald E. Yett, *An Economic Analysis of the Nurse Shortage,* (Lexington, MA: Lexington Books, 1975).

All RNs and for Hospital RNs. With respect to Teachers, the Hospital RN ratio was similar to what had existed in the 1940s.

Based on the above data on relative wages, it would appear that there was a relative *surplus* rather than a relative shortage of nurses before 1966. An RN surplus would be characterized by RN supply increasing faster than demand for RNs, leading to falling relative wages (RNs to other female workers) and a declining relative rate of return to a nursing career. Comparing data on relative rates of return to a nursing education to "females with 1 to 3 years of college training" again appear to indicate that RNs were in surplus. From 1946, the relative rate of return to nursing declined, reaching a low in 1961, indicating women could receive a higher rate of return by entering an occupation other than nursing. By the late 1960s and early 1970s, however, the relative rate of return to nursing had increased.

Of interest is that in the period before 1966, nurse wage increases were not uniform according to place of nurse employment. Wages (nominal) increased much more rapidly between 1946 and 1966 for nurse education (224 percent) and school nurses (215 percent) than for hospital-employed nurses (157 per-

cent). After 1966, the opposite occurred as hospital nurses experienced the largest percent increase in their wages.

Consistent with these RN wage increases by place of employment, the number of nurses employed in nonfederal hospitals increased by 109 percent between 1949 and 1966. However, the increase in the number of nurses employed in nurse education positions and in other areas that had larger percent wage increases was much greater, 254 percent.

Relatively large increases in nurses' wages in nonhospital markets led to correspondingly large increases in nurse supply. The percent increase in nurse employment was greater in the non-hospital sector which, at that time, employed only 23 percent of all nurses. Surprisingly, if there were no barriers to RNs moving between the hospital and non-hospital sectors and if the training costs were similar, one would expect wage increases to be similar in both sectors, yet nurses in the non-hospital sectors received higher wage increases.

Although the relative salary differential of RNs to other nurses (i.e., LPNs and aides) changed very little (until the mid 1980s), a great deal of substitution occurred (as shown in Table 16-3). From 1949 to 1966, the ratio of RNs to LPNs decreased, from 6.25 in 1949 to 2.22 in 1966. Substitution would be expected if salary differentials increased or if there was a change in relative productivity (changes in productivity should be reflected in changes in relative salaries). There was, however, virtually no change in their relative salaries over this period. The downward trend in the use of RNs relative to LPNs began to reverse itself beginning in the early 1970s with the use of RNs relative to LPNs increasing from 1.96 in 1970 to 2.70 in 1980 to 4.8 in 1990 and to 7.7 by 2000. (The decline in the use of LPNs continued into the 1990s even though their wages relative to RNs also declined; this change in staffing pattern is discussed later.)

Based on the above data, what can one conclude about how well the market for RNs was performing? Beginning in the late 1940s, the base period for comparison with changes over time and with other occupations, nursing appeared to be a relatively attractive profession from a financial standpoint. Its rate of return was slightly higher than comparable professions. From that base period to the mid 1960s, however, the relative financial attractiveness of a nursing career declined. With a smaller increase in wages and a decline in relative rates of return, fewer persons would be expected to enter nursing. This data would be more indicative of an RN surplus (i.e., demand increasing less rapidly than supply, resulting in a decline in the relative wage of nurses) rather than a shortage.

The common belief during this period, however, was that there was an RN shortage; practical nurses were being substituted for RNs, and RN vacancy rates in hospitals were increasing. Contrary to a shortage, however, RN wages (and their rates of return) were not rising relative to comparable professions or to practical nurses.

Throughout this period, hospital associations complained about the shortage of registered nurses. The evidence used to support such claims was data on vacancy statistics of unfilled nursing positions in hospitals and studies using the ratio of registered nurses to the population. For example, in 1956, it was estimated that there was a shortage of 70,000 nurses in the United States and (in 1963) that by 1970 the magnitude of the shortage would reach 200,000 nurses. Vacancy rates increased from between 13 and 16 percent in the mid 1950s to 23 percent by 1962.

As a result of these claims of a shortage of RNs, the U.S. Congress in 1964 passed the Nurse Training Act (NTA) which provided $300 million over a 5-year period to alleviate the alleged shortage. (The NTA was subsequently renewed and amended many times. Periodic concerns of RN shortages led to almost $3 billion being authorized by the U.S. government to alleviate various nurse shortages.)

A static shortage was the only type of market situation that logically incorporated the contradictory data of falling relative RN wages and increasing vacancy rates. The nurses' market was essentially in equilibrium during the period 1946 to 1949, as shown by the intersection of the demand and supply curves D_1 and S_1 in Figure 16-2. As the demand for hospital care increased bringing with it an increased demand for RNs, the demand curve shifted to D_2. If hospital RN wages were kept below the new equilibrium wage, Q_1–Q_2 would represent the size of the shortage (i.e., vacancies in hospitals). Hospitals would have had to substitute toward greater use of practical nurses because they could not employ all the RNs they wanted at the RNs' wage. Similarly, hospital RNs' wages, relative to those of RNs in other nursing employment, would increase less rapidly if wages were held down in the hospital

Table 16-3. Ratio of RNs to LPNs in Nonfederal Short-Term General and Other Special Hospitals

Year	Employment	Year	Employment
1949	6.25		
1955	3.45	1975	2.17
1959	2.70	1980	2.70
1960		1985	3.70
1962	2.50	1990	4.76
1963		1995	6.20
1966	2.22	2000	7.70
1968	2.00		
1969			
1970	1.96		
1972	2.00		

Source: 1949–1978: U.S. Department of Health and Human Public Health Services, Health Resources Administration, *The Recurrent Shortage of Registered Nurses: A New Look at the Issues,* DHHS Publication (HRS), pp. 3 and 6. Years 1980–2000: derived from data in American Hospital Association, *Hospital Statistics,* (Chicago: AHA), various editions.

sector but not in other nurse employment sectors. As hospital RN wages were prevented from increasing, RN wages and relative rates of return fell behind those in comparable occupations.

A static shortage where RN wages increased in an absolute amount but fell relative to non-hospital employed RNs and comparable professions also explains why hospital nurse employment increased less than in the non-hospital sector.

Given that the data appears consistent with a static shortage in the hospital market prior to Medicare, it is necessary to explain how such a static shortage could have persisted. Namely, what mechanism would have prevented nurses' wages from reaching the equilibrium level, and second, why did the static shortage disappear in the period after 1966?

Hospital Market Power in the RN Labor Market

Prior to 1966, hospitals acted as a cartel in setting RN wages. By acting collusively, hospitals set RN wages below the equilibrium level thereby creating a static shortage. At that time, hospitals employed 75 percent of all RNs (both hospital based and private duty nurses). With relatively few hospitals in an area, it was relatively easy for them to collude in setting RN wages and to monitor whether each hospital was adhering to the agreement.

When there are many small firms in a competitive industry, it is both difficult to organize a cartel and, if successful, for the cartel to monitor firms to ensure that they do not violate the collective agreement. It is in each firm's interest to cheat because they can attract nurses from other hospitals by slightly raising their RN wages. Hospitals, however, can quickly find out whether or not another hospital in the area has changed its wage policy. Also, because hospitals employ almost all of the active nurses, it is difficult to attract nurses from other, non-hospital firms.

Hospitals decided to hold down nurses' wages because they believed that the short-run supply of nurses was relatively inelastic (i.e., increasing the wage would result in small, if any, increases in the number of nurses seeking work, either through a change in their status from inactive to active or from in-migration from other areas). RN wages also represented a significant portion of a hospital's budget; increasing the wage rate to attract new nurses would have required an increase in the wage paid to all existing RNs as well.

To test the hypothesis of hospital collusion in setting RN wages, Donald Yett conducted a survey of the thirty-one largest hospital associations to determine whether or not they had wage stabilization programs. Fourteen of the fifteen hospital associations that responded reported that they did have such programs. (The one hospital association that did not asked how it could start one.) Additional evidence of the attempt by hospitals to fix nurses' wages in their area is the following statement that appeared in the *Los Angeles Times*: "The majority of hospitals fix wages for nurses on recommendations from the Hospital Council of Southern California. The Council's recommendations have always been accepted and are based on recommendations from the management consulting firm of Griffenhagen-Kroeger Inc." (4).

As hospitals found it difficult to hire more nurses during the pre-1966 period and vacancy rates continued to increase, they began recruiting foreign-trained nurses and lobbied for federal legislation to subsidize an increase in the number of registered nurses.

The Market for RNs in the Post-Medicare Period

After the passage of Medicare and Medicaid, the market for RNs changed. The demand for hospital care increased as the aged and the poor were provided with hospital coverage. At the same time, hospitals were reimbursed on a "cost-plus" basis (in addition to their costs of caring for an aged person, hospitals received 2 percent for growth and development). Hospitals increased their demand for RNs and because the hospital's costs of more RNs and higher RN wages could be passed on to the government, their demand became inelastic with respect to the RNs' wage.[3]

---

3. During the 1960s, hospitals did not have good accounting systems. Thus to calculate their payment from the government for caring for Medicare patients, the hospital's total charges were divided by the proportion of charges to Medicare patients. That ratio was then assumed to equal the proportion of costs of caring for Medicare patients, hence the phrase, "ratio of charges to charges to cost." Depending upon what portion of their hospitalized population was covered under some form of cost reimbursement (e.g., government, Blue Cross, or other third-party reimbursement), hospitals were relieved from pressures to contain their costs.

Wage increases to hospital-employed nurses increased rapidly in the post-Medicare period, more rapidly than wage increases to non-hospital-employed nurses and to persons working in non-health occupations with comparable training. Hospital RN wages, which had been held down for a number of years, were allowed to rise. Thus by 1969, rates of return to hospital-employed RNs were comparable to other occupations.

To sum up, hospitals were no longer inclined to act collusively in holding down RN wages after 1966 because Medicare and Medicaid reimbursed hospitals for the costs of caring for the aged and poor, regardless of the cost of that care. RN wages consequently increased at a rapid rate and, as a result, RN participation rates rose, hospitals were able to hire more nurses, and the vacancy rate decreased; by 1971 the vacancy rate dropped to 9.3 percent from its high of 23 percent in 1962.

The static shortage of RNs before 1966 was caused by hospital collusion to keep RN wages from rising. The appropriate public policy would have been enforcement of the anti-trust laws against anti-competitive behavior to allow RN wages to rise, which would have increased hospital costs—a normal occurrence in an industry experiencing a rising demand for its services and facing a rising supply curve for its factor inputs. Claims of a "shortage" in this type of situation are merely a matter of employers not wishing to pay higher prices for their inputs. Allowing nurses' wages to rise would have brought forth an increase both in the stock of nurses and in their participation rate. Federal legislation to increase the supply of nurses was not necessary.

The Market for RNs in More Recent Years

As RN wages increased in the mid to late 1960s, vacancy rates declined, nurse participation rates increased, and nursing school enrollments increased. There is always a time lag as prospective students learn of the nursing profession's changing prospects and adjust their career plans. Enrollments were sharply increasing by the early 1970s, resulting in large increases in the supply of RNs (see Figure 16-4). There no longer appeared to be concern with a nurse shortage. In 1975, President Ford vetoed Congressional renewal of federal funding for nurse education (but Congress overrode the veto).

The basis for another nurse shortage, however, began in 1971 when President Nixon imposed wage and price controls on the economy. Although these controls were removed from all other industries in 1972, they remained in effect for health care until 1974. The effect of these wage controls, together with the increased supply of RNs, began to have it effect by the late 1970s. Demand for RNs continued to grow throughout the 1970s, however, the wage controls led to lower relative wages for RNs. The government created a static shortage. By the late 1970s nursing school enrollments began to decline, and vacancy rates reached 14 percent by 1979.

The 1979 to 1980 shortage was short lived. As shown in Figure 16-5, RN wages sharply increased at the same time the economy entered a severe recession in the early 1980s. The rising national unemployment rate caused more nurses to seek employment and to increase their hours of work. Since 70 percent of RNs are married, the loss of a job by a spouse—or even the fear of losing a job—is likely to cause RNs to increase their labor force participation rate to maintain their family income. Rising wages and the rising unemployment rate increased nurse participation rates from 76 percent in 1980 to 79 percent by 1984. As a consequence of these forces, nurse vacancy rates declined to a low of 4.4 percent by 1983, indicating that was no longer a shortage.

The (dynamic) nursing shortage of the late 1970s was once again resolved through a combination of rising wages, an increase in the nurse participation rate, and a high national unemployment rate (2).

As nurse wages remained stable (and actually declined in real dollars) between 1983 and 1985 and the vacancy rate declined, nursing school enrollments began a sharp decline through the late 1980s.

Starting in the mid 1980s, the market for hospital services underwent dramatic changes that affected the market for nurses. The trend by Medicare, private insurers, and HMOs to reduce the use of the hospital led to shorter hospital lengths of stay. Patients required more intensive treatment for the shorter time they were in the hospital. Hospitalized patients were more severely ill, a greater number of transplants were being performed, and there was an increase in the number of

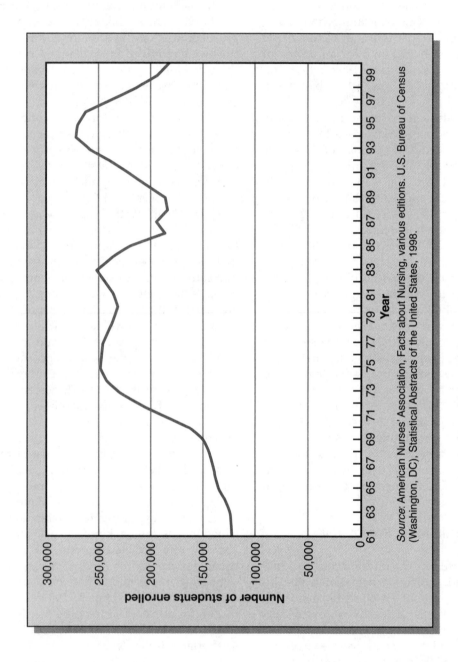

Source: American Nurses' Association, Facts about Nursing, various editions. U.S. Bureau of Census (Washington, DC), Statistical Abstracts of the United States, 1998.

Figure 16-4. Nursing school enrollments, 1961–1999.

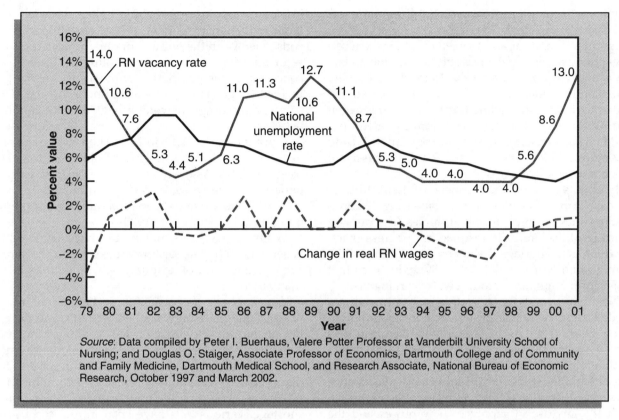

Figure 16-5. RN vacancy rates, annual percent changes in real RN wages, and the national unemployment rate, 1979–2001.

low birthweight babies. (The Medicare patient case-mix index for all hospitals increased from 1.17 in 1985 to 1.39 by 1992.) The recovery period, which requires less intensive care, was occurring outside the hospital. As a result, hospitals began to use a greater number of RNs per patient. The greater demand by hospitals for RNs during this period is indicated by the following: in 1975 there were 0.65 RNs per patient, it increased to 0.88 by 1980, to 1.31 by 1990, to 1.63 by 1995, and to 1.98 in 2000. The percent increase in RNs per patient exceeded the decline in patient days.

There was also an increase in the demand for nurses in outpatient and non-hospital settings. As the use of the hospital declined, use of outpatient care, nursing homes, home care, and hospices for termi-

nally ill Medicare patients increased. Between 1980, 1991, and 1999, outpatient visits (ambulatory care visits to physicians' offices, hospital outpatient, and emergency departments) increased from 262 million to 400 million to 944 million. Use by Medicare patients of skilled nursing homes increased from 8.645 million days in 1980 to 24.126 million in 1991 to 50.1 million days in 1999. Home health visits increased sharply from 22.4 million in 1980 to 78 million in 1991 to 258 million in 1997 (then declining to 113 million in 1999), and hospice admissions increased from 2,200 (in 1984 when it became a Medicare benefit) to 112,595 in 1991 to 700,000 by 2000 (3). In addition to providing care in these alternative settings, there was an increased demand for registered nurses by cost-containment companies to conduct utilization review and case management.

As the demand for nurses in all these different settings increased faster than supply in the mid to late 1980s, nurses' wages were slow to respond, nursing school enrollments had been falling, and the national unemployment rate declined as the economy began improving. As a consequence, vacancy rates once again began to rise, going from 5.1 percent in 1984 to 12.7 percent in 1989. By the late 1980s there was again concern over a shortage of nurses.

Hospitals again lobbied Congress for subsidies to increase nurse education and for an easing of immigration rules on foreign-trained nurses. The nursing shortage of the late 1980s resulted in Congress enacting the Nurse Shortage Reduction Act (1988) and the Immigration Nurse Relief Act (1989), which made it easier for foreign nurses to receive a working visa.

Neither of the above legislative acts, however, was needed since economic incentives once again eliminated the shortage. As the economy weakened in 1990 and the unemployment rate began to rise, nurse participation rates increased to 82 percent by 1992. Nursing school enrollment had begun increasing 2 years after nurse wages and the vacancy rate began their increase. With the increase in supply of new nurses and the higher participation rate, vacancy rates declined to 4 percent by 1994. The nursing shortage ended.

As the nurse shortage was over by the mid 1990s, one could have forecast that another shortage would occur by the end of the decade. As shown in Figure 16-5, starting in 1994, nurses' real wages (adjusted for inflation) declined and were negative for 4 years. It was during this time that hospitals were trying to reduce their costs to be price competitive so as to be included in managed care's provider networks. It was not until recently that nurse wage increases finally increased faster than inflation.

The national unemployment rate also declined throughout the late 1990s since the U.S. economy was doing very well. Nursing school enrollments typically decline several years after a decline in wages and vacancy rates. As shown in Figure 16-4, nursing school enrollments peaked at 270,000 in 1993 and then declined for the remainder of the 1990s. The reduction

in nurse wages during the mid to late 1990s led to a large reduction in nursing school enrollments and, consequently, in the number of nurse graduates.

In addition to declining enrollments, there was concern that the population of nurses was aging (4). In 1980, 25 percent of RNs were under the age of 30 compared to only 9 percent in 2000. And the number between 35 to 54 years of age increased by more than 50 percent between 1980 to 2000. The average age of a nurse was 37.9 in 1980, 42.4 in 2000, and is expected to be 45.4 in 2010. As the nurse population ages, participation rates decrease as does the number of hours worked. (The nurse participation rate began to show a slight decline in the late 1990s.)

Within a few years, one would have expected to observe newspapers writing articles about the shortage of nurses and of hospitals paying bonuses to attract nurses (5).

As expected, the years of declining real nurse wages, falling nursing school enrollments, and the aging of the nurse population led to another nursing shortage. After years of low vacancy rates, the vacancy rate began increasing from 4.0 percent in 1998 to 5.6 percent in 1999, and quickly rose to 13 percent by 2001.

And, as expected each time there is a new nursing shortage, various bills have been introduced in the Congress that attempt to address different aspects of the nursing shortage.

Of serious concern to hospitals, who already have great difficulty in filling nurse vacancies, is legislation recently enacted in California supported by the California Nurses Association that sets minimum nurse-to-patient staffing ratios. These mandated ratios, which vary by hospital department, are higher than current staffing levels. The proponents of mandated minimum ratios claim that RN staffing had fallen behind the needs of the increasing severity of hospitalized patients, and higher RN ratios will increase patient safety and quality of care.

Minimum staffing ratios were mandated in California without any conclusive empirical evidence as to which RN ratios, either by type of nursing unit or type of patient, produces the best outcomes (6).

Other states are waiting to see how the new staffing ratio law works before deciding to imitate California.

While it is uncertain as to what staffing ratio in different hospital departments would produce an increase in patient outcomes, it is clear that an increase in staffing ratios will increase hospital costs. These increased costs will be passed on in the form of higher health insurance premiums, which will increase the number of uninsured since their insurance becomes too expensive. It is unfortunate that the new California law does not require a monitoring system to determine whether the higher ratios improve patient care and, if so, by how much.

Since the end of government wage and price controls in the mid 1970s, the recurrent shortages of RNs were caused by increased demands for RNs and hospitals' failure to immediately recognize that, at the higher demand, nurse wages must be increased. Once hospitals realized that the market for RNs has changed, the adjustment process to eliminate that shortage begins, namely, increased RN wages. The disequilibrium in RN labor markets is the result of dynamic rather than static shortages. With higher wages, the supply of RNs increased, by increases in nurse participation rates and, over time, through increased nursing school enrollments. These recurrent shortages were resolved through the workings of the market; federal subsidies to support nurse education were unnecessary. The most appropriate response to recurring dynamic nurse shortages is to facilitate the market's adjustment process. Better information to hospitals and to prospective nursing students about nurse labor market conditions would improve performance of both the RN labor market and the education market and dampen the severity of the recurrent RN shortages.

The current nurse shortage, however, may take longer than usual before equilibrium is once again achieved because of both the aging of the nurse population and the legislated higher nurse staffing ratios.

THE REGISTERED NURSE EDUCATION MARKET

The number of RN graduates plus immigration of foreign trained RNs less retirement of RNs from the labor force determine changes in the long-run supply of nurses. The nurse education sector is the most important determinant of the future stock of RNs and has been the recipient of large federal subsidies. Thus, a better understanding of the responsiveness of nurse enrollment to economic incentives can clarify both the effectiveness of federal subsidies to increase the number of RNs as well as the role of nurse enrollment in exacerbating as well as alleviating recurrent dynamic shortages.

Nursing education is typically provided in one of three types of settings: 3-year diploma schools associated with hospitals, community colleges offering a 2-year associate degree, and 4-year colleges offering a baccalaureate (B.S.) degree.[4] While attending classes, students in diploma schools worked in hospitals and received a stipend. Hospitals subsidized the cost of their diploma schools to assure themselves a supply of nurses upon graduation. However, as the mobility of nurses increased, hospital diploma schools became a diminishing source of nurses for the particular hospital subsidizing them. Hospitals were no longer assured that their subsidies to such schools would be repaid when the nurses left to work elsewhere. As tuition costs to the students in diploma schools rose, enrollments declined.

After World War II, diploma schools of nursing declined rapidly. In 1950, there were 1,314 state-approved schools of nursing. Of these, 1,118 were diploma schools, 195 were B.S. programs, and 1 was an associate program. By 1966 there were 1,266 programs; of these, 788 were diploma schools, 280 were B.S. schools, and 198 were associate degree schools. By 2002, the total number of programs increased to 1,462; of these, only 89 were diploma schools, 587 were B.S. schools, and 786 were associate degree schools (7).

Although the number of diploma school programs declined, graduates from these programs still made the largest contribution to the number of new active nurses until 1972. Since 1972, more nurses have graduated from associate degree programs; these graduates

---

4. Of the approximately 2.2 million employed RNs in 2000, 26 percent graduated from diploma nursing schools, 43 percent from associate degree programs, 25 percent graduated from a 4-year baccalaureate degree program; and 6 percent graduated from masters and doctorate programs.

represented 3 percent of graduates in 1960, 9.6 percent in 1965, 31 percent by 1970, and 60 percent in 2000. The large growth in associate degree programs began before federal subsidies for nurse education became available. The percent of graduates from each of these programs is shown in Figure 16-6.

To understand the probable intent of federal subsidies to support nurse training and how effective it was in achieving its stated goals of increasing the supply of RNs, it is worthwhile to examine the original Nurse Training Act.

The stimulus for the Nurse Training Act of 1964 was the 1963 report by the Surgeon General's Consultant Group on Nursing, appointed in 1961, that there was a serious shortage of nurses. Evidence for the shortage was the very high nurse vacancy rate in the early 1960s (see Table 16-1) and an estimate of the number of RNs needed based on the ratio technique (thus unrelated to any economic definition of shortage). The forecast of a shortage was also unrelated to any analysis of the performance of the nurse labor market.

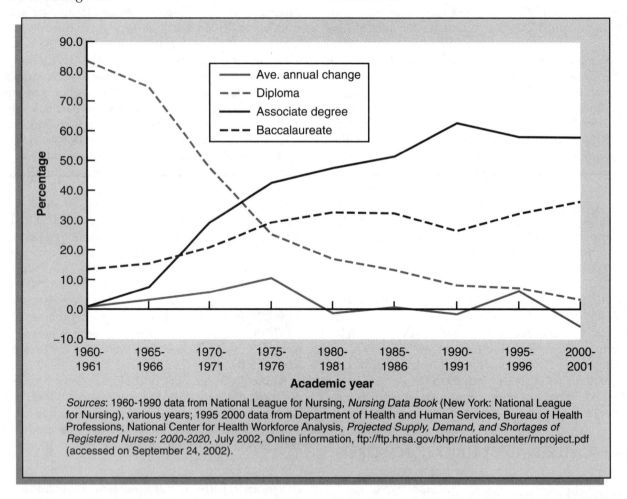

Sources: 1960-1990 data from National League for Nursing, *Nursing Data Book* (New York: National League for Nursing), various years; 1995 2000 data from Department of Health and Human Services, Bureau of Health Professions, National Center for Health Workforce Analysis, *Projected Supply, Demand, and Shortages of Registered Nurses: 2000-2020*, July 2002, Online information, ftp://ftp.hrsa.gov/bhpr/nationalcenter/rnproject.pdf (accessed on September 24, 2002).

Figure 16-6. Percent distribution of nursing graduates by type of nursing school program and average annual change in total graduates, 1960–2001.

Support for federal legislation to subsidize nurse training came from several groups: Congress recognized the potential political rewards of backing health legislation; the federal bureaucracy—specifically, the Division of Nursing in the U.S. Public Health Service—helped to justify the need for the legislation with an eye toward an expanded role in administering it; hospitals favored it because they wanted an increased supply of nurses, thereby slowing down the rate of increase in nurses' wages. Hospitals wanted the federal subsidies to be used to increase the number of nurses graduating from diploma schools of nursing. Sufficient capacity existed in those schools to accommodate increases in enrollment.

The American Nurses Association (ANA) also favored the legislation, but with different expectations than hospitals as to its effects. As a professional association, an important goal of the ANA is to increase its members' incomes. If the legislation were to have the effect desired by hospitals, namely an increase in the supply of nurses, then the subsidy would limit the rise in nurses' wages, which would be contrary to the ANA's objective. Instead, the ANA envisaged the educational subsidies as an opportunity to change the role of registered nurses. Nursing leaders saw the transfer of nursing education from non-college settings into universities as important to the advancement of nursing as a profession (recognizing that economic advancement would follow). The ANA wanted the educational subsidies to be redirected toward producing fewer but more highly trained nurses who could increase their productivity by undertaking additional responsibilities. The effect of fewer nurses with more training would be an increase in nurses' wages.

From the ANA's perspective, unless B.S. graduates were subsidized, fewer prospective nurses would choose a 4-year school. A graduate from a baccalaureate school spends more time in school compared with graduates from associate degree or diploma schools, yet the wage differential does not compensate baccalaureate graduates for the additional training time or forgone income. Studies confirm that the rate of return to the nurse with a baccalaureate degree working

in a hospital setting is less than for a nurse with only a 2-year associate degree (8).[5]

The growth in demand for associate degree education was related to its relatively high rate of return compared with comparable occupations. Associate degree programs would have grown without federal subsidies.

Thus the reasons for federal nurse education subsidies varied. Hospitals wanted cheaper inputs, and the ANA wanted to change educational requirements and graduate fewer nurses capable of performing more tasks. Neither outcome would have improved the functioning of the market for nurses, consequently there was no economic justification for the federal legislation.

By analyzing its implementation and its effects, it becomes possible to evaluate the legislation.

The two broad purposes stated in the Nurse Training Act (NTA) of 1964 were: to increase the quantity of nurses and to improve their quality, matched the separate interests of the ANA and AHA. To achieve these goals, the two most important areas for federal funding (receiving over 90 percent of the total funds expended on nurse training and which were continued in subsequent renewals to that legislation) were grants to schools of nursing for distribution in the form of scholarships and loans to students and grants to the nursing schools for construction, planning, or initiating programs of nursing education, or for general financial support.

Numerically, the legislation was to increase the number of nursing school graduates to 53,000 a year by 1969, a 75 percent increase over 1961. However, the

5. To further make the B.A. degree a more attractive option to prospective nurses, the ANA has proposed a two-tier licensure system, one for graduates with a B.A. degree and the other for associate and diploma school graduates. Nurses graduating from two-year programs would only receive a technical nursing license. If the ANA were successful in changing state educational requirements for nurses in this manner, there would be a sharp reduction in the number of new graduates each year. Currently, graduates with a B.S. degree represent only 32 percent of new nurse graduates; thus this policy would result in a loss of two-thirds of nursing graduates.

number of graduates produced by schools of nursing in 1969 was only 1,196 more graduates than what the government estimated would have been the case without any federal legislation.

In administering the NTA, no attempt was made to maximize the number of nurse graduates. If that had been the goal, the funds would have been allocated differently according to the types of nursing schools. Instead, there appears to have been a conscious decision to favor growth in the number of nursing graduates from baccalaureate degree programs, which coincided with the ANA's goals. The National League for Nursing (NLN) was designated as the accrediting agency for dispensing federal support to schools of nursing; its goals were, of course, similar to those of the ANA. Until 1968, payment to diploma and associate degree schools under the NTA received much fewer funds than what Congress authorized, while payments to baccalaureate programs were approximately equal to what was authorized.

Although federal funding of nursing schools and students did not achieve the increase in graduates its proponents claimed would occur, a large increase in the number of employed nurses did occur. An increase in the number of RNs employed can occur in one of three ways: (a) an increase in the number of nursing graduates, (b) an increase in the nurse participation rate, and (c) an increase in immigration of foreign-trained nurses. The federal program was directed exclusively at increasing the number of nursing graduates.

Using an econometric model to simulate the nursing market over time, the authors concluded that the achievement of the increase in number of RNs was primarily the result of increased nurse participation rates rather than the federal subsidy program, which resulted in a very small increase in graduates compared to what would have otherwise occurred (9).

Paradoxically, the more successful the federal government is in increasing the number of nursing graduates, the lower will be the increase in nurses' wages. An increased supply of new nurses would hold down potential increases in nurses' wages; this dampening effect would have an adverse impact upon the participation rate (10). Thus the subsidy to nursing schools could well have been self-defeating!

Important to the discussion of federal subsidies for nurse education is whether the nurse education market responds to changes in the demand for RNs. If the education market is responsive to changes in the RN labor market, then again there is little justification for federal subsidies. As shown in Figure 16-4, over the period 1961 to 2000, nursing enrollments have, at different times, sharply increased and decreased. While the size of the age cohort is an important factor influencing nurse enrollments, other factors also influence the attractiveness of a nursing career, such as changing career opportunities for women. However, a number of prospective students who are undecided between different career options will be influenced by the financial attractiveness of a nursing career.

There is a relatively close relationship between changes in nurse enrollments with changes in RN (real) wages, shown in Figure 16-5. As discussed previously, RN wages increased rapidly in the period after Medicare and Medicaid were enacted in the mid 1960s. Accordingly, nurse enrollments sharply increased several years afterward. Nurse enrollments were constant during the period in the early to mid 1970s when wage and price controls were imposed on hospitals, and hospitals could not increase nurse wages; consequently, a nursing shortage occurred, and the vacancy rate rose. Nurse enrollments thus declined from the end of the 1970s through the 1980s.

RN wages increased in the early 1980s and increased, on average, through the 1980s (Figure 16-5), however, it was not until the end of the 1980s before nurse enrollments increased. During the time nurse enrollments were increasing in the early 1990s, RN wages were declining. After several years of declining wages, nurse enrollments once again fell.

There is a time lag between changes in the financial attractiveness of a nursing career and prospective students' decision to enroll in a nursing school. It is likely that current decline in nurse enrollments will not reverse its trend until several years after the long decline in nurse wages during the 1990s have risen.

Proposals for continued federal subsidies to increase the supply of nurses ignore the important role played by higher wages in increasing both the short-

and long-run supply of nurses. In contrast to the time required for federal subsidies to have their impact on increasing the supply of nurses, the adjustment process by existing and prospective nurses to increased wages has been relatively quick.

AN ECONOMIC ANALYSIS OF COMPARABLE WORTH

Nurse Associations have made numerous proposals affecting either the demand for RNs or the supply of RNs whose intended outcome would be an increase in RN wages. Examples of demand-increasing programs are to legally permit RNs to perform more highly valued tasks, thereby increasing their productivity and second, mandating minimum RN staffing ratios in hospitals (minimum ratios that are higher than existing ratios). Supply-side examples have been limits on immigration of foreign-trained RNs and the American Nurses' Association's efforts to change state licensure requirements for becoming a nurse, requiring a professional nurse receive a B.S. degree. The following section discusses an additional proposal for increasing RN wages, using the concept of comparable worth to calculate nurse wages. The effect of these policies is to increase RN salaries, while their higher costs would, in part, be shifted to patients, government, and other third-party payers.

Nursing associations, whose members are predominately female, have been in the forefront of the movement to legislate "comparable worth" since it was seen as a way to raise nurses' wages. Although these political efforts have not been successful to date, it is instructive to examine this concept since it clarifies the determination of wages in a market system. The crux of the debate regarding comparable worth is over the appropriate mechanism for setting wages.

According to the 1964 Civil Rights Act, a person must receive equal pay for performing equal work; discrimination in employment is illegal. Comparable worth goes beyond that concept; its proponents want *equal pay for work of comparable value.* Two people performing different jobs should receive the same pay if a government agency determines that their work is of equal value. The proponents of comparable worth base their argument on the empirical observation that certain jobs that are filled predominately by women are paid less than jobs that are filled predominately by men. Accordingly, the value of each job should be determined not by the marketplace, but by fact-finding commissions.

Comparable worth is analyzed by first reviewing how wages are determined in a competitive market and, second, the effects on wages and employment of noncompetitive restrictions. Two alternative theories are then used to explain observed wage disparities between males and females. Next, the consequences of using comparable worth to achieve pay equity are discussed, and finally, alternative strategies to increase nursing salaries are presented.

The Determination of Wages in Competitive Markets

In a competitive market, wages are determined by the interaction of the firm's demand for employees and by the supply of those employees. The wage is the equilibrating mechanism; it is the price of labor. At higher or lower wages, the firm would be willing to hire fewer or more persons, respectively. Also, the higher the wage or income, the greater are the number of people willing to enter that occupation or profession. (A change in the wage represents a movement along the firm's demand curve and a movement along the supply of labor curve.)

The firm's demand for labor is also determined by the value of an employee's output which consists of two parts: the productivity of the employee (i.e., how much output each additional worker can produce), and the price at which that output can be sold in the marketplace. (Changes in either employee productivity or the price of the output cause *shifts* in the demand for labor.) Employee productivity is affected by education/training, skill, experience, and the amount of invested capital or equipment per employee. Thus, even within a given profession, differences in income exist because of differences in productivity. The higher the price at which the output can be sold, the greater is the market value of the employee producing that output. For example, if a nurse practitioner is reimbursed for performing a physical exam at a lower fee than a family practitioner, the value of the output produced by the nurse practitioner is lower.

In a competitive market, therefore, a person's income depends on three factors: their productivity, the price at which that service is sold in the market, and the number (supply) of people in the profession.

Market restrictions may either increase or decrease employees' incomes. Limiting entry into the profession will increase the incomes of those in the profession while shifting supply into those occupations without entry barriers, thereby decreasing their incomes. Entry barriers are either sanctioned by the government (as occurs with licensing) or by non-government groups such as unions when limits are placed on the number of unionized plumbers. The effect of these entry restrictions is to have a smaller supply of professionals in the restricted market and a larger supply in the unrestricted market, causing a wage differential between the two markets.

Restrictions on the tasks that health professionals may perform have similar effects. A health professional is often capable of performing certain tasks (either by experience or training) but is prohibited from doing so by state practice acts. Prohibiting a professional from performing highly remunerative tasks reduces the economic value of their output (the demand for their services is shifted to the left).

When hospitals colluded in setting nurses' wages (as apparently occurred in the 1950s and early 1960s), these anti-competitive restrictions by the purchasers of nurses' services were able to limit the rate of increase in nurses' wages.

Finally, if a firm does not face competition in the sale of its product and the firm is non-profit, then the firm does not have to be as concerned with its costs of production (i.e., the wage rates they pay or whether they employ the best people for the job). Examples of this behavior may be found in regulated companies (such as utilities) or in state and local governments. Prior to enactment of prospective payment legislation (DRGs) in 1983, non-profit hospitals were not constrained to produce in cost-minimizing ways. Heavily subsidized medical schools with excess demand for their spaces can also be less efficient.

A firm that is a non-profit or regulated monopolist in the sale of its product can pass on higher wages and the additional costs of hiring less competent personnel. It is precisely in such situations that firms can also practice discrimination in hiring. In a competitive industry, if a firm paid higher wages or hired less competent workers than its competitors, its costs would be higher. The firm could not compete on price and would either be forced to go out of business or to change its employment practices. Discriminatory practices are therefore more likely to occur in industries or among firms that are less concerned with their costs (11).

Theories to Explain Wage Disparities

Women, on average, earn less than men. Some occupations are also filled predominately by women. Why does this occur?

According to the "crowding" theory, women are channeled by either their own expectations or by those of others into certain professions that are predominately female. The exclusion of women from higher-paying male dominated jobs causes a surplus of women within particular jobs, thereby leading to lower wages in the female-dominated jobs. Little evidence, however, exists to support the premise that women's occupations, such as nursing or clerical work, are more crowded than men's occupations. Moreover, for the crowding theory to be a valid explanation of differences in male/female wages, the market would have to be non-competitive in some manner, otherwise some women would enter male-dominated professions to receive a higher rate of return. The mobility between occupations would equalize wages.

The most accepted explanation by economists for wage disparities is based on the theory of human capital (12). There are non-monetary reasons why people select certain jobs; preferences as to the type of work and location may have an influence on a person's employment preferences. Wages reflect these differences in preferences. Second, individuals have different abilities resulting in different incomes. However, an individual's productivity is not fixed; it can be increased with additional training and education. Therefore, wages also differ according to the individual's investment in education, training, and experience. Thus if females anticipate leaving the work force, they may invest less in education; married women who have undertaken traditional home responsibilities have found this to be an obstacle in making a full commitment to their careers.

How well does the above explain male/female wage differentials? According to empirical studies, most of the differences in male/female wage ratios can be explained by differences in the total number of years of work experience, the years of tenure on the current job, and the pattern or continuity of previous work experience (13). These studies do not deny that discrimination may exist; however, it is not an important determinant of observed wage differences.

As differences in human capital between males and females lessen, so should differences in their wage rates. Career patterns and expectations have changed significantly since the 1960s. For example, in 1970 females represented 9.4 percent of medical school applicants and 8.4 percent of the graduates. In 2001–2002, 48.0 percent of the applicants were female as were 44.1 percent of the graduates. This percentage should continue to increase. As educational levels, work roles, and work expectations of males and females become similar, so should their relative wages.

Determination of Wages Through Comparable Worth

What are the likely consequences if wages were based on comparable worth instead of the marketplace? Consultants and committees would be used to conduct job evaluations on each position within an organization or firm. These evaluations would involve assessment of the relative worth of each position according to skill required, effort involved, working conditions, and level of responsibility. Points would be assessed for each of these factors, and salaries would be determined by the total number of points in each position.

A comparable worth based wage determination system would result in a number of problems. First, the complexity of categorizing people would be tremendous, particularly if one were trying to establish a nationally applicable system affecting tens of thousands of jobs in hundreds of thousands of places. Further, these job evaluations would have to be updated as tasks and job conditions change. The implementation cost of such a system would be enormous, not only in terms of the time involved but also the cost of hiring the consultants and establishing job evaluation committees. An additional very large cost would result from the resolution of identified pay inequities, which will be in the billions of dollars.

Second, wage equity under comparable worth would not be achieved by lowering wages in job classifications in which job evaluations indicated that certain groups were being overpaid. Individuals in those groups would protest. Instead, occupations in which employees were currently being underpaid would have their wages increased. When the employer is a state government, the state can increase taxes to pay the increased costs; however, if taxpayers or their legislators were unwilling to vote for higher taxes, less money would be available for other programs or the employer would be forced to reduce employment in those occupations where wages were raised. Moreover, it is in female-dominated occupations that wages would be increased and, consequently, where fewer people would be hired. Although those remaining on the job would receive higher wages, some would be let go.

Third, wages determined by a commission would not reflect supply and demand conditions. Visualize a market with shifting demand and/or supply curves. The result would be shortages and surpluses of workers in different occupations and regions. How would these shortages and surpluses be resolved? How will it be possible to increase wages in male-dominated occupations (e.g., firemen) experiencing shortages? Jobs in surplus professions will have to be rationed since the wage would be above the equilibrium level. What criteria will be used for selecting employees when the wage exceeds the equilibrium wage? Rationing provides an opportunity for discrimination, as has previously been the case with medical school admissions.

In summary, while comparable worth may be conceptually appealing to those that distrust the market, its implementation would be costly and unlikely to achieve the goals its proponents desire. Problems that would emerge are politicization of wage determination, a large bureaucracy for evaluating all positions in the economy, lower levels of employment for women in those occupations in which wages have been increased artificially, increased costs of services and a smaller output in those industries with a greater portion of women, a decreased incentive for women to move into other professions, and no mechanism for eliminating shortages and surpluses.

Alternative Strategies for Increasing Wages

Alternative strategies should be pursued to achieve greater pay equity. The first is the enforcement of current laws against discrimination; females desiring to enter male-dominated professions should be able to do so. A shift in the number of females from female-dominated professions to male-dominated professions would increase the wage in the former and depress wages in male-dominated professions. Differences in wages would more closely reflect either preferences for some types of occupations or differences in investment in human capital.

Next should be the elimination of the many restrictions that prevent labor markets from operating competitively. Legal restrictions that prohibit trained professionals from undertaking tasks even though they are qualified to perform them result in higher prices to society and in lower wages to those who are prohibited from performing them. For example, a nurse could receive increased income as a nurse-midwife. However, when an insurance company refuses to provide malpractice coverage to obstetricians working with the nurse-midwives or if an insurer refuses to pay the nurse-midwife unless the bill is submitted by a physician, access by patients to nurse-midwifery services is limited and nurses are prevented from increasing their incomes. In many instances, restrictive nurse practice acts unnecessarily limit the nurse's ability to perform certain functions.

Competition in the delivery of health services is beneficial to the career goals of nurses. Managed care organizations must be price competitive if they are to survive and grow. The managers of such organizations are more willing to look for less expensive methods of providing services, more willing to innovate, more responsive to patient concerns, and less bound

to traditional tasks and roles than were not-for-profit hospitals reimbursed on a cost basis and state medical societies concerned with protecting their members' incomes. In a price-competitive system, nurses are moving into such new areas as utilization review, case management for catastrophic care, and home health services, and are performing additional tasks previously denied them.

The marketplace does not place the same value on certain workers or services as some would prefer. However, years of experience with trying to regulate the market through wage and price controls have demonstrated that it is costly and eventually ineffective to try to do so. Alternatively, to increase nurses' wages the market's criteria for wage determination must be understood and relied upon. Enforcing current laws on discrimination, removing economic restrictions, and providing access to educational and training opportunities would increase job opportunities and incomes for women while benefiting society through increased availability of services.

SUMMARY

In the late 1940s, the nursing market appeared to have been in equilibrium. However, up until the mid 1960s there was a shortage; the demand for nurses by hospitals exceeded the supply of nurses at the market wage. Based upon an analysis of relative wages of hospital-employed nurses relative to other nurses, it appeared that a static shortage was created by hospitals colluding to prevent nurses' wages from rising. In an attempt to limit the increase in their nursing costs and a belief that increased wages would not increase the number of employed nurses, hospitals instead intensified their recruiting of foreign-trained nurses and substituted nurses aides for RNs. Hospitals also lobbied for federal subsidies to increase the supply of nurses.

The static shortage disappeared after Medicare and Medicaid were enacted. As the demand for hospital care (and the consequent demand for nurses) increased, hospitals were able to pass on to the government the increased costs of higher wages and the increased number of nurses. Nurses' wages in the post-Medicare period increased rapidly, as did nurse participation rates. In both the short and long run, nurses' employment and career decisions were more responsive to higher wages than hospitals believed. The high rate of return to nursing led to increased enrollments in associate degree programs. The rate of return to nursing again became comparable to other occupations. (The rate of return varied, however, depending upon the type of degree received by the nurse.)

Federal legislation to support nurse training started in 1964 and continued for many years. The original manpower goals underlying the 1964 Nurse Training Act were achieved, although they would have been achieved without the federal subsidy program. In fact, had the federal subsidy program been very successful in increasing the number of nurse graduates, the increased supply of nurses would have led to a lower rate of increase in nurse wages, hence a smaller increase in the nurse participation rate.

Reliance on market mechanisms rather than on federal subsidies to solve nurse shortages is likely to bring about a quicker resolution of that shortage. First, future demand increases for nurses can be met by increasing the number of hours that part-time nurses work. Almost 30 percent of all employed nurses (more than 625,000) work part time. Increased wages that induce these nurses to increase their hours of work can result in large increases in the supply of nursing time. Second, higher wages for nurses will cause hospitals and other demanders of nurses to rethink how they use their nurses. As nurses become more expensive to employ, hospitals use nurses in higher-skilled tasks and delegate to lesser-trained nursing personnel, such as licensed practical nurses, certain housekeeping and other tasks currently performed by registered nurses (a significant percentage of nurses' time is spent on tasks that can be delegated to others). Third, higher wages and new roles for nurses make nursing a more attractive profession. Lastly, nursing has been a female profession. There is no reason why more males (6 percent of all RNs) and minorities (14 percent of all RNs) cannot be attracted to a nursing career. Higher wages (annual average earnings of registered nurses employed full time were

$46,782 as of 2000) and new nursing roles will increase the attractiveness of nursing to a larger segment of the population.

No economic justification for the government to subsidize nurse education exists. If RNs desire to undertake additional roles and responsibilities, it is not the government's role to subsidize their education to enable them to achieve their objectives any more than for any other professional group. Revision of state practice acts to permit nurses to undertake additional tasks for which they are trained and qualified to perform will result in an increased return from doing these tasks, which would justify increased investment by nurses for this training. Eliminating anti-competitive restrictions is a more appropriate policy. The goals used by the nursing profession to justify subsidies to nursing education should be explicit so that it can be determined whether it is a goal agreed to by the rest of society and whether the proposed approach is the least expensive way to achieve it.

Recurrent claims of a shortage of nurses have been temporary or dynamic and have been resolved through market forces without government intervention.

Nurse associations have sought various types of legislation to increase the roles, responsibilities, and incomes of nurses. These legislative remedies have included federal subsidies to nursing schools, comparable worth for setting nurse wages, minimum nurse staffing ratios in hospitals and other care settings, as well as efforts to prevent the merger and closure of hospitals.

Nurse aspirations of greater responsibilities and independence, along with higher incomes, are, however, more likely to be achieved in a competitive market than through government regulation. In their search for lower costs and increased quality in a competitive environment, managed care organizations and group practices are less bound by traditional dividing lines between nurses and physicians. The demand for different types of nurse education will be market driven, determined by the types of roles nurses will be engaged in, such as caring for more severely ill patients, greater responsibilities in primary care settings, as well as increased managerial responsibilities in managed care organizations.

APPENDIX: MARKET STRUCTURE AND NURSE WAGES AND EMPLOYMENT

The earlier discussion on RN shortages was based on either hospital collusion (static shortage) or information lags on the part of both hospitals and RNs that demand and supply conditions had changed (dynamic shortages). Separate from the above types of shortage, a shortage of RNs can occur because hospitals are monopsonists or oligopsonists in their demand for registered nurses. In monopsony or oligopsony markets, high vacancy rates will persist, and hospitals will not be able to hire all of the nurses they want at the going wage rate, *even though the market is in equilibrium.*

For the RN market to be characterized by monopsony or oligopsony there is only one or just a few hospitals hiring RNs. As the major demanders of RNs in a market, the hospital faces a rising (less elastic) supply curve for RNs. (For other types of labor, such as computer programmers, hospitals may represent a small portion of the total demand for such personnel, therefore the hospital faces a more elastic supply curve.) Non-hospital settings (physician offices, outpatient clinics, etc.) employing RNs are small purchasers of RNs. These firms face a much more elastic supply curve for RNs, and RNs represent a small portion of their total cost. These employers would therefore be able to hire all the RNs they want at or slightly above the prevailing wage.

Further, when nurses have limited mobility, the nurse supply curve will be less elastic, otherwise they would move to those markets where wages are highest and nurse labor supply curves would be more elastic. Particularly in previous times, diploma school graduates, married nurses who considered themselves secondary wage earners, and nurses with young children who preferred to work part time were likely to be less mobile.

Thus monopsony and oligopsony market structure is an additional explanation of the existence of nurse vacancy rates and why hospitals claimed there was a shortage of nurses. Hospitals will demand more RNs than will be supplied at the going wage rate. Hospitals will therefore report RN vacancies and claim there is a shortage.

Monopsony also results in lower wages and employment of RNs compared to a competitive market. (If input supply curves were elastic to hospitals, then hospitals would be able to hire all the RNs demanded at the going RN wage; hospitals would not report vacancies nor claim a shortage of RNs exist. The difference between a monopsonist and a competitive hospital when both face an elastic RN supply curve is that the monopsonist would hire fewer RNs because the monopsonist's demand for RNs would be its marginal revenue product curve.)

The following discussion explains why a monopsonist reports vacancies and claims there is a shortage when an equilibrium situation exists.

A monopsonist, with a demand curve D_1, will face a rising supply curve for nurses described by S_1 in Figure 16-7. The hospital will have to raise the wage rate to hire an additional nurse; however the monopsonist cannot pay a higher wage just to that additional nurse. It must pay the same, higher, wage to all of its currently employed nurses. Thus the cost of hiring an additional nurse is not just the wage that nurse re-

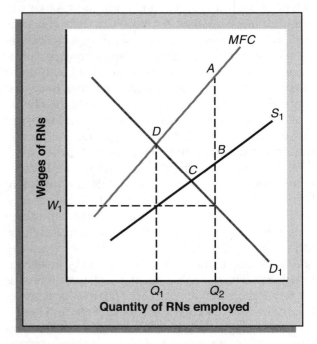

Figure 16-7. An illustration of a monopsonistic market for registered nurses.

ceives but also the wage increase that all currently employed nurses receive. Thus the monopsonist faces a marginal factor cost (MFC) curve that lies above the supply curve. The MFC curve represents the cost to the monopsonist of hiring an additional nurse. At each point on the supply curve, the MFC curve indicates the additional cost in terms of higher wages that must be paid to all nurses hired previously. Thus the equilibrium quantity of nurses the firm will hire and the wage it will pay under such circumstances are given by the intersection of the demand curve and the MFC curve. Drawing a line down to the supply curve will indicate the wage the firm would pay and the quantity of RNs employed.

At the equilibrium wage, W_1, the monopsonist would be willing to hire Q_2 quantity of nurses, which is the intersection of the wage and the firm's demand curve. However, if the firm were actually to hire Q_2 number of RNs, it would have to pay a wage much higher than W_1 to attract them. The new wage would be at that point on the supply curve above Q_2 shown by B. The cost to the firm of that wage and Q_2 number of nurses would be Point A *on the MFC curve*. Since Point A on the MFC curve exceeds the firm's demand, the firm would not want to hire Q_2 nurses at a wage represented by Point B on the supply curve. Thus W_1 and Q_1 are equilibrium points for the monopsonist. However, at that wage, W_1, the firm will report Q_1–Q_2 vacancies for nurses. These are the number of nurses it would be willing to hire at wage W_1.

Vacancies are thus expected and are consistent with an equilibrium position in a monopsony situation, even though the hospital will claim it faces a shortage of nurses.

The effect of unionization in a market dominated by a monopsonist will be to eliminate the monopsonist's "shortage," since a prevailing wage will be established whereby the hospital could hire all the nurses demanded at that wage. The vacancy rate should decrease. Hospital monopsony power over nurses' wages is weakened by the growth (both actual and expected) of a nurse's union.

For example, if a union were formed and set a minimum (prevailing) wage for its employees, the supply curve for nurses would change. It would become horizontal up to the point of the minimum wage on the

original supply curve. This would indicate that under the collective bargaining agreement, nurses could not be paid below a certain minimum union wage. The hospital can hire all the nurses it wants at that wage. The MFC curve would also change. It would become equal to the new minimum wage since there is no additional cost to the hospital as it hires an additional nurse; that is, it does not have to increase the wages of those nurses currently employed. Up to the point where the negotiated wage intersects the original supply curve, the hospital can hire all the nurses it wants at the negotiated wage. Beyond that point the hospital will again face a rising supply curve and a rising MFC curve; the hospital will have to increase its wages and also pay higher wages to its existing nurses.

In situations involving a monopsony purchaser and a union representing the employees, it is possible for the union to set a wage that is higher than the previous wage and also increases employment (see Figure 16-8). If the union sets a wage rate anywhere between A and B, it will raise the wage (since the current wage is W_1),

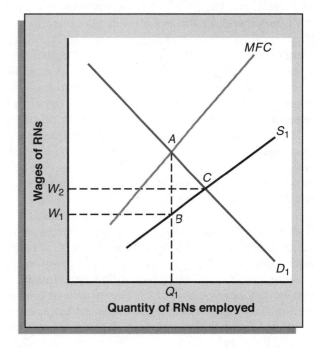

Figure 16-8.   Collective bargaining and a monopsony market for registered nurses.

and it will increase the number of nurses hired. Any wage between A and B will make the supply curve and the MFC curve horizontal up to that point. For example, a wage rate of W_2 is the point where employment of RNs is greatest. The new wage rate intersects the demand curve at the same point that the supply curve does. Therefore the wage rate (W_2) is the new MFC and supply curve up to the point where it intersects the original supply curve. To hire more nurses after that point, the firm will have to pay a higher wage and thus face a rising MFC and rising supply curve.

Point A on the demand curve is the highest union wage that can be set without decreasing employment of RNs.

With a union, nurse wages should increase and possibly employment. Whether or not increased employment will occur will depend on the union's objectives. If the union seeks to maximize wages for current union members, then there will be no increased employment of RNs.

Registered nurses employed in non-profit hospitals were expressly exempt from the legal provisions of the National Labor Relations Act between 1947 and 1974 and therefore did not have legal protection of their rights to organize or support a union. Hospitals were under no obligation to engage in collective bargaining with their employees. (In 1974, an amendment to the Taft-Hartley Act repealed hospitals' exempt status.) Collective bargaining on behalf of hospital nurses therefore started slowly. In addition to the impediments to collective bargaining contracts that legally permitted hospitals to refuse to bargain with unions representing hospital employees, the American Nurses' Association (ANA) had not been a strong proponent of unionization.

In 1970, approximately 38,000 RNs were included under collective bargaining agreements, representing about 5 percent of employed RNs. By 1977, 200,000 RNs (more than 20 percent of employed nurses) were included under collective bargaining agreements, a substantial increase over 1970. The growth in unionization has lagged behind the increased number of RNs, in 2000 representing only 19 percent of employed RNs (14).

The effects of collective bargaining agreements, however, are felt beyond the numbers of nurses cov-ered. To forestall such agreements, hospitals are likely to offer higher wages to RNs.

A number of studies have attempted to estimate the degree of monopsony (or oligopsony) power in nurse labor markets (15). These studies generally found evidence supporting hospitals' monopsony power. It is likely that monopsony power was more prevalent in earlier periods. A greater percentage of nurses graduated from diploma schools and were more closely tied to the hospitals where they were trained. Also many nurses who were married and who had families considered themselves to be secondary wage earners and were therefore less mobile.

The increased number of hospital mergers and consolidation that has been occurring increase hospitals' monopsony power and can result in lower RN wages and employment. RNs should therefore favor the application of anti-trust laws to hospital mergers.

REVIEW QUESTIONS

1. Various measures have been used to indicate that there has been a shortage of nurses. Evaluate the use of such measures to indicate the existence of a shortage. Second, what information would you use to indicate whether or not a shortage exists? Third, distinguish between a dynamic and a static shortage.
2. Contrast the market for registered nurses during the periods before and after Medicare. How well did the market for hospital-employed nurses perform in each of these two periods?
3. How have the last several shortages of nurses been resolved? How does an increase in nurse wages affect both hospitals' demand for nurses and the supply of nurses?
4. Why was the shortage of nurses that occurred before Medicare different from subsequent shortages?
5. Contrast the following two approaches for eliminating the shortage of nurses:
   a. Federal subsidies to nursing schools.
   b. Providing information on nurse demand and supply to prospective nursing students

and to demanders of nursing services, such as hospitals.

6. Nurses are restricted in the tasks they are permitted to perform. Also, certain nurse specialties (e.g., nurse-midwives) would like to bill for their services on a fee-for-service basis rather than work for obstetricians. Using the theory of the demand for labor, explain how changes in each of the above would affect the demand for registered nurses.

7. You are an economic consultant to the American Nurses' Association. What would you expect the effects of changes in the healthcare markets, such as prospective payment for hospitals, growth in HMOs, the increased supply of physicians, and so on, to be on the employment and earnings of RNs? In your answer, trace through the effects you expect on both the product and factor markets.

8. "Comparable worth" proponents seek equal pay for work of comparable value. What are the consequences of setting nurses' wages according to the concept of comparable worth? Describe the factors that determine wages in a competitive market (including those factors that cause shifts in the demand for labor). What are noncompetitive situations that have resulted in lower nurses' wages?

9. Nursing associations have proposed increasing the educational requirements to a 4-year B.S. degree for all persons desiring to become professional nurses. What are the economic consequences of instituting such a change? Who would be expected to favor it, and who would be expected to oppose it?

10. How would unionization in a monopsony market for nurses' services increase both nurses' wages and hospital employment?

REFERENCES

1. The discussion of the RN market in the period before and after the start of Medicare and Medicaid is based on Donald E. Yett, *An Economic Analysis of the Nurse Shortage*, (Lexington, Mass: D.C. Health, 1975).

2. Peter Buerhaus, "Capitalizing on the Recession's Effect on Hospital RN Shortages," *Hospital and Health Services Administration*, 39(1), Spring 1994, 47–62.

3. U.S. CDC, National Center for Health Statistics, Advance Data, 320, 321, 322, June 25, 2001, June 26, 2001, July 10, 2001 [online information], http://www.cdc.gov/nchs/express.htm; based on 1999 National Hospital Ambulatory Medical Survey.

4. Peter Buerhaus, Douglas Staiger, and David Auerbach, "Implications of an Aging Registered Nurse Workforce," *Journal of the American Medical Association*, 283(22), June 14, 2000, 2948–2954.

5. Buerhaus, P. I. "Is Another RN Shortage Looming?," *Nursing Outlook*, 46, May/June 1998, 103–108.

6. The most recent study on nurse staffing and patient outcomes is Jack Needleman, Peter Buerhaus, Soeren Mattke, Maureen Stewart, and Katya Zelevinsky, "Nurse-Staffing Levels and the Quality of Care in Hospitals," *New England Journal of Medicine*, 346(22), May 30, 2002, 1715–1722.

7. Data for 1950 is from *Source Book of Nursing Personnel*, (Bethesda, MD: U.S. Department of Health, Education, and Welfare, Division of Nursing, DHEW Publication (HRA), 75-43, December 1974); Data for subsequent years is from *Nursing Data Review*, (National League for Nursing: New York), various years and http://www.discovernursing.com.

8. Evelyn Lehrer, William White, and Wendy Young, "The Three Avenues to a Registered Nurse License," *Journal of Human Resources*, 26(2), Spring 1991 362–379. This study also contains reviews of previous research in this area.

9. Robert T. Dean, "Simulating an Econometric Model of the Market for Nurses," unpublished doctoral dissertation, Department of Economics, University of California at Los Angeles, 1971: 218. A further discussion of the ineffectiveness of the Nurse Training Act (NTA) may be found in Robert Deane and Donald Yett, "Nurse Market Policy Simulations Using an Econometric Model," in Richard M. Scheffler and Louis Rossiter, ed., *Advances in Health Economics and Health Services Research*, vol. 15, (Greenwich, Conn. JAI Press Inc.), November 1995.

10. Based on data from the 1984 National Sample Survey of Registered Nurses, Buerhaus estimated the elasticity of the participation rate with respect to nurse wages to be 0.49 for all RNs and 0.88 for unmarried RNs. See Peter I. Buerhaus, "Economic Determinants of the Annual Number of Hours Worked by Registered Nurses," *Medical Care*, 29(12), 1991, 1181–1195.

11. Gary Becker, *The Economics of Discrimination,* 2nd ed. (Chicago: University of Chicago Press, 1971).

12. Gary Becker, *Human Capital,* (New York: Columbia University Press, 1964).

13. F. Levy and R. Murnane, "U.S. Earnings Levels and Earnings Inequality: A Review of Recent Trends and Proposed Explanations," *Journal of Economic Literature,* 30(3), September 1992, 133–1381 and F. Blau and L. Kahn, "Rising Inequality and the U.S. Gender Gap," *American Economic Review,* 84(2), May 1994, 23–33.

14. *The Union Membership and Earnings Data Book: Compilation from the Current Population Survey,* (Washington DC, The Bureau of National Affairs), Fall 2000; and *Union Organizations in the Health Care Industry,* (Washington, DC, The Bureau of National Affairs), Fall 2000.

15. Using data from 1979 to 1985, one study concluded that hospitals have a substantial degree of monopsony power, the labor supply curve is upward sloping with an elasticity of +1.25 in the short run (one year) and about +4.0 in the long run. Daniel Sullivan, "Monopsony Power in the Market for Nurses," *Journal of Law and Economics,* 32(2), Pt.2, October 1989, pp. 135–178. Another study, using data from 1985 to 1993 does not find empirical support for the monopsony model; nurses' wages are found not to be related to hospital density and decrease rather than increase with respect to labor market size. Barry T. Hirsch and Edward J. Schumacher, "Monopsony Power and Relative Wages in the Labor Market For Nurses," *Journal of Health Economics,* 14(4), October 1995, 443–476.

CHAPTER

17

The Role of Government in Health and Medical Care

KEY TERMS AND CONCEPTS

- Consumer sovereignty
- Economic efficiency
- Externalities
- Market failure
- Market imperfections
- Externalities in consumption
- Direct and indirect subsidies
- In-kind subsidies
- Optimal level of output with externalities

Learning Objectives

Upon completing this chapter, the reader should be able to:

- Understand the economist's definition of an optimal rate of output.
- Discuss economic inefficiencies in the market for medical services.
- Explain why consumption externalities are a justification for government health insurance subsidies.
- Contrast the direct and indirect effects of in-kind demand versus in-kind supply subsidies.

GOVERNMENT INTERVENTION IN MEDICAL CARE

Government, particularly at the federal level, has a significant role in the financing, provision, and regulation of health and medical services. Federal expenditures for personal medical services have risen sharply since the passage of Medicare and Medicaid in the mid 1960s. Various levels of government are also suppliers of medical services: the Veterans Administration's system of hospitals and medical services supplied to military dependents in military facilities under the auspices of the Department of Defense. Different levels of government also provide indirect subsidies for medical services in the form of subsidies for medical research, for hospital construction (under the former Hill-Burton Act), for health manpower under federally supported programs, and state subsidies for health professional education.

At least as important as this financial involvement of government in medical service is the less obvious role of government in setting the rules under which medical services are paid for, organized, and produced, and the protection provided to patients through mechanisms such as licensing. Although government has long been involved in establishing the rules of the game for medical care, its role in financing medical care, particularly with regard to national health insurance, has been more controversial.

Some people view this increasing involvement of government in the medical sector as inevitable and beneficial; to others it is improper and the cause of inefficiencies. To clarify the debate over the expanding role of government in medical care, it is useful to review the traditional economic criteria for the functions of government in a market system and to apply this criteria to medical care. Disagreements over the role of government in medical care can then be separated into differences regarding (1) whether the traditional criteria for government involvement is appropriate, and (2) given the appropriateness of the criteria, whether such criteria warrant government involvement in medical care.

The appropriate criteria for justifying government intervention involves value judgments over the role

of government. The sooner these differences are recognized as such, the sooner the participants will be able to focus the debate on whether there are more appropriate alternatives to the traditional criteria for government involvement. Then, given an agreed upon set of criteria for government intervention, the government role can be more easily resolved because the existence of certain situations in medical care can be determined empirically. The evaluation of government's role in medical care, therefore, depends both upon appropriate criteria for government involvement and upon the applicability of such criteria to medical care.

There are two traditional areas where government is acknowledged to have a role in a market-oriented system (1). Each of these areas is briefly discussed.

MARKET IMPERFECTIONS

Inefficiencies in the Medical Marketplace

In a competitive market, economic efficiency on the demand and supply sides cannot be achieved when the assumptions underlying competitive markets are violated. The most important assumptions that are not fulfilled in medical care are: consumers and providers (physicians) have perfect information, there is complete mobility of resources,[1] and patients and providers have an incentive to minimize their costs of purchasing and providing medical treatment.

Consumers have insufficient knowledge regarding their medical diagnosis, treatment needs, the quality of different providers, and the prices charged by different providers. Patients' ignorance as to their med-

---

1. Another imperfection would be with respect to the capital markets. If full-cost tuition were charged to medical students, students would not be able to borrow from banks based solely upon their prospective earnings and without collateral. This type of market imperfection exists for all forms of higher education and is not peculiar to medical or dental education. At present, however, other market imperfections in the health education market, such as barriers to entry, are of greater overriding concern since they prevent full-cost tuition from being instituted.

ical needs, diagnosis, and treatment requirements have enabled physicians to induce demand for their services. The empirical evidence indicating demand inducement consists, for example, of differences in rates of specific surgical procedures according to methods of physician payment. The agency relationship between patients and their physicians has not always worked well. Different mechanisms have arisen to compensate for supplier-induced demand, such as utilization review by managed care organizations (MCOs). However, problems regarding the agency relationship still exist under both fee-for-service and capitation.

Lack of provider information is indicated by wide geographic variations in use rates unrelated to differences in physician payment (discussed in the chapter on the Physician Services Market). (Studies on appropriateness of care for different diagnoses, undertaken by MCOs and also funded by the government, are an attempt to increase physician knowledge.)

There are several different types of barriers or restrictions on the mobility of resources. There are limits on entry into health manpower professions as a result of non-profit medical schools and the accreditation criteria for those schools enforced by the Liaison Commission on Medical Education. The continual excess demands by applicants for a medical (and dental) education, continually high rates of return to the medical profession, and the willingness of U.S. citizens to bear higher costs and study for a longer period in foreign medical schools to become a U.S. physician are indications of barriers to entry. Second, many states still have Certificate of Need laws that bar entry by institutions and even home health agencies from entering and competing in various markets within their state. And third, restrictions exist, unrelated to quality, on the tasks various personnel are permitted to perform.

Tax-free health insurance purchased by employers on behalf of their employees lessened patient concerns with their costs of medical care; it created a moral hazard problem. The continued existence of tax-free health insurance continues to distort employees' choice of health plan and patients' use of medical services. Provider incentives to be concerned with

their costs were lessened by the previous use of cost-based payment by third-party payors, including government.

Lack of consumer and provider information, barriers to entry and restrictions on tasks, and tax-free employer-paid health insurance resulted in prices that exceeded average costs and large variations in medical use rates. Excess insurance for patients and the previous cost-based payment to providers resulted in inappropriate utilization, excessive duplication of facilities, rapidly rising medical costs, and inefficiency in production, namely, costs of producing medical services that exceeded the minimum costs of providing that care.

Thus it is apparent that there were (and still are) imperfections in the market for medical services. The government itself has been responsible for many of these inefficiencies. To discuss the appropriate role of government in the face of these imperfections on both the demand and supply sides of the medical services market, it is first necessary to understand why many of these imperfections were originally instituted.

The tax exemption for employer-paid health insurance is a federal tax subsidy to increase the demand for health insurance. Instituted during World War II to prevent a strike for higher wages when there was a wage and price freeze on the economy, tax-free employer-paid health insurance was based on expediency; it was not an explicit redistributional policy to help those with lower incomes. Instead, its effect was the opposite. The main beneficiaries of this tax subsidy, as discussed in the chapter on The Demand for Health Insurance, are those with higher incomes who are in higher tax brackets.

The Goal of Consumer Protection

The *ostensible* reason for placing restrictions on entry, information, and price competition was to provide consumer protection. Given the technical nature of medical services and the potential harm that may be inflicted upon an uninformed patient by an incompetent provider, the government, working through the health professions and health institutions, placed its emphasis for consumer protection on nonprofit providers and on the process of becoming a health professional. Training requirements in nonprofit institutions were specified; licensure, carried out by the health professions, placed strong restrictions on who was permitted to practice and on who was responsible for performing medical services; information on prices, quality, and accessibility was prohibited to prevent unethical providers from misleading the sick. Thus the very imperfections that prevented the medical sector from performing more efficiently were instituted under government auspices.

How can the demand for consumer protection[2] be achieved while eliminating the inefficiencies caused by policies to achieve that goal? The U.S. Supreme Court ruling that the anti-trust laws apply to the health field has eliminated restrictions on advertising and price competition. Large employers and employer coalitions are pressuring competing health plans and providers to gather data and publish outcome, rather than process, measures of quality. Once licensed, physicians are *not* required to be re-examined. Only if they want to be board certified are they re-examined. Relying more on examinations rather than standardized educational requirements, re-examination, and monitoring the quality of care provided are examples of outcome approaches. The competitive market, with its emphasis on monitoring physician behavior and practice patterns and providing outcomes information to improve consumer choice, is a move in the direction of greater consumer protection.

Consumer protection can be achieved more directly and more efficiently by an approach that actu-

ally monitored the quality of care provided. It would no longer be necessary to rely solely on proxy methods to accomplish this objective.

Often government provides subsidies to alleviate the consequences of imperfections of the type discussed, rather than eliminating the imperfections themselves; such subsidies cannot be justified as a means of improving market efficiency. Entry and practice barriers decrease the availability of medical care by increasing its price. Government construction or manpower subsidies, which have as their stated goal an increase in availability of medical resources, merely mask the effects of the market imperfections. These subsidies would have to be justified on grounds other than as a means of improving market efficiency.

When faced with imperfections in the marketplace, the appropriate role of government should be to eliminate restrictive practices and directly address the need that the restrictions were ostensibly imposed to meet (i.e., consumer protection).

Many people (particularly providers) oppose eliminating restrictions on information and on medical practice. Such persons also oppose a market approach for determining the quantity and quality of medical care to be provided. Their opposition to market competition is not based on grounds of greater economic efficiency but is, instead, a result of a value judgment that such criteria is inappropriate in medical care. Patients, in their opinion, do not have sufficient information, nor are they rational enough to make competent choices as to the appropriate providers and correct amounts of medical care when they are ill. Such a decision should not involve the consumer at all but should be determined professionally; the professional determination, or allocation, of medical care should be based on medical need and not on consumer choice.

Difference in Value Judgments

Consumers (in general) are believed to make cost-benefit decisions in determining the quantity of a good or service to buy. According to consumer de-

---

2. A demand for consumer protection might be considered an externality; namely, if the government or some agency were to ensure that all providers are competent, all consumers would benefit from the lower risks and lower search costs when seeking a provider. The reason for including a discussion of consumer protection in this section rather than in the following one (which discusses externalities) is that whether or not externalities are in fact the real reason for the market imperfections mentioned, the proposed policy prescriptions are similar to what would be the situation if such imperfections were simply a result of monopoly behavior on the part of the providers.

mand theory, consumers will use a service until the price they pay for the last unit purchased (their marginal cost) equals the additional value they receive from it. When the marginal utility of the last unit consumed equals the price paid, consumers are maximizing their utility. Since the price they must pay represents forgone utility that could be received from other goods and services, consumers adjust their utilization when prices change so that the marginal value of their last unit equals the new price. Consumers use different quantities of services even though they face the same prices because the marginal utilities to them of additional units differ. Each consumer, however, is assumed to match the marginal utility of that last unit to the forgone utility of other goods and services. Further, when the consumer is the sole beneficiary of his or her purchases, it is said that his or her marginal private benefit is equivalent to marginal social benefit.

The demand curve is determined by the consumer's cost-benefit calculation of price and quantity at different market prices.

If consumers are not assumed to be rational or if persons do not believe that consumer choice should prevail, the traditional demand curve does not represent marginal social utility. Under such circumstances, traditional economic policy, which favors removing imperfections so as to satisfy consumer wants, will not achieve the goals of those persons who do not believe in consumer choice and sovereignty in determining the amount of medical care to be provided.

Typically, those who oppose consumer sovereignty in medical care favor medical determination or prioritization of need for determining access to medical services. These approaches are difficult to operationalize. The criteria that government agencies would use for placing a marginal value on services to allocate resources would be very controversial. Not everyone would agree with the value judgment that a person should be prohibited from consuming something that he or she is willing to pay for (as long as it does not impose any negative effects on other persons). Based on their valuation of their time, some people may prefer to pay a higher price rather than wait for the receipt of a service. Substituting collective judgment for an individual's judgment to determine how much medical care is to be available represents a difference in values and is unrelated to whether a market system will be more efficient than an alternative system for achieving the same set of values.

This difference in values regarding how much medical care should be available and to whom is also related to another set of values. Those opposed to the use of consumer sovereignty in the demand for medical care are also opposed to the use of competition on the supply side. The proponents of market competition assume that when providers compete for consumers, they will minimize their costs in order to better compete on price and provide the services that consumers most desire. Persons who do not believe that providers should be responsive to consumer demands express similar disbelief in the ability of suppliers to compete with one another without harming patients; their preference is to substitute regulation and monopolization for competition.

Regardless of differences in values regarding who should determine the quantity and quality of medical services, it should be possible to allow different delivery systems to compete on the supply side. Allowing competition to exist and to be an alternative to a more controlled delivery system (e.g., a system of VA hospitals) would provide a fairer test of which approach is more efficient at achieving a level of output, whether it is established by government agencies or by consumers.

The reason for this discussion of differences in values in medical care is because the appropriate role of government is continually debated with regard to the values and criteria that underlie a market system. Much of the criticism of a market approach is not based upon the market's ability to achieve the specified economic criteria. Instead, the disagreement is a result of differences in values and unspecified criteria, thus the discussion on the role of government and public policy alternatives would be sharpened if these distinctions were more explicitly defined.

MARKET FAILURE

Divergences From A Competitive Market

There are certain situations where price-competitive markets will not produce the optimal amount of output, which is defined as price equaling marginal cost. A "natural" monopoly in the provision of a particular service is one such situation. When economies of scale are very large for a given size of market, it is less costly to have one firm produce that service. If multiple firms competed, one of the firms would be able to lower its costs by increasing its scale of production, thereby driving other firms out of business. Price competition cannot exist under natural monopoly, and the output is likely to be less than optimal because the monopolist will price according to where marginal revenue equals marginal cost. Consequently, price will exceed marginal cost.

Natural monopolies, however, are relatively rare in the health field. Relatively good substitutes exist for most medical services at a local level. Even in a rural area, patients will have to travel to urban areas for complex procedures. While services such as transplant units may be subject to relatively large economies, these services serve a much larger market than is served by the hospital in which they are located. Thus the regional market served by such specialized facilities and services is sufficiently large for several units to compete with one another. Because few services in medical care appear to have the characteristics of a natural monopoly, the natural-monopoly argument has not been an important justification for government intervention in medical care.

Although price-competitive markets may not fulfill the assumptions of a textbook model of competition (namely, many firms and a homogeneous product), workable competition can exist as long as entry is possible and the firms are prohibited by the antitrust laws from engaging in anti-competitive behavior, e.g., boycotts, price fixing, and other forms of monopolizing the market. Competing firms are not perfect substitutes for one another, consequently each firm will have a downward-sloping demand curve (hence price will exceed marginal cost) because each

provider is somewhat different given their location, services available, etc. In these competitive situations, government intervention is not necessary since it has not been shown that regulation can improve market performance without imposing greater economic inefficiency.

Externalities

An important reason for market failure is the existence of externalities. Externalities occur when an action undertaken by an individual (or firm) has secondary effects on others, which may be favorable or unfavorable. Externalities result in a non-optimal amount of output being produced because individuals or firms consider only their own benefits and costs when making a production or consumption decision. If others receive costs or benefits as a result of someone's private decision, the level of output produced in the market will be based upon either too small a level of benefits (i.e., positive external benefits) or too small a level of costs of production (i.e., positive external costs).

For example, as shown in Figure 17-1B, when there are external benefits (MEB) these will not be taken into account by an individual when (s)he makes a decision based on their own calculation of the (marginal private) benefits (MPB) expected from a purchase. The resulting output level is determined by the intersection of the marginal private benefit (MPB) schedule and the marginal private costs (MPC) of producing that service. (The marginal private benefit curve is the demand curve for that service.) The resulting level of output, Q_0, would be smaller than if the external benefits to others (MEB) were included. If the marginal private benefits and the marginal external benefits were added together (to result in the marginal social benefits (MSB) curve), the resulting level of output would be Q_1, which is greater than Q_0.

A similar approach would be used for determining the optimal level of output when there are external costs, although the effect would be opposite that of external benefits. A firm deciding how much output to produce would consider only the marginal private benefits (demand for its product) and marginal

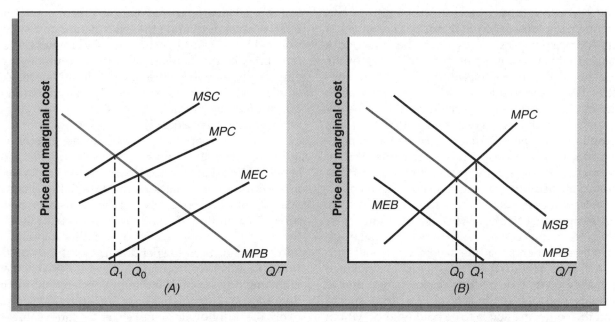

Figure 17-1.   Externalities in production and consumption: (A) a case of external cost; (B) a case of external benefits.

private costs (its costs of production); it would not take into account any costs imposed on others, such as air pollution. If the marginal costs imposed on others (MEC) were added to the firm's costs of production (MPC), the resulting cost of producing that output, the marginal social cost curve (MSC), would represent the full costs of production. The level of output that would then be produced would be smaller, Q_1, than when the external costs were not considered, Q_0.

Individual consumers and producers in a competitive market do not take into consideration the external benefits or costs imposed on others as a result of their decisions. When such external costs and benefits are not incorporated into the private decision-making process, the resultant output level is not optimal. Some persons receive benefits for which they would be willing to pay but do not, whereas others bear additional costs for which they did not receive any benefits. (In the case of external costs, the persons

purchasing that good or service pay a price that is less than the full cost of producing that service; they should bear the full cost (MPC + MEC) of their consumption decisions.)

Externalities therefore have two effects. The first is on economic efficiency: it is only when all the marginal benefits (MSB) equal all the marginal costs (MSC) that the optimal level of output is determined. The second effect is redistribution: some persons receive an external benefit for which they do not compensate those providing it, or a cost is imposed on them for which they are not reimbursed.

The reason externalities occur is because of a lack of ownership or property rights. If someone owned the air or stream that is polluted as a result of a firm producing that product, the polluter could be charged for the pollution, and that charge would become part of the cost of producing that product. Similarly, if persons who receive an external benefit could be charged for their benefit, then the appropriate level of output would occur.[3] At times, the cost of monitoring and collecting from those who impose or receive an externality (transactions costs) exceeds the benefits of doing so, in which case it is not done. (The size of the transactions costs in relation to the size of the externalities is an important reason why compensation does not occur for many externalities. When the extent of the externality increases over time (such as occurred with air pollution) and exceeds the transactions costs, that compensation arrangements occur.)

Because of the lack of ownership rights, collective, non-market, decision making is needed to incorporate external costs and benefits into the private decision-making calculus. When large numbers of persons are involved, it becomes difficult to make voluntary arrangements that are satisfactory to all concerned. Group or collective decision making in which all persons must abide by the decision is required to determine both the optimal level of output and to whom the compensation is to be paid (and on whom the taxes should be assessed). It is a legitimate role for government to serve as the group's agent in a non-market situation.

The Role of Government When Externalities Occur

The existence of externalities legitimizes a role for government in health care, but of what should that role consist? It is not sufficient merely to claim that externalities exist and then justify all types of government intervention and financing of health and medical care.[4] The proper role of government is twofold. First, it must determine the exact nature and size of external benefits and costs. The measurement of externalities is a difficult task, both conceptually and empirically, as will be discussed below. Non-market studies, referred to as cost-benefit analysis, are important for determining the optimal level of output when externalities exist (2).

It is not appropriate, however, for the government to undertake *any* program that has "favorable' cost-benefit ratios. For example, with respect to personal medical programs that have no external effects, the analyst may propose government subsidies based solely on a finding of a favorable cost-benefit ratio. If there are no external effects and the individuals involved do not wish to spend their own funds on the program, it is inappropriate to have the government intervene unless one is willing to declare that the individuals making the decision are not rational. More likely, the individuals do not share the same values or perception of benefits as does the analyst.

The second appropriate role of government when externalities exist is to determine how the externalities should be financed—who will be compensated and who will be taxed. For example, air pollution is an external cost imposed on others. The government should determine the magnitude of the external costs and then place a unit tax (equivalent to the size of the external costs) on those who are producing the particular product that is causing the pollution. The per-unit tax will cause an increase in the polluters' costs of production and a consequent decrease in production and pollution (as shown in Figure 17-1A). The proceeds of the tax can then be used to reimburse those who bear these external costs. Similarly, when there

---

3. R. Coase, who received a Nobel Prize in economics for his work, stated that when there is an external cost, regardless of how property rights are assigned to the opposing parties, the outcome will be the same, assuming very low transactions costs. For example, if the party bearing the external cost were assigned the property rights, they could then sue the party creating the external cost; if the property rights were assigned to the party creating the external cost, the party bearing that cost would be willing to pay to prevent the external cost from being imposed on them. In each case, both parties would presumably calculate the marginal benefits and marginal costs to themselves of either paying to prevent the lawsuit or paying the producer of the external cost to eliminate that external burden; the outcome would be the same.

Ronald Coase, "The Problem of Social Cost," *Journal of Law and Economics*, 3(2), October 1960, 1–45.

---

4. Not all externalities require government intervention. Externalities may exist in a market, however they may be relatively small so that when the MEB is added to the MPB curve, the sum of the two curves intersect at a point to the left of the intersection of the MPB and MPC curves. Thus the optimal rate of output is unaffected by including the MEB. When the market produces more than the amount demanded by the MEB, then this is referred to as "inframarginal" externalities. This subject is discussed in the chapter on The Market for Medical Education with reference to whether medical education should be subsidized.

are external benefits, as in the case of medical research, then those receiving the external benefits should be similarly taxed and the proceeds used to subsidize an increase in medical research.

The principal underlying financing should attempt to affix the taxes and subsidies to those who generate the external costs and benefits. A system of financing based on ability to pay would be inappropriate unless such a system reflected the extent of the external benefits and costs. Further, not all non-market decision-making should be at a federal level. For some health programs the benefits and costs are purely local in character (e.g., water fluoridation); the appropriate level of financing, therefore, should be local.

Situations involving externalities do not necessarily require government production or provision of particular services. If a particular service does not have the characteristics of a natural monopoly, there is no reason why there could not be competition in the provision of that service. Medical schools and other research institutions could compete for research grants. Research is not necessarily produced more efficiently if undertaken solely by federally employed researchers. The criterion for whether the service should be governmentally or privately provided should be efficiency; there is nothing inherent in the nature of externalities that suggests that services should be publicly provided.[5]

---

5. Using the criterion of efficiency, is there any reason for allowing the federal government to have a monopoly on the provision of medical care for veterans? Presumably, the government could determine how much it was willing to spend on medical care for a specific class of veterans (those with a service-connected disability) and then allow them a choice as to whether they wished to purchase care in the private medical sector or in the government's Veterans Administration hospitals. Such potential competition would be threatening to the Veterans Administration bureaucracy. Prohibiting competition for the provision of governmentally financed services often has less to do with efficiency and choice considerations than with the survival of an entrenched government agency. It would also reduce the size of the VA organization since many of its beds are filled with veterans who do not have a service-connected disability. (Instead of reducing the size of its bureaucracy and budget as the number of veterans of the type for whom it was originally established to provide medical care decreases, the VA would prefer to maintain its institutions and budget by expanding the eligible class of veterans.)

Externalities in Health Care

Several types of situations in the health and medical fields give rise to externalities. The first type may be referred to as the "consumer protection" argument discussed previously. Given the technical nature of medical care and the patient's lack of knowledge regarding diagnosis, treatment needs, and the provider's competence, consumers might benefit from the establishment of certain minimum standards and the provision of information. If the private market did not provide minimum standards (possibly through monitoring of providers and malpractice actions) or the necessary information required by consumers, or if all consumers desired the government to ensure some minimum standards, consumer protection would become an externality and hence a legitimate role of government. The methods by which the government could fulfill this public demand for protection would be similar to those discussed previously, i.e., using outcome rather than process measures.

Another externality with regard to personal medical services is what may be referred to as "externalities in consumption." If healthier and wealthier individuals do not want to see persons less fortunate than themselves go without necessary medical care and are willing to contribute to their medical care, an externality in consumption is said to exist. This is because the utility of individuals depends not only upon the quantity of goods and services they themselves purchase, but also upon the amount of certain goods and services (such as medical care) purchased by others. Under such circumstances, if some contribute to the medical services of the less fortunate, then other persons who similarly would have been willing to contribute receive an external benefit; everybody receives the benefit of seeing the less fortunate receive medical care, even though everybody did not necessarily contribute. Theoretically, each person who receives an external benefit should contribute according to the size of the external benefit. Unless there is some form of non-market decision-making, it will not be possible to collect from all the persons who receive an external benefit.

Donor Versus Recipient Preferences

The implications from the preceding discussion are twofold. First, government, acting as the agent for the collective desires of those wishing to contribute, should tax those persons (assuming the government knows the amount each person is willing to spend on those less fortunate than themselves) and provide a subsidy to the desired recipients equivalent to the magnitude of the collected tax. Second, the form of that subsidy (e.g., medical services) and the determination of its method of distribution (possibly an income-related determination of recipients) should represent the desires of the *donors*, not those of the recipients (3). This is because some donors may be willing to contribute (and thereby receive an external benefit) only if their contributions go to a particular income group, for a particular type of service, and are distributed in a certain manner.

There are a number of ways in which subsidies could be provided to help those who are ill or who have low incomes. These persons could be given an income supplement rather than just an increase in their medical services. With an increase in their incomes, they could spend those funds on housing, nutritional foods, or medical services. If it were a lack of access to medical services that the more fortunate wish to redress, it would be inappropriate, from the donor's perspective, to allow those funds to be spent on goods and services other than medical care. Under circumstances of externalities in consumption, in-kind subsidies are efficient.

The justification for national health insurance and other forms of in-kind subsidies (to be discussed more completely in Chapter 18) is presumably based on the assumption that there are externalities in consumption; otherwise, proposed in-kind subsidies would not be efficient. If the objective of the subsidies were the redistribution of income, direct cash supplements would be a more efficient means to this end. The recipients of the subsidy would always prefer cash which can be used to satisfy their most important needs, rather than a subsidy that can be used for only one of their needs, a need which may not represent their highest priority (4).

For in-kind subsidies to be efficient, therefore, the intent must be to satisfy the preferences of the *donors* rather than the recipients. When an in-kind subsidy is called for (as in the case of externalities in consumption), the type of person the donors are willing to subsidize and the amount of subsidy to be provided to each person are most likely inversely related to the recipient's income: the lower the recipient's income, the greater will be the donor's willingness to provide a subsidy. It is unlikely that a person will receive an external benefit from seeing a person with a possibly higher income than themselves receive a subsidy. These aspects of in-kind subsidies should be kept in mind when national health insurance and other in-kind subsidies are discussed.

Requiring everyone to purchase at least catastrophic health insurance can be justified on grounds of externalities. If a person who can afford it decides not to buy insurance, then other persons are bearing part of the cost of that decision. If the person who self-insures is unfortunate enough to incur catastrophic medical expense that he or she is unable to pay, the community (through welfare payments) will have to reimburse the medical providers for that person's medical services. The rest of the community will have to bear part of the cost (in terms of higher taxes) of that individual's decision to self-insure (or purchase less than catastrophic insurance). It would be more equitable, therefore, if these costs were borne in full by individuals at risk, similar to an uninsured motorists fund.

The third type of externality that occurs in the health field is usually associated with public health programs rather than with personal medical services. Vaccination programs, clean water supplies, air pollution abatement, and medical research are examples of goods that result in large external benefits. It has generally been with respect to these types of programs that a great many cost-benefit studies have been undertaken.

REDISTRIBUTION USING IN-KIND SUBSIDIES

There are many types of in-kind subsidies in medical care. Some of these are demand subsidies, others are supply subsidies; some are indirect with regard to the beneficiary groups they hope to affect, others are direct. National health insurance would be classified as a direct demand subsidy. Before discussing national health insurance, it would be instructive to discuss the different types of in-kind subsidies in medical care, their magnitude, their probable effects, and their probable beneficiaries. With a better understanding of in-kind subsidies, their actual as compared to their stated purpose becomes clearer, and a context within which national health insurance can be analyzed is provided. If national health insurance is enacted and designed as an efficient in-kind subsidy, then it is questionable whether other in-kind subsidies should be continued.[6]

In-Kind Demand Subsidies

The major in-kind subsidies on the demand side are Medicare, Medicaid, the tax exemption of employer-paid health insurance, and the tax deductibility of medical expenses in excess of 7.5 percent of adjusted gross income. Expenditures under Medicare and Medicaid (excluding other direct government subsidies on the demand side such as maternal and child health care) were $491 billion in 2002 (5). The exclusion from taxes of employer-paid health insurance premiums were estimated to cost the federal government $120 billion a year in lost federal income and Social Security taxes in 2001 (excluding lost state income taxes)(6).

On the supply side there are (and have been) both direct and indirect subsidy programs. Subsidies are provided for health manpower education, graduate medical education, for hospital construction, provision of medical services through the Veterans Administration and state and local government hospitals, as well as numerous indirect subsidies, such as those that grant tax-exempt status to nonprofit hospitals and state assistance in financing hospital bond issues.

The magnitude of these direct and indirect demand and supply subsidies has been—and still is—very large; it is clear that the role of government in the financing and provision of personal medical services has been substantial.

Given the significant role of government in financing personal medical services, it is important to determine who are the beneficiaries of these subsidies and the efficiency with which they are being distributed. These two issues are interrelated; as discussed previously, the argument for in-kind subsidies is based upon externalities in consumption. As such, the primary recipients should be those persons with low incomes and/or poor health. If the subsidies are distributed in such a way as to benefit higher-income groups or provide them with a greater proportionate share of the subsidy, then the distribution of the subsidy is inefficient; that is, the desired beneficiary group (low-income persons) could receive a greater amount of the subsidy if it were provided in a different, presumably more direct manner.[7]

It is generally easier to determine the beneficiary groups under demand rather than supply subsidies. Under the Medicaid program, for example, the designated beneficiaries are the medically indigent. Since Medicaid is a federal-state matching program, the definition of medical indigency and the benefits provided under the program vary by state. However, as shown in Table 17-1, expenditures under Medicaid go

---

6. Regardless of their stated intent, in-kind medical care subsidies do not have as their actual objective an increase in health status. Instead, their goal appears to be an increase in use of medical services. For example, total public spending on medical services for those 65 years of age and older were $3,823 per person in 2000; for those 19 to 64 and under 19, the equivalent figures were $446 and $224. If the actual purpose of government medical care expenditures were to achieve an increase in health levels, these expenditures might well have been allocated to different population groups, disease categories, and to non-medical-care programs. Even if it were agreed that the in-kind subsidy was to be provided to the aged alone, a different allocation of funds for non-medical-care services would be called for. An equivalent cash supplement to the aged to enable them to increase their consumption of food, housing, and heating would probably contribute more to their health than a subsidy restricted to medical services alone. http://www.meps.ahrq.gov/mepsnet/hc/mepsnethc.asp

---

7. This assumes that the method of distribution is not prescribed by the same externalities argument that gave rise to the subsidy in the first place.

predominantly to those with low incomes. Since Medicaid is funded by general income taxes, those with low incomes receive a subsidy financed by those with high incomes.

When indirect demand subsidy programs are examined, it becomes less obvious that the subsidies are going to those persons with the lowest incomes and/or greatest medical needs. Under Medicare, because the beneficiary group is defined by age rather than income level, the subsidy is more evenly distributed across income levels. Not all aged persons have lower incomes than non-aged persons. Although per capita Medicare expenditures decrease with higher income levels (because older aged have lower incomes), the percentage of total Medicare expenditures going to each income level is more evenly distributed. Those aged with low incomes received 36 percent of total Medicare expenditures as compared to the high-income aged group, who received 31 percent. The redistributional effects of Medicare are small.

When tax subsidy programs, such as the exclusion of employer-provided health insurance premiums from taxable income and the deduction of medical expenses are examined, higher-income groups are the major beneficiaries (48 percent). Middle-income and high-income groups together receive 81 percent of those subsidy dollars.

It would thus appear that the more directly the demand subsidy is aimed at a designated low-income population group, the more likely it is that the intended recipients will receive a larger proportion of that subsidy. Direct subsidy programs of this sort would be more in accordance with the stated goals of the legislation. Indirect demand subsidy programs (such as Medicare, which is based on age) are a less efficient way of subsidizing those with low incomes. If in-kind medical subsidies are justified on grounds of externalities, the beneficiaries should presumably be those with lower incomes and/or greater needs for medical care. Direct demand subsidies are both a more obvious and a more direct means of assuring that this objective is achieved.

It is perhaps an indication of what is the true, as compared to the stated, intent of the legislation that

Table 17-1. Major Federal Government Expenditures on Health Services, 2003 (in percentages)

Family Income	Medicare(a)	Medicaid(b)	Health Benefits Tax(c)
Low Income	36	84	19
Average Income	33	14	33
High Income	31	2	48

Sources: Data on Medicare from C. Eugene Steuerle and Adam Carasso, The Urban Institute, 2002, personal correspondence, February 12, 2004.

Data on Medicaid based on Gail R. Wilensky, "Government and the Financing of Health Care," *American Economic Review,* 72(2), May 1982, pp. 202–207, table 2.

Data on Health Benefits Tax from John Sheils and Randall Haught, "The Cost of Tax-Exempt Health Benefits in 2004," *Health Affairs—Web Exclusive,* February 25, 2004, W4-110, Exhibit 3, http://content.healthaffairs.org/cgi/content/abstract/hlthaff.w4.106 (accessed on February 25, 2004.)

(a) Data on Medicare lifetime benefits minus taxes for two earner couple who turns 65 in 2000.
'Low income' refers to a family with two wage earners one earning a low and the other earning an average wage. 'Average Income' refers to a family with two earners each earning an average wage. 'High Income' refers to a family with two earners one earning a high and the other earning an average wage.
Low wage is 45% of the Social Security average wage, in the year 2000 it was $14,470 for an individual; Average wage in the year 2000 was $32,155 for an individual; High wage is 160% of the Social Security average wage, in the year 2000 it was $51,448 for an individual. The percent of families in each of the three income categories is 60, 25, and 15 respectively.

(b) 'Low Income' includes those whose family income was less than 200 percent of the 2003 poverty level. 'Average Income' is 200 to 400 percent of the poverty level, and 'High Income' is 4.01 times the poverty level or more. For a family of four in 2003, these three groups distribute as follows: less than $40,000, $40,000 to $74,999 and equal to or greater than $75,000.

(c) 'Low Income' category includes family income lower than $40,000, 'Average Income' includes family income between $40,000 and $74,999, 'High Income' includes family income equal to or higher than $75,000.

The percent of the population age 15–65 in each of the income categories is 34, 32, and 34 respectively.

in-kind subsidies are indirect, such as the tax subsidy programs. The legislation's real goal is not to just assist the poor, but to provide a benefit to those in the middle- and high-income groups as well.

Demand subsidies impose costs on those persons not receiving them in two ways. First, those persons must pay increased taxes to pay for the subsidy program. Second, an increase in demand by the recipients of the subsidies results in an increase in the price of medical services which (depending upon the price elasticity of demand and supply) increases the cost and decreases the use of medical services of those who are not being subsidized. After Medicare and Medicaid were introduced, prices in the medical sector more than doubled, as shown previously.

The demand subsidy will have secondary effects throughout the entire medical sector. A demand subsidy will cause an increase in demand in the different institutional markets: hospitals, physician services, and so on. How large the increase in demand will be in each of the separate institutional markets will depend, in part, upon the type of demand subsidy (i.e., how much price is reduced to the beneficiaries) in each of the institutional settings and the elasticity of supply in that market. An inelastic supply will result in greater price increases which will tend to reduce demand in both the beneficiary and non-beneficiary groups.

As demand increases in each of the institutional settings, there will be an increase in the derived demand for the inputs (different types of health manpower and non-labor inputs) used in that setting. With increased demands for health manpower, wages and incomes in the manpower markets will increase, together with participation rates. In the long run, an increase in the incomes of health personnel will result in increased demands for a health professional education and, if the health education market responds, there will be an increase in the stock of trained health manpower.

How much of the demand subsidy ends up in higher prices rather than in increased services will depend upon the elasticity of supply in the various medical markets. The greater the number of restrictions on entry into the health professions and on the tasks that different health personnel can perform and the greater the lack of efficiency incentives in methods of provider payment, the greater the inelasticity of supply and the higher will be the increases in medical prices.

Supply Subsidies

Supply subsidies may also be classified according to whether they are directly targeted to a beneficiary group or whether their benefits are diffused among many population groups. An example of a direct supply subsidy to a designated beneficiary group is the provision of funds to establish a clinic in a low-income neighborhood. Even if there is no corresponding demand subsidy, the new clinic will result in an increased use of medical services by those with low incomes because it will decrease the patients' cost of travel to the facility. Most direct supply subsidies are not of this type; the major direct supply subsidies are the Veterans Administration hospitals and state and local government hospitals.

The Veterans Administration medical system is fairly extensive, consisting of 162 hospitals, 864 outpatient clinics, 137 nursing homes, a $27.5 billion 2004 budget, and 188,217 employees. Although the major stated role of the VA is to provide medical care to veterans with a service-connected disability, only 10 percent of the veterans in VA hospitals are there for that purpose. The remaining 90 percent have low incomes and receive care for illnesses unrelated to their military service (7).

State and local government hospitals account for approximately 17 percent of all admissions to short-term general hospitals and approximately 17 percent of all hospital outpatient visits. These hospitals have served as important sources of medical care for the indigent and have relieved the private hospitals and physicians of the financial risk of caring for these patients.

In view of the amounts being spent on Medicare and Medicaid, which are targeted to similar population groups served by the VA and other government hospital systems, what is the justification for these government providers? If the medically indigent were to receive a demand subsidy with benefits at least as complete as those presently available to them in the VA and other government hospitals, the demand for care in these institutions is likely to decline sharply. State and local government hospitals have had a reputation for providing lower quality care and/or lower patient satisfaction than that provided by community nonprofit hospitals. VA hospitals are inconveniently located in relation to their beneficiary population (there are only 162 VA general and psychiatric hospitals as opposed to more than 5,000 community hospitals).

If all providers, including the VA and the other government hospitals, had to compete for patients under a targeted demand subsidy to these patient populations, the VA and governmental hospitals would either have to adapt or they would not be able to survive in a competitive environment. For the VA system to compete for the 90 percent of its population who use the VA because they are medically indigent, it would have to provide ambulatory services, change its organizational and reimbursement arrangements with its physicians, increase its relative efficiency by lowering lengths of stay and use less costly substitutes for inpatient care, and compete on a more local basis for patients since patient travel costs and time are likely to be significant determinants in choosing medical delivery systems. If the VA cannot survive under competitive conditions where patients are provided with a demand subsidy and are free to choose, what economic justification is there for providing additional large subsidies to enable the VA to maintain its current role?

State and local governmental hospitals in many states are being forced to compete with HMOs and other providers as more of the Medicaid population is being enrolled in capitated managed care systems. If everyone were enrolled in either private or public insurance programs, then it would not be necessary to separately subsidize local governmental hospitals. Unfortunately, not everyone is covered by private insurance or eligible for demand subsidies, such as the uninsured and illegal immigrants. Local governmental hospitals will continue to remain as the providers of last resort, requiring a supply subsidy. Under a competitive system, the existence of public hospitals

would be an indication that either the size of the direct demand subsidies is insufficient for the private sector to serve these population groups or that certain groups are ineligible for subsidized medical care.

Indirect supply subsidies, the other major type of in-kind supply subsidy, are exemplified by funds for training additional health manpower and capital grants to hospitals. These indirect supply subsidies have their initial effects on a particular medical market. For the subsidy to increase medical services, its effect must eventually be transmitted through several medical markets. For example, when a subsidy is given to medical schools to increase the number of physicians, several years pass before there is an increase in the number of additional graduates. These graduates will then work in a number of settings, ranging from hospitals to physicians' offices.

The increase in the amount of services eventually received by the members of a particular beneficiary group (i.e., those with low incomes) will depend upon their elasticity of demand for those services. (The increased supply of services is a downward shift along a patient's demand curve for that service.) If demand by members of the beneficiary group is relatively inelastic (i.e., not very responsive to changes in the price of the service), there will be relatively little increase in their use of medical services. Since indirect supply subsidies are not generally targeted to particular beneficiary groups, the beneficiaries will be everyone using the service; they will be paying a lower price than before the subsidy. Because low-income persons do not use medical services as much as those with high incomes, they are likely to receive less benefit than high users from such subsidies; the high users may also have relatively higher incomes.

In addition to being inefficient in that the greatest portion of the supply subsidy does not go to those with low-incomes, general supply subsidies present further problems. When only one input into the process of producing medical care is subsidized, a manager who is attempting to use the lowest-cost combination of inputs will tend to use more of the subsidized input because its cost has been artificially reduced. For example, a subsidy to train additional registered nurses will, if it is successful, result in a greater increase in the supply of nurses and a relatively lower wage for them. Because the wage of nurses is lowered, hospitals will substitute away from other nursing personnel toward more registered nurses in providing patient care.

Subsidizing a specific input is less efficient than if the hospital were merely awarded an equivalent unrestricted subsidy. In the latter case, the hospital would use a combination of registered and non-registered nurses and other inputs based on their relative prices and productivities. Consequently, the hospital would use fewer registered nurses than if only RN wages were artificially reduced through a subsidy. Subsidies that increase the supply of a particular input are therefore less efficient (more costly) than an equivalent dollar subsidy.

It is also often difficult to determine what additional services have been produced as a result of a supply subsidy. Although one might be able to count the number of additional persons trained as a result of the subsidy (which is not as easy as it might appear), it is more difficult to calculate the net increase in services resulting from the additional health manpower. Without additional nurses, the wage rate of existing nurses would have risen more rapidly thereby causing an increase in the nurse participation rate. In the long run, higher wages would cause an increase in the number of persons seeking a career in nursing. Similarly, without a subsidy to increase the number of physicians, the productivity of existing physicians might be greater. To assume that the additional services provided by the subsidized manpower are the net benefits of the supply subsidy greatly overstates its benefits.

To understand exactly what impact supply subsidies have on increased use of services and for which beneficiary groups, it is necessary to use a complex econometric model of the medical sector. For example, a subsidy to increase the number of registered nurses will have its initial impact on the nursing education market. How many additional nurses will be graduated as a result of that subsidy will depend, in part, on the objectives of the different types of nursing schools and on which schools receive the subsidies. The number of nurses will also depend upon the elasticity of demand for a nursing education by prospective nurses since the subsidy will reduce their educational costs.

The impact of additional nurses on the market for nurses will affect nurses' wages, participation rates, and nurse employment. How many additional nurses will be employed in the various institutional settings will depend upon the elasticity of demand for nurses in each of the different settings and the new wage for nurses. (The determination of wages and employment will, of course, be a simultaneous process.) The greater the substitutability of registered nurses for other types of nursing personnel, the higher will be the elasticity of demand and the greater will be the decrease in demand for non-registered nurses. Each of the institutional settings that employ registered nurses will have a slightly lower cost for its nursing personnel; the cost of care in each institutional setting will also be lower. How much lower will depend upon how many registered nurses are employed and the elasticity of the demand for nurses (i.e., whether many more nurses are hired as a result of their relatively lower wage).

The effect of the nurse subsidy on cost of care will vary for each institutional setting; hospitals, which hire the majority of nurses, would receive the largest cost reduction. Since the relative cost of the different institutional settings has changed, how much the price of care will be reduced in each of the institutional settings as a result of a lowering of costs will depend upon the elasticity of demand for services and the market in which an institution competes. If there are no competitive pressures on the institution or if the institution attempts to maximize its prestige, it is less likely that the cost savings will be passed on to patients and other third-party payors.

As seen from the above discussion, it is much more difficult to determine the end result of supply subsidies compared with the impact of demand subsidies. It is equally difficult to determine which consumer or payor group receives the major benefit, if any, of the supply subsidy.

When the government has served as the supplier of medical services, e.g., state hospitals, such supply subsidies have generally had a direct impact on low-income persons. When supply subsidies have been indirect, in-kind subsidies have provided benefits to all those persons who use medical services; but as with the Hill-Burton program for hospital construction, nothing was done to help those who could not afford to use the hospital. A demand subsidy was still required for the medically indigent.

In-kind supply subsidies take longer than direct-demand subsidies to provide greater access to medical services to a beneficiary group. They are also economically inefficient either because patients have no choice as to provider (as under the VA system), or because the relative cost of inputs is distorted. Further, the benefits of indirect supply subsidies are overstated since employee participation rates and productivity increases are, in fact, likely to be lower than what they would otherwise have been.

If the funds used to provide general supply subsidies were instead provided as a direct demand subsidy to low-income groups, this targeted group would receive a greater benefit than the portion they would receive from a general supply subsidy.

Although direct-demand subsidies would appear to be a more efficient method of providing an in-kind subsidy, supply subsidies are legislatively popular. The probable reason is not that legislators are necessarily unaware of which is the more efficient subsidy method, but rather that the providers of medical care and manpower education are important beneficiaries of such proposals. Such supply subsidies are generally the direct result of lobbying by these interest groups.

The intent of the preceding discussion on existing in-kind subsidies in medical care was to provide both an indication of the magnitude of such subsidies and criteria by which to judge the efficiency of alternative types of in-kind subsidies. If national health insurance were enacted, many of the demand and supply (direct and indirect) subsidies could be eliminated; the funds saved could be used to lessen the cost of national health insurance.

SUMMARY

Poor performance may occur when the assumptions of a competitive market are not fulfilled. Such market imperfections may be the result of a lack of consumer information, inadequate purchaser and supplier incentives to be efficient, and barriers to the mobility of resources. When such market imperfections exist, there may be a role for government. Unfortunately, government itself has created many of these market imperfections, such as entry barriers and lack of patient and provider incentives.

The appropriate role of government when such market imperfections exist should be to eliminate them and directly address the stated purpose for which they were imposed, namely, consumer protection. That the stated goal of such restrictive practices can be achieved more directly and more efficiently and are not suggests that the intended objective is different from the stated goal.

A second justification for government intervention is the existence of externalities. Individual consumers and producers do not take into consideration the external benefits and costs imposed on others as a result of their actions. When externalities exist, the appropriate role of government is to calculate their magnitude and use a system of taxes or subsidies to achieve the optimal rate of output. One such externality, to provide medical care to the poor, is an important justification for in-kind demand and supply subsidies.

Indirect subsidies are less efficient (more costly) than direct subsidies since many who are not part of the intended beneficiary group also benefit. Direct-demand subsidies are both the fastest and most efficient means for increasing the use of services by a designated beneficiary group.

REVIEW QUESTIONS

1. Explain the economist's definition of the correct or optimal rate of output.
2. Define externalities. Why do they occur? What are examples of externalities in the health field? Explain why the presence of externalities will, in

the absence of some collective action, lead to a sub-optimal rate of output. What type of collective action is called for?

3. Is there an optimal amount of pollution? What would occur if government were to mandate the elimination of all pollution?

4. If a cost-benefit analysis is "favorable," does this suggest that the government should always undertake such an expenditure? In your answer, discuss the criteria that should be used or who should undertake such projects, and how they should be financed.

5. What are the economic rationales for different types of government intervention in health care?

6. Explain the rationale for requiring everyone who can afford it to purchase, at a minimum, catastrophic health insurance.

7. What economic arguments support government financing of personal health services to certain population groups?

8. If the objective is one of redistribution, what are the welfare implications of achieving this redistribution by providing cash supplements versus medical care to the desired beneficiary group?

9. "We all benefit by having physicians available in case we need them. Therefore the government should subsidize medical education." Critique this justification of government subsidies based on an externalities argument.

REFERENCES

1. For a complete discussion of the role of government, see Richard A. Musgrave and Peggy B. Musgrave, *Public Finance in Theory and Practice*, (New York: McGraw-Hill, 1989). Musgrave categorizes government programs into those that affect the allocation of resources, those that alter the distribution of incomes, and stabilization programs (i.e., those that regulate the level of economic activity).

2. For an extensive discussion of cost-benefit analysis, see Edward M. Gramlich, *A Guide to Benefit-Cost Analysis,* 2nd ed. (Englewood Cliffs, N.J.: Prentice-Hall, 1990).

3. For a more extended discussion of this proposition, see Paul Feldman, "Efficiency, Distribution, and the Role of Government in a Market Economy," *Journal of Political Economy,* 79(3), May–June 1971: 508–526.

4. A proof of this statement may be found in a number of texts on microeconomics. See, for example, Robert H. Frank, *Microeconomics and Behavior,* 2nd ed., (New York: McGraw-Hill, Inc. 1994): 89–91.

5. Centers for Medicare and Medicaid Services, Office of the Actuary: National Health Statistics Group, [online information, 2004], http://www.cms.gov/statistics/nhe (accessed on January 8, 2004).

6. For 2001 estimates on the cost of employment-based health insurance subsidies, Congressional Budget Office, Budget Options, February 2001, http://www.cbo.gov/bo2001/bo2001_showhit1.cfm?index=REV-12 (accessed on September 2, 2003).

7. Data from Department of Veterans Affairs, http://www.va.gov (accessed on January 15, 2004).

CHAPTER

18

Health Policy and the Legislative Marketplace

KEY TERMS AND CONCEPTS

- Public interest theory of government
- Government policy objectives
- Government policy instruments
- Economic theory of government
- Price of legislation
- Concentrated interests
- Diffuse costs
- Regressive taxes
- Visibility of legislation's effects
- Five types of producer legislation

Learning Objectives

Upon completing this chapter, the reader should be able to:

- Contrast two competing theories of government behavior, the Public Interest and the Economic Theory.

- Understand why those having a "concentrated" interest are more likely to represent their interests than those who have a "diffuse" interest.

- Discuss each of the five types of demand increasing legislation favored by health associations.

- Explain how political markets differ from economic markets, thereby enabling organized interests to benefit at the expense of majorities.

THE LEGISLATIVE MARKETPLACE

There has been and (continues to be) extensive government intervention in the financing and delivery of medical services. For example, on the demand side of the market, there are substantial government subsidies such as Medicare, Medicaid, and the exclusion from taxable income of employer-purchased health insurance. On the supply side, government subsidizes medical schools, nursing schools, and other health professional educational institutions; state licensing boards establish barriers to entering the various health professions and define the tasks permitted to various health professionals. Some states subject health facilities' investment to state review and determine which benefits must be offered under health insurance plans. And the federal government regulates hospital and physician prices for Medicare patients. These are just some of the more significant examples of government involvement in health care.

To gain a better understanding of the reasons for the extensive government intervention, which at times may seem contradictory in its effects, it is necessary to develop a framework within which to view government behavior. Different theories of legislative outcomes exist. At opposite ends of the theory spectrum are the "public interest" and "economic" theories.

THE PUBLIC INTEREST VIEW OF GOVERNMENT

The traditional or Public Interest view of government assumes that legislation is enacted to serve the public interest. To accomplish this, the public interest theory assumes that there are two basic objectives of government: to improve market efficiency and, second, to redistribute income in a more equitable manner.

The efficiency objective of government is to improve the allocation of resources. Inefficiency in resource allocation can occur, for example, when firms in a market have monopoly power or when externalities exist. A firm has monopoly power when it is able to charge a price that exceeds its cost by more than a normal profit. Monopoly is inefficient because it produces too small a level of service (output). The addi-

tional benefit to purchasers (as indicated by its price) from consuming a service is greater than the cost of producing that benefit; therefore more resources should flow into that industry until the additional benefit of consuming that service equals the additional cost of producing it.

The bases of monopoly power are several: there may be only one firm in a market, such as when there is a natural monopoly (e.g., an electric company); there may be barriers to entry in a market; firms may collude on raising their prices; or, because of a lack of information, consumers are unable to judge price, quality, and service differences among different suppliers. In each of these situations, the prices charged will exceed the costs of producing the product (which includes a normal profit). The appropriate government remedy to decrease monopoly power is to eliminate barriers to entry into a market, prevent price collusion, and to improve information among consumers.

The second situation where the allocation of resources can be improved is when there are "externalities" which occur when someone undertakes an action and in so doing affects others who are not part of that transaction. The effects on others could be positive or negative. For example, a utility using high-sulfur coal to produce electricity also produces air pollution. As a result of the air pollution, residents in surrounding communities may have a higher incidence of respiratory illness. Resources are misallocated since the cost of producing electricity excludes the costs imposed on others. As a result, too much electricity is being produced. If the costs of producing electricity also included the costs imposed on others, the electricity price would be higher and, consequently, its demand would be less. The allocation of resources would be improved if the utility's cost included both types of costs. The appropriate role of government in such a situation is to determine the costs imposed on others and to tax the utility an equivalent amount.

Redistribution, the second objective of government, causes a change in wealth and is based on the values of society, namely, how equitable should be the distribution of resources? If society decides that medical services should be more equitably distributed, then those with lower incomes would be expected to receive net benefits (their benefits exceed their costs or taxes), and those with higher incomes should incur net costs (their taxes exceed their benefits) from the legislation. Crucial to the evaluation of redistributive legislation is which population groups are eligible for the benefits and the types of taxes imposed to finance those benefits. When eligibility is by income and income taxes are used to finance the program's benefits, it is likely that redistribution occurs from high- to low-income groups. Two large redistributive programs are Medicare for the aged and Medicaid for the medically indigent. The benefits and costs of a redistributive medical program, such as Medicaid, are shown in Table 18-1.

These traditional objectives of government—redistribution and efficiency—can be achieved by using one or more of the following policy instruments: expenditures, taxation, and/or regulation (1). These policy objectives and instruments are shown in Table 18-2. The policy instruments can be applied to either the purchaser (demand) or the supplier side of the market. For example, the government has subsidized (expenditure policy) medical schools to increase the number of physicians (supply side) and has also subsidized the purchase of medical services by the aged (demand side). Tax policy has benefited employees by excluding employer-paid health insurance from taxable income (demand side) and enabled nonprofit hospitals to pay lower interest costs by issuing tax exempt bonds (supply side). State government regulations specify which medical services and practition-

Table 18-1. Determining the Redistributive Effects of Government Programs

	Low Income	High Income
Benefits	X	
Costs		X

ers must be included in health insurance sold in that state (demand side), and some states require government approval if a health provider, such as a hospital or home health agency, wants to enter a market (supply side).

According to the Public Interest theory, all health policies using the different policy instruments (on both the demand and supply sides of the market) should be able to be categorized according to whether the policy objective is to increase efficiency or redistribution; and if it is redistribution, then the net benefits and costs should be distributed as shown in Table 18-1.

AN ECONOMIC THEORY OF GOVERNMENT

Dissatisfaction with the Public Interest theory occurred for several reasons. Instead of just regulating natural monopolies, government has also regulated competitive industries such as airlines, trucks, taxicabs, as well as various professions. Further, nonregulated firms always want to enter regulated markets. To prevent entry into regulated industries, the government established entry barriers. If the govern-

Table 18-2. Health Policy Objectives and Interventions

Government Policy Instruments		Government Objectives	
		Redistribution	Improve Efficiency
Expenditures	Demand side		
	Supply side		
Taxation (±)	Demand side		
	Supply side		
Regulation	Demand side		
	Supply side		

ment supposedly reduced prices in regulated markets (hence the firm's profitability), why would firms want to enter a regulated industry?

With regard to the redistribution objective, why was it necessary to enact both Medicare and Medicaid? Why was Medicare financed by both a payroll and an income tax? And why do those with higher incomes gain the most from tax-exempt employer-paid health insurance?

To reconcile these apparent contradictions with the Public Interest view of government, an alternative theory of government behavior, the Economic Theory of Regulation, was developed (2). The basic assumption underlying the economic theory is that political markets are no different from economic markets; individuals and firms seek to further their self interest. Firms undertake investments in private markets to achieve a high rate of return. Why wouldn't the same firms invest in legislation if it also offered a high rate of return? Organized groups are willing to pay a price for legislative benefits. This price is political support, which brings together the demanders and suppliers of legislative benefits.

The suppliers of legislative benefits are legislators, and their goal is assumed to be to maximize their chances for re-election. As the late Senator Everett Dirksen said, "The first law of politics is to get elected, the second law is to be re-elected." To be re-elected requires political support which consists of campaign contributions, votes, and/or volunteer time. Legislators are assumed to be rational, to make cost-benefit calculations when faced with demands for legislation. However, the legislator's cost-benefit calculations are not the costs and benefits to society of enacting particular legislation. Instead, the benefits are the additional political support the legislator would receive from supporting the legislation. The costs are the lost political support they would incur as a result of their action. When the benefits to the legislators exceed their costs, they will support the legislation.

Concentrated Interests

Those who have a "concentrated" interest (that is, the effect of the legislation will have a large impact on their profitability by either affecting their revenues or their costs) are more likely to be successful in the legislative marketplace. It becomes worthwhile for the group to organize, to represent their interests before legislators, and to raise political support to achieve the profits that favorable legislation can provide. It is for this reason that only those with a concentrated interest will demand legislative benefits.

Whenever legislative benefits are provided to one group, others must bear those costs. When only one group has a concentrated interest in the legislation, they are more likely to be successful if the costs to finance those benefits are not obvious and can be spread over a large number of people. When this occurs, then the costs are said to be "diffuse."

For example, assume that there are ten firms in an industry and, if they can have legislation enacted that would limit imports that compete with their products, they would be able to raise their prices and thereby receive $280 million in legislative benefits. These firms have a concentrated interest ($280 million) in trying to enact such legislation. The costs of these legislative benefits are financed by a small increase in the price of their product amounting to $1 per person. It is often not obvious to consumers that the legislation increases their costs. Further, even if consumers were aware of the legislation's effect, it would not be worthwhile for them to organize and represent their interests so as to forestall a price increase that will decrease their income by $1 a year. The costs of trying to prevent the cost increase would exceed their potential savings.

It is easier (less costly) for providers rather than consumers to organize, provide political support, and impose a diffuse cost on others. It is for this reason that there has been so much legislation affecting entry into the health professions, which tasks are reserved to certain professions, how (and which) providers are paid under public medical programs, why subsidies for medical education are given to the school and not to the student (otherwise they would have to compete for students), and so on. Most health issues have been relatively technical, such as the training of health professions, certification of their quality, methods of payment, controls on hospital capital investment, etc. *The higher medical prices resulting from regulations that benefit providers have been diffuse and not visible to consumers.*

Understanding Contradictions of the Public Interest Theory

The economic theory of legislation provides an explanation for the above dissatisfactions with the public interest theory. Firms in competitive markets seek regulation in order to earn higher profits than are available in competitive markets. Prices in regulated markets, such as interstate airline travel, were always higher than non-regulated markets, such as intrastate air travel, thereby enabling regulated firms to earn greater profits. These higher prices provided non-regulated firms with an incentive to try to enter regulated markets. Government, on behalf of the regulated industry, imposed entry barriers to keep out low-priced competitors. Otherwise the regulated firms could not earn more than a competitive rate of return.

Through legislation, firms try to receive the monopoly profits they are unable to achieve through market competition.

When only one group has a concentrated interest in the outcome of legislation and the costs are diffuse, legislators will respond to the political support the group is willing to pay to have favorable legislation enacted. When there are opposing groups each with a concentrated interest in the outcome, legislators are likely to reach a compromise between the competing demanders of legislative benefits. Rather than balancing the gain in political support from one group against the loss from the other, legislators prefer to receive political support from both groups and impose diffuse costs on those unable to offer political support.

When the beneficiaries are specific population groups, such as the aged, the redistributive effects of the legislation are meant to be very visible. An example of this is Medicare. By making it clear which population groups will benefit, legislators hope to receive their political support. The costs of financing such visible redistributive programs, however, are still designed to be diffuse so as not to generate political opposition from others. A small diffuse tax imposed on many people, such as a payroll tax, is the only way large sums of money can be raised with little opposition to finance visible redistributive programs.

Payroll taxes that include a maximum wage level to which the tax applies, such as the one used to finance Medicare, were regressive. The tax represented a greater portion of income from low-income employees. Economists have determined that payroll taxes, even when imposed on the employer, are borne mostly by the employee. However, the advantage of imposing part of the tax on the employer is that it appears that employees are paying a smaller portion of it than they really are. The remainder of the tax is shifted forward to consumers in the form of higher prices for the goods and services they purchase.

Differences in the sources of political support are important for understanding our two main redistributive programs. Medicaid is a means tested (income-related) program for the poor and is funded from general tax revenues. Since the poor (who have low voting participation rates) are unable to provide legislators with political support, the support for Medicaid comes from the middle class, who must agree to higher taxes to provide the poor with medical benefits. The inadequacy of Medicaid in every state, the conditions necessary for achieving Medicaid eligibility, the low levels of eligibility, and their lack of access to medical providers are related to the generosity (or lack thereof) of the middle class. The beneficiaries of Medicare, on the other hand, are the aged themselves who (together with their children) provide the political support for the program. As the cost of Medicare has risen, government has raised Medicare payroll taxes and reduced payments to providers rather than reducing benefits or beneficiaries from this politically powerful group.

Provider organizations also have a concentrated interest in redistributive programs. When Medicare and Medicaid were enacted, physician and hospital associations were concerned with how their members would be paid by the government. These provider associations were also interested in precluding competition by competitive industries, such as HMOs, nurse practitioners, psychologists, etc. Given their concentrated interest in these issues, physician and hospital associations were important contributors of political support for the purpose of defining the regulations determining provider payment and eligibility of providers to participate in these programs.

The political necessity of keeping costs diffuse explains why the financing of both Medicare and producer regulation relies upon regressive taxes, either payroll taxes or higher prices for medical services. Spreading the costs over large populations keeps those costs diffuse. The net effect is that low-income persons pay the costs and higher income persons, such as physicians or high-income aged, receive the benefits. According to the economic theory, those receiving the benefits and those bearing the costs are not based on income, as shown in Table 18-1, but instead according to which groups are able to offer political support (the beneficiaries) and which groups are unable to do so (they bear the costs). Regressive taxes are typically used to finance producer regulation as well as provide benefits to specific population groups.

Why Health Policies Change

Health policies change over time because groups who previously bore a diffuse cost develop a concentrated interest. Until the 1960s, medical societies were the main group with a concentrated interest in the financing and delivery of medical services. Thus the delivery system was structured to benefit physicians. Increases in the physician-to-population ratio remained constant for 15 years (until the mid 1960s) at 141/100,000, state restrictions were imposed on HMOs to limit their development, advertising was prohibited, and restrictions were placed on other health professionals to limit their ability to compete with physicians. Financing mechanisms also benefited physicians; until the 1980s, capitation payment for HMOs was prohibited under Medicare and Medicaid, and competitors to physicians were excluded from reimbursement under public and private insurance systems.

As the costs of medical care continued to increase rapidly to government and employers, their previously diffuse costs became concentrated. Under Medicare, the government was faced with the choice of raising taxes or reducing benefits to the aged, both of which would have cost the Administration politi-

cal support. Successive administrations developed a concentrated interest in lowering the rate of increase in Medicare expenditures. Rapidly rising Medicaid expenditures forced states to reduce Medicaid eligibility and provider payments, otherwise the states would have had to raise taxes or reduce expenditures for politically popular programs, such as prisons and education. Similarly, large employers were concerned that rising medical costs were making them less competitive internationally. The pressures for cost containment increased as the "costs" of an inefficient delivery and payment system grew larger. Rising medical expenditures are no longer a diffuse cost to large purchasers of medical services.

Other professional organizations, such as psychologists, chiropractors, and podiatrists saw the potentially greater revenues their members could receive if they were better able to compete with physicians. These groups developed a concentrated interest in securing payment for their members under public and private insurance systems and expanding their scope of practice. The rise in opposing concentrated interests weakened the political influence of organized medicine.

Evaluating Opposing Theories of Government Behavior

The Public Interest and economic theories of government provide opposing predictions of the redistributive and efficiency effects of government legislation, as shown in Table 18-3. To determine which of these contrasting theories is a more accurate description of government, it is necessary to match the actual outcomes of legislation to each theory's predictions. Do the benefits of redistributive programs go to those with low incomes? Are they financed by taxes that impose a larger burden on those with higher incomes? Does the government try and improve the allocation of resources by reducing barriers to entry and, when information is limited, monitoring and publishing quality measures of physicians' and other medical services?

The economic theory of regulation provides greater understanding of why health policies are enacted and why they have changed over time than alternative theories. The economic theory predicts

Table 18-3. Health Policy Objectives under Different Theories of Government

	Objective of Government	
Theories of Government	Redistribution	Improve Efficiency
Public Interest Theory	Assist those with low incomes	Remove (and prevent) monopoly abuses and protect environment (externalities)
Economic Theory of Regulation	Provide benefits to those able to deliver political support and finance from those having little political support	Efficiency objective unimportant; more likely to protect industries in order to provide them with redistributive benefits

that government is not concerned with efficiency issues. *Redistribution is the main objective of government, but it is to redistribute wealth to those who are able to offer political support from those who are unable to do so.* Thus the reason medical licensing boards are inadequately staffed, have never required re-examination for relicensure, and have failed to monitor practicing physicians is that organized medicine has been opposed to any approaches for increasing quality that would adversely affect physicians' incomes. Regressive taxes are used to finance programs such as Medicare, not because legislators are unaware of their regressive nature, but because it was in the economic interest of unions to ensure that all their members would be eligible for Medicare (3).

The structure and financing of medical services is rational; the participants act according to their calculation of costs and benefits. Viewed in its entirety, however, health policy is uncoordinated and seemingly contradictory. Health policies are inequitable and inefficient, low-income persons end up subsidizing those with higher incomes. These results, however, are the consequences of a rational system. The outcomes were the result of policies intended by the legislators.

THE DEMAND FOR LEGISLATION BY HEALTH ASSOCIATIONS

Producer-type regulation has affected the structure and efficiency of the healthcare market. While it has not been as visible as redistributive legislation, such as Medicare and Medicaid, producer regulation has influenced the costs of these programs. It has also affected the performance of each of the medical markets. The following discussion provides an analysis of the different types of producer regulation demanded together with past examples of their use. Understanding the types of regulation demanded by health associations provides insights into the types of legislation health associations will favor or oppose in the years ahead.

Although differences existed in the objectives of health associations representing health professionals, hospitals, medical and dental schools, and Blue Cross and Blue Shield plans, the members of these associations all tried to make as much money as possible. They would then retain it for themselves, as did health professionals, or spend it to achieve prestige goals, as did nonprofit hospitals and medical schools; the incomes of employees of prestigious institutions are likely to exceed those of less prestigious institutions. Thus the objective underlying the demand for legislation is the same for each health association.

Each association attempts to achieve for its members through legislation what cannot be achieved through a competitive market, namely, a monopoly position. Increased monopoly power and the ability to price as a monopolist seller of services was—and is—the best way for the associations to achieve their goals.

There are five types of legislation that health associations demand on behalf of their members. As government policy shifted from increasing to decreasing health expenditures (given the concern over the budget deficit) the emphasis devoted to each of these types of legislation by health interest groups has changed over time.

Demand-Increasing Legislation

An association favors demand-increasing legislation since an increase in demand with a given supply will result in an increase in price, an increase in total revenue, and consequently an increase in incomes or net revenues.

The most obvious way to increase the demand for the services of an association's members is to have the government subsidize the purchase of insurance for the provider's services. Health providers, however, do not want the government to become the insurer for everyone. Instead, the providers' demand for insurance subsidies was always discussed in relation to specific population groups in society, i.e., people with low incomes.

The reason for selective government subsidies is twofold: first, people with higher incomes presumably have private insurance coverage or can afford to purchase the provider's services. The greatest increase in demand would result from extending coverage to those unable to pay. Second, extending government subsidies to those currently able to pay for the services would greatly increase the cost of the program to the government. A greater commitment of government expenditures would result in the government developing a concentrated interest in controlling the provider's prices, utilization, and expenditures. Thus when health associations favored demand subsidies, they were always in relation to specific population groups or services rather than to the population at large.

Examples of the above approach were the AMA's position on national health insurance, Medicare, and Blue Shield. The AMA successfully defeated President Truman's national health insurance proposal in 1948 because subsidies would have been provided to all regardless of income level. The AMA's opposition to Medicare was also based on the fact that all aged, regardless of income, were to be subsidized. Instead, the approach favored by the AMA was a system of tax credits for the purchase of private health insurance which would decline as a person's income rose.

In more recent years, as concern with the federal deficit increased and federal funds to subsidize those with low incomes were unlikely to be available, the AMA has favored an employer mandate whereby employers are required to purchase health insurance on behalf of their employees. An employer mandate would increase the demand for physician services by requiring the working uninsured to have private coverage. It would also move low-income employees and their families off Medicaid onto private insurance which reimburses providers at a higher rate.

The American Dental Association's (ADA's) major demand-increasing effort has been to expand private insurance coverage for dental services. Insurance is generally purchased for events that are very expensive, such as hospital care and in-hospital physician services, and that have a low probability of occurring. Dental expenditures, which are relatively small, expected, and not catastrophic, are therefore not insurable in the same sense as hospital or surgical services; in fact, dental prepayment is not really insurance but a form of forced savings.

If special incentives to purchase dental insurance did not exist, most people would just pay for dental care when they needed it. The use of dental services is also highly related to income. Thus a major reason for the growth in dental insurance has been the favorable tax treatment of employer-paid health insurance premiums. Such contributions are not considered part of the employee's income; the employee does not have to pay federal, state, or Social Security taxes on employer-paid health benefits.

Eliminating or "capping" the amount of employer-paid health benefits that are excluded from taxable income has been proposed in some health care reform proposals as a means of raising revenues to finance health benefits for those with low incomes.

The ADA's major legislative strategy has been to defeat any such tax cap. If a tax cap were passed, employees would want less comprehensive health benefits because they would have to pay for additional benefits with after-tax dollars. The ADA believes, and rightly so, that if the tax discount for purchasing dental insurance were eliminated, the incentive for employees to purchase such insurance would decline. With less dental insurance, consumers would have to pay the full price of dental care. The demand for dental care would decline, and consumers would be more inclined to "shop" among dentists for the lowest price (4).

The American Nurses Association has favored three types of demand-increasing legislation. The first are proposals that increase the demand for medical services. An example is the ANA's support for national health insurance. Increases in demand for medical services would increase the demand for institutions in which RNs are employed, thereby increasing the demand for RNs. However, since health insurance coverage for hospital care is more extensive than for any other delivery settings (and two-thirds of nurses work in hospitals), nurse associations have also favored other demand-increasing proposals. The ANA has favored requiring minimum nurse staffing ratios in hospitals, nursing homes, and home health agencies. In California, the nurse association was successful in having the state implement by the year 2003 minimum nurse-to-patient staffing ratios that are higher than current hospital staffing ratios.

Second, nurse associations have opposed hospital attempts to substitute lower-paid nurse aides to perform more of the RNs' tasks, which would decrease the demand for RNs. For example, California nurses were successful in enacting legislation prohibiting hospitals from assigning unlicensed personnel to perform nursing functions, such as administering medications.

A third type of demand proposal favored by nurse associations is one that widens the nurse's role, that is, increases the number of tasks nurses are legally able to perform. The nurses' value to the institution increases as they are permitted to perform more—and higher valued—tasks. The demand for their services will increase, with a consequent increase in their incomes. In attempting to increase their tasks, nurses have come in conflict with the AMA. The AMA is fearful that changing state laws that limit the scope of what nurses with advanced training can do would decrease the demand for physicians (5).

As nurses work to increase their roles, they wage a struggle in the legislative marketplace to prevent other health professionals, such as licensed practical nurses (LPNs) from performing tasks previously reserved to RNs. The ANA is also in competition with physician assistants (PAs) over which profession will be able to perform tasks previously reserved to physicians.

The health professional association that is successful in enabling its members to increase their role while preventing other health professionals from encroaching upon their own tasks will be able to increase the demand, hence the incomes, of its members. Examples of the legislative conflict over state practice acts are the attempts by optometrists to increase their role at the expense of ophthalmologists—as well as the struggles of psychologists versus psychiatrists, obstetricians versus nurse midwives, and podiatrists versus orthopedic surgeons.

The initial approach used by hospitals to increase the demand for their services was their establishment and control of Blue Cross. When hospitals started Blue Cross, Blue Cross only paid the costs of hospital care. Even if it was less costly to perform diagnostics in an outpatient setting, for the patient with Blue Cross coverage it was less expensive to have it performed in the hospital. The patient with Blue Cross did not have to pay any additional out-of-pocket hospital payments, thus high-cost hospitals were not at a price disadvantage with low-cost hospitals, thereby precluding price competition for Blue Cross patients. Further, every Blue Cross plan had to have at least 75 percent of the hospitals in its area participate in Blue Cross. This requirement precluded Blue Cross from contracting with only a lower-cost panel of hospitals. (The 75 percent rule also meant that Blue Cross would not have to compete with another Blue Cross plan in its area.)

As the price of hospital care became free to the Blue Cross subscriber, hospital use increased. Blue Cross reimbursed hospitals generously for their services.

Legislatively, the American Hospital Association favored government subsidies to stimulate the demand for hospital services by the aged and the poor. Medicare, which provided generous hospital coverage for the aged, increased the demand for hospitals by a high user group with generally low incomes. Hospitals have been in the forefront of lobbying efforts to receive federal subsidies for "uncompensated care," that is, the provision of hospital care to the poor for which they are not reimbursed. In the 1990s debate over national health insurance, the AHA had favored an employer mandate which would increase the demand for private health insurance by those who were uninsured and by those whose hospital bills were paid by Medicaid.

The Association of American Medical Colleges had favored legislation at both state and federal levels that provided such schools with unrestricted operating subsidies. Such subsidies would increase the demand for medical and dental schools by enabling them to set tuition levels greatly below the actual costs of education. With artificially low tuition levels and limits on the number of students they would accept, there would be an excess demand for their spaces. As long as there is an excess demand for a medical education—and the schools do not willingly expand their spaces to satisfy this demand—then the schools can determine the type of educational curriculum that comes closest to meeting their (and the AMA's or ADA's) preferences.

Securing the Highest Method of Reimbursement

The method of reimbursement (or the method used by the provider to charge for their services) has been crucial to understanding provider economic behavior.

Health associations have used two basic approaches to achieve the highest possible reimbursement for their members. The first has been to try and eliminate price competition. The ability to engage in price competition is more important to new practitioners or firms desiring to enter a market. New competitors must be able to let potential patients know (through advertising) they are available, and new surgeons must be able to provide primary care physicians with an incentive (fee splitting) to switch their surgical referrals away from established surgeons.

To prevent price competition from occurring, health associations have termed the elements of price competition, such as advertising and fee splitting, "unethical behavior" and have prohibited such be-

havior in their state practice acts (6). The medical and dental professions have used strong sanctions against practitioners who engaged in unethical behavior. A physician could have had his or her license suspended and be assessed financial penalties. Previously, medical societies were able to deny hospital privileges to physicians who advertised or engaged in price competition (7). Without hospital privileges, a physician could not offer patients complete medical service. Since physicians new to an area had the greatest incentive to engage in such "unethical" behavior, they were given probationary membership in the local medical society. They were thereby placed on notice that they could lose their hospital privileges if they engaged in such behavior. (Since the application of the anti-trust laws to health care in 1982, such anti-competitive behavior by medical societies is no longer permitted.)

A more recent example of the AMA's attempt to eliminate price competition among physicians has been the AMA's lobbying of Congress for an exemption from the anti-trust laws to allow competing physicians to collectively negotiate prices for their services with insurers. Currently, such price fixing is illegal but does not apply to employees or union members or merged corporations that no longer operate as competitors. If the AMA was successful, physicians would be able to establish a cartel and set their own prices. For example, all the anesthesiologists in a market could get together and decide upon the prices they wanted to charge.

The second approach used by health providers to secure the highest possible payment for their services was to engage in price discrimination, which means charging different patients or payers different prices for the same service. These different prices do not result from differences in costs, but from the patients' or their payers' abilities to pay. Charging according to ability to pay results in greater revenues than a pricing system that charges everyone the same price.

The desire by organized medicine to maintain a system whereby physicians could price discriminate influenced the financing and delivery of medical services for many years. Once medical insurance was introduced, organized medicine attempted to retain the physician's ability to price discriminate. For example, when medical societies started Blue Shield plans, the physician's fee was paid in full for those subscribers whose incomes were below a certain level. Physicians were permitted to charge higher-income patients an amount in addition to the Blue Shield payment. The Blue Shield income limits were eventually eliminated as the large majority of subscriber's incomes exceeded the income limit. Blue Shield insurance was not worth as much to high-income people if they had to pay a significant amount each time they went to the physician, in addition to the annual premium. As Blue Shield organizations dropped their income limits in order to be able to enroll more high-income subscribers, some medical societies dropped their sponsorship of the Blue Shield plans.

Once the income limits were removed, physicians could still maintain some ability to price discriminate by deciding when they wanted to participate in Blue Shield and when they wanted to charge the patient directly (referred to as "balance billing"). In the latter case, the patient would then receive payment from Blue Shield for an amount less than the physician's charge. For persons with higher incomes, physicians would charge the patient directly, which would provide them with a higher payment than if the physician participated in Blue Shield.

The physician payment system under Medicare was based on the same principle. Physicians decided whether to participate in Medicare on a case-by-case basis. If they thought they could make more money by charging the patient directly, they would do so. When they accepted the Medicare fee, the patient was responsible for a 20 percent co-payment. When the physician chose not to participate, the patient had to pay the physician's fee, which was greater than the Medicare fee, and the patient was responsible for the difference in the fees as well as the co-payment. By having the option of participating when they wanted to, physicians were assured of payment from low-income persons while still being able to charge a higher price to the higher-income patient. The method of pricing and flexibility of physician participation under Blue Shield and Medicare was crucial to their acceptance of these plans.

Organized medicine's desire to maintain a physician's ability to price-discriminate limited the growth of prepaid health plans (precursors to the HMO). HMOs charge patients the same premium regardless of income level. When fee-for-service physicians charge higher-income patients a higher fee, then an HMO that charges all persons the same premium is a form of price competition; it limits the physician's ability to price discriminate. When physicians moved into an area with the intention of joining a prepaid plan, local medical societies prevented them from receiving hospital privileges. Unless the plan had its own hospital (which was unlikely), this effectively eliminated competition. Medical societies were subsequently successful in having restrictive legislation enacted at a state level that effectively limited the growth of these plans.

In the mid 1980s, the AMA was opposed to the federal government allowing Medicare enrollees to voluntarily join an HMO which would then be paid an annual capitated price for each Medicare enrollee (referred to as Medicare Risk contracts).

Dental societies have acted similarly with respect to advertising and price competition. Until the successful FTC suit against the AMA, dental societies included bans on advertising in their state practice acts.

An important legislative activity of many state medical and dental societies in more recent years has been to enact "Any Willing Provider" legislation which seeks to ensure that all patients have free choice of any provider. Providers included in closed provider panels established by HMOs and PPOs are willing to discount their fees and practice cost effectively in return for receiving a greater volume of patients. HMOs and PPOs are thereby able to offer their services to employers at premiums lower than those prevailing in the area. Providers who are not a part of these closed panels do not have access to the HMO's and PPO's patient population. Providers in closed panels are engaged in price competition with providers who are not in the closed panels.

By enacting "Any Willing Provider" legislation, medical and dental societies remove providers' financial incentive to discount their fees in return for more patients. If providers in closed panels have to share their patients with providers who are not in closed panels, providers are unlikely to join closed panels and discount their fees.

To enable dentists to charge what the market will bear, the American Dental Association (ADA) has opposed the use of insurer fee schedules. Several years ago, Pennsylvania Blue Shield (PBS) won an anti-trust suit against the Pennsylvania Dental Association (PDA) on grounds that the PDA boycotted PBS because the Blue Shield dental plan paid dentists according to a fee schedule. The PDA wanted dentists to be able to charge the patient an additional amount if they so desired.

Similar to the above, the ADA has also opposed the practice of insurance companies reimbursing a patient a lower amount if they go to a nonparticipating dentist. The ADA has called for legislation prohibiting insurance companies from this payment approach. (The dentist is not prohibited from participating with the insurance company. However, they would prefer not to participate, to receive the same amount as participating dentists, as well as to be able to charge the patient an additional amount.)

The American Nurses Association has long been in favor of permitting advanced practice nurses to bill fee for service. Against the opposition of the AMA, registered nurses are striving to become independent practitioners, such as nurse practitioners and nurse midwives, who will then be able to bill the patient on a fee-for-service basis. Fee-for-service payment to a health professional, which in most cases is reimbursed by the government or private insurance, is the most direct way for a health professional to increase their income and to work independently of physicians.

Nurse practitioners have been able to work independently and be reimbursed by many state Medicaid programs that serve low-income people and by Medicare for patients in rural areas. The numbers of independent nurse practitioners are likely to increase as a result of a decision in 1997 by the federal Department of Veterans Affairs to formally accept nurse practitioners without links to physicians and of a federal law (effective 1998) allowing Medicare to pay nurse practitioners directly who work in cities and suburbs, not just in rural areas.

The American Hospital Association was, until the 1980s, successful in eliminating any incentive for hospitals to engage in price competition. When hospitals started Blue Cross, the plans were required to offer their subscribers a service benefit plan which provides the hospitalized patient with services rather than dollars, a characteristic of an indemnity plan. By guaranteeing payment to the hospital for the services used by the patient, the service-benefit policy removes any incentive the patient (or the hospital) may have regarding the cost of hospitalization. Since the patient does not have to make any out-of-pocket payments, the prospective patient has no disincentive to enter the most expensive hospital, which may or may not be the highest-quality hospital. Under a service-benefit policy, hospitals cannot compete for patients on the basis of price.

When Medicare was enacted, the AHA proposed a method of hospital payment adopted by the government that paid hospitals for providing care to Medicare patients based on each hospital's costs plus 2 percent. Once the patient paid a deductible, they were not assessed any co-payments. Not only did this method of payment eliminate any incentive for patients to select less costly more efficient hospitals, but it provided hospitals with an incentive to increase their costs. (Further, hospitals were not permitted to compete for Medicare patients by offering to reduce the hospital deductible.)

Hospitals have also tried to price discriminate. When hospitals started Blue Cross they gave Blue Cross a 20 percent discount compared to what commercial insurers were charged. This discount enabled Blue Cross to offer a more expensive policy (a service benefit) that was in the hospitals' interest. The discount was also a competitive advantage for Blue Cross and enabled them to increase their market share over the commercial insurers.

Hospitals did very well financially under the initial Medicare payment policy. The government was anxious for hospitals to participate in Medicare and therefore accepted many of the AHA's payment proposals. Not only were hospitals able to negotiate a 2 percent addition to their costs of serving Medicare patients and receive favorable treatment for depreciating their assets, but the manner in which hospital costs were calculated gave hospitals additional payment. Hospitals could not separate the actual costs of serving Medicare patients from those of other patients. The method used to calculate Medicare costs was to use the ratio of what hospitals charge for Medicare patients to the charges for non-Medicare patients. That ratio was then used to determine the portion of the hospitals' total costs that should be paid by Medicare. The effect of this policy was to provide hospitals with an incentive to raise charges on those services used predominantly by the elderly, such as bed rails. By increasing the proportion of their charges for the aged, a greater portion of the hospitals' total costs were paid by the government. The hospital would then be able to make a higher profit on its charges to commercial insurers.

Hospitals were also able to price discriminate by setting a higher price-to-cost ratio for those services for which there was a greater willingness to pay, that is, services that were less price-elastic. Ancillary services, such as lab tests and x-rays, had higher price-to-cost ratios than the hospital's basic room charge. Once a patient was hospitalized they had little choice on the use or price of ancillary services. Patients who paid part of the hospital bill themselves could, before they entered a particular hospital, more easily compare charges for obstetric services and room rates. The charges for these services were much closer to their costs.

The method by which public medical and dental schools are subsidized is very important. Subsidies go directly to the school, as do government funds distributed for loans and scholarships. Under this arrangement, the student receives a subsidy (tuition less than costs) only by attending a subsidized school. This method requires that students compete for medical and dental schools. *If government subsidies went directly to the student, then the schools would have to compete for students.* As with subsidies, medical and dental schools prefer to distribute loans and scholarships themselves rather than have students apply directly to the government for such financial assistance. If the students received the subsidies and loans directly, then they would have an incentive to shop and select a school based on its tuition rates and reputation. The

current system provides a competitive advantage to schools receiving subsidies. Needless to say, private schools would prefer that the subsidies go directly to the students.

The methods used by health professionals and health institutions for pricing their services has enabled these providers to maximize their revenues. The health associations representing each provider group have had, in negotiating with the government, in establishing their own insurance organizations, and in proposing legislation, a clear appreciation for which pricing strategies are in their members' economic interest.

Legislation to Reduce the Price and/or Increase the Quantity of Complements

A registered nurse may be a substitute or a complement to the physician. It is difficult to determine when an input, such as a nurse, is a complement or a substitute based only on the task performed. A nurse may be as competent as a physician in performing certain tasks. If the nurse works for the physician and the physician receives the fee for the performance of that task, then the nurse has increased the physician's productivity and is a complement. If, however, the nurse performs the same task and is a nurse practitioner billing independently of the physician, then the nurse is a substitute for the physician providing that service. *The essential element in determining whether an input is a complement or a substitute is who receives the payment for the services provided by that input.* Whoever receives the payment controls the use of that input.

The state practice acts were the legal basis for determining which tasks each health profession can perform and under whose direction health professionals must work. A major legislative activity for each health association was to ensure that the state practice acts worked to their members' interests. Health associations that represent complements, e.g., nurses and denturists, attempt to have their members become substitutes. Health associations whose members control complements seek to retain the status quo.

In the past, almost all the health professions and health institutions were complements to the physician. That situation has changed. The physician is no longer the sole entry point to the delivery of medical services. HMOs, for example, may use nurse practitioners to serve their enrollees. The AMA has continued to oppose the use of independent nurse practitioners and has lobbied against state laws that allow advance practice nurses to provide medical care without the supervision of a physician. The American Academy of Family Practitioners (who would be most adversely affected by independent nurse practitioners) has stated that such nurses should only be paid by insurers when they work in a "collaborative" relationship with physicians.

Providers can increase their incomes if an increase in demand for their services is met through greater productivity than through an increase in the number of competing providers. The providers' income can be increased still further if their productivity increases are subsidized and they do not have to pay the full cost of the increased productivity.

The following are several examples of legislation that has subsidized providers' productivity. The American Hospital Association lobbied for passage of the Nurse Training Act in the belief that federal educational subsidies would increase the supply of RNs available to hospitals. With a larger supply of nurses, nurses' wages would be lower than they otherwise would have been. The AHA was a strong proponent of the Hill-Burton program, which provided capital subsidies to modernize hospitals. The AHA opposed legislation that would have increased the cost of inputs to hospitals. It opposed the extension of minimum wage legislation to hospital employees and called for a moratorium on the separate licensing of each health professional. (Separate licensing limits the hospital's ability to substitute different health professionals in the tasks they perform and to use such personnel in a more flexible manner.) Conversely, separate licensing is demanded by each health professional association in order to increase the demand for its members' services by restricting the tasks that other professions can perform.

The AMA has favored internship and residency programs in hospitals. Interns and residents are excellent complements for physicians; they can take care of the physician's hospitalized patients and relieve the physician from serving in the hospital emergency room and from being on call. The more advanced the resident is, the closer the resident is to being a potential substitute for the physician. Residents, however, are complements since the physician bills for the service. For this reason the AMA has favored the use of foreign medical graduates to serve as interns and residents. Once they graduate, however, they become substitutes to existing practitioners. The AMA has, therefore, favored the return of foreign medical graduates to their home country once their residencies are completed. (The AMA advocated a time limit on how long foreign medical graduates can remain in the United States, as well as the requirement that they be out of the country two years before returning.)

The main concern of the AMA toward emerging health professionals, such as physician assistants, was to ensure that these types of personnel become complements to, not substitutes for, the physician. Thus, whether there is direct or indirect supervision of the PA by the physician is less important to the AMA's political position than who receives the fee for the PA's service.

The legislative attempt by physicians and dentists to lower the cost of their inputs has been action at both the federal and state level to limit increases in malpractice premiums. There are many reasons why malpractice premiums have risen (8). Professional associations have been more willing to seek legislation to place limits on the size of malpractice awards and restrict the percentage of awards to attorneys than to make a concerted effort to eliminate unqualified practitioners.

Up until the mid 1980s (at which time large employers placed pressure on insurance companies to reduce their premiums), the Blue Cross premium consisted almost entirely of the costs of hospital care. Its main cost, therefore, has been the cost and quantity of hospital care used by its subscribers. Commercial insurance companies had broader coverage (although it included deductibles and cost sharing), and therefore hospital care was a smaller portion of the total premium. Thus to remain competitive against commercial insurance companies, Blue Cross had to keep the cost of hospital care (both hospital use and cost per unit) from rising so rapidly. Under the service-benefit policy, however, patients, their physicians, and the hospital had no incentive to be concerned with cost or use. In fact it was in the hospital's interest to add facilities and services and pass the costs on to Blue Cross. As more hospitals added facilities and services in a race to determine who could be more prestigious, there was a great deal of duplication of costly facilities and services and, consequently, low use rates of these costly facilities. Blue Cross, however, was committed to pay. To limit the increase in these costly facilities, Blue Cross favored legislative restrictions on hospital investment.

Given the control hospitals had over Blue Cross, Blue Cross was not aggressive in trying to limit the rapid rise in hospital costs such as by limiting what they would pay hospitals. Blue Cross and large hospitals favored an indirect approach that prevented smaller hospitals from expanding their beds and facilities and the entry of new hospitals. To receive Blue Cross (and Medicare) reimbursement for capital expenditures, a hospital had to receive the approval of a planning agency for its investment. Existing large hospitals either had the latest facilities or were the likeliest candidates to receive approval from the planning agency whose criteria favored large, full-service hospitals. These large institutions also favored the development and strengthening of planning agencies because it limited competition.

Blue Cross relied on controls to hold down hospital investment and rising Blue Cross premiums. All studies have shown that controls on capital investment were not effective in holding down either hospital investment or the rise in hospital costs (9). It was not until Blue Cross began to experience strong competitive pressures sufficient to affect its survival that it finally undertook more direct means of lowering the costs of its major input. Blue Cross began including lower-cost substitutes to hospitals as part of its benefits, instituting utilization control programs, and changing the method by which it pays hospitals.

Legislation to Decrease the Availability and/or Increase the Price of Substitutes

All health associations try to increase the price of services that are substitutes to those provided by their members. (Similar to increasing the price of a substitute is decreasing its availability.) If the health association is successful in achieving this, then the demand for its members' services will be increased.

Health associations use three general approaches to accomplish this. The first is to simply have the substitute declared illegal. If substitute health professionals are not permitted to practice or if substitutes are severely restricted in the tasks they are legally permitted to perform, then there will be a shift in demand away from the substitute service. The second approach (used when the first approach is unsuccessful) is to exclude the substitute service from payment by any third party, including government health programs. This approach raises the price of the substitute. (The out-of-pocket price to the patient of the uninsured service is thus much greater than the service for which it is a substitute.) The third approach is to try and raise the costs of the substitutes who must then raise their own prices if they are to remain in business. The following examples illustrate the behavior of health associations for each of these approaches.

For many years the AMA regarded osteopaths as "cultists." It was considered "unethical" for physicians to teach in schools of osteopathy. Unable to prevent their licensure at a state level, the AMA tried to deny osteopaths hospital privileges. (A physician substitute is less than adequate if that substitute cannot provide a complete range of treatment.) As osteopaths developed their own hospitals and educational institutions, medical societies decided the best approach to controlling the increase in supply of these physician substitutes was to merge with the osteopaths, make them physicians, and then eliminate any future increases in their supply. An example of this approach, which was used in California until it was overturned by the state Supreme Court, was to allow osteopaths to convert their D.O. degree to an M.D. on the basis of twelve Saturday refresher courses. After the merger between the two societies occurred in California, the Osteopathic Board of Examiners was no longer permitted to license osteopaths.

Medicare has been the vehicle for much legislative competition. The AMA lobbied for only covering physician services under Medicare Part B while excluding non-physician services. By including only physician services, the prices of substitute providers to the aged are effectively increased relative to those of physicians. For example, optometrists and chiropractors are potential substitutes for ophthalmologists and family physicians. By including physician services under Medicare but excluding payment for non-physicians, the price of non-physicians is increased relative to physicians. An aged person with Medicare Part B pays less for a physician's services since the out-of-pocket price to the aged of physician services has been lowered. The AMA has similarly opposed direct payment of nurse anesthetists and nurse practitioners under Medicare.

In one case, the intervention of the courts prevented physicians from artificially raising the price of a substitute. In Virginia, Blue Shield did not reimburse psychologists as providers of psychotherapy. Psychiatrists' services were therefore less expensive than psychologists' to a patient with Blue Shield. The psychologists brought a successful antitrust case against Blue Shield in 1980 claiming discrimination of non-physician providers.

An example of the legislative behavior of dental societies toward substitute providers is illustrated by dentistry's actions toward denturists. Denturism is the term applied to the fitting and dispensing of dentures directly to patients by people not licensed as dentists. Independently practicing denturists are a threat to dentists' incomes since they provide dentures at lower prices. Denturists are legal in most of Canada. As a result of their political success in Canada, denturists in the United States became bolder by forcing referendums on the issue and by lobbying for changes in the state practice acts. Several states subsequently enacted laws legalizing denturism.

Occasionally denturists have sold dentures directly to patients illegally. To eliminate this competition and to prevent its increase, local dental societies such as in Texas, responded in two ways: first, they offered to provide low-cost dentures to low-income persons; second, they pressured state officials to enforce the state laws against illegal denturists.

It was only the threat of competition that resulted in the dental profession's offer to provide low-cost dentures to the indigent or near-indigent. Once the denturist's competitive threat is eliminated through

dentistry's use of the state's legal authority, the poor will once again pay higher prices for dentures.

The ADA is also concerned that dental hygienists remain complements to, not become substitutes for, dentists. Several state dental hygienist associations have attempted to change the state practice act to permit hygienists to practice without a dentist's supervision and to become independent practitioners. In 1986, despite being opposed by the ADA, the hygienists were successful in achieving this goal in Colorado.

One of the most important substitutes for registered nurses is foreign-trained registered nurses. Nurses' salaries are considerably higher in the United States than in other countries, providing a financial incentive for foreign nurses to enter the country. The ANA has tried to decrease the availability of a low-cost substitute for U.S. registered nurses by making it more difficult for foreign-trained RNs to enter this country. For example, the ANA has proposed that foreign RNs desiring to enter the United States be screened by examination in their home country before being allowed to immigrate. If the screening exam were administered only in the United States, then foreign-trained RNs could still work in some nursing capacity in this country even if they did not pass the exam. The foreign-trained nurse could then retake the exam in the future. As it is, the screening exam is an additional barrier for foreign nurses to pass before they can enter the United States; if they do not pass the exam, they are unlikely to emigrate.

An additional legislative approach used by the ANA is to prevent other personnel from performing tasks performed by the RN. The ANA has opposed permitting physicians to decide which personnel can perform nursing tasks; the ANA has opposed permitting LPNs to be in charge of skilled nursing homes, otherwise there would be substitution away from RNs (who receive higher wages) currently performing such functions. The California Nurses Association opposed a bill that would have authorized firemen with paramedic training to give medical and nursing care in hospital emergency departments. As a means of preventing physician assistants from assuming a role that the RN would like, the ANA has favored a licensing moratorium. A moratorium would prevent any new health personnel from being licensed to perform tasks that RNs do or would like to perform.

The American Hospital Association opposed the growth of freestanding ambulatory surgicenters. Surgicenters are low-cost substitutes for hospitals; performing surgical procedures in a surgicenter decreases the use of the hospital and its revenues. To limit the availability of these low-cost substitutes, hospital associations argued that surgicenters should be permitted only when they are developed in association with a hospital. Denying Blue Cross reimbursement to freestanding surgicenters and including surgicenters under certificate-of-need (CON) legislation (making it difficult for them to enter a market) were approaches favored by hospital associations. Health maintenance organizations were also included in state CON legislation for the same reason since they decrease the use and revenues of hospitals.

Hospitals have been concerned in recent years by the growth of physician-owned specialty hospitals. Physician specialists, such as cardiovascular and orthopedic surgeons, while remaining on the staff of an acute general hospital, have invested in a specialty facility and referred some of their patients to their own facility for surgery. General hospitals have claimed that these specialty hospitals decrease the demand for their own facilities and take the more profitable, less severely ill patients. Hospital associations were successful in eliminating competition from these specialty hospitals by including in the 2003 Medicare Prescription Drug Act, a provision placing an 18-month moratorium on the development of new physician-owned specialty hospitals.

Hospital associations have used several approaches to raise the price of their competitors—for-profit hospitals. For example, hospitals opposed granting for-profit hospitals Blue Cross eligibility. Being ineligible for Blue Cross payment precludes the use of the for-profit hospital by patients with Blue Cross coverage.

Substitutes for American medical and dental schools are foreign schools whose graduates (who may be U.S. citizens) want to practice in the United States. To reduce the likelihood that foreign medical schools will substitute for U.S. medical schools, the AAMC has been a strong proponent for eliminating Medicare graduate medical education payments for residents trained in foreign medical schools. This reduction to teaching hospitals would be a strong incentive for these hospitals not to accept foreign trained graduates.

The American Dental Association and the Association of American Dental Schools have been more successful in reducing the attractiveness of a foreign dental education. Practicing dentists do not use residents as do physicians. Therefore their interest is solely with decreasing the supply of dentists. There are increased time requirements for a foreign-trained dentist wishing to practice in the United States. A minimum number of years of training in the foreign country is required, as well as a license to practice in that country. (For a U.S. citizen, this would mean learning a different language.) And once foreign-trained dentists enter the country, additional requirements are then imposed upon them. They are required to take the last 2 years of dental school in an accredited U.S. dental school. They may also be required to take additional examinations before the licensing exam. To date, such restrictive practices have raised the cost of a U.S. dental license for foreign-trained dentists (both U.S. and non-U.S. citizens). The consequence has been a decreased demand for a foreign dental education as a substitute for a U.S. dental education. The measure of how successful the dental profession and the dental schools have been is that less than 5 percent of all practicing dentists in the U.S. are foreign trained.

Legislation to Limit Increases in Supply

Essential to the creation of a monopoly are limits on the number of providers of a service. Health associations, however, have justified supply control policies on grounds of quality. Restrictions on entry, they maintain, ensure high quality of care to the public. These same health associations, however, oppose quality measures that would have an adverse economic effect upon existing providers (their members).

This apparent anomaly—stringent entry requirements and then virtually no quality assurance programs directed at existing providers—is only consistent with a policy that seeks to establish a monopoly for existing providers.

If health associations were consistent in their desire to improve and maintain high quality standards, then they should favor all policies that ensure quality of care, regardless of the effect on their member's incomes. Quality control measures directed at existing providers, such as re-examination, re-licensure, and monitoring of the care actually provided, would adversely affect the incomes of some providers. More importantly, such "outcome" measures of quality assurance would make entry or "process" measures less necessary, thereby permitting entry of a larger number of providers.

As previously discussed in the chapter on Physician Manpower, a test of the hypothesis that entry barriers are primarily directed toward developing a monopoly position rather than improving quality of care would be as follows: Does the health association favor quality measures regardless of the effect on its members' incomes, or does it only favor those quality measures that either enhance or do not affect their members' incomes? If the health association only favors those quality measures that do not affect or favorably impact its members' economic position, then it can be concluded that the real intent of those quality measures is the improvement of its members' competitive position rather than the assurance of quality care in the most efficient manner.

In recent years there has been a growing concern among dentists (as well as among other health professions) that there are too many practitioners. As would be expected, rather than relying on market forces to determine the number of dentists, the ADA approach is to reduce the number of dental school spaces. Indicative of this approach is the ADA's statement, "Resolved, that public statements made by the American Dental Association . . . include the recognition that a surplus of dentists does exist to meet the current demand for dental services, . . . [and that] the ADA encourage and assist constituent societies in

preparing legislation that may be used to petition state legislatures and governmental bodies with respect to private schools to adjust enrollment in dental schools" (10).

Optometrists have also followed the same supply control policies as previously discussed for medicine and dentistry. Similarly, as educational requirements were increased, existing members of the profession were grandfathered in. By the early 1900s, optometrists were able to secure licensure in all states. However, there were many private schools for training optometrists. By the 1920s, the American Optometric Association was successful in disqualifying twenty of the thirty optometric schools and in raising educational requirements. Optometry requires 6 years of education in an approved optometric school and at least 3 years (most applicants have completed 4 years) of traditional undergraduate college education (11). Increasing educational requirements for a profession involves not just increasing the number of years of professional training but also requiring more years of undergraduate training.

Nursing also tried to impose stringent educational requirements. The ANA has proposed and has lobbied their state legislatures that nursing education occur only in colleges that offer a BS degree (12). Only 4-year nurse graduates would be referred to as professional nurses, otherwise the nurse would be a technical nurse. By proposing an increase in the educational requirement of two-thirds of the nurse graduates, the ANA must be well aware that the result will be a decrease in the number of nurse graduates. The effect of increased education and an increase in nursing tasks would be an increase in the incomes of existing nurses who would be grandfathered in as professional nurses.

It is unlikely one would ever observe a health association proposing increased educational requirements that are then applied to its existing members. Only to forestall more stringent requirements proposed by others would a health association favor additional training requirements for its existing members. Health associations do not favor re-licensure or re-examination requirements for their current members, even though increased knowledge is the basis for requiring additional training for those entering the profession. Re-examination and re-licensure would lower the incomes of their members since they would have to take the time to study for the exam. Current practitioners also may not be able to pass the exam. No health association proposes that the time required to prepare a person to enter their profession be reduced.

As knowledge increases and educational requirements for new graduates in the health professions lengthen, the public is led to believe that all persons in a profession are equally (or at least minimally) qualified. This is unlikely to be the case, particularly for those practitioners who were trained 30 years ago and have not maintained their knowledge.

At times the profession has imposed requirements on new entrants that are blatant barriers. For example, foreign medical and dental graduates were required to be U.S. citizens before they were allowed to practice in some states (13). Further, a dentist desiring to practice in Hawaii, for example, no matter how well-trained or how long in practice in another state, is required to complete a 1-year residency requirement before being allowed to practice (14). Foregoing income for a year before they can practice is a high cost for entering a new market. Such requirements cannot be remotely related to the profession's concern with quality.

If the members of a profession are concerned with quality, then they should favor monitoring quality among themselves. Yet associations have opposed any attempts by others to review the quality of care practiced by their members. Health associations that have proposed continuing education for their members have done so in response to demands by those outside the profession. These requirements are made easy to achieve and at low cost to the members of the profession.

SUMMARY

Health professionals and health institutions do not exhibit characteristics of a natural monopoly, that is, large economies of scale for a given size of market sufficient to preclude entry of competitors. Because these professionals and institutions cannot achieve a monopoly position through the normal competitive process, they seek to achieve it through legislation. The first step toward increasing their monopoly power is to erect barriers to entry. The next is to limit competition among their members. They then attempt to improve their monopoly position by further demanding legislation that will increase the demand for their services, permit them to price as would a price-discriminating monopolist, lower their costs of doing business, and disadvantage their competitors either by causing them to become illegal providers or by forcing them to raise their prices.

Health professionals, particularly physicians and dentists, have been successful in the legislative marketplace as evidenced by the design of public programs to pay for their services and by their relatively high incomes. However, three types of "costs" are imposed on the rest of society as a result of the restrictions that cause a redistribution of wealth to members of health associations that have achieved legislative success.

The first is higher prices. The more successful a health association is in achieving their members' goals, the higher will be the price of their members' services. However, once price competition occurs between members of different health associations, the lower will be the prices of both groups' services. Allowing freestanding surgicenters to compete with hospitals lowered the cost to the patient for surgical procedures (through reduced insurance premiums). Other tactics used by health associations to prevent price competition among their members included prohibitions against advertising, limiting productivity increases to prevent excess capacity, preventing physicians in HMOs from having hospital privileges, and requiring free choice of provider under both public and private insurance plans. These restrictions have resulted in health care prices being higher than they would be otherwise.

The second implication of successful legislative behavior by health associations is that the public is provided with a false assurance with respect to the quality of the medical care it receives. The state delegated its responsibility for protecting the public to the individual licensing boards, which in turn have been controlled and operated in the interests of the providers themselves. The approach toward quality assurance used by both the profession and by licensing boards is needlessly costly and inefficient. It has been more concerned with the process of becoming a health professional, such as entry into the profession, than with monitoring the care provided. As such, state licensing boards have devoted too few resources to investigating complaints against and removing incompetent or unethical providers. Too rarely do state licensing boards take disciplinary actions against their members.

The movement toward a competitive market in medical services has resulted in a new emphasis on quality of care. Large employers are pressuring HMOs to provide information on their enrollees' medical outcomes, preventive measures undertaken, and health status indicators of their enrollees. It is through actions by such large purchasers that HMOs are developing "report cards." Employer emphasis on "outcome" measures is forcing HMOs and medical groups to re-examine how medical care is provided. It is doubtful that this new approach toward quality would have occurred had market competition not developed (15).

The third effect of legislative success by a health association is that innovation in the delivery of medical care was inhibited. Innovation provides benefits to consumers; they have greater choice, higher quality, and lower costs. Innovation, however, threatens the monopoly power of a protected provider group, and is therefore opposed. Medical and dental societies have been protectors of the fee-for-service delivery system. These organizations have delayed the introduction of alternative delivery systems, such as HMOs and preferred provider organizations.

Rather than being pro-competitive, "Any Willing Provider" laws and "free choice of provider" have been used by the professions to eliminate competition from "closed" provider panels. HMOs and PPOs cannot negotiate volume discounts with closed panels of providers if they have to offer their subscribers free choice of any provider. HMOs and managed care organizations are able to offer lower premiums than traditional insurance because they are able to impose restrictions on the types of participating providers and by instituting medical management programs.

Legislative restrictions against closed panels, such as by requiring free choice of provider, has prevented managed care organizations from successfully competing against traditional insurance plans.

Medical and dental societies have inhibited the development of new types of health personnel (such as nurse midwives, nurse practitioners, and expanded function dental auxiliaries) because they might become substitutes. The determination of which tasks a health professional is able to perform is related more to their economic effects on another health profession than to the professional's qualifications and training.

Hospital associations have sought, through certificate-of-need legislation, to stifle innovations such as the growth of freestanding surgicenters. It was the commercial insurance companies that introduced major medical insurance, a distinct innovation that also increased their share of the health insurance market. The process of receiving a professional education (medical, dental, and optometric) has changed little over time (except for an increase in years required) because it has remained under the auspices of accredited schools and their professions. It is highly likely that the necessary knowledge could be provided to students in a shorter period of time, thereby decreasing the total cost of such an education.

Innovation offers the hope of greater productivity, lower costs, and an increase in quality. The political activities of health associations should be viewed in their proper perspective, namely, to benefit their members while imposing a cost on the rest of society. Past reliance on professional regulation to protect the patient has reduced incentives for innovation.

The usefulness of the different theories of government should be judged by their predictive ability. While it is unlikely that any one theory will be able to explain all or even a very high percentage of all legislation, a theory is necessary for trying to understand why certain types of legislation were passed and why others were not, unless one believes that all legislation is ad hoc. It is natural to try to organize what we observe in some meaningful manner. The criteria for selecting one theory over another should be based upon pragmatic grounds: which approach is better at explaining events under a broad range of circumstances? To reject a theory, it is necessary to have a better theory.

The economic theory of government assumes that human behavior is no different in political than in private markets. Individuals, groups, firms, and legislators seek to enhance their self interests. They are assumed to be rational in assessing the benefits and the costs to themselves of their actions. This behavioral assumption enables us to predict that firms in private markets will try to produce their products and services as efficiently as possible to keep their costs down and that they will set their prices so as to make as much profit as possible. They will be motivated to enter markets where the profit potential is greatest and, similarly, to leave markets where the profit potential is low.

It is merely an extension of the above discussion to include political markets. Individuals and firms use the power of the state to further their own interests. Firms try to gain competitive advantages in private markets by investing in technology and advertising. Why shouldn't firms also make political investments to be able to use the powers of government to increase or maintain profit?

The actions of organizations of individuals are no different from those of firms. Many people would like to use the power of the state to assist them in what they cannot otherwise achieve. For some, this may mean using the state to help them impose their religious or social preferences on others. Still other groups would like to use the state to provide them with monetary benefits that they could not earn in the market and that others would not voluntarily provide to them, such as low-cost education for their children, pension payments in excess of their contributions, and subsidized medical benefits.

It is usually with regard to our public "servants" that the assumption of acting in one's self interest becomes difficult to accept. After all, why would a person run for office if not to serve the public interest? However, to be successful in the electoral process requires legislators to behave in a manner that enhances their re-election prospects. Political support, votes, and contributions are the bases for re-election. Legislators must therefore be able to understand the sources of such support and the requirements for receiving it. A hungry man quickly realizes that if money buys food then he must have money to eat. Legislators act no differently than others.

Political markets have several characteristics that differentiate them from economic markets. These differences make it possible for organized interests to benefit at the expense of majorities. First, individuals are not as informed about political issues as they are about the goods and services on which they spend their own funds.

Second, in private markets individuals make separate decisions on each item they purchase. They do not have to choose between sets of purchases, such as between one package that may include a particular brand of car, a certain size house in a particular neighborhood, several suits, and a certain quantity of food. Yet in political markets their choices are between two sets of votes by competing legislators on a wide variety of issues.

Third, voting participation rates differ by age group. The young and future generations do not vote, and yet policies are enacted that impose costs on them. Future generations depend on current generations and voters to protect their interests. However, as has been the case many times, such as with respect to the federal deficit, Social Security, and Medicare, their interests have been sacrificed to current voters.

Fourth, legislators use different decision criteria from those used in the private sector. A firm or an individual making an investment considers both the benefits and the costs of that investment. Legislators, however, have a different time horizon that not only affects the emphasis they place on costs and benefits, but also on when each is incurred. Since members of the House of Representatives run for re-election every 2 years, they are likely to favor programs that provide immediate benefits (presumably just before the election) while delaying the costs until after the election or years later.

Further, from the legislator's perspective, the program does not even have to meet the criterion that the benefits exceed its costs, only that the immediate benefits exceed any immediate costs. Future legislators can worry about future costs.

It is for these reasons that organized groups are able to receive legislative benefits while imposing the costs of those benefits on the remainder of the population. For those bearing the costs of legislative benefits that others receive, it may be perfectly rational not to oppose such legislation. As long as the cost of changing political outcomes exceeds the lost wealth imposed by legislation, it is rational for voters to lose some wealth rather than to organize and bear the cost of changing the legislative outcome.

At times, self-interest legislation may be in the "public interest." When this occurs, however, it is because it is a byproduct of the outcome rather than its intended effect.

REVIEW QUESTIONS

1. Describe the economic theory of regulation. Contrast its predictions to the public interest theory of regulation with respect to certificate of need legislation. What evidence leads you to select one theory over the other?
2. Predict which organizations would oppose and support:
   a. Subsidies for the training of nurse midwives.
   b. State mandates requiring all health insurers include chiropractic services in their benefits.
   c. Inclusion of psychologists as a covered provider under Medicare.
3. Why are concentrated interests and diffuse costs important in predicting legislative outcomes?
4. Contrast the benefit-cost calculations of legislators under both the public interest and economic theories of government.
5. Evaluate the following policies according to the public interest and economic theories:
   a. The performance of state licensing boards in monitoring physician quality.
   b. Medicare reform.
6. There are a number of restrictions in the methods by which medical care is organized and provided. With regard to restrictions on entry, on tasks performed, and (previously) on information, contrast the reasons for such restrictions in terms of improved quality versus enhancement of provider incomes.
7. Apply the theoretical model of the demand for legislation to predict legislation demanded by the American Medical Association (AMA) or the American Dental Association (ADA). Be explicit regarding the objective of the AMA or ADA, and justify the choice of that objective.
8. What are some practices in medical care that are purported to result in higher standards of quality that are in effect restrictive devices intended to confer monopoly power on the practitioners of the profession? What are alternative ways of achieving the goal of higher quality without the restrictive element?

REFERENCES

1. In his review article, Barr uses a different classification of government interventions, regulation, which can apply to quality, quantity, or price of a product or service; a price subsidy, which can be direct or through the tax system; public production, such as when the government is the supplier of the service; and income transfers, which can be tied to specific products, such as food stamps or general, as with Social Security. Nicholas Barr, "Economic Theory and the Welfare State: A Survey and Interpretation," *Journal of Economic Literature*, 30(2), June 1992, pp. 741–803.
2. The Economic Theory of Regulation was first proposed by G. J. Stigler, "The Economic Theory of Regulation," *The Bell Journal of Economics*, 2, Spring 1971, 3–21. For additional references and a more complete discussion of this theory and its applicability to the health field, see P. J. Feldstein, *The Politics of Health Legislation: An Economic Perspective*, 2nd ed. revised, (Chicago, Illinois: The Health Administration Press, 2001).
3. For a more complete discussion of the reason for financing Medicare Part A through the use of payroll taxes, see P. J. Feldstein, *The Politics of Health Legislation: An Economic Perspective, op. cit.*
4. One demand-increasing proposal is reputed to have had an adverse effect on patients' oral health. In 1974, the Federal Social Court in Germany ruled that false teeth should be included in the country's compulsory health insurance programs. "Fillings went out of fashion and prevention was ignored as vast quantities of teeth were pulled and replaced. By 1980, German dentists were using 28 tons of tooth gold a year, one-third of the world total." Dentists' incomes soared, exceeding those of physicians by 30 percent. The sickness funds reported a huge deficit, forcing them to raise the level of

compulsory contributions. "Dentists Gnashing Teeth in West Germany," *The Wall Street Journal*, December 26, 1985, p. 11.

5. "Doctors Group Denounces Nurses' Demand for Power," *The Washington Post*, December 7, 1993, p. A3.

6. Fee splitting occurred when a physician referred a patient to a surgeon and in return received part of the surgeon's fee; surgeons would compete amongst themselves on the size of their fee to be given to the referring physician. Fee splitting is an indication that the surgeon's fee is in excess of his or her cost; the surgeon can still make a profit rebating part of the fee. If the fee were not in excess of the costs (including the opportunity cost of the surgeon's time), the surgeon would be unwilling to split the fee. The state practice acts permitted surgeons to act as a cartel by preventing any one surgeon from engaging in this form of price competition. Fee splitting was a way of eroding the surgeons' monopoly power. Surgeons opposed to fee splitting consider it unethical because the referring physician has a monetary incentive to select the surgeon. Any concern the medical profession had with the quality of surgeons or with the ethical behavior of physicians should have been addressed directly through examination and monitoring procedures and not by prohibiting price competition. Unfortunately, the medical profession has opposed re-examination and monitoring. For a more complete discussion of fee splitting, see Mark V. Pauly, "The Ethics and Economics of Kickbacks and Fee Splitting," *The Bell Journal of Economics*, 10(1), Spring 1979, 344–352.

7. Reuben Kessel, "Price Discrimination in Medicine," *The Journal of Law and Economics*, 1, October 1958, 20–53.

8. Danzon, P., "Liability for Medical Malpractice," pp. 1341–1404, in Culyer, A., and Newhouse, J., editors, *Handbook of Health Economics*, Vol. 1b, (North-Holland Press: New York), 2000.

9. David S. Salkever and Thomas W. Bice, *Hospital Certificate-of-Need Controls: Impact on Investment, Costs, and Use*, (Washington, D.C.: American Enterprise Institute, 1979).

10. 1984 House of Delegates Resolutions, October 25, p. 537. This resolution follows a previous one (124H-1981) where the ADA was to encourage their "constituent dental societies to utilize these reports (on dentist supply) in petitioning their legislative bodies to consider by lawful means the number of dentists that should be trained." Transactions, 125th Annual Session, October 20–25, 1984, (Chicago: American Dental Association, 1984).

11. James W. Begun, *Professionalism and the Public Interest: Price and Quality in Optometry*, (Cambridge, MA: The MIT Press, 1981). Also see, James W. Begun and Ronald C. Lippincott, "A Case Study in the Politics of Free-Market Health Care," *Journal of Health Politics, Policy and Law*, 7(3), Fall 1982, 667–685.

12. For a more complete discussion of this proposal, see Andrew K. Dolan, "The New York State Nurses Association 1985 Proposal: Who Needs It?," *Journal of Health Politics, Policy and Law*, 2(4), Winter 1978, 508–530.

13. Many states adopted the citizenship requirement for foreign medical graduates after the AMA's House of Delegates passed such a resolution in 1938. Five states continued such a requirement as late as 1975. Citizenship is no longer required in any state.

14. Another entry barrier used in dentistry is restrictions on interstate mobility. Various studies have shown that dentists graduating from a dental school within a state have a greater chance of passing that state's licensing exam than dentists from other states. Unlike medicine, most states do not permit reciprocal licensing for dentists. See, for example, Lawrence Shepard, "Licensing Restrictions and the Cost of Dental Care," *The Journal of Law and Economics*, 21(1), April 1978, 187–201. See also, B. Friedland and R. Valachovic, "The regulation of Dental Licensing—The Dark Ages," *American Journal of Law and Medicine*, 17(3), 1991, 249–270.

15. For an excellent discussion of licensure, quality, and the production of information concerning comparative performance of physicians and hospitals, see Lee Benham, "Licensure and Competition in Medical Markets," in H. E. Frech, *Regulating Doctors' Fees*, (Washington, D.C.: American Enterprise Institute), 1991.

C H A P T E R

19

National Health Insurance:
An Approach to the Redistribution
of Medical Care

KEY TERMS AND CONCEPTS

- Value judgment of minimum provision
- Equal financial access
- Equal treatment for equal needs
- Negative prices
- NHI evaluation criteria
- Incidence of the payroll tax
- Medicare's redistributive effects
- Equity and efficiency of Medicaid
- Tax-exempt employer-paid health insurance
- Mandated employer health insurance
- Canadian-type health system
- Medical savings accounts
- Refundable tax credits
- Concentrated interests in health reform

Learning Objectives

Upon completing this chapter, the reader should be able to:

- Understand how the different values underlying national health insurance affect both the type and size of government subsidies.
- Discuss the criteria for evaluating different national health insurance proposals.
- Explain who bears the burden of a payroll tax.
- Evaluate the redistributive and efficiency effects of government subsidies for Medicare, Medicaid, and tax-exempt employer-paid health insurance.
- Explain the advantages and disadvantages of a Single Payer system, an Employer Mandate, and Refundable Tax Credits.
- Understand why the U.S. is unlikely to have national health insurance in the near future.

National health insurance (NHI) has been a highly visible political issue many times. Each time its proponents have been disappointed. It is an issue that is unlikely to go away. To understand the issues surrounding NHI requires both an economic and political framework. The latter explains why efficiency and equity criteria are unlikely to be the basis of any NHI plan.

This chapter begins with a theoretical framework that can be used to analyze various NHI proposals in terms of the efficiency with which they achieve the different values that underlie proposals for NHI. No attempt will be made to select one set of values over another; instead, the analysis will be concerned with the most efficient means for achieving a given set of values. Some empirical evidence based on Medicare will be used to support the theoretical conclusions. This theoretical discussion will then be used as a basis for developing a set of criteria for evaluating alternative health insurance proposals. The current system of financing medical care and several suggested NHI proposals will then be discussed according to the criteria developed. No attempt will be made to provide a detailed discussion of various legislative proposals (1). The chapter concludes with a discussion of why the U.S. has not enacted NHI.

ACHIEVING EFFICIENCY FOR DIFFERENT VALUES UNDERLYING NATIONAL HEALTH INSURANCE

A Theoretical Discussion

National health insurance (NHI) may be viewed as an in-kind demand subsidy based on the argument that there are externalities in consumption. Assuming the non-poor wish to subsidize the poor, this will result in a demand for government subsidies. The non-poor benefit by knowing that the poor receive medical services when ill. Unless the government were to tax the non-poor for this benefit, some non-poor would "free ride," i.e., receive the benefit without contributing to assist the poor with their medical care.

The extent of government subsidization will differ depending upon the values held by the non-poor

with respect to redistribution of medical care services. One set of values may be termed minimum provision, meaning that no person in society, when ill, should receive less than a certain quantity of medical care. A second set of values might be called equal financial access to medical care. If these values were the basis for the externalities in consumption, they would suggest an NHI plan that would equalize the financial barriers to all persons. The third set of values that people may share with respect to redistribution of medical services goes beyond equal financial access to require equal treatment for equal needs—in other words, equal consumption of medical services regardless of economic or other factors affecting utilization.

The different demands for government subsidies reflect varying sets of values that are believed to exist in the population. The first set of values would require the smallest level of subsidization; the third set of values would be the most expensive to achieve.

It is not possible for an economist to state which set of values is most appropriate; whichever set of values the population selects would be the proper basis for the level of government subsidies under NHI. Although it is not possible to determine a priori the set of values that is likely to be chosen by the population, it is possible to determine the most efficient (least costly) approach for achieving each of the three sets of values. Thus it is possible to state which types of NHI proposals will be more efficient than others, regardless of the set of values one selects.

Minimum provision may be achieved in one of two ways: those persons whose consumption of medical care is below the minimum may be subsidized to bring their consumption up to the minimum or, alternatively, a subsidy can be provided to *everyone* so that at the resulting new, lower (subsidized) price, no person's consumption would be below the minimum specified by society. These two alternatives are shown in Figure 19-1. Assuming that there are three different income groups—high incomes (HY), middle incomes (MY), and low incomes (LY)—their demands for medical care would be shown by the three demand curves, HY, MY, and LY, respectively. The aggregate demand curve of all three income groups (which is summed horizontally) is shown by HYMYLY.

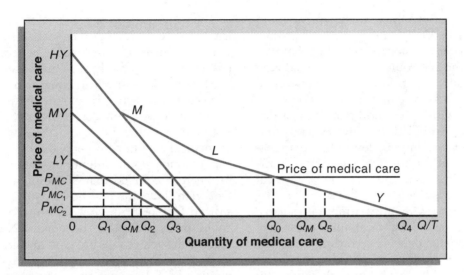

Figure 19-1. Demand curves of different income groups.

The reason the three demand curves do not result in the same consumption of medical care at zero price is that there are factors (other than financial ones) that result in differences in demand between different income groups. For example, low-income groups may incur greater costs in traveling to providers than do higher-income groups; differences in attitudes may also affect their utilization. Provider preferences in dealing with different income groups may also play a role. If the current price of medical care is P_{mc}, the utilization of the three income groups would be Q_1, Q_2, and Q_3, and their aggregate utilization would be Q_0, which is the intersection of the aggregate demand curve and the supply of medical care (assuming, for simplicity, perfect elasticity).

If society wanted to assure that no one received less than a minimum amount of medical care, Q_m, a national health insurance system could use one of two approaches to achieve this goal. A system of subsidies that lowered the price of medical care just to those whose consumption is less than the minimum would be one approach. Alternatively, a "universal" program that reduced the price of medical care to everyone (or set the price to zero for everyone) would also achieve this goal. If medical care were free, everyone's consumption would increase, with the total going

from Q_0 to Q_4. If, instead, a subsidy were provided to just those persons whose consumption was below the minimum (i.e., by lowering the price to lower-income persons to P_{mc1}), the aggregate increase in use of medical care would be from Q_0 to Q_{mo}.

The cost to society of achieving minimum provision by just subsidizing those whose use is below the minimum amount would be the subsidized price required to increase the low-income group's utilization, which is $P_{mc}-P_{mc1}$, multiplied by that group's utilization, Q_m. The cost of making medical care free to all would be the price of medical care multiplied by the new and greater quantity that would result when the price was reduced to everyone, which is P_{mc} multiplied by Q_4.

Both approaches (subsidies to lower income persons and the universal program) would achieve the goal of minimum provision. However, providing a subsidy just to the lower-income group would be less costly, hence more efficient.

The second value with respect to redistribution of medical care is that all persons should have equal financial access to medical care. This value could again be achieved by using two different approaches. First, by establishing a universal program, i.e., a free medical care system (or a subsidized low price) to all persons, as in the previous illustration, which would equalize financial barriers among different income groups. Alternatively, a system of subsidies that varied according to income could be used. Subsidizing the price of medical care to low-income persons so that it is reduced to zero would increase their consumption to Q_3. A subsidy to middle-income groups equal to $P_{mc}–P_{mc2}$ would also increase their consumption to Q_3. At consumption level Q_3, the utilization of medical care for the three income groups would be equal. The aggregate increase in medical care use would go from Q_0 to Q_5.

Equal financial access requires a more expensive subsidy than for achieving minimum provision. However, providing this subsidy according to income ($Q_3 \times P_{mc}$ for the low-income group, plus $Q_3 \times (P_{mc}–P_{mc2})$ for the middle-income group), would still be less costly than a medical care system that eliminated all financial barriers for everyone (a universal program).

Based on the value that there should be equal financial access, it is unlikely that the external demand for subsidization would include the value judgment that the demands of higher-income persons should be increased beyond levels that they currently spend, and that this increase should be financed through higher taxes. If such persons are currently purchasing Q_3 amount of medical care, then the value to them of additional units of care is less than the price they would have to pay to consume it. It would be illogical for people to vote for an additional tax on themselves to purchase additional units of medical care when they were previously not willing to pay the equivalent amount of money to purchase those same units.

Equal treatment for equal needs expresses the third set of values that give rise to a demand for medical care subsidies. Since demands for medical care vary for more reasons than just financial ones, merely making the price of medical care free to all will not result in equal consumption. As shown in Figure 19-1, high-income groups would still consume more medical care at zero price than would those with middle and lower incomes. Thus a free medical care system would *not* be able to achieve the set of values defined as equal treatment for equal needs.

The value likely to be achieved through a free medical care system would be equal financial access which, as we have shown, could be achieved at lower cost by a system of subsidies that varied by income.

The only way in which equal treatment for equal needs could be achieved would be through differential subsidies, varying according to income level. For example, as shown in Figure 19-2, lowering the price of medical care to zero for both low- and middle-income groups would still not increase their utilization to where it equaled that of the high-income group. Only if the low- and middle-income groups were subsidized further through a system of negative prices could their utilization be equal. (Negative prices mean that such groups are paid to increase their use.) How large the negative prices would have to be would depend, in part, upon the consumption levels of the high-income groups.

Legislation would not be enacted that would actually pay people to increase their use of medical care. Instead, a negative price would be paid by means of a direct in-kind supply subsidy to low-income groups.

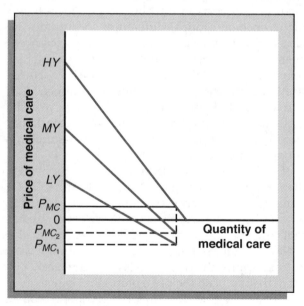

Figure 19-2. Equal treatment for equal needs through a system of negative prices.

For example, although the price of medical care to a low-income person would be zero, substantial travel and access costs might deter that person from using more medical services. Establishing clinics and neighborhood health centers in low-income areas and providing incentives for health personnel to practice there would increase access and decrease travel costs, thereby increasing use.

The cost in resources and the consequent increase in taxes required to achieve each of the three sets of values are even greater when the more realistic assumption is made that the supply of medical care is not perfectly price elastic but is, instead, relatively price inelastic. Figure 19-3 is similar to Figure 19-1 except that the supply of medical care is less price elastic. The consequence of a rising supply curve is that as demand is subsidized, the cost of a subsidy will be greater than if supply were more elastic. The cost of the subsidy necessary to achieve minimum provision is the utilization of the low-income group multiplied by the higher price of medical care (Point A on the supply curve). This higher price will also be borne by those persons in society who favor medical

care subsidies to low-income groups.[1] The taxes required to fund equal financial access will be greater than those required to achieve minimum provision.

As might be expected, as the price to those who are not being subsidized rises and the cost of achieving a given set of values increases, the amount that they are willing to subsidize others will decline.

For national health insurance to have the redistributive effects desired by society, increased utilization must occur; it will most easily occur when there is a high price elasticity of demand for medical services by those persons receiving subsidies. However, the greater the price elasticity of demand, the greater will be the increase in demand along an inelastic supply; the consequence will be rapidly increasing prices and total expenditures.

It is precisely because of these expected higher expenditures that proposals for national health insurance have also included approaches for changing the delivery system. In evaluating alternative national health insurance proposals, demand proposals should be analyzed separately from supply proposals. Presumably, proposals to enhance efficiency on the supply side (which were discussed in a previous chapter) can be incorporated into any NHI plan. A supply proposal becomes an integral part of the demand proposal only when its proponents are not willing to accept the criterion of economic efficiency in supply.

Under one NHI approach, a Canadian-type system that would make medical care free to all, a great deal of emphasis is placed upon how the supply side will be financed and organized. Expenditure limits by region and by type of provider would be established. As shown in Figure 19-3, total expenditures and prices would increase sharply under a free medical care system. Arbitrary establishment of dollar limits is an outgrowth of a political process and is unrelated to underlying supply and demand conditions.

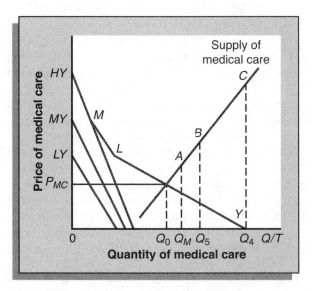

Figure 19-3. The cost of different demand subsidies when supply of medical care is relatively inelastic.

---

1. Because the supply of medical care is not very price elastic, it is necessary to think in terms of the post-subsidy market price that an income group will face when the price of medical care is subsidized. National health insurance based on a tax credit is one way of achieving this.

Expenditure limits would serve as a cost-control mechanism, but if cost control is the consequence of this approach, either intended or otherwise, the proponents of a free medical care system should be more explicit in defining the set of values that underlie this approach. They should also demonstrate how arbitrarily determined expenditure limits on the supply side would achieve these values.

The advocates of a free medical system might argue that it would still be possible to achieve, through greater efficiency, the program's stated goals at a lower expenditure level than indicated by the supply curve in Figure 19-3. Single-payer proponents are basically opposed to market competition for determining the most efficient providers and delivery system. Instead, they prefer to rely upon government to manage the medical system and to bring about greater efficiency in supply.

Previous attempts by government to regulate or manage the supply of a good or service (both outside and within the medical care field) lend little credibility to the belief that the government can be as efficient and innovative as a competitive system.

It is more likely that under a free medical system the medical care delivery system would be frozen in existing patterns. The government has not been able to close Veterans Administration, Public Health Service, or any municipal hospitals when it wanted to do so on grounds of efficiency; political pressure from employee groups and the constituencies of these facilities have prevented such closures. (The same has been true of military bases.) It is likely that each provider group within each region would attempt to protect its expenditure allocation each year; such actions would prevent changes in methods of delivery when dollar allocations to providers are affected.

The use of managed care techniques used so widely in the private sector has not been adopted in Medicare or the Canadian health system. Management performance in a government system is unlikely to be as high as in a competitive health care system because a government-run system would not have a point of reference outside itself by which managers could be evaluated. There are also no incentives for managers to be innovative in a government system since the financial rewards for risk taking are lacking. In the medical system, too, unions would become more powerful in the decision-making process and, as in the postal service, might inhibit the introduction of labor-saving innovations and flexibility in use of personnel.

For each set of values examined—minimum provision, equal financial access, and equal treatment for equal needs—it was shown that these values can be achieved more efficiently when the subsidy varies by income level rather than through a universal system that either provides an equal price reduction to all or makes medical care free to everyone regardless of income level. Although this analysis was theoretical, empirical data support these conclusions.

Empirical Evidence on Achieving a Given Set of Values: Medicare

Medicare is an existing in-kind demand subsidy to the aged. (Part A of Medicare provides hospital coverage, while Part B is a voluntary program primarily for physician services, with 75 percent of the premium being subsidized by the government.) All of the aged beneficiaries under Medicare receive the same set of benefits, and all pay the same reduced (subsidized) price for the services they receive. To use physician services (Part B of Medicare), an aged person was initially required to pay a $50 deductible (since increased to $100) and a 20 percent co-payment.

It would appear that Medicare's subsidized pricing mechanism was designed to ensure that all the aged either had equal financial access to medical care or equal treatment for equal medical needs.

As long as demand for medical care among the aged differs according to income and accessibility, then, as shown in Figure 19-1, a similar price to all persons, such as charged the aged under Medicare, would result in differences in utilization. Setting the same price to all the aged will result in higher-income aged having higher use rates than lower-income aged. The reduced price would represent a smaller financial burden to higher-income aged. Also higher-income aged are likely to have lower travel costs since they are likely to live in areas that are closer to medical providers.

According to data shown in Table 19-1, in 1968, higher-income aged were more likely than lower-income aged to pay the deductible and use the Part B coverage under Medicare; the ratio of high-income to low-income persons using Part B was 1.28. Medicare services used by the higher-income aged also cost the government more; the ratio was 1.48 per reimbursable service. (These higher prices represent higher prices for the same services as well as possibly higher-quality services, as when specialists are used.) Medicare reimbursement per person enrolled was more than twice as high for the higher-income aged; the ratio was 2.04.

If Medicare were based on the assumption of equal treatment for equal needs, one would expect to observe an equal number of physician visits according to level of medical need. When all aged recipients face the same price but differ according to income and other characteristics such as location, equal treatment for equal needs is unlikely to occur. As shown in Table 19-2, regardless of health status, aged persons with higher incomes had more physician visits than did aged with lesser incomes. Of those aged who are classified as being in poor health, in 1969 low-income aged had 10.47 physician visits per year compared to 16.98 visits per aged person with a high income.

By 1977, differences in visit rates among the aged in different income groups were smaller; further, visit rates among the high-income aged decreased. Between 1969 and 1977, the "real" price (adjusted for inflation) declined for the low-income aged, hence increasing their visit rates, while the "real" price faced by the high-income aged increased, thereby decreasing their visit rates. Physicians serving low-income aged were likely to accept Medicare assignment; that is, they were willing to accept the Medicare fee as the price for their services. Medicare fee increases were limited by the Medicare Economic Index, which increased much more slowly than the rate of inflation. Thus, to low-income aged, the "real" price of a physician visit (the 20 percent co-payment of a physician's fee which had not been permitted to rise rapidly) declined. The physician assignment rate, those physicians participating in Medicare, declined after Medicare started, reaching a low of 50.5 percent in 1977.

Table 19-1. Medicare Reimbursements for Covered Services Under the Supplementary Medical Insurance Program and Persons Served, by Income, 1968 and 1977

Income Group	Persons Receiving Reimbursable Services per 1,000 Medicare Enrollees	Medicare Reimbursement per Reimbursable Service	Medicare Reimbursement per Person Enrolled
		1968	
Under $5,000	431.7	$7.02	$78.77
Over $15,000	552.3	10.40	160.30
Ratio, over $15,000 to under $5,000 incomes	1.28	1.48	2.04
		1977	
At or near poverty line	773.4	6.43	60.32
High-income	801.7	5.82	57.72
Ratio, high income to at or near poverty line	1.04	.91	.96

Source: For 1968 data: Karen Davis, "Equal Treatment and Unequal Benefits: The Medicare Program," *Milbank Memorial Fund Quarterly/Health and Society,* 53(4), p. 457, Table 1, Copyright Milbank Memorial Fund. For 1977 data: G. Wilensky, L. Rossiter, and L. Finney, "The Medicare Subsidy of Private Health Insurance," Rockville, MD: National Center for Health Services Research, *National Health Care Expenditure Survey,* 1983.

Table 19-2. Average Physician Visits for the Elderly, by Health Status and Family Income, Adjusted for Other Determinants, 1969 and 1977

| | Health Status(a) | | |
	Good	Average	Poor
		1969	
Family Income:			
Under $5,000			
No aid(b)	2.78	5.64	10.47
Aid	3.86	7.52	13.42
$5,000–9,999	3.14	6.60	11.70
$10,000–$14,999	3.75	7.27	12.98
$15,000 and over	5.35	9.53	16.98
		1977(c)	
At or near poverty line			
No Medicaid	3.72	6.56	9.06
Medicaid	5.89	7.36	10.46
Middle-income	4.21	7.31	10.66
High-income	4.34	7.30	—(d)

Source: 1969 data are from Karen Davis, *National Health Insurance: Benefits, Costs, and Consequences* (Washington, D.C.: Brookings Institute, 1975), p. 85. The 1977 data are from G. Wilensky, L. Rossiter, and L. Finney, "The Medicare Subsidy of Private Health Insurance," National Center for Health Services Research, *National Health Care Expenditure Survey*, 1983.

(a) Good health status is defined as absence of any chronic conditions, limitations of activity, or restricted activity days. Average and poor health are defined at the mean and twice the mean level, respectively, of the three morbidity indicators used.

(b) Aid indicates public assistant recipients.

(c) For 1977 data, respondents are asked to characterize their own health status relative to people of the same age.

(d) Cell size too small to estimate.

Physicians were also less likely to take assignment for those aged that had higher incomes. All aged were required to pay a deductible and a co-payment. However, a high-income aged person going to a nonparticipating physician also had to pay the full difference between what Medicare reimbursed as the physician's fee and the physician's actual fee. Physicians not accepting assignment were also able to raise their fees more rapidly than the increases permitted under the Medicare Economic Index. Thus high-income aged, using nonparticipating physicians, experienced an increase in the "real" prices they paid for physician visits.

The 1969 data is therefore consistent with the expectation that visit rates will differ when different income groups face the *same* price. The 1977 data (and the change from 1969) is also consistent with what would be expected when different income groups pay *different* prices for physician visits. (Since the early 1990s, physicians must either participate for all Medicare patients or for none. Thus once again both high- and low-income Medicare patients pay the same physician fees.)

Based on the Medicare experience, it is obvious that a reduced but similar price to all aged persons will achieve neither equal financial access nor equal treatment for equal needs. As could have been hypothesized based on the earlier theoretical discussion, *Medicare is an inefficient approach for achieving either of the foregoing sets of values;* higher-income persons use a greater number of services than do lower-income persons, and the services they use are more costly.

If the Medicare subsidy varied according to income level, the same services could have been provided to lower-income aged at a lower total cost. Not only would the overall level of utilization under Medicare be less with a subsidy that varied by income, but with a smaller overall increase in demand, the rise in medical prices would also have been less. The record of the Medicare program should be kept in mind when specific proposals for national health insurance are analyzed.

SPECIFIC CRITERIA FOR EVALUATING NATIONAL HEALTH INSURANCE PLANS

Before discussing specific proposals for national health insurance, it would be useful to have a common set of criteria by which these alternative plans may be evaluated.

The Beneficiaries

Based on the previous discussion of the different sets of values held by society regarding redistribution of medical care, the primary recipients of national health insurance should be those who are or might become medically indigent. The medically indigent are those persons who have low incomes and cannot buy as much medical care as society would prefer them to have. Another category of beneficiaries are those persons who are potentially medically indigent—those whose medical expenses are large in relation to their incomes. Even persons with middle incomes may be hard pressed to pay their medical bills if they have a chronic or pre-existing medical condition requiring large expenditures.

Subsidies under national health insurance, therefore, should vary according to income (decline as income increases). An upper limit on liability for medical expenses should be available to protect even higher-income persons from suffering an undue financial hardship. *Everyone should, therefore, be required to have, at a minimum, catastrophic health insurance coverage.*

The primary beneficiary groups included under national health insurance should be categorized according to both income and the size of the medical bill in relation to income. Categorizing population groups by age is an indirect approach for determining current medical need and potential financial hardship. Although many aged are low income, not all of them require the same degree of financial subsidy; many younger persons have greater medical and financial needs than some of the aged.

The size of the medical subsidy for low-income persons is basically a value judgment. Some persons would prefer that the poor receive all their medical care without any payments; others would prefer a less generous subsidy. Any plan for national health insurance should be able to incorporate either of these conflicting values by varying the degree of subsidization in relation to income levels.

Incentives for Efficiency

A second criterion by which alternative health insurance plans should be judged is whether there are incentives to encourage the efficient and appropriate use of medical resources by both demanders (the moral hazard problem) and suppliers (supplier-induced demand issue). These efficiency incentives may be accomplished in several ways. The moral hazard issue, namely the patient's desire to use more services when the price is decreased, may be resolved by placing incentives on either the patient or the provider to limit use of services. When the financial incentives are placed on the consumer, as is done in indemnity or catastrophic type of insurance plans, then deductibles and co-payments are used to control patients' use of services. Deductibles and co-payments provide consumers with an incentive not to "overuse" services as well as to select providers on the basis of price, as well as other attributes.

When the financial incentive to control moral hazard is placed on the provider, then the insurer or provider of service has the incentive to limit the patient's use of services and to deliver the appropriate level of care. Examples of such provider techniques are utilization management, selecting providers for the insurer's provider network who are more appropriate prescribers of medical services, and the insurer monitoring provider behavior. These types of managed care techniques are also useful for reducing the extent of supplier-induced demand.

The financial incentive to control moral hazard and supplier-induced demand is shifted to the insurer and/or provider when consumers have a choice of managed care plans and they must pay the additional cost (co-premium) of more expensive plans. Consumers then have an incentive to weigh the benefits and the costs of the competing health plans based on premiums and other attributes of the plan. Price competition among health plans provides those plans with an incentive to be responsive to consumer demands as well as to be efficient so as to be price competitive. Health plans will therefore select those providers believed to be appropriate users of medical services and employ monitoring mechanisms to ensure that appropriate guidelines for delivery of medical services are used.

Equitable Financing

A third criterion for evaluating alternative NHI plans is the equitability of their financing. Any one or combination of the following taxes could be used (and have been suggested) to finance NHI. An income tax would place the greater cost burden on those with higher incomes, which is the most equitable method of financing a redistributive program. A disadvantage of an income tax is that it is highly visible and therefore likely to generate political opposition from middle- and high-income groups. Further, while income tax financing is generally regarded as being more equitable, it is a tax on work effort and may therefore cause a decrease in the supply of such effort.

Deficit financing, whereby the government borrows the money to subsidize different population groups, shifts the cost burden to future generations. Therein lies both its political advantage and its inequity. Future generations do not vote on current policies, thereby enabling politicians to provide benefits without imposing costs on current recipients and voters.

A sales tax, particularly if it does not exclude such expenditures as food, could be regressive in that those with lower incomes contribute a higher percentage of their incomes than those with higher incomes. A small increase in a sales tax typically generates a great deal of tax revenue and is not as visible a tax as income or property taxes; property taxes are paid in a lump sum making their magnitude very visible to voters. "Sin" taxes, such as taxes on alcohol and cigarettes, are also regressive but are economically efficient when the beneficiaries of such goods are required to pay the full costs of their consumption.

The equity and efficiency aspects of payroll taxes, which are used for financing Medicare Part A and have been proposed as part of an Employer Mandated NHI plan, are discussed more completely.

The two major financing approaches previously used have been an income tax, which funds Medicaid and (75 percent of) Medicare Part B (physician and non-hospital services), and a separate Medicare payroll tax, which pays for Medicare Part A (hospital services). In 1965, the Social Security tax paid by both employee and employer was 3.625 percent (for a total of 7.25 percent) of the employee's wage up to a maximum annual wage of $4,800. To finance Medicare Part A, the Medicare Trust Fund was established and funded by a separate payroll tax of 0.35 percent on the employee and employer for a total of 0.70 percent. The total payroll tax was therefore increased to 4.2 percent (a total of 8.4 percent) on an increased wage base of $6,600.

The Medicare Trust Fund is a "pay as you go" fund rather than a "true" trust fund. Medicare payroll taxes contributed by *current employees* are used to fund Medicare Part A expenses incurred by *current Medicare beneficiaries*. The payroll taxes contributed by current employees are not invested and used to pay for their own Medicare expenses when they become eligible for Medicare, as would occur under a typical trust fund. Instead, to remain solvent, the Medicare Trust Fund requires that current contributions be sufficient to pay current expenditures. Whenever the Trustees estimate that current Medicare payroll taxes will be insufficient to pay Medicare expenditures, Congress increases both the Medicare payroll tax and the wage base to which it applies.

Since the start of Medicare, rapidly increasing hospital costs for Medicare beneficiaries (primarily the result of new technology) has continually resulted in increased Medicare payroll taxes and the wage base to forestall the Medicare Trust Fund from going bankrupt. The Medicare payroll tax is currently 1.45 percent on the employee and employer for a total of 2.9 percent and it applies to *all* earned income (unearned income is excluded from the tax). (The combined Social Security and Medicare tax on both the employee and employer is currently 7.65 percent, a total of 15.3 percent.) Thus, Medicare is now financed by an almost proportional tax rather than the regressive tax with which it started (Social Security still has a maximum wage base of $87,900 as of 2004).

The large amount of funds required to fund NHI would likely necessitate an increase in either income or payroll taxes. Although the most equitable method of financing a redistributive program would be an income tax, the size of the income tax required would require imposing higher taxes on the middle class as well as those with high incomes, making such a tax increase politically difficult. Although a payroll tax would likely be regressive, it has many proponents. And, unlike an income tax, a payroll tax would not affect the budget deficit nor would it place an additional burden on those employees and employers who have employer-paid health insurance, namely those with middle and high incomes.

The payroll tax used to finance Medicare and, as has been proposed, to finance NHI would be imposed on both the employer and employee (some proposals suggest 80 percent of the tax be imposed on the employer). Imposing all or part of the payroll tax on the employer makes it appear that those who must pay the tax actually bear the burden of the tax. The magnitude of the tax on the employee becomes less visible since it is believed by many to be borne by the employer, not the employee.

In actuality, the incidence of the tax (who bears the burden of the tax) is determined by the elasticity of the demand and supply curves for labor. Assume that the initial wage rate is $10 an hour, as shown in Figure 19-4A. If the government were to impose a $2-an-hour tax on the employee, the new labor supply curve would be ST, which is equal to the initial labor supply curve, S, plus the tax of $2 an hour. The new equilibrium wage

will rise to $11 an hour. However, the employee would have to pay $2 of the $11 an hour to the government. The employees' net wage is $9 an hour, $1 less per hour than their previous earnings. The employer pays $1 an hour more than previously. Thus in the above example, even though the employee is required to pay the $2 tax, the employee pays 50 percent of the $2-an-hour tax, while the employer pays 50 percent.

Assume that instead of placing the tax on the employee, the $2-an-hour tax is placed on the employer. As shown in Figure 19-4B, the size of the tax is indicated by the vertical distance between the two equilibrium points. (The employer's demand for labor shifts down with a per-unit tax because the initial demand curve represents the maximum amount of labor the firm will hire at any given wage.) The burden of the tax when it is imposed on the employer is the same as when it was imposed on the employee. The employee receives $9 an hour (one dollar less than previously), the employer pays the government $2 per hour, and the employer ends up paying $11 an hour, $1 an hour more than previously. In both cases less labor is hired.

Thus it does not matter who is required to pay the tax, the employee or the employer, the incidence of the tax will be the same.

Figure 19-5 shows who bears the burden of a tax on labor when the demand for labor is less elastic (Figure 19-5A) and more elastic (Figure 19-5B). The elasticity of labor supply is the same in both cases.

When the demand for labor is less elastic (Figure 19-5A), a greater portion of the tax is borne by the employer. The greater the elasticity of demand for labor (Figure 19-5B), the greater will be the burden of the tax on the employee. The demand for unskilled labor is believed to be more elastic than the demand for skilled labor.

Figure 19-6 describes the tax burden under differing elasticities of labor supply. When the tax is imposed on business, as shown by a downward shift of $2 an hour in the demand for labor, and the labor supply is completely inelastic with regard to the wage (Figure 19-6A), a tax on labor is shifted entirely onto labor. As the labor supply becomes more elastic (Figure 19-6B), the employer pays a portion of the tax.

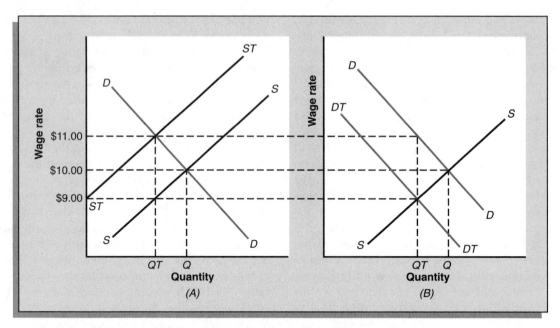

Figure 19-4. The burden of a tax on labor is the same regardless of who pays the tax: (A) employees pay the tax; (B) employers pay the tax.

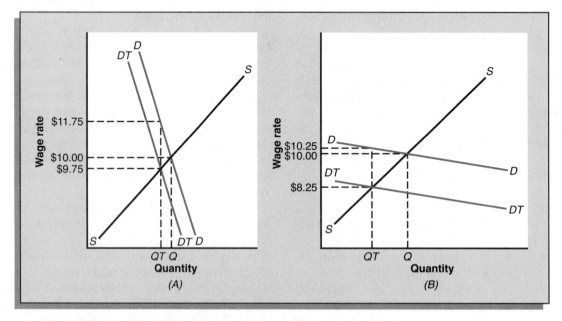

Figure 19-5. The burden of a tax on labor according to different elasticities of demand for labor: (A) less elastic demand for labor; (B) more elastic demand for labor.

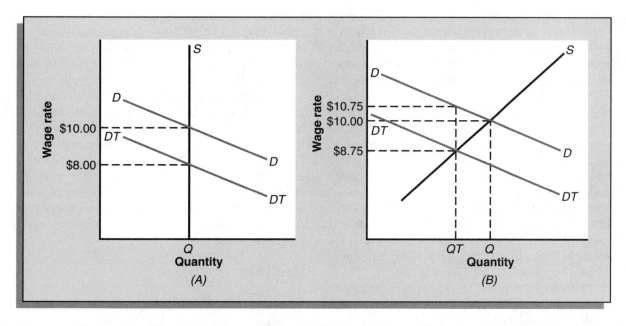

Figure 19-6.   The burden of a tax on labor according to different elasticities of labor supply: (A) inelastic supply of labor; (B) more elastic supply of labor.

As shown above, the burden of the payroll tax is determined by the elasticity of the demand and supply for labor and not on who is obligated by the government to pay the tax. (Although the net wage received by labor is shown to decrease as a result of the tax, in a dynamic economy increases in the payroll tax may result in wages not rising as much as they would otherwise.)

A crucial issue, therefore, for determining the burden of a payroll tax is the wage elasticity of the supply of labor. Economists believe that the supply of labor facing any one industry is relatively elastic since labor can move to other industries. *The aggregate supply of labor to the economy, however, is believed to be relatively inelastic with respect to the wage rate,* similar to that shown in Figure 19-6A.

Most people believe that only one-half of the payroll tax is imposed on labor. Thus the size of the tax on labor appears smaller than it is. The main advantage of placing half of the payroll tax on the employer is political. It is not obvious to the employee who bears the true burden of the entire tax.

There are two additional effects of a payroll tax that should be considered. When business bears a portion of the tax, as shown in Figure 19-4, the prices of the firm's goods and services are increased. (An increase in the wage results in an increase in the firm's marginal and average total cost curves.) Those industries most adversely affected by the tax on labor are those that are more labor intensive and those that face increased price competition from foreign competitors. Second, when the price of labor is increased, employers will hire fewer employees. The decline in the demand for labor is greater, the greater is the employer's elasticity of demand for labor; this is shown in Figure 19-5. The lower the skill level of labor, the greater is their elasticity of demand.

An increase in the income tax (to raise an equivalent amount of money as a payroll tax) will not cause the firm to raise its prices or decrease its demand for labor. This is because the firm's cost of labor is not affected by an income tax.

One other issue to be considered in evaluating payroll taxes as a method for financing medical services is which income groups will bear the greatest burden of the tax. If all employees must pay 7.65 percent of their wages, up to a maximum of $87,900, then a person with $87,900 of income as well as a person with $200,000 of income each pays $6,724 a year (plus the employer's contribution of $6,724). The $6,724 payment represents a greater proportionate tax on a low-income than on a high-income employee. For this reason the Social Security tax is referred to as a "regressive" tax. As the Social Security wage base has increased over time, the Social Security tax has become more of a proportionate tax. While low-income individuals may have too low an income to pay any income taxes, they still have to pay Social Security taxes on their earnings.

To the extent that not all of the tax is shifted and employers must pay part of it, the prices of goods and services will increase. These price increases are also regressive in their effect; they represent a greater portion of a low-income person's income.

An analysis of the Social Security tax is important not only for understanding the financing of the original Medicare legislation, but also for determining who bears the burden of NHI proposals that require regressive payroll taxes be used to finance employee health benefits.

In addition to these three criteria—the population group to be covered, incentives for efficiency, and the method of financing—two other supplementary goals are usually mentioned. First, should NHI be administered by the government or by private insurers? The concern with having the government administer the NHI plan is that the government is likely to control the prices they pay for medical services. Second, the NHI plan should be politically acceptable to the public, the providers, insurers, and the government. Political acceptability includes such issues as methods of reimbursing providers, whether there is a role for insurance companies, how large a tax increase would be necessitated by the program, and the impact on the federal budget.

THE CURRENT SYSTEM FOR FINANCING MEDICAL SERVICES

Using the above criteria, a brief evaluation of the current system for financing care is presented, along with proposals for improving the current system, and then several types of NHI proposals are discussed.

There are a myriad of government subsidies, direct and indirect, to decrease the price of medical services to various population groups. For example, there is the Veterans Administration, Civilian Health and Medical Program for Uniformed Services (CHAMPUS), the Indian Health Services, state and county health services, State Children's Health Insurance Program (SCHIP), as well as Medicare, Medicaid, and the exclusion from employees' taxable income employer-paid health insurance (to be referred to as employer-paid health insurance). Since these last three programs comprise the largest portion of demand subsidies, each will be briefly discussed.

Medicare

Medicare, a federal program to cover the medical expenses of those aged 65 years and older, started in 1966. It was extended in 1974 to cover all persons with chronic renal disease. All aged, regardless of their income levels, are presently included. There are two main parts to Medicare; Part A primarily covers hospital care as well as skilled nursing facilities and hospice care and is funded by the Medicare Trust Fund. The aged pay a large deductible ($879 in 2004) for each hospital admission. The Trust Fund is financed by a Medicare payroll tax. Medicare Part B (generally non-hospital services, such as physician services, hospital outpatient care, and home health services) is voluntary, and to participate the aged must pay a monthly premium which only covers 25 percent of the costs of the program; the remainder is funded from general federal tax revenues, a large portion of which comes from income taxes. Since Part B is not funded by an earmarked tax, these federal subsidies contribute directly to the budget deficit.

The growth in Medicare Part A expenditures has been dramatic, increasing from $5.3 billion in 1970, to $25.6 billion in 1980, to $67.0 billion in 1990, and $152.5 billion in 2002, as described in Figure 19-7. The growth in Part B expenditures has similarly been rapid, also shown in Figure 19-7.

The benefits and the prices the aged must pay, including the monthly premium for Part B (physician

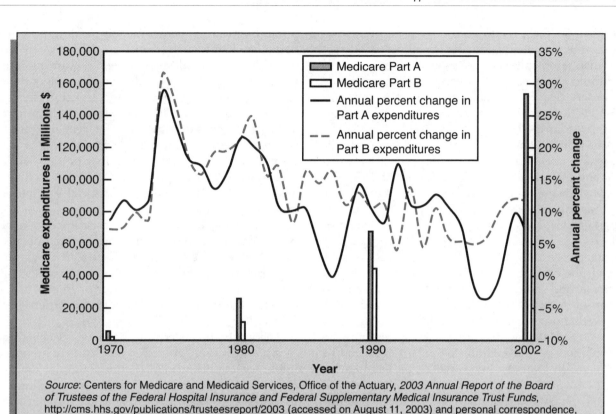

Figure 19-7. Medicare Part A and Part B expenditures, 1970–2002.

and non-inpatient services), as well as the deductibles and co-payments for both hospital and physician services, are "regressive" since they are the same for each aged person regardless of their income.

Medicare's benefit coverage has severe limitations: it does not provide catastrophic protection; the financial liability of the aged for co-payments, deductibles, and services not covered by Medicare is open-ended. Medicare does not cover outpatient prescription drugs, which are particularly important for those aged with chronic illnesses who are treated as outpatients. This results in a financial hardship to many aged. (Medicare also does not cover long-term nursing care.) Higher-income aged can afford to purchase more medical services and to buy supplementary

coverage for service gaps (such as prescription drug coverage) not covered by Medicare.

Because Medicare benefits are *not* income related, many aged find it difficult to pay for the gaps in benefit coverage and co-payments and deductibles. Consequently, about 12 percent of the aged must rely on Medicaid.

Traditional Medicare lacks efficiency incentives. Medicare patients face a 20 percent co-payment for use of physician services, and if they have supplementary (Medi-gap) private insurance, they may face no out-of-pocket expenses when seeing a physician. Similarly, physicians have limited incentives not to induce demand for their services since Medicare pays them fee for service. Managed care techniques prevalent in the private sector, such as utilization management, are not used in traditional Medicare since neither hospitals nor physicians have an incentive to be concerned with overuse or inappropriate use of services. Only a small percentage (16 percent in 1998) of Medicare beneficiaries are enrolled in managed care plans.

As a consequence, per capita Medicare expenditures have risen almost 7.4 percent per year between 1990 and 2000, reaching $266 billion in 2002 (2). Per capita Medicare expenditures have risen more than 2 percentage points a year faster than per capita private expenditures. These differences in annual rates of increase are believed to be the result of growth in managed care in the private sector.

The method used to finance Medicare is inequitable and results in large intergenerational transfers from the working population to the aged (3). A couple that turned 65 in 1980 could expect Medicare to spend $114,000 on them during their lifetime. The total lifetime estimate climbs to $232,000 for a couple turning 65 in 1995. By the year 2020, the estimate increases to $428,000. These couples will have contributed much less than the costs of those benefits. Also, higher-income aged tend to live longer and therefore receive several times the lifetime benefits compared to those with low incomes.

To forestall the Medicare Trust Fund from going bankrupt, Congress, in 1997, made the Medicare payroll tax applicable to all earned income; home health care was removed from Medicare Part A (thereby reducing Part A expenditures) and placed into Medicare Part B, which is funded by general income taxes rather than the Trust Fund. Further, reductions were made in the rate of increase in hospital payments. The aged were then provided with additional preventive services under Medicare Part B. Congress' method for resolving Medicare's financial crisis (and which groups are likely to bear the largest burden of resolving the crisis) should be kept in mind the next time the Medicare Trust Fund approaches bankruptcy.

Medicare faces several major problems: how to make Medicare financially stable, how to improve its efficiency, and how to make it a more equitable redistributive program. The focus of current public policy, however, is devoted to providing the aged with additional Medicare benefits, namely, adding an outpatient prescription drug benefit. Adding a new drug benefit to traditional Medicare will require enormous federal subsidies, worsen the federal budget deficit, reduce incentives for the aged to switch from traditional fee-for-service Medicare into Medicare managed care, and exacerbate the intergenerational inequity of Medicare. Current policy, however, is based on which political party can gain a political advantage (the political support of the aged) rather than on an attempt to solve Medicare's financial, efficiency, or inequitable financing issues.

Medicare's insolvency has been postponed by hospital payment reductions and the shifting of benefits from Medicare Part A to Medicare Part B. Previous approaches used to stave off the Trust Fund's bankruptcy, such as reducing provider payments and increasing the payroll tax, will not be sufficient in the future. The problem will be too great.

The impending Medicare financial crisis is driven by a baby boomer generation that starts to become eligible for Medicare in 2011, the continual development of expensive medical technology, an aging population with greater medical needs, unlimited access to medical services by the aged under traditional Medicare, and lower birth rates.

In 1945, there were 42 workers for each retiree. As shown in Figure 19-8, by 1960 that number had declined to 5.1 workers per retiree. The number of workers per retiree continued to decline to 3.4 by 2000. By 2020, it is estimated that there will be only 2.6 workers per retiree. As the ratio of workers per aged person continues to decline, a greater financial burden is placed on each worker to pay the Medicare expenses of an aging population. The decline in the ratio of workers per aged beneficiary is leading to a huge financial burden on future generations. The working population will begin to experience that financial burden when the baby boomers begin to retire, starting in 2011.

As the very large number of baby boomers (born between 1946 and 1964) start becoming eligible for Medicare, it will become increasingly difficult to make drastic reductions in their benefits on the eve of their retirement. Given the timing of presidential elections every four years and congressional elections

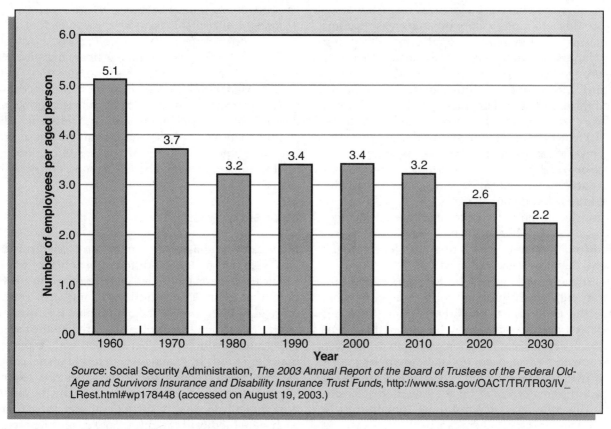

Figure 19-8.   Number of employees per aged person, 1960–2030.

every two years, there are few non-election years for Congress to reform Medicare before the baby boomers retire. It is unlikely that a presidential (or congressional) candidate will campaign on a platform of decreasing benefits to those population groups who have the highest voting participation rates. Further, candidates would likely be willing to lose the votes of the aged's children, who would then have to shoulder an increased financial responsibility for their parent's medical expenses.

Any long-run solution to the Medicare crisis will have to be gradually phased in, otherwise political opposition by those groups adversely affected will make an equitable solution more difficult to achieve.

Given the huge needs for additional funds to keep the program solvent, the longer the delay before solu-

tions are implemented, the more costly each of the options become, the more taxes required, the larger the benefit reductions, and the steeper the reductions in provider payments.

A number of proposals have been made to maintain Medicare's solvency; the following are several such options which are not mutually exclusive. The first is to phase in an increase in the eligibility age (one month each year) to age 67 so that it will eventually be similar to the eligibility age for Social Security, which is also being increased.

Second, an increase in the Medicare payroll tax is likely, however, too large an increase would further add to the financial burden on the working population, particularly those with low incomes. Given the decline in the number of workers per aged beneficiary, a large payroll tax would have to be imposed on each worker to raise sufficient funds to support an increasing number of aged. The employed population will oppose such a large tax burden to pay for the medical services of many aged who are financially well off.

Third, Medicare expenditure increases can be reduced through reduced payments to the suppliers of Medicare services, such as hospitals and physicians. While Medicare has previously used this approach, too great a reduction in provider payments will reduce provider participation in Medicare, reduce patients' access to medical services, and eventually result in reduced quality of care.

A fourth option is to make Medicare an income-related program. Higher-income aged can be required to pay a larger Part B premium (currently 25 percent) than lower-income aged.

A fifth approach would be to change Medicare from an entitlement program with defined benefits where the government pays the cost of providing mandated benefits regardless of the cost of those benefits, to a defined contribution program where the government pays a fixed dollar amount toward a health plan (perhaps equal to the average cost of all the health plans or based on the lowest cost health plan). This approach (referred to as "premium-support") is similar to a voucher plan; health plans would compete for Medicare beneficiaries, and the aged would have an incentive to choose less costly health plans since they would have to pay the additional cost of choosing more expensive plans.

A defined contribution, as discussed above, could also be income related whereby the government pays the entire premium for those with low incomes and the contribution declines the higher the beneficiary's income.

Merely making the health care system more efficient will not solve the long-run financial burden of achieving Medicare solvency. Further, reducing benefits for all the aged (such as increasing deductibles, co-payments, premium increases, and increasing the eligibility age) will adversely affect low-income aged. Instead, to make the Medicare system more efficient and more equitable (both across generations as well as redistributing subsidies toward low-income aged away from high-income aged) *Medicare reform should*

be based on two principles: income related subsidies (or a declining contribution as income rises) and to allow Medicare beneficiaries a choice of health plans.

These principles of equitable financing and efficient provision of services raise the question, "Why should Medicare and Medicaid be maintained as a separate systems?" *Both programs are welfare programs in that the beneficiaries are heavily subsidized.* Why should there not be just one system for those both over and under 65 years of age based on income-related subsidies and choice of competing health plans?

Medicaid

Medicaid was enacted the same time as Medicare but was designed to serve a different beneficiary group. Medicaid is a means-tested welfare program for the poor that provides medical and long-term care to more than 15 percent of the population. It is administered by each state, but policy is shared by the federal government which pays between 50 and 76 percent matching funds based on each state's financial capacity (per capita income). While the states may expand eligibility beyond the groups mandated by the federal government, to qualify for federal matching funds, each state Medicaid program must cover three federally mandated population groups.

The first—and largest—of the federally mandated population groups are those receiving cash assistance, including single-parent families eligible for Aid to Families with Dependent Children (AFDC) and low-income aged, blind, and disabled persons who qualify for Supplemental Security Income (SSI). The second mandatory eligibility group are low-income pregnant women and children who did not qualify for cash assistance, as well as those considered to be "medically needy," those who do not qualify for welfare programs but who have high medical or long term care expenses. The third group consists of low-income Medicare beneficiaries who cannot afford the deductibles, cost sharing, premiums for Medicare Part B, or the cost of services not covered by Medicare.

States may enroll additional groups (and add additional services above those mandated by the federal government). Those groups typically added at the state's option include medically needy individuals, pregnant women and children at a higher percentage in excess of the federal poverty level, e.g., 200 percent, and expanded Medicaid eligibility to include all uninsured persons with incomes below a certain level. However, the percent of the population covered by Medicaid that is Poor (less than 100 percent of the poverty level) varies greatly by state, between 33 and 65 percent. Just being poor is insufficient to qualify for Medicaid. *On average, only 40 percent of those classified as Poor are enrolled in Medicaid.* The percentage of Near-Poor (100 to 199 percent of poverty) enrolled by states varies from 7 to 28 percent, or 16.5 percent.

In recent years, Temporary Assistance to Needy Families (TANF) was enacted to replace AFDC. This new program, TANF, retains the same eligibility rules as previously. Before welfare reform, many poor children automatically qualified for Medicaid because their families were receiving Aid to Families with Dependent Children (AFDC), the national cash benefits program for poor children. Welfare reform ended that link because it abolished AFDC, but Congress did not want anyone to lose Medicaid eligibility as a result of welfare reform. Thus Congress decreed that states should continue using their old AFDC rules for determining Medicaid eligibility, such as pregnant women, the medically needy, and children if their parents would have qualified for AFDC under the old law. The children of women who leave welfare for work are still eligible for Medicaid because of low family income.

As part of the 1997 Balanced Budget Act, Congress also enacted the Children's Health Insurance Program (CHIP). This program provided the states with federal matching funds to initiate and expand health care assistance for uninsured low-income children, up to age 19, with family incomes as high as 200 percent of the federal poverty level. (Federal matching funds may be as high as 85 percent.) States may purchase health insurance coverage for eligible children in the private market or they may be included in the state's Medicaid program. Medical benefits for children are considered to be relatively inexpensive as compared to uninsured adults. Politically, children are considered to be a more deserving group than other uninsured groups, consequently this program

expansion received bipartisan support. Further, providing coverage to children was viewed as an expansion of existing Medicaid policies which expanded Medicaid coverage to infants, younger children, and pregnant women in the late 1980s.

As of 2002, approximately 41 million people were on Medicaid. Broadened eligibility requirements for Medicaid have caused the number of recipients to sharply increase (from 22 million in 1988 to 41 million), however, the distribution of beneficiary groups has stayed roughly constant over this time period. Most of the enrollment growth resulted from federal and state expansions in coverage of low-income children and pregnant women. Currently, the major beneficiary groups consist of low-income children (51 percent), non-disabled low-income adults (pregnant women and adults in families with children receiving cash assistance) (21 percent), aged persons receiving Medicare that need Medicaid to pay for their deductibles, cost sharing, premium for Medicare Part B, and other services not covered by Medicare (10 percent), and acute medical and long term care services for the blind and disabled (18 percent).

As shown in Figure 19-9, the distribution of Medicaid expenditures does not match the distribution of Medicaid enrollees. Although about 73 percent of Medicaid recipients are low-income parents and children, they account for only 27.5 percent of Medicaid expenditures. The remaining 72.5 percent of Medicaid expenditures are for medical services and institutional care for the aged, disabled, and mentally retarded (27 percent of Medicaid recipients).

State and federal Medicaid expenditures have been rapidly increasing and are expected to continue to sharply rise over the next decade. Congressionally mandated benefit and eligibility expansions, along with an increase in the number of uninsured, have been important reasons for these rapid increases. As shown in Figure 19-10, federal and state Medicaid expenditures were $5.3 billion in 1970, $26 billion in 1980, $73.6 billion in 1990, rising to $224 billion in 2001, and are expected to reach $446 billion by the year 2010. The federal share of Medicaid expenditures is expected to more than double over the next 10 years, from $130 billion in 2001 to $312 billion by the year 2011. The remaining expenditures represent the

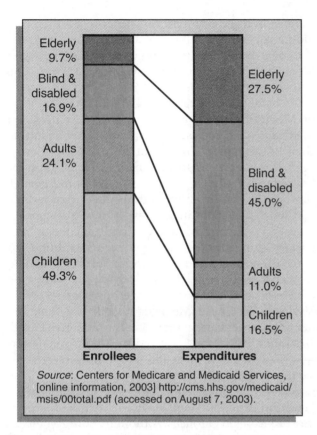

Enrollees:
Elderly 9.7%
Blind & disabled 16.9%
Adults 24.1%
Children 49.3%

Expenditures:
Elderly 27.5%
Blind & disabled 45.0%
Adults 11.0%
Children 16.5%

Source: Centers for Medicare and Medicaid Services, [online information, 2003] http://cms.hhs.gov/medicaid/msis/00total.pdf (accessed on August 7, 2003).

Figure 19-9. Percent distribution of Medicaid recipients and Medicaid vendor payments by eligibility status, 2000.

state's financial burden. During this same time period, however, the number of beneficiaries is expected to increase by 11 percent.

As in the case with Medicare, although the direct beneficiaries of Medicaid have been helped, there are equity and efficiency concerns with the current program.

Because Medicaid is administered by each state, there are wide variations in eligibility requirements and in services covered. In some states, people may lose all of their eligibility if their income rises slightly above the cutoff level; in other words, eligibility is not graduated according to income level. Although the beneficiary group is the poor, only about one-half of the population below the poverty level is eligible for Medicaid benefits. No state covers all those whose incomes are below the federal poverty level. Even within a state there are variations in access and use of services between white and nonwhite persons and between urban and rural dwellers.

Medicaid is financed through a state's general tax revenues and from federal income taxes, which is typical of programs whose beneficiaries are those with low incomes.

An important policy concern with regard to increased Medicaid eligibility is whether the new beneficiaries dropped their private insurance because Medicaid became available as a lower-cost substitute. The large increase in the non-elderly population on Medicaid since 1987 is partly attributed to individuals who dropped their private coverage. Cutler and Gruber estimate the magnitude of this effect and propose that a preferable approach would be to subsidize the purchase of private insurance for those with low incomes with a subsidy that decreases as income increases (4).

States are under pressure to reduce their share of rising Medicaid costs since it is their fastest increasing expenditure. States have attempted to reduce these expenditure increases by limiting eligibility of other groups, reducing benefits, and by paying medical providers less. This latter approach has reduced access to medical care by the poor; lower reimbursement levels have limited the willingness of many providers to serve Medicaid patients. With the difficulties that states have in meeting projected increases in Medicaid expenditures, the gaps in Medicaid are unlikely to be resolved and are likely to worsen.

Various proposals have been made to improve both the efficiency and horizontal equity (treating similar persons the same across states) of the Medicaid program. One approach is to have uniform eligibility standards across states. Second, as mentioned above, subsidies (in the form of a voucher for a health plan) could be provided to low-income people on a decreasing scale; the size of the premium subsidy would decline with higher income levels. Providing a declining subsidy has a number of advantages. The benefits are directed to those with lowest incomes; there is a gradual decline in benefits as income rises in order to provide an incentive to earn

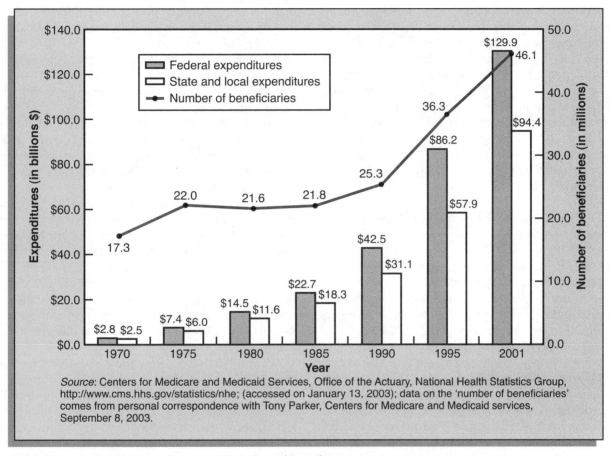

Figure 19-10. Medicaid expenditures and number of beneficiaries, 1970–2001.

more income; the financing is based on general tax revenues, which raises more funds from those with higher incomes; and the eligibility and benefits are uniform across the states, thereby eliminating any incentive for those with low incomes to move to states with higher eligibility criteria.

There are, however, a number of problems with an income-related subsidy for Medicaid. The first is political. Medicaid beneficiaries have low incomes, both the young and those aged who are in nursing homes; thus, their voting participation rates are lower than other population groups. It is for these reasons that states have been reluctant to raise taxes on the middle class to adequately fund Medicaid.

Second, states could still reduce their Medicaid expenditures by reducing payments to providers and/or making the value of the voucher too low for health plans to participate. Inadequate hospital and physician payments and/or capitation payments to health plans decrease provider participation and thereby decrease access to care by the poor. Unless Medicaid payments were competitive, providers and health plans would be unwilling to serve the Medicaid population.

To improve provider participation and to increase the efficiency of Medicaid expenditures, many states are contracting on a capitation basis with managed care organizations. In contrast to past practices,

Medicaid patients enrolled in a managed care health plan are no longer able to go to an emergency room for non-emergent services; the health plan has to arrange with its providers to be able to respond to the Medicaid patient's needs for service. Crucial to the success of Medicaid managed care plans is the state's willingness to monitor the quality, outcomes, and patient satisfaction of the care provided. Access to care and the quality of those services are more easily monitored in a managed care system than in a fee-for-service system. Provider efficiency incentives are also greater.

The Tax Treatment of Employment-Based Health Insurance

Employer-purchased health insurance on behalf of their employees is not considered part of the employee's taxable income. This exclusion is equivalent to a discount or a subsidy on the purchase of insurance equal to the employee's marginal tax rate. It is through this favorable tax treatment that the federal government subsidizes the purchase of medical care and insurance by the non-poor. Tax-free employer-purchased insurance increases employee demands for insurance and results in more comprehensive insurance as well as coverage for additional benefits, such as vision and dental coverage. It has been estimated that the cost of these subsidies in terms of lost federal income, Social Security, and state income taxes was approximately $120 billion in 2001 (5).

The beneficiaries of these subsidies are those who are employed and who file tax returns, but the major beneficiaries are those in highest income tax brackets. A deduction from income is worth more to a person in a higher-income bracket than to a person with a lower income. For example, the after-tax cash equivalent of an employer-paid premium for health insurance totaling $1,000 would be $850 for a person in a 15 percent tax bracket, whereas it would be $666 for a person in the 33 percent bracket. (It would be even less than $666 since employer-purchased health insurance is not subject to either Social Security or state taxes.) If the true actuarial value of that premium is $900 (the remaining $100 going for administrative cost), the person in the 33 percent tax bracket will de-

mand more insurance because the after-tax cost of that insurance is much *less* than the actuarial value of that insurance.

As shown in Table 19-3, both the percentage of households receiving employer contributions and the average employer contribution increase with higher household incomes.

Up until the 1980s, tax brackets were much higher, up to 70 percent (plus state and Social Security taxes). At that time, the incentive was even greater for high-income persons to have their employers purchase their health insurance.

The consequences of these tax subsidies were (and are) that higher-income persons receive greater benefits than lower-income persons and that the higher-income person purchases "too much" health insurance coverage. It becomes worthwhile for higher-income persons to insure (through their employer) against small, routine medical expenses. This is because the cost of the insurance is less than the cost of those services if high-income persons were to pay for it with after-tax dollars.

Economists have often proposed that employer contributions toward their employees' insurance become completely taxable or, to make it more politically acceptable, that a "cap" or dollar limit be established, above which employer contributions become taxable. Depending upon where the cap was set, it could increase federal tax revenues by $50 billion a year. Equity would be improved; those with the highest incomes would receive less of a tax subsidy for the purchase of health insurance. Importantly, a cap would make employees more price sensitive to alternative health plans; they would either join managed care plans or they would purchase less health insurance, namely, policies with larger deductibles. Greater competition among managed care plans and increased patient sensitivity to medical prices would lead to greater efficiency in the provision of medical services.

There are, however, political difficulties in placing a limit on the employer's contribution. Unions that have bargained for and received generous health benefits have opposed making such contributions taxable; their members' taxes would be increased. Raising the after-tax price of insurance would decrease the demand for

Table 19-3. Employer Contributions to Health Benefit Plans and Employee Tax Benefits, 1994

Family Income(a)	Families Receiving Contributions		
	Percentage Receiving Employer Contribution	Average Employer Contribution	Average Subsidy
$1 – 9,999	8	$1,519	$ 190
$10,000 – 19,999	34	1,896	450
$20,000 – 29,999	62	2,587	800
$30,000 – 39,999	78	3,066	900
$40,000 – 49,999	85	3,758	1,090
$50,000 – 74,999	89	4,420	1,320
$75,000 – 99,999	91	5,229	1,740
$100,000 – 199,999	89	5,641	1,910
Over 200,000	76	4,922	1,830

Source: The Tax Treatment of Employment-Based Health Insurance, (Washington, D.C.: Congressional Budget Office, 1994), p. 30, Table 4.

Note: The table excludes families in which all members are covered by Medicare or Medicaid.

(a) Adjusted gross income reported on tax returns plus certain nontaxable forms of income including employers' contributions to the cost of health insurance premiums and tax-exempt interest.

health insurance, thereby generating opposition from health insurers. Provider interest groups, such as the American Dental Association, are opposed to eliminating (or limiting) the tax subsidy since it would reduce insurance coverage for their members' services, which are highly income elastic.

Limiting the tax exclusion has desirable consequences, but it is not NHI. Equity would be improved as the tax subsidy for those with high incomes is reduced; greater efficiency would also be introduced into the system as employees become more price sensitive in their choice of health plans. Thus limiting the tax exclusion is worthwhile in and of itself. However, such a proposal must be combined with another proposal if NHI is to be a universal program and cover those with low incomes and the unemployed. Limiting or ending the tax exclusion would generate additional tax revenues that could be used to finance medical services and/or insurance to those with low incomes.

NATIONAL HEALTH INSURANCE PROPOSALS

Many proposals have been made to increase access to care by those with low incomes. Each of the major types of proposals is described, together with an evaluation of their redistributive and efficiency effects.

A Canadian-type Health System

The most far reaching of all NHI proposals is to introduce a system similar to the Canadian health system (referred to as "Single Payer") (6). Universal coverage would be achieved since the entire population would be covered. Further, the benefits would be uniform for all and there would be no out-of-pocket expenses ("zero" price) for basic medical services.[2] An important characteristic of this plan is that private insurance for hospital and medical services is not permitted. In

2. Although Canada's basic medical services are free, public sector funding represents about 69 percent of total health expenditures, with the remaining 31 percent financed privately though independent insurance plans or directly out of pocket. (Private insurers are restricted from offering coverage that duplicates that of the government.) Supplementary health insurance is widely available in Canada to cover non-insured health benefits such as prescription drugs, dental and vision care, durable medical equipment such as wheelchairs and prostheses, costs of full-time care in a nursing home or in the patient's own home, as well as the services of allied health professionals including chiropractors and podiatrists. http://www.hc-sc.gc.ca/datapcb/iad/insurance-e.htm

other words, it is not possible to "buy out" of the system.

The proposed method of financing would be a combination of employer taxes, Medicare and Medicaid expenditures, private insurance payments, and a tax to raise the equivalent amount consumers currently spend out-of-pocket and on health insurance premiums.

To prevent expenditures from rising rapidly, regional expenditure limits would be imposed on hospitals and physicians. Since new technology is an important determinant of rising health care costs, regional boards would determine the introduction and financing of high-technology equipment and services.

The main advantages of the Canadian system, according to its proponents, is its universal coverage and its ability to control rising health care expenditures; Canada spends a smaller percentage of its GDP on health care than the U.S.

A single-payer system is but one NHI proposal, thus it should not be compared to the current U.S. health care system but to other NHI proposals to achieve universal coverage and methods to limit rising health care expenditures.

Proponents of a Canadian system point to two cost savings. The first is lower administrative costs; the second is a lower rate of increase in health care costs achieved by imposing expenditure limits on providers. Each approach is discussed.

Administrative Costs: Advocates of the Canadian system claim that if the United States adopted the Canadian system, it could greatly reduce its administrative costs since insurance companies would no longer be necessary, thereby financing universal access at no additional cost (7). Reducing administrative costs produces a one-time savings in the rate of increase; increasing access to all the uninsured, however, is an ongoing annual increase.

More importantly, simple comparisons of administrative expenses between the two countries are misleading (8). Administrative and marketing costs could be reduced if the United States were willing to eliminate choice of health plans and agree to a standardized set of health benefits. The United States has a wide variety of health plans, such as HMOs, point-of-service plans (POS), and PPOs offering different benefits with different cost-sharing levels and different access to providers. Competition among health plans offers consumers greater choice at different premiums.

Choice is costly. However, without choice there would be less innovation in benefit design, patient satisfaction, and competition on health plan premiums. The diversity of insurance plans reflects differences in subscribers' preferences and how much they are willing to pay for those preferences.

Lower administrative costs are not synonymous with greater system efficiency. A system in which physicians and hospitals send their bills to the government and the government simply pays them will have very low administrative costs. Health care expenditures, however, will be higher because inappropriate use and overuse of services will not be detected nor deterred. A trade-off exists between having lower administrative costs versus higher health expenditures due to insufficient monitoring of physician and hospital behavior. For example, the U.S. Medicare system, which has a similar design as the Canadian system, has much lower administrative costs than private managed care plans. However, the U.S, Government Accounting Office has criticized Medicare for having "too low" administrative costs; billions of dollars could be saved "... by adopting the health care management approach of private payers to Medicare's public payer role" (9). Studies have shown that cost-containment approaches, such as pre-authorization for hospital admissions, utilization review for hospitalized patients, catastrophic case management, and physician profiling for appropriateness of care performed by private health plans save money.

The health insurance industry in the United States is very price competitive and would only increase administrative costs if the benefits from doing so exceeded their costs. Any savings in administrative costs by eliminating cost-containment techniques and patient cost-sharing would be more than offset by the increased utilization that would occur. If higher administrative costs resulting from cost containment programs did not pay for itself by reducing medical expenses and over-utilization, managed care plans would not perform them.

Expenditure Limits: The lower rate of increase in per capita health expenditures (adjusted for inflation) in Canada than in the U.S. throughout the 1980s is an oft-cited measure of the success of Canada's health system which has been achieved through government-imposed expenditure limits. (Apparently the rate of increase was too low since for the past five years, 1997 to 2001, Canada's rate of growth has been *higher* than in the U.S. The Canadian government was likely compensating for the serious lack of funding in previous years. See Figure 19-11.)

Government expenditure limits are necessary in the Canadian system because patients incur zero out-of-pocket expense for hospital and physician services; patients will use additional services until the marginal benefit of those additional services equals their marginal cost (travel and waiting costs). At zero out-of-pocket price, the actual resource costs of those services exceeds its additional benefits. Further, Canadian providers are paid fee for service thereby eliminating any incentive for them to be concerned with limiting patients' use of services. No government can fund all the medical services demanded at zero price, thus the government resorts to arbitrarily imposed expenditure limits. In the U.S., the moral hazard problem is addressed through the use of co-payments, utilization management, or incentives placed on the provider, such as capitation and insurers profiling providers for inclusion in a PPO.

New Technology: Any comparison of the Canadian health system and alternative NHI plans should consider *who will decide* the rate at which new technology

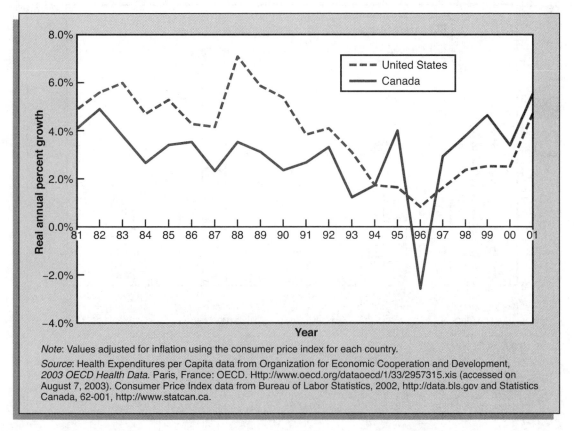

Figure 19-11. Annual percent growth in real per capita health expenditures in Canada and the United States, 1980–2001.

is adopted and made available to patients. Major advances in diagnostic and treatment procedures have occurred. Imaging equipment has improved diagnostic accuracy and also reduced the need for exploratory surgery. New technology has resulted in less invasive procedures, quicker recovery times, as well as improved treatment outcomes. Technological advances have increased the survival rate of low-birthweight babies and permitted an increasing number and types of organ transplants.

In Canada, the availability of capital to invest in both cost-saving and benefit increasing technology, as well as for developing new delivery systems, is determined by the government, not providers. Providers are not rewarded for risk taking, thus have little incentive to innovate in developing new delivery systems. Given their budget constraints and their reluctance to raise taxes, governments are less likely to provide capital for new technology and for as many units as would health plans competing for subscribers. The adoption of new technology under managed care competition is different from what a government (or quasi-governmental agency) would use since the government would be concerned with losing political support if it had to raise taxes or incur large budget deficits to increase access to new technology.

Examples of differences in availability of technology (per million persons) between Canada and the United States are shown in Figure 19-12. There are 8 times more lithotripters available per person in the

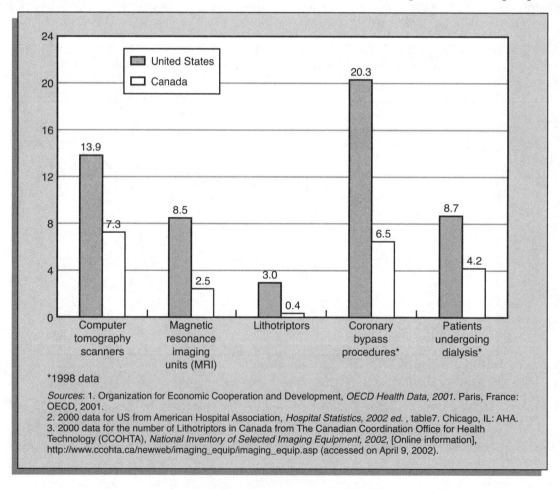

*1998 data

Sources: 1. Organization for Economic Cooperation and Development, OECD Health Data, 2001. Paris, France: OECD, 2001.
2. 2000 data for US from American Hospital Association, Hospital Statistics, 2002 ed. , table7. Chicago, IL: AHA.
3. 2000 data for the number of Lithotriptors in Canada from The Canadian Coordination Office for Health Technology (CCOHTA), National Inventory of Selected Imaging Equipment, 2002, [Online information], http://www.ccohta.ca/newweb/imaging_equip/imaging_equip.asp (accessed on April 9, 2002).

Figure 19-12. Indicators of medical technology per million people, 2001.

U.S. than in Canada, 2.4 times as many MRI units, and 1.4 times as many CT scanners per person. In Canada, about 58 percent of the patients with end-stage renal failure undergo dialysis compared to 73 percent in the U.S. It is clear that the likelihood of a patient in the United States receiving any of the services listed in Figure 19-12 is much greater than a similar patient with equal needs but living in Canada. (How successful would a health plan in the U.S. be if it used similar access criteria as used in Canada?)

Patient Access To Care: Decreased access to patient care is another consequence of a government-imposed lower per capita expenditure growth rate. At a zero price, patient demand will exceed supply; waiting time is used to ration non-emergency care. According to a Fraser Institute report on the Canadian health care system, Canadian patients in 2003 had to wait, on average, 12.7 weeks for an MRI (the range was 8 to 24 weeks depending on the Province), 5.5 weeks for a cat scan (the range being 4 to 8 weeks), and 3.6 weeks for an ultrasound (the range was 2 to 8 weeks) (10). The long waits for first-time mammograms virtually eliminate this screening mechanism as a preventive method.

Acknowledging these long waits and their adverse effects on patients, at least two Canadian provinces pay for heart surgery in the United States. Almost 12 percent of all British Columbians (13.3 percent of those residing in NewFoundland) requiring radiation oncology treatment have been sent by the Canadian government to the United States, which is Canada's safety valve. Ontario has contracted with hospitals in Buffalo and Detroit for MRI services.

Quebec sent more than 250 cancer patients to the U.S. in 1999 for treatment; 350 cancer patients have waited more than 8 weeks for radiation or

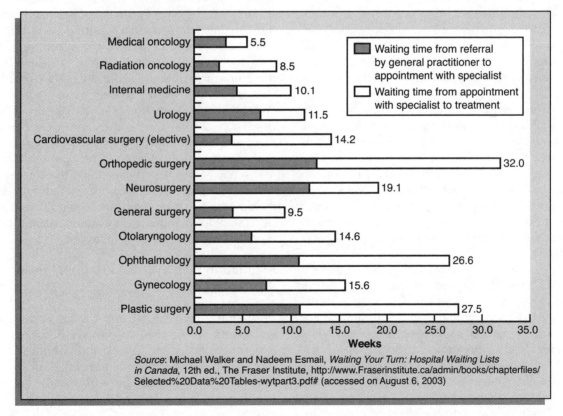

Figure 19-13.   Canada hospital waiting lists. Total expected waiting time from referral by general practitioner to treatment, by specialty, 2003 (in weeks).

chemotherapy (more than 4 weeks waiting time is considered medically risky) (11).

The Fraser Institute performs annual surveys on waiting times from referral by the general practitioner to an appointment with a specialist and then the waiting time from appointment with a specialist to treatment. These surveys are by medical specialty and for each Canadian Province. Figure 19-13 describes the waiting time in weeks for treatment by specialty. For example, for orthopedic surgery (e.g., hips and knees), a person would have to wait on average 32.2 weeks in 2003 to receive treatment; in some provinces, however, the wait may be as short as 23 weeks or as long as 63 weeks to have the surgery performed. (Previously, in 1991, aged patients had to wait up to 4 years for a hip or knee replacement in some provinces.) Ophthalmology (e.g., cataract removal) requires a wait, on average, of 30 weeks, but this can vary by province between 14 to 52 weeks.

After an appointment with a specialist, a patient would have to wait 18 weeks for a coronary artery bypass operation (urgent) in one province, but only one week in another province. For radiation oncology for prostate cancer, the wait can be as long as 16 weeks or as short as 1.8 weeks depending upon the province.

The Fraser Institute also asks not only how long patients wait but also asks the specialists how long a patient *should* wait before they receive the recommended treatment. For example, the actual waiting time for cardiovascular surgery (urgent) in Alberta after they have seen a specialist is 11.2 weeks while specialists believe that the reasonable waiting time should not exceed 1.7 weeks; for cardiovascular surgery (elective) the actual waiting time is of course much greater.

The value of time spent in waiting is lost; there is also the discomfort involved in waiting for procedures, such as hip replacements; elderly patients must forego driving while they wait months for cataract surgery; further, some patients will die while waiting for heart operations. Proponents of the Canadian system ignore these implicit costs. These patients are clearly worse off if the system does not permit them to pay a monetary price which would enable them to have access to the latest technology, to forego their waiting, their pain, and possible death.

The failure to consider the higher patient time costs in the Canadian system understates health expenditures in Canada. Canadians are legally prohibited from insuring against the risks of not receiving timely care when they require it.

Canada does not have an egalitarian system. Access to care depends not only on the province in which one lives, but also whether a person can afford to pay for their care in the U.S.

According to various surveys, Canadians are more pleased with their health system than are Americans. But it is important to keep in mind that Canadians share a set of egalitarian values with respect to access to care and to technology that are not shared by a majority of Americans. These differences in values are important for understanding why the United States is unlikely to adopt the Canadian system.

Limiting health expenditures to a certain percent of GNP or rate of growth in GNP is controversial. (Changes in the rate of growth in GNP itself would arbitrarily limit the growth in health expenditures.) In a competitive medical market, the appropriate rate of growth in medical expenditures is determined by the amount people are willing to pay (directly and through taxes). There are legitimate reasons for increased health expenditures such as an aging population, more chronic illness, increased technology, new diseases, shortages of personnel (thereby requiring wage increases), etc. If expenditure growth is held below what would otherwise occur, the consequences will be shortages of services and technology and reduced access to care. Arbitrary expenditure limits are unrelated to changes in consumer demands or to economy-wide input price increases.

Mandating Employer-Paid National Health Insurance

Presidents Nixon, Carter, and Clinton each proposed employers be required to provide health insurance benefits to their employees and families. An employer mandate typically requires that all employers offer a health insurance plan with specified minimum health benefits to their employees or else pay an employee tax, hence the name "pay or play." (It is less expensive for the employer to pay than play under several of the proposed plans.) The employer is generally required to pay a major portion of the premium (as high as 80 percent) with the employee responsible for the remaining 20 percent. A tax credit may be provided to small firms to help the employer and employee defray part of the costs of the mandated insurance.

The employer mandate typically covers all employees who work more than half time and firms with more than a minimum number of employees, such as five to twenty-five employees. (The minimum number of employees is very controversial; the Pepper Commission suggested that 100 employees be the minimum number.) Large firms and unions are typically unaffected by mandated insurance since they already have employment-based health insurance and their coverage exceeds the specified minimums.

Important to any analysis of a mandated employer proposal is a determination of who are the uninsured and the characteristics of employees and firms (with fewer than fifty employees) that would be most affected by this approach.

The Uninsured: As shown in Table 19-4, for those under 65 years of age, almost 69 percent have private health insurance; 65 percent have employment-related insurance. The government covers 12.2 percent of the under-65 population through such programs as Medicaid. Approximately 19 percent of the under-65 population (about 45.7 million) do not have any health insurance. Persons in a family with a working adult are more likely to have insurance (72.7 percent) than persons in a family without a working adult (28.8 percent). However, because there are so many more working than non-working adults, most of the uninsured (89 percent) are in families with working adults. Another characteristic of the uninsured is that 54 percent of the uninsured are working adults and 21 percent are children of working adults. Thus almost 75 percent of the total number of uninsured is employed or dependents of someone employed.

Selected characteristics of the uninsured are shown in Table 19-5. Those more likely to be uninsured are young adults, 19-24 years of age (31.4 percent);

Table 19-4. Health Insurance Coverage and Employment Status of the Civilian Noninstitutionalized Population Under Age 65, 2001

Employment status of adults in family	Total population in thousands	Private		Public only	Uninsured	Percent distribution of uninsured
		Total private	Employment-related(a)			
		Percent distribution				
Total	241,762	69.3	65.2	12.2	18.9	100.0
Persons in families with a working adult	222,652	72.7	68.6	9.1	18.2	88.6
Working adult	134,296	78.1	74.1	3.5	18.5	54.3
Nonworking adult	21,106	58.5	53.3	11.9	29.6	13.7
Child	67,250	66.4	62.4	19.6	14.1	20.7
Persons in families without a working adult(a)	20,110	28.8	23.8	45.3	25.9	11.4
Nonworking adult	14,710	34.8	28.3	37.4	27.8	8.9
Child	5,400	12.4	11.4	66.9	20.7	2.4

Source: Agency for Healthcare Research and Quality, Center for Cost and Financing Studies, Medical Expenditure Panel Survey, personla correspondence with Jeffrey Rhoades, February 24, 2003.

(a) Employment-related includes insurance acquired through employer/union and holder outside the household.

Note: Percents may not add up to 100 due to rounding.

Table 19-5. Total Population of Workers Ages 16–64 and Uninsured Workers: Percent Distribution by Selected Characteristics, United States, 2001

Characteristic	Working population in thousands	Percent distribution of workers	Percent uninsured	Percent distribution of uninsured workers
Total(a)	136,979	100.0	18.4	100.0
Age in years				
16–18	4,871	3.6	18.2	3.5
19–24	17,038	12.4	31.4	21.2
25–29	14,973	10.9	26.5	15.7
30–34	16,513	12.1	18.4	12.1
35–44	37,807	27.6	16.0	24.0
45–54	31,339	22.9	13.3	16.5
55–64	14,438	10.4	12.1	6.9
Race/ethnicity				
Total Hispanic	14,937	10.9	38.8	23.0
Total black	15,788	11.5	21.7	13.6
Total white	99,792	72.9	14.7	58.3
Total other	6,461	4.7	19.7	5.1
Self-employed	15,702	11.5	31.1	19.4
Size of establishment(b)				
Less than 10 workers	32,005	25.6	30.8	45.5
10–24 workers	18,372	14.7	23.0	19.5
25–49 workers	13,487	10.8	14.9	9.3
50–99 workers	14,495	11.6	13.4	9.0
100–499 workers	25,218	20.2	8.6	10.0
500 or more workers	21,504	17.2	6.7	6.7
Hours of work				
Less than 20 hours	7,603	5.8	19.9	6.5
20–34 hours	17,176	13.1	27.1	20.1
35 or more hours	106,664	81.1	16.0	73.4
Hourly wages(b)				
Less than $5.00	2,993	2.7	25.9	4.5
$5.00–$9.99	32,367	29.7	29.7	55.9
$10.00–$14.99	33,687	29.7	14.3	28.0
$15.00–$19.99	16,476	15.1	6.4	6.2
$20.00 or more	23,551	21.6	3.9	5.4

Source: Agency for Healthcare Research and Quality, Center for Cost and Financing Studies, Medical Expenditure Panel Survey, personal correspondence with Jeffrey Rhoades, February 24, 2003.

(a) Excludes persons with unknown self-employment status, hours of work, hourly wages, and size of establishment.

(b) For wage earners only.

Note: Restricted to civilian non-institutionalized population. Percents may not add up to 100 due to rounding.

persons in this age group are usually excluded from their parent's employment-related coverage and unless they are full-time students are likely to have jobs that do not provide insurance. A higher percentage of blacks (21.7 percent) and Hispanics (38.8 percent) are likely to be uninsured than whites (14.7 percent). However, due to the greater size of the white population, the majority of the uninsured (58.3 percent) are white.

Examining the insurance status of the employed population, one finds that 31 percent of the self-employed are uninsured. Further, the smaller the size of firm, the greater the likelihood of the employee being uninsured; 30.8 percent of employees in firms with less than 10 employees are uninsured. In firms having between 10 and 24 employees, 23.0 percent are uninsured; 65 percent of all uninsured employees are working in firms with fewer than 25 employees. Proposals for mandated coverage that exclude small firms also exclude an important segment of the working uninsured. Thus the Pepper Commission's proposal to mandate coverage for firms with more than 100 employees would only affect a small portion of the uninsured.

Those who are uninsured are also low-wage employees, most likely because they are also young (19 to 24 years) with low skill levels. As of 2001, 56 percent of the uninsured workers were earning less than $10 an hour. Further, those working less than full time are more likely to be uninsured.

Proponents of mandated employer coverage point out that 88.6 percent of the uninsured are employed or are dependents of an employee. Requiring employer coverage for all employees and their dependents would eliminate 88.6 percent of the uninsured without increased federal or state spending. A large portion of the working uninsured, however, are low-wage employees who cannot afford to buy insurance for themselves or for their family. Further, mandated coverage, by itself, *would not achieve universal coverage* since it would still leave 11.4 percent of the uninsured population without insurance.

Interest Group Positions: Important interest groups favor employer-mandated NHI. For example, Congress would not have to pass a special tax to finance a mandated NHI program. Thus it offers the illusion that federal expenditures are unaffected or even reduced. State governments would be able to reduce their Medicaid expenditures by shifting those medical costs onto small employers and their low-wage employees. Medical services for low-income employees and their dependents would be paid by private insurance rather than Medicaid or through bad debts. Hospital, physician, and dental associations favor this approach since it would increase the demand for their services without disrupting the current practice of medicine or payment systems. Similarly, insurance companies favor this approach since it would increase the demand for insurance. In fact, associations representing health insurers, hospitals, physicians, and dentists have each proposed an employer mandate as their NHI plan.

Mandating a minimum set of insurance benefits does not affect large employers and their employees and permits unions and higher-income employees to retain their current negotiated benefits, which are generally greater than the mandated benefits. The political support for an employer mandate is importantly related to large firms and union self-interest. An employer mandate would require employers to cover union members' working spouses, thereby enabling their members to reduce spousal medical benefits; the wages of their union members would increase as the costs of their medical benefits decrease. Many large employers (and unions) believe that an employer mandate would increase labor costs (and prices) of low-cost competitors and thereby increase the demand for their services (and increase the derived demand for their employees).[3] As Robert

---

3. When employers negotiate with unions or determine their labor costs, they are concerned with the total compensation costs of their employees, which consists of fringe benefits and wages. Because of tax considerations, employees prefer part of their compensation in the form of non-taxable fringe benefits. An increase in health insurance costs, therefore, results in a decrease in the wage portion of their total compensation. Thus employer-paid health insurance is unlike other costs incurred by the firm, such as raw materials or an increase in the cost of supplies, since higher health insurance costs are offset by a reduction in wages. For example, Gruber found that the increased cost of mandated maternity benefits were offset by a reduction in wages. Jonathan Gruber, "The Incidence of Mandated Maternity Benefits," *American Economic Review,* 84 June 1994, 622–641.

For an excellent economic discussion of who bears the burden of mandated employer health insurance, business' attitudes on the incidence of the tax, together with an analysis of the mandated employer portion of President Clinton's health reform proposal, see Mark V. Pauly, *Health Benefits At Work: An Economic and Political Analysis of Employment-Based Health Insurance,* (University of Michigan Press: Ann Arbor, Michigan), 1997.

Crandall, Chairman and Chief Executive of American Airlines, stated in 1987:

> At American, we spend about $1,666 per employee per year—that's more than $80 million this year alone—on medical benefits for active employees and dependents. And we're spending $16 million a year for medical benefits for retirees.
>
> Yet Continental doesn't provide any medical benefits for retirees at all—and its active employees pay for most of their own health insurance. As a result, Continental's unit cost advantage versus American's is enormous—and worse yet, is growing!
>
> . . . which is why we're supporting Sen. Edward Kennedy's legislation mandating minimum benefit levels for all employees (12).

Although employer-mandated NHI has political support from important groups, the main opposition has come from small employers who employ low-wage labor and who would be most affected by this approach. The trade association of small employers (National Federation of Independent Business) played an important role in defeating President Clinton's health care reform proposal, which relied on an employer mandate.

Problems With An Employer Mandate: Relying on an employer mandate as a vehicle for NHI has several problems. First, the federal government will lose tax revenue as more employers and employees purchase tax-exempt employer-paid health insurance; the employee's taxable income is reduced and employers are able to deduct their payments as a business expense, which reduces the firm's taxable revenues.

Second, requiring firms to purchase insurance for each employee is equivalent to placing a tax on each employee. Assuming the supply of labor in aggregate is inelastic, then labor will bear the full amount of the tax in the form of reduced wages. However, large firms with higher-income employees already have insurance and would therefore be unaffected by this tax. The employees most affected by this tax are those working for small firms, earning low wages, and without health insurance. The labor supply curve fac-

ing these industries is elastic; labor could move to other industries or leave the workforce. *The tax would only affect those firms without insurance.* Thus an analysis of the tax must examine just those firms without insurance; these firms have elastic demand and supply curves for labor, consequently, only part of the tax will be shifted by the firm onto the employee by lowering their wages. (See the earlier discussion on who bears the burden of an increase in the Social Security tax.) To the extent that the cost of the insurance is shifted to the employee, low-wage employees will receive reduced wages. An employer mandate requires workers to trade some of their taxable income for nontaxable health insurance coverage. Because the entire mandate is not shifted to the employee, there will also be a decreased demand for labor, and unemployment will occur.

For those employees who are at or near the minimum wage, it will not be possible for the firm to shift the cost of insurance to them, and these employees will also be laid off.

Further, to the extent that small firms are unable to shift the entire burden to their employees (because of an elastic labor supply curve), there will be increased costs to the employer and, consequently, lower profits. Facing higher marginal costs, the firm will increase the prices of their goods and services. Consumers will thus bear part of the costs of mandated insurance since the increased prices are equivalent to a regressive tax on consumers.

As the firm's prices increase, there will be a decrease in demand for those goods and services and, consequently, a decrease in the demand for labor. With an increase in prices, the demand for substitutes will increase for products in the U.S. and for firms producing the same product located overseas. U.S. firms will have an incentive to shift their production to other countries. The decrease in demand for labor should be greater among unskilled workers whose wages may be close to the minimum wage. Skilled labor is unlikely to be affected since their benefits are typically greater than those mandated. As their relative wages change, substitution toward skilled labor and capital away from unskilled labor is likely to occur (another reason it is favored by unions). Unemployment among unskilled labor near the minimum wage will increase. (Thus, while states will benefit by a decrease in their Medicaid expenditures, they will experience an increase in unemployment compensation and welfare payments.)

Typically, the benefits and financing mechanisms of a mandated employer program are not income related.[4] As part of such a mandate, some form of assistance is usually proposed for small employers (but not for low-income employees in large firms). Unless such subsidies are income related, small law firms may also receive subsidies.

Mandated employer insurance does not result in universal coverage. To cover the entire population, it must be combined with government subsidies to individuals since part-time employees and those who do not work would not be eligible. These groups, unless subsidized, would still have to rely on Medicaid.

The middle class is unlikely to oppose an employer mandate as a means of providing medical care to those with low incomes as long as they are not required to pay additional taxes. It would appear to be a means of shifting the cost onto employers even though, in actuality, the low-wage employee is being taxed to bear most of the burden of their own insurance.

Mandated employer health insurance, while politically attractive to many groups with a concentrated interest is, however, not NHI. Most importantly, *it does not provide the middle class with any visible net benefits.* It was for this reason that President Clinton combined an employer mandate with regulatory controls on increases in medical expenditures. Under the Clinton proposal, health insurance premiums and out-of-pocket expenses of the middle class would presumably have risen less rapidly; part of the costs of their care would be borne by the providers, who would be paid less. In this manner, the middle class would have received the visible benefits of being assured of their choice of provider at lower prices; they would not be required to make any sacrifices.

The Clinton health plan was not enacted for a variety of reasons. Important among those reasons was the lack of political support by the middle class (and opposition by small businesses). As more information became available on the Clinton health plan and on its cost, its complexity, and the higher premiums that were to be required, the middle class' interest in having such a radical plan enacted diminished.

The structure and financing of NHI proposals generally reflect the economic interests of politically powerful groups, including those of the middle class. More equitable forms of taxation, incentives for more efficient delivery systems, economy-wide employment effects, etc. are secondary considerations to political feasibility. Given the diverse economic interests, it is not surprising how difficult it is to devise a politically acceptable NHI plan.

Health (Medical) Savings Accounts

A relatively new proposal for financing medical care is the use of Health Savings Accounts (HSAs) in conjunction with a catastrophic health insurance plan. Federal legislation enacted in 1996 provided for a pilot Medical Savings Account (MSA) program for the self employed and for employees of small firms with the same favorable tax treatment as employer-paid health insurance. Under the pilot MSA program, growth of MSAs was limited since the legislation placed severe restrictions on who could own them and on the number of policies that could be sold; the pilot program was also set to expire in 2003. As a result of these restrictions, many insurers did not offer MSAs. However, the Medicare Prescription Drug bill, enacted in November 2003, included a provision to permit the non-aged to have Health Savings Accounts (HSA) which are a new and improved version of MSAs. The new HSAs were not subject to the previous restrictions placed on MSAs.

The basic idea behind an HSA is to combine an inexpensive high deductible insurance policy with a tax-free savings account.

An HSA plan works as follows: a person (or their employer acting on their behalf) annually contributes a specified tax-free amount, e.g., $5,000, into their HSA. Part of these funds, $2,000, must be used to

---

4. To finance his health care reform plan, President Clinton proposed a proportional tax on wages, 12 percent. This would have greatly benefited unions such as the United Auto Workers whose benefits were costing about 15 to 18 percent of payroll. The difference would have been returned to union members in the form of increased wages.

purchase a catastrophic health insurance policy. (A high-deductible catastrophic policy has a much lower premium than a comprehensive health insurance policy.) The person then has $3,000 remaining in their HSA. The person's total out-of-pocket expenses, including the deductible, are then limited to $4,500. The person would be at risk for the difference between the out-of-pocket maximum ($4,500) and the remaining funds in their HSA ($3,000), which is $1,500. (The numbers in the above example are merely illustrative.) The money in the HSA can be spent on medical services or it can be allowed to grow so the money will be there for retirement purposes or for their long term care needs. If the HSA funds are spent on non-medical services before retirement, the funds taken out are taxed together with a 15 percent penalty.

HSA advocates claim that individuals will have a financial incentive to be concerned with the costs of medical care, the prices they pay for services, and their use of services. Medical expenditures would increase at a slower rate. A fundamental problem with tax-exempt employer-paid health insurance is that the amount that can be tax exempt is unlimited, leading to comprehensive policies and a lack of patient incentives to be concerned with the price and use of services.

Opponents criticize the HSA approach on several grounds. First, they claim that savings would be relatively small because once the out-of-pocket maximum has been reached, the patient has no incentive to spend less. Second, it is the adoption and availability of new technology, typically used in an inpatient setting, that determines medical expenditure increases, not spending on outpatient services. Further, HSA critics believe that HSAs will split the risk pools, with the healthier risks choosing HSAs (thereby gaining financially) while the higher risks remain with more comprehensive health plans. The consequence of this adverse selection, if it occurred, would be that premiums for the traditional plan would sharply increase. To eliminate risk selection, employers are likely to offer only one plan to their employees. In the individual insurance market, HSAs would also effectively segment the market with higher-risk individuals paying much higher premiums than if the low- and high-risk groups were combined.

HSA proponents respond that once the patient's out-of-pocket maximum has been reached, the incentive to be concerned with medical costs shifts to the insurer who will manage the patient's catastrophic expenses. The insurer will also have an incentive to use less costly settings to provide care and to undertake studies on appropriateness of care.

HSA proponents disagree that HSAs would split the insurance market according to low and high risks, arguing that higher risks would also benefit from and choose HSAs because their out-of-pocket expenses, such as prescription drugs, would be subject to a limit. Those with chronic conditions or the aged, for example, would spend less on prescription drugs and other medical expenses under an MSA because of the stop loss limit; Medicare does not have an out-of-pocket maximum.

Limited empirical evidence regarding the expected performance of HSAs exists. Several employers have adopted HSAs for their employees and report large reductions in annual rates of increase in employees' medical expenditures. However, there have been no control groups to match with these companies; thus their performance may have been affected by factors other than the adoption of HSAs. For example, annual rates of increase in medical expenditures were declining for many companies during this same period.

Two studies have estimated the effect of MSA adoption. Keeler, et al., simulated the effects of several scenarios regarding MSAs concluding that while the MSA approach is unlikely to produce the large reduction in health care costs its advocates anticipate, neither is it likely to result in the adverse selection problem expected by its critics (13). The second study investigated whether those who are sick in one year also tend to be sicker on average throughout their lives. If this were the case, then MSAs would only benefit the healthy while those who are sick would not accumulate any assets in their MSAs (although they would limit their losses). The authors find that health care spending of employees with the sickest families tends to diminish over time, thus even the sickest may accumulate some savings in their MSAs (14). It is estimated that only about 20 percent of the employees would have saved less than half of their contributions while fully 50 percent of employees would have kept more than 70 percent of their contributions. This conclusion is based on the very restrictive assumption that spending one's own money would have no effect on a person's spending for medical services. If people do in fact spend less, then the accumulated savings would be much greater.

Its proponents view HSAs as an alternative to the current system, which relies on employer-paid health insurance. HSAs would place much greater responsibility for medical expenses on the individual, providing them with financial incentives for efficiency in use of medical services. As providers compete on price and managed care plans become responsible for catastrophic services, there would also be incentives for efficiency in the delivery of services. HSAs will not assist those with low incomes who cannot currently afford health insurance; to achieve universal coverage, these individuals would require government subsidies.

An Income-Related NHI Proposal: A Refundable Tax Credit

The following illustrative type of tax credit proposal attempts to achieve universal coverage in an equitable manner while providing incentives for efficiency in the use and delivery of medical services (15).

To achieve universal coverage, the government must ensure that the two groups without insurance—those who can afford insurance but refuse to purchase it and those who cannot afford insurance—have a minimum level of health insurance. To do so, the federal government should, first, *require* everyone to have a minimum level of health insurance (an "individual mandate") which could be a catastrophic policy for higher income persons. Many uninsured are financially able to purchase health insurance but choose not to do so. Mandatory catastrophic coverage for those who can afford it is justified on the basis of externalities. If someone who can afford insurance does not have catastrophic coverage and suffers a large medical expense that has to be subsidized by the community, that person is shifting the risk (hence the cost of catastrophic coverage) to the rest of the community.

Proof of insurance would be attached to the person's federal income tax form (or employers could indicate on the individual's annual W-2 tax statement whether an amount has been deducted for health insurance). Lack of such evidence would result in the government collecting the appropriate premium as it would if the individual paid insufficient income taxes. The government would then assign the person to a health plan in their area, which the person could change at the open enrollment period. Thus everyone who could afford health insurance will not become a burden to others if they incur a serious illness or accident.

The second important role of government in ensuring universal coverage is to provide a "refundable tax credit" (subsidies) for the purchase of health insurance to those with low incomes. The refundable tax credit would work as follows: A taxpayer would be allowed to subtract from their income tax liability the tax credit to purchase health insurance. For example, if a person's income tax liability was $7,000 and the tax credit was $4,000, then the tax liability would be reduced to $3,000. Individuals whose tax credit exceeded their tax liabilities would receive a *refund* for the difference; if the tax liability was $1,000 and the tax credit were $4,000, the person would receive a refund of $3,000. Thus, if a person's income were too low to pay taxes, the full amount of the credit would be used to provide them with a voucher. As a person's income increased and they have an income tax liability, the tax credit would offset part of the tax liability, leaving them with part of the tax credit to be used toward the purchase of a health insurance voucher.

The tax credit must be refundable, otherwise the benefits will go only to those who pay taxes, thereby excluding those with low incomes.

The full tax credit subsidy would be equal to the premium of a managed care plan. (These refundable tax credits are essentially vouchers for a health plan for persons with little or no tax liability.) The tax credit could be an equal dollar amount for all families, such as $4,000), or it could decline with higher incomes. Under a refundable tax credit that declines with higher income, the subsidy would primarily go to those with the lowest incomes. At which income levels the tax credit became zero is a political decision to be determined by Congress. However, providing a tax credit of an absolute dollar amount to all would be more politically acceptable in that those with higher incomes would also receive some benefit (although it would be more costly).

The value of the voucher could equal the premium of the lowest cost managed care plan in the market. (This latter approach is used by an increasing number of employers.) In this manner, the preferences of the non-poor for what they want to purchase from a managed care plan will determine the benefits to be offered to those with low incomes. (Those receiving a full or partial voucher could choose a more expensive health plan by paying the additional cost themselves.)

The current unlimited exclusion from the employee's taxable income of employer-purchased health insurance would be removed as the tax credit is substituted in its place. The lost tax revenues from this open-ended subsidy (approximately $140 billion in lost federal, state, and Social Security taxes) would be an important revenue source to offset the new tax credit to those with low incomes. No longer would there be the horizontal inequity of two persons with the same income receiving different size subsidies because one person is self-employed while the other is an employee of a large firm whose employer purchases insurance. (For political reasons, the tax subsidy for employer-purchased health insurance may be phased out over time or amounts above a certain limit could be subject to income taxes.)

The financing of a tax credit proposal would be from general income taxes and would thus be financed in an equitable manner for a redistributive policy.

The obligation to purchase insurance under the above refundable tax credit proposal is placed on the individual ("Mandated Individual Health Insurance") and not on the employer. The effects on the demand for labor and the unemployment effects discussed above with respect to mandated employer insurance would therefore not occur. It is likely, however, that most employers would continue to purchase health insurance for their employees because group insurance is less expensive than if each employee did so on their own. Further, benefit managers could act as efficient agents in screening health plans and in providing information to the employees. Individuals could work for firms that did not provide

health insurance as long as they purchased coverage themselves.

Because the insurance mandate is on the individual, employees would be able to change jobs without fear of losing insurance or being denied coverage because of a pre-existing condition. Further, an employer should be willing to hire those with pre-existing conditions because there would be no additional health insurance cost to the employer and/or other employees.

The refundable tax credit could partially replace Medicaid (likely excluding those in nursing homes) using expenditures currently spent on Medicaid to partially offset the costs of the tax credit. Those eligible for Medicaid would be entitled to receive a voucher equal to the premium in a managed care plan. As a person's income increased, there would no longer be a sharp cutoff of Medicaid benefits (the "notch" effect) with the previous disincentive to work; the person would still be able to deduct from their tax liability the tax credit. Those eligible for Medicaid and others who do not file income taxes could register at their local Social Security or welfare office to receive their insurance voucher.

Medicare could be included in the tax credit proposal or, for political feasibility, it could be phased in for those not yet eligible for Medicare. It would be politically difficult to apply the proposed system to current Medicare beneficiaries, particularly if it is an income-related refundable tax credit. Thus all current Medicare beneficiaries (and those close to the Medicare eligibility age) would receive a fully subsidized voucher in a managed care plan. Those who are 55 to 60 years of age could receive a partially subsidized voucher related to their Medicare contributions, and the Medicare system could be phased out for those under a certain age. If Medicare and Medicaid are kept separate from the refundable tax credit system, then the gaps and problems in these programs would have to be remedied.

As part of any private NHI plan, including an individual mandate, provision must be made for those individuals who do not have health insurance and who have pre-existing conditions that would make them uninsurable. Government subsidized high-risk pools would have to be established. Over time the need for a high-risk pool would decline as everyone has private insurance.

There would be no need for state health mandates, such as requiring all insurance plans to include chiropractic services or hair transplants. Eliminating the more than 1,500 state mandates across the 50 states would reduce the cost of health insurance.

The refundable tax credit, particularly if it is income related, meets the efficiency and redistribution criteria in the following ways: everyone is obligated to have a minimum set of health insurance benefits. Those with the lowest incomes would be assured of adequate health insurance and would receive the largest net benefits under the proposed plan. The size of the subsidy would decline as income increases. Employer-purchased health insurance (perhaps above a certain dollar amount) would become part of the employee's taxable income. The resulting increased tax revenues, together with funds from the income tax system and from Medicaid, would provide the funding for the income-related subsidies. Thus the financing source is based on progressive taxation. And the requirement of universal coverage means that cost shifting by those who do not purchase insurance to those who do will no longer occur.

Employees would have incentives to make cost-conscious choices. With the removal of the current unlimited employer-paid tax subsidy, persons desiring to spend more than the tax credit would be able to do so, but only with after-tax dollars. Those with high incomes would purchase less comprehensive insurance and have a greater incentive to be concerned with the prices and premiums they pay and the health plans they select.

Lastly, a refundable tax credit provides an incentive for increased efficiency in the provision of medical services. A competitive health insurance market would be relied on for achieving efficiency and quality. Managed care plans competing for price (premium) sensitive employees (and employers acting on their behalf) will have an incentive to be concerned with the providers they use, provider fees, physician practice patterns, medical outcomes, as well as patient satisfaction. Unless health plans are responsive to consumers at a premium the consumer is willing to

pay, the health plan will not be able to compete in a price-competitive market.

A national health insurance system based on an income-related refundable tax credit would achieve both increased equity and economic efficiency in the use of medical services.

WHY THE U.S. HAS NOT HAD NATIONAL HEALTH INSURANCE

To understand why the U.S. has not had NHI, it is first necessary to understand the actual rather than the stated goal of NHI. Further, the debate over the structure and financing of NHI actually represents the controversy over the underlying objective that is to be achieved by NHI. Discussing the possible goals of NHI therefore clarifies both the design features of different NHI proposals as well as providing insights as to why this country has not had NHI.

The Conflicting Goals of National Health Insurance

Increase Medical Services to Those With Low Incomes: While many individuals support increased services to the poor, this is not, nor has it ever been, the driving force behind NHI. *Medicaid is NHI for the poor.* To use the power of government to achieve one's objectives requires political power. The structure and funding of Medicaid is indicative of the limited political power of the poor and of their advocates. Medicaid's inadequacies are not the actions of a few miserly bureaucrats or legislators but are instead reflective of the resources that society—the middle class—is willing to devote to the poor. The states vary in their generosity and in the criteria they use for determining eligibility for Medicaid. No state reaches the federal poverty level in determining Medicaid eligibility, and some states are only at 25 percent of the federal poverty level. How much the non-poor are willing to spend on charity depends on how much the non-poor themselves have, on how culturally similar the poor are to the non-poor, and on how much it costs to provide for the poor.

Since it is the non-poor who have the political power to determine the allocation of resources to the poor, one must assume that the inadequacies of Medicaid reflect insufficient interest or desire among the non-poor to improve Medicaid and increase funding for the poor. *If society is unwilling to improve Medicaid, why would they be willing to tax themselves to enact NHI for the poor?*

The Use of Government to Benefit Politically Powerful Groups: Another view of NHI is that since legislators respond to politically powerful groups, these groups seek to use the power of government to provide themselves with net benefits they would not otherwise receive from the marketplace.

Politically influential groups are those who have a "concentrated" interest in a particular issue and who are able to organize themselves so as to provide legislators with political support, i.e., campaign contributions, votes, and/or volunteer time. A group is said to have a concentrated interest when some regulation or legislation has a sufficiently large effect on that group to make it worthwhile for them to invest resources to either forestall or promote that effect. The potential legislative benefits are greater than the group's costs of organizing and providing political support to achieve their legislative objectives.

Implicit in this discussion of concentrated interests is the assumption that legislators respond to political support since their objective is to be re-elected. Legislators, similar to the other participants in the policy process, are assumed to be rational; they undertake cost/benefit calculations of their actions. The costs and benefits of their legislative decisions, however, are not the legislation's effect on society but instead are the political support gained and lost by the legislator's actions.

In the health field, physicians and hospitals were initially the major groups with a concentrated interest in health legislation. Payment systems under both public and private insurance systems had a large effect on their revenues. Subsidies to increase the demand by those with low incomes also increased hospital and physician revenues. The availability of competitors, such as HMOs, PPOs, outpatient surgery centers, foreign-trained physicians, etc., adversely affected hospital and physician revenues.

Given their financial interest in issues affecting their demand for services, methods of pricing, availability of substitutes to their services, and their overall supply, physician and hospital associations represented their concentrated interests before both state and federal legislatures. The defeat of President Truman's proposed NHI plan by the AMA was a demonstration of the AMA's political power and demonstrated to legislators opposed to its economic interests that the AMA was a force to be reckoned with at election time.

The consequences of these legislative actions by physician and hospital associations were neither very obvious nor initially very costly to consumers of medical services. Medical prices were higher than they would otherwise have been and fewer alternatives, such as managed care, were available to the fee-for-service system. These costs were not sufficiently large to make it worthwhile for consumers to organize, represent their interests before legislatures, and offer political support to legislators.

The concentrated interests of medical providers and the consequent diffuse (small) costs imposed on consumers explains much of the legislative history on the financing and delivery of medical services until the early 1960s. The design of payment systems for physicians and hospitals and the structure of the medical services delivery system were economic benefits provided to medical providers as a result of government legislation.

The AFL-CIO unions had a concentrated interest in their retirees' medical costs that placed them in opposition to the American Medical Association (AMA) throughout the 1950s and early 1960s. Employers that paid for union retirees' medical costs did not pre-fund these liabilities, instead they were paid as part of current labor expenses. If union retirees' medical expenses could be shifted away from the employer, then those same funds would be available to be paid as higher wages to union employees. The union's attempt to shift these costs onto others became the basis of the debate over Medicare. The Democratic Party was on the side of the unions, and the Republicans favored the AMA.

To ensure that their union retirees would be eligible for Medicare, the unions insisted on granting eligibility to all retirees who contributed to Social

Security; a separate Social Security (payroll) tax would then be used to finance Medicare. The AMA was willing to have government assistance go only to those unable to afford medical services which would have increased the demand for physicians. Thus the AMA favored a means-tested program funded by general tax revenues. The AMA was concerned that subsidies to the non-poor would merely substitute government payment for private payment. Such a program would cost too much, leading to controls on physicians' fees.

Thus the real fight over Medicare was whether Social Security eligibility would determine eligibility for Medicare.

With the landslide victory of Democratic President Johnson in 1964, the unions were able to achieve their objective of Social Security eligibility and payroll tax financing. Once eligibility for Medicare was determined and financed by a separate Social Security tax, Part B was added, which was voluntary and financed by general tax revenues.

Although the unions won on the eligibility and financing issues, the Congress acceded to the demands of the medical and hospital associations on all other aspects of the legislation. A payment system to hospitals and physicians was implemented that promoted inefficiency (cost-plus payments to hospitals) and restrictions were placed on alternative delivery systems (HMO-type plans) that limited competition.

The outcome of this historic conflict in medical care between opposing concentrated interests left them both victorious. The power of government was used to economically benefit politically important groups.

As a result of Medicare, a massive redistribution of wealth occurred in society. The beneficiaries were the aged, union members, and medical providers; it was financed by a diffuse payroll tax over a large group, the working population, who also paid higher prices for their medical services.

Medicare was designed to be both inefficient and inequitable because it was in the economic interests of those with concentrated interests.

This brief discussion of Medicare illustrates the real purpose of NHI. It is to redistribute wealth, i.e., to increase benefits to politically powerful groups without them having to pay the full costs of those benefits or, similarly, to shift costs from the politically powerful to those who are less so.

Groups Having a Concentrated Interest in Change

An important reason why health policies change is that groups that previously had a diffuse interest develop a concentrated interest in the policy's outcome. For example, the potential benefits to unions of having their retiree's health benefits shifted from the employer to the government (via the taxpayer) under Medicare became sufficiently great as to provide them with a concentrated interest in this issue. Thus groups with a diffuse interest may develop a concentrated interest as the potential benefits or costs to their members increase. As diffuse costs become "concentrated" there is greater incentive for a group to organize and represent its interests.

There are many more groups today with a concentrated interest in health legislation. To understand the conflicting forces pressuring for change and NHI, however, one has to examine the objectives of several of the more important groups.

The Federal Government: Since Medicare and Medicaid were enacted in 1965, every Administration has been faced with the problem of rapidly rising Medicare and Medicaid expenditures. As expenditures greatly exceeded projections, an initial diffuse cost became a concentrated cost to successive Administrations. Each Administration faced choices that were politically costly. To prevent the Medicare Trust Fund from going bankrupt, the Administration could reduce benefits (or increase costs) to the aged, increase the Medicare payroll tax, or pay hospitals less. All three choices were politically costly, however it was less politically costly to increase the payroll tax and to place limits on how much hospitals were to be paid than reduce benefits to the aged.

To limit rapidly rising Medicaid expenditures which are funded from general tax revenues, the states chose to restrict Medicaid eligibility and reduced their payments to health providers rather than reduce other politically popular programs or increase taxes. The percent of the poor served by Medicaid declined, as did the participation of physicians and hospitals.

Medicare Part B, funded by general tax revenues, contributes to the federal budget deficit. As these expenditures began to increase, each Administration's choices were limited; an increase in taxes or a larger deficit are both politically costly; increasing the aged's contribution (they currently pay 25 percent of the premium) is also politically costly; the only alternative was to pay physicians less and place them under an overall expenditure limit.

State and federal administrations developed a concentrated interest in holding down the rise in government expenditures, placing them in conflict with hospital and physician organizations. Only under Medicaid are the politically weak beneficiaries also adversely affected.

Employers: Employers and their employees are interested in reducing the rise in their employees' insurance premiums. Rising employee medical expenses became a concern to employers in the 1980s because of intense import competition. Many employers believe that they bear part of the cost of rising insurance premiums. More importantly, the stimulus for several large corporations promoting national health insurance, such as Chrysler, was a ruling by the Financial Accounting Standards Board (FASB) requiring employers who provide their early retirees with medical benefits and retirees who receive Medicare supplementary benefits to add that liability to their balance sheet (as of 1993). This estimated liability had to include their retirees' future medical expenses, as well as the retiree benefit liability for their current employees. Retiree medical benefits had been an unfunded liability to those large corporations that provide such benefits. Previously, the employer paid retiree medical costs as they occurred; they were treated as a current expense. To place this entire liability on the balance sheet reduced the net worth and equity per share of many major corporations by a significant amount. In addition, corporate earnings declined since a portion of this retiree liability for medical benefits (for both retirees as well as current employees) had to be expensed annually.

Any NHI plan that restricts the growth of medical expenditures provides a direct economic benefit to large corporations by limiting the size of their obligation for their (current and future) retirees' medical expenses.

Unions: The percent of the working population that is unionized has been declining. Only about 13 percent of employees are unionized, down from 25 percent in 1972. The wages earned and medical benefits received by union members vary widely, from those engaged in manufacturing to those employed in the retail and construction businesses. Because unions are organized, several of the larger unions have been able to provide legislators with political support to exercise political influence greatly in excess of their proportion to the total working population.

The economic interests of the major unions, such as the UAW, have not changed since the enactment of Medicare. At that time they were successful in shifting part of the cost of their retirees onto the general working population. Since then they have been trying to reduce the costs of their employees' medical benefits (which are among the most expensive of all employees) by limiting provider price increases. If the unions can limit cost increases for their benefits without increasing their members' cost-sharing, the savings could go toward increased wages. (Unions would also like to increase the cost of low-wage labor thereby increasing the demand for unionized workers by favoring mandated employer health insurance.)

Physicians and Hospitals: As other groups with a concentrated interest in limiting medical expenditures (federal and state governments, employers, and unions) developed, the influence of physician and hospital associations declined. Also adding to their loss of political influence was the inability of their national organizations to represent the interests of their diverse constituencies under "budget neutral" federal programs. When Medicare and Medicaid had to make expenditure choices between their constituencies (urban versus rural hospitals, teaching versus non-teaching hospitals, surgical specialties versus primary care physicians, etc.), these provider coalitions split apart, each trying to gain at the expense of the other by providing political support to further their own interests. Their national associations were unable to favor one constituency over another during these debates, consequently their political influence declined.

The years of excessive provider payments ended. Hospitals and physicians are striving to limit further deterioration in their financial wellbeing. Their objective, as opposed to other concentrated interest groups, is increased medical expenditures. The strongest lobbyists for financing medical care to the poor today are hospitals since it is in their economic interest; they stand to gain additional revenues.

The Aged: Although the aged have NHI for acute care (Medicare), they would like lower out-of-pocket payments for their medical expenses, particularly for outpatient prescription drugs. Given the high voting participation rate of the aged, the closeness of the last presidential election (2000), and the electoral significance of Florida with its many elderly voters, both political parties are competing to provide the aged with a prescription drug benefit. Even though Medicare is financially unsustainable, very expensive prescription drug benefits are being proposed (between $400 and $800 billion over 10 years or upwards of $3 to $5 trillion by 2030). Regardless of the impact any new drug benefit would have on the already large federal deficit, both political parties continue to favor a new drug benefit for the aged in fear of losing their political support.

A new drug benefit covering all the aged will enable the middle- and high-income aged to shift part of their costs to other population groups. Low-income aged would continue to fall back on Medicaid.

The Middle Class: The middle class (those in the middle income group) has a disproportionate amount of political power since they are the median voters; it is difficult to form a majority of voters without those in the middle. If national health insurance were a highly visible issue and strongly supported by the middle class, legislators would respond to the political support that would be forthcoming from them. It is instructive therefore to consider why the middle class has not been a strong supporter of NHI.

Rapidly rising medical costs have, until recently, been a diffuse cost to the middle class. Tax-free employer-paid health insurance insulated employees and their families from the rising costs of medical care. Until the last several years, employees have had unlimited choice of providers, limited cost sharing, and small, if any, co-premiums. *Tax-free employer-paid health insurance has been the middle- and high-income group's NHI.* The value of this tax subsidy exceeds $140 billion in foregone federal, Social Security, and state taxes. Given the significant tax advantages of employer-paid premiums and the fact that increased employer-paid premiums has not visibly lowered their wages, middle- and high-income employees have been insulated from rising medical costs; NHI has not been an important financial issue. Employees have probably been at greater financial risk for the prescription drug costs and long term care needs of their aged parents than for their own acute care needs.

The middle class' dissatisfaction with our current system is increasing because they are being required to pay higher co-payments, forced into more restrictive health plans, and cannot have the free access to specialists as they once did. However, they are unwilling to pay higher co-premiums for health plans that allow for greater provider choice. Basically, the public would like unrestricted access (traditional fee-for-service insurance) for HMO premiums. They are also unwilling to pay higher taxes for NHI. They would like someone else, either government or employers, to pay for their health care.

Other groups, such as insurance companies, also have a concentrated interest in any NHI plan; they do not want to be displaced by a government agency.

These conflicting objectives by powerful interest groups explain why there has not been (nor is there currently) consensus on NHI. The federal and state governments, as well as large employers, want to limit the rate of increase in medical expenditures. The previously politically powerful physician and hospital associations want increased medical expenditures. The aged, who have national health insurance, want a new drug benefit; the unions and the middle class want unrestricted access and at a lower cost, presumably by shifting those costs to others, either different population groups or to the providers by paying them less.

As long the public is led to believe that it is possible for them to have all the care they want without paying for it, serious discussions of the trade-off between access and cost are unlikely to occur. From a legislator's perspective, responding to enrollees' desire to have unlimited access cost the legislator and the government very little since they do not have to vote to increase taxes. Instead, a less visible cost is imposed on enrollees in terms of higher insurance premiums. Unfortunately, the indirect, long-run consequences of these actions are ignored.

Recent Legislative Developments In Lieu of NHI

Several types of legislation have been enacted since the failure of President Clinton's ambitious health care reform plan in 1994. The first was health insurance reform. The Health Insurance Portability and Accountability Act (HIPAA) of 1996 benefited, to a large degree, those who have health insurance. By guaranteeing renewability of their coverage and making insurance "portable" (employees changing jobs do not have to undergo another pre-existing condition waiting period with their new insurer), Congress removed a middle class concern regarding losing their insurance.

Second, by regulating managed care plans, Congress and the states moved into new territory, in some cases regulating the practice of medicine. In the 1990s, managed care competition and low inflation rates reduced the rate of increase in medical expenditures, prices, and health insurance premiums. Middle class concerns over rapidly rising medical expenses declined. Instead, they became concerned with the cost-containment approaches used by managed care plans. Anecdotal stories of HMO enrollees being denied access to specialists and to experimental treatments, of not being permitted to have an overnight stay for normal deliveries, "drive-through" mastectomies, and HMO "gag" orders on physician communication with their patients, led state legislatures and Congress to enact legislation prohibiting such actions.

The use of regulation in response to the media attention given to anecdotal instances of inadequate care is a new role for government. Regulation prescribing the practice of medicine has the potential for increasing the cost of treatment, hence the cost of managed care and, consequently, decreasing the demand for insurance.

In the late 1990s, huge federal budget surpluses were projected. Federal funds were available to expand health insurance to the uninsured without having to raise taxes on the middle class. However, Congress could only agree on assisting low-income children who, along with pregnant women and infants, are considered a deserving group. The Children's Health Insurance Plan (CHIP) was enacted in 1997. With regard to adults, however, the emphasis has been on assisting only a portion of the uninsured, those who lose their health insurance when they lose their job, not those who are employed but never had insurance. And even with regard to this smaller group, Congress could not agree on how the recently uninsured should be assisted. Republicans favored refundable tax credits to buy insurance while the Democrats supported making them eligible for (thereby expanding) existing public programs, such as Medicaid, or enabling them to keep their employer paid insurance.[5]

In 2003, Congress enacted the Medicare Prescription Drug Act providing the aged with subsidies to purchase prescription drugs. The Act was very controversial regarding whether all of the aged should benefit, the size of the subsidies to be provided, and whether the subsidies should be administered by private programs or by the government. The Act also established a program of Health Savings Accounts (HSAs), similar to MSAs, for the non-aged. The HSA provision was not intended to subsidize those with low incomes, but instead to promote greater individual decision-making in the use of medical services. HSAs are very controversial since they threaten the goal of those desiring a single-payer system.

There is an important ideological difference among the political parties regarding the direction of this

---

5. The Trade Adjustment Assistance program (2002) applied to a relatively small number of employees (about 250,000) and was a political compromise that permitted refundable tax credits but required that they could only be used for former workers who are eligible for COBRA (Consolidated Omnibus Reconciliation Act) and for former workers not eligible for COBRA who purchase from state plans (not Medicaid or SCHIP). The first category of workers could not use their 65 percent subsidy to buy individual insurance even though it may be less expensive than an employer's expensive COBRA health plan.

country's medical system. This debate affects federal policies on tax-exempt health savings accounts ("Consumer Directed Health Care"), regulation of managed care, methods to assist the uninsured, and the design of a prescription drug benefit for the aged. There are those who favor expanding public programs, particularly Medicare, as a way of moving toward a "Single Payer" health system; a universal Medicare system would be a single-payer system. It is for this reason that they favor approaches, such as proposed by President Clinton, to allow those age 55 to 65 to buy into Medicare. They also favor expanding the current employer-paid health insurance system (such as an employer mandate) not only because the unions have it, but also it would be easy to transfer all employer-paid health insurance contributions to fund a single-payer system. A new tax would not have to be imposed on the middle class; the funds would just be collected from their employer. (It would be politically difficult for the government to legislate transferring funds that are in individual or HSA accounts.)

Single-payer proponents also oppose approaches, such as refundable tax credits and Medicare reform ("premium support") since these approaches would strengthen a private medical system and move the medical care system away from the direction they favor. Similarly, they favor proposals that increase the cost of the private system, such as regulating managed care to increase its costs (hence premiums) which will cause the public to demand an alternative system, namely, a publicly financed system such as Medicare (or a single-payer system) for everyone.

The opportunity to help the uninsured was lost. Now that the projected surpluses have disappeared, it is even less likely major new programs to help the uninsured will be enacted, funded by increasing the federal deficit or raising taxes.

Until NHI becomes a visible political issue for which the middle class would be willing to provide its political support, NHI is unlikely to be enacted. And given the close division of the Congress and its large ideological differences, there is a fundamental disagreement on the approach to be used to help the uninsured. Although the number and percentage of the uninsured are increasing, there seems to be little interest by the middle class (and consequently by the

Congress) to move quickly and increase their tax burden to enact such a program.

As Victor Fuchs stated, "Major changes in health policy are political acts undertaken for political purposes. The political nature of such changes was apparent when Bismarck introduced national health insurance to the new German state in the 19th century. It was apparent when England adopted national health insurance after World War II; and it will be apparent in the United States as well. National health insurance will probably come to the United States after a major change in the political climate—the kind of change that often accompanies a war, a depression, or large scale civil unrest" (16).

SUMMARY

Different values underlie the extent to which government would subsidize care for the poor under any national health insurance plan. These values range from Minimum Provision to Equal Treatment for Equal Needs. Each set of values can be achieved more efficiently (at lower cost) when the subsidy varies (inversely) with income. The Medicare program was used to illustrate these theoretical conclusions.

Several criteria were specified for evaluating all NHI plans. These included defining the beneficiaries by income, providing beneficiaries and suppliers with incentives for the efficient use of resources, and that the method of financing be equitable, namely, a greater cost burden should be placed on those with higher incomes.

Current subsidies for financing medical services were evaluated according to the above criteria, together with proposals for improving each of these programs. Several proposals for NHI, such as a Canadian-type system, an employer mandate, medical savings accounts, and a refundable tax credit were also evaluated.

The goal of a single-payer health system is not obvious. If the purpose is equal financial access, then this could be achieved more efficiently by a system of subsidies that varies inversely with incomes. A Canadian-type system cannot achieve equal treatment for equal needs, even though the price of medical care is the same for all income groups (zero). Differences in use of services will exist, owing to the value of waiting time, the Province one lives in, and whether the patient can afford to buy care in the United States.

Efficiency and innovation are determined by incentives; it is difficult for a government bureaucracy to outperform competitive markets in this regard. Consumers are unable to leave a monopolized health system when they are dissatisfied as they can when there are competing health plans. Adjustments to changes in supply and demand are also more rapid in a competitive market than in a system where financial incentives are lacking. Further, a competitive health care market is more likely than is a government-controlled system to achieve a rate of growth in expenditures that is appropriate, that is, where the benefits are equal to the amount consumers are willing to spend to receive those benefits.

The Canadian system should be compared not to the current U.S. system, but to one where the goal is universal coverage, such as using income-related refundable tax credits within a competitive managed care system. This approach is more likely to achieve the equity and efficiency criteria.

Rather than assuming that the intended goal of NHI is to assist those with low incomes, an alternative assumption benefiting politically powerful constituencies was used to explain why this country has not had NHI. This alternative hypothesis provides a more useful explanation why many health programs are inefficiently designed and inequitably financed.

Economic analysis can be a powerful tool in the analysis of alternative proposals for national health insurance in that it can sharpen the debate by providing information as to the redistributive and efficiency consequences of alternative proposals. If economists can clarify the issues by separating those that involve differences in the values underlying various goals of NHI from issues of efficiency with regard to achieving a given set of NHI goals, they will have served an important policy role.

REVIEW QUESTIONS

1. What criteria is most appropriate for evaluating a government's health insurance scheme?
2. Describe the characteristics of the uninsured.
3. A payroll tax imposed one-half on both the employer and the employee is used to finance Medicare Part A. Using supply and demand diagrams for labor, show how the elasticity of supply and demand for labor determines who actually bears the burden of the payroll tax.
4. If society were to establish as a principle for national health insurance that everyone should have equal consumption of medical care for equal needs, explain why a policy that established the same price to everyone for medical care (or makes medical care free to all, i.e., zero price) will not achieve society's goal.
5. Assume that in country X where medical care was privately paid for, a new government was elected, with one of its policies being free medical care for all. As the new Minister of Health, what are the various actions you would have to undertake to ensure that at a zero price for all medical care services, an efficient and adequate supply will be available in the future?
6. One approach that has been proposed for national health insurance is a system whereby all employers would be required to provide their employees with a minimum set of health insurance benefits ("An Employer Mandate"). Evaluate this proposal in terms of the demand for different types of labor, the effects on federal revenues, the effects on the prices of goods and services produced by different types of industries, and the effect on imported goods. How equitable do you believe such a proposal to be? Be explicit regarding any assumptions you make.
7. Compare an income-related refundable tax credit NHI plan to the current tax-exempt employer-purchased health insurance system in terms of their likely effects on efficiency in

delivery and equity with respect to government subsidies.

8. Which groups would be expected to favor and oppose an employer-mandated health insurance plan?

9. National health insurance can be financed by either a payroll or an income tax. Compare the equity and economic efficiency effects of each of these methods of financing.

REFERENCES

1. The May 15, 1991, issue of the *Journal of the American Medical Association*, 265 (19), which is devoted to issues of the uninsured, contains a number of proposals for national health insurance.

2. Centers for Medicare and Medicaid Services, 2003 Annual Report of the Boards of Trustees of the Federal Hospital Insurance Trust and Federal Supplementary Medical Insurance Trust Funds, http://cms.hhs. gov/ publications/trusteesreport/ (accessed on August 18, 2003.)

3. For an excellent and comprehensive discussion of this issue, together with estimates of the intergenerational transfer, see: Ronald J. Vogel, "An Analysis of the Welfare Component and Intergenerational Transfers Under the Medicare Program," in Mark Pauly and William Kissick, eds., *Lessons From The First Twenty Years of Medicare*, (University of Pennsylvania Press: Philadelphia), 1988. Also see, Ronald J. Vogel, *Medicare: Issues in Political Economy*, (University of Michigan Press: Ann Arbor), June 1999 and Mark McClellan and Jonathan Skinner, "Medicare Reform: Who Pays and Who Benefits?" *Health Affairs*, 18(1), January/February 1999, 48–62.

4. David Cutler and Jonathan Gruber, "The Effect of Medicaid Expansions on Public Insurance, Private Insurance, and Redistribution," *American Economic Review*, 86(2), May 1996, 378–383.

5. For a more complete discussion of this and related proposals, see *The Tax Treatment of Employment-Based Health Insurance*, (Washington, D.C.: Congressional Budget Office, Congress of the United States), March 1994. For 2001 estimates on the cost of employment based health insurance subsidies, Congressional Budget Office,

Budget Options, February 2001, http://www.cbo.gov/bo2001/bo2001_showhit1.cfm?index=REV-12 (accessed on September 2, 2003.).

6. The Physicians' Working Group for Single-Payer National Health Insurance, "Proposal of the Physicians' Working Group for Single-Payer National Health Insurance," *Journal of the American Medical Association*, 290(6), August 13, 2003, 798–805.

7. Steffie Woolhandler, and David Himmelstein. "The Deteriorating Administrative Efficiency of the U.S. Health Care System," *The New England Journal of Medicine*, 324(18), May 2, 1991: 1253–1258. More recently, Steffie Woolhandler, Terry Campbell, and David Himmelstein, "Costs of Health Care Administration in the United States and Canada," *The New England Journal of Medicine*, 349(8), August 21, 2003, 768–775.

8. Patricia M. Danzon, "Hidden Overhead Costs: Is Canada's System Really Less Expensive?" *Health Affairs*, 11(1), Spring 1992, 21–43.

9. *Medicare: Rapid Spending Growth Calls for More Prudent Purchasing*, (Washington, D.C.: United States Government Accounting Office), GAO/T-HEHS-95-193, June 28, 1995.

10. The Fraser Institute website: http://www.fraserinstitute.ca/shared/readmore.asp?snav=nr&id=550

11. Steven Pearlstein, "Health Care on the Critical List: Canada's Public System Is Overwhelmed, and Under Attack," *The Washington Post*, December 18, 1999, p. A20.

12. As quoted in "Notable & Quotable," *The Wall Street Journal*, August 8, 1987: 16.

13. Emmett B. Keeler, et al., "Can Medical Savings Accounts for the Nonelderly Reduce Health Care Costs?," *Journal of the American Medical Association*, 275(21), June 5 1997, 1666–1671.

14. Mathew Eichner, Mark McClellan, and David Wise, "Insurance or Self-Insurance? Variation, Persistence, and Individual Health Accounts," in David A. Wise, ed., *Inquiries in the Economics of Aging*, (The University of Chicago Press: Chicago, Ill.) 1998.

15. The following is an example of a proposal for national health insurance based on tax credits and catastrophic coverage. Mark Pauly, Patricia Danzon, Paul Feldstein, and John Hoff, "A Plan for 'Responsible National Health Insurance,'" *Health Affairs*, 10(1), Spring 1991: 5–25. Also see Mark Pauly and John Goodman, "Tax Credits for Health Insurance and Medical Savings Accounts," *Health Affairs*, 14(1), Spring 1995, 125–139,

and Mark Pauly and Brad Herring, "Expanding Coverage Via Tax Credits: Trade-Offs and Outcomes," *Health Affairs*, 20(1), January/February 2001, 9–26.

16. Victor R. Fuchs, "What's Ahead for Health Insurance in the United States?," *New England Journal of Medicine*, 346(23), June 6, 2002, 1822–1824.

CHAPTER
20

Concluding Comments on the Economics of Health Care

The purpose of this book has been to demonstrate how the tools of economics can be applied to the study of medical care issues. Economic concepts define and clarify the different aspects of medical care, making them more susceptible to analysis. Differences in values among persons on particular issues can be separated from differences in the efficiency with which various approaches can achieve a specified set of values. In addition, economics offers criteria for determining whether particular policies increase or decrease *efficiency* and *equity* in medical care. Of course, economic analysis cannot resolve all of the concerns that health professionals and the public have with regard to medical care—different problems require different training and analytical expertise. Particularly suited to economic analysis are problems that relate to issues of scarcity. Economics can illustrate the choices a society can make when its resources are insufficient to achieve everything it desires.

THE TOOLS OF ECONOMIC ANALYSIS

The two economic tools used throughout this book are marginal analysis, which underlies all optimization problems, and supply and demand analysis, which is used for predicting new equilibrium situations. These two tools are interrelated in that supply and demand analysis assumes that individuals or firms are attempting to maximize some goal (e.g., utility or profits) subject to certain budget constraints. The welfare criteria we have been concerned with are the equity effects resulting from different policies, both government and private, and the implications of different market structures, such as competitive and monopolistic markets.

The use of our economic tools may lead to predictions that turn out to be different than what we observe. One such example is that high rates of return to a medical education should have led to an increase in the supply of physicians during the 1960s. When predictions differ from what we observe (there were very small increases in the supply of physicians during the 1960s), it does not mean that the theory is wrong or not useful. Instead, the theory suggests which assumptions should be examined that may have been violated. In the physician example cited above, the assumption of free entry in medical education was incorrect, enabling high rates of return to persist. When the underlying assumptions are different from the assumptions of a competitive market, there is a possible role for public policy.

Medical care markets differ from competitive markets and other industries in several ways. Lack of consumer information, uncertainty of a medical expense and the outcome of a treatment, tax-exempt employer-paid health insurance, the existence of moral hazard for the insured, the dual role of the physician as the patient's agent and the supplier of a service, the large number of not-for-profit firms, payment of providers (in the past) on a cost basis, limitations on entry into the professions and on tasks that different professionals may perform, and the desire by society to provide all its members with a minimum level of medical care are some of the characteristics of this market. Although many of these characteristics might exist in other sectors, together they give medical care a certain uniqueness.

Important policy differences occur with respect to this set of unique characteristics. Should the medical care sector be made to conform to more traditional economic markets (e.g., competitive pricing with its attendant incentives), or should medical care be insulated from traditional market forces? Public policy regarding the organization of medical services has changed over time.

THE THREE BASIC DECISIONS OF ANY MEDICAL CARE SYSTEM

Public policy has been directed at the three basic questions that any economic system or industry must resolve.

How Much To Spend On Medical Care

How much of its limited resources should society spend on medical care? The choice is *not* how much to spend on health, but how much to spend on medical services. People do not desire increased health at any cost, as evidenced by their refusal to stop smoking, wear seat belts, and change their personal health habits. Medical services expenditures serve, to some extent, as a substitute for undertaking other activities to enhance health; part of the costs of neglecting these activities are borne by the population at large through taxes and higher medical care prices. While the decision of how much to spend on health may be more relevant, the emphasis of the U.S. medical system and government financing is to provide more medical services, which is only one approach, and perhaps one of the most costly, for improving health.

Before it can be determined how much should be spent on medical care, it must be decided whether consumers or government will make the necessary decisions. It should again be recognized that this basic decision, which will determine the size and growth of the medical sector, depends upon resolving the issue of whose values are to dominate medical care. Are consumers to determine how much of their income is to be allocated to medical care, or is that decision to be made by a government agency? The answer will determine whether the consumer or an agency's preferences will dominate.

A market approach for allocating resources to different goods and services maximizes the consumer's preferences. Opponents of consumer decision-making argue that the uniqueness of medical care make a market approach inapplicable: first, consumers may not be aware of their medical needs; second, they may not spend as much as some persons believe they should on their medical needs; and third, because they do not have sufficient information to judge different providers. Under such circumstances, opponents of a market approach propose substituting another mechanism for making the necessary allocation choices in medical care, but they do not explicitly state the criteria by which such a system of decision-making should be judged. Proponents of relying on consumer preferences recognize the limitations of the current medical system and how they affect consumer ability to make choices, and seek to improve the consumer's decision-making process.

The amount, type, and quality of medical services provided have not represented either consumer or third-party preferences. Consumer demands for medical care have been distorted both by their excess health coverage resulting from tax subsidies for the purchase of health insurance and by the lack of information on which to base their choices. The most knowledgeable purchaser in the medical market—the patient's physician—lacked the fiscal responsibility to be concerned with medical costs and also had a financial interest in the service that he or she provides. These distortions in the medical care market resulted in the provision of either too many or too few of certain types of services.

Public and private policy during the 1980s sought to improve the consumers' ability to make choices, make consumers bear more of the costs of their choices, and change the incentives facing the providers. In the private sector, employees pay higher premiums for more costly health plans and increased deductibles and cost sharing in indemnity plans. Both Medicare and Medicaid are increasing their use of managed care programs. Consumers are being given financial incentives to limit their use of medical services or choose more restrictive plans for a lower premium.

How To Best Produce Medical Services

The second basic decision to be made in any medical system is how medical services should be produced to ensure that output is provided at lowest cost. Until the 1980s, rapidly increasing medical costs, duplication of expensive facilities and services, provision of unnecessary services, excessive testing, and unnecessary use of expensive settings were all indications that the efficiency with which medical care was provided could be improved. The alternatives were to rely on greater regulation and controls implemented by government agencies, or reliance on competitive market pressures to achieve greater efficiency.

Many have a basic distrust of a market system; they are concerned that the patient would not be adequately protected when providers are motivated by profits. Concern for consumer protection resulted in many restrictions which were promoted by health associations. However, restrictions on who can perform certain tasks, who may enter the health professions, and who may be reimbursed for providing medical services did not alleviate the public's concern that incompetent and unethical health providers still practice. Instead, these restrictions reduced competition in the provision of medical services.

The movement to a price competitive market in medical care started in the early 1980s. The Supreme Court ruled in 1982 that the antitrust laws were applicable to the health professions. As anti-competitive restrictions, such as prohibitions on advertising and provider boycotts of insurers promoting cost containment methods, were eliminated and efficiency incentives increased, the health sector underwent a major restructuring. Under the pressure by business and government to reduce their medical expenditures, providers began to take advantage of economies of scale in the provision of services; hospitals merged and large multi-hospital systems came into being. Physicians joined group practices to achieve economies of scale and to have more market power when negotiating with insurers. Managed care increased and insurers consolidated to take advantage of economies of scale and to have greater market power over hospitals and physicians.

A great deal of regulation still exists in medical care. Many states rely on CON laws. DRGs are a system of regulated prices. And many states restrict the tasks that different professionals may perform. Since the 1980s, the trend has been toward a more price-competitive system. As provider incentives change, so does the structure of the medical system. Under a price-competitive system, the organization of medical services will reflect the most efficient methods of delivery.

Efficiency in the provision of medical services and containment of rapidly escalating medical expenditures are important public policy issues. Unless the rise in medical expenditures can be limited, benefits and beneficiaries of current public programs will be reduced, and new programs are unlikely to be initiated. Raising taxes to continue funding existing programs for the poor has limited political appeal. Thus efficiency in the provision of services and rapid increases in medical expenditures influence the degree to which society is willing to expand access by the poor.

The Distribution of Medical Services

Equity concerns, namely how much medical care should be redistributed to different population groups and by what mechanisms, is the third basic decision that must be made in medical care. The choice of how much medical care to provide to particular population groups is affected by the costs of such programs. Proposals to restructure medical care or to change Medicare and Medicaid are often justified as much by their ability to contain costs as for their success in redistributing medical services.

All health policy has redistributive effects. Explicit redistributive programs, such as Medicare, Medicaid, care for the uninsured, tax subsidies for the purchase of health insurance, and financing medical (and other health professional) education, involve raising funds and distributing benefits. However, some types of taxes and methods of distributing benefits result in greater equity than others. If low-income persons pay more in taxes than they receive in benefits, that health policy makes them worse off. Similarly, when high-income groups receive more in benefits than they pay in taxes, they are made better off. Both types of situations exist in medical care. Unless the costs and benefits of public programs (including tax policies) by income group can be directly measured, such perverse redistributive situations are likely to continue.

Concern over the rise in medical expenditures and greater equity in financing medical services are major health policy issues today. Depending on the policy selected to achieve each of these objectives, the redistributive effects may have positive or negative effects on those with low incomes. The uninsured can be provided for by an employer mandate, expanding Medicaid, refundable tax credits for an HMO voucher, or by paying hospitals for uncompensated care. Limiting the rise in medical expenditures can be achieved by relying on competitive markets, such as increasing patient sensitivity to prices and premiums, or through regulation by setting expenditure limits on hospitals and physicians (as is done under Medicare). Each of these alternative approaches for achieving greater equity and limiting expenditure increases impose burdens and provide benefits to different groups. As such, the policy mix is as likely to be guided by the benefits and burdens imposed on politically influential groups as it is by the efficiency and equity of specific approaches.

How efficiently each of our current (and proposed) subsidy programs redistributes medical services to those least able to afford them is questionable. Tax subsidy programs, such as employer-paid health insurance, generally benefit those with higher incomes. Medicare results in huge inter-generational subsidies, with the current aged benefiting from taxes imposed on the working population, many of whom have low incomes. Those who come from higher-income families and who subsequently enter professions whose incomes are among the highest in the country have received the majority of subsidies to health professional education. Recognizing the redistributive benefits that these huge subsidy programs provide to different income groups is the first step in deciding whether the resulting redistributive effects are desirable. It should then be determined whether such subsidies could be provided more efficiently so that those in greatest financial need receive them.

Implementing redistributive programs involves providing benefits (in excess of their costs) to one group by imposing costs (in excess of the benefits they receive) on other groups. To anticipate which groups will receive net benefits and which groups are likely to bear those costs requires a theory of legislation. According to the economic theory of legislation, legislation is provided in return for political support by those who have a concentrated interest. Within such a framework, it is unlikely that redistributive legislation will be provided or financed in as equitable a manner as possible unless those groups able to offer the greatest amount of political support are favorably disposed toward that approach.

Funding for redistributive programs could be reduced if government subsidies were targeted directly to desired beneficiary groups. However, the political feasibility of achieving an efficient strategy for redistribution is questionable. Each subsidy program creates a distinct constituency. Attempts to change the current distribution of subsidies will encounter strong political opposition from the beneficiaries of current subsidies. The potential beneficiaries of a more direct subsidy system, namely the poor, are not well organized to engage in the political process, as is indicated by the very fact of their need for such subsidies. Economic analysis of current as well as of proposed subsidy programs can indicate who is likely to receive such subsidies and whether the stated objectives of such subsidies can be achieved in a more efficient manner. Although such information may not determine the outcome of legislation, it is an input into the political process and raises the political costs to those who might otherwise benefit from less efficient subsidy schemes.

THE YEARS AHEAD

Forecasting the future is perilous. When one looks back at how the financing and delivery of medical services has changed from the 1960s, few have anticipated the changes that occurred. Hospital and physician payment changed several times under both public and private programs. The organization of hospitals and physicians changed from being independent providers to being part of hospital systems and the development of large physician groups. Health insurers changed from being passive payers of provider claims to interfering in the physician-patient relationship. Few controls were initially placed on rapidly rising health care costs, regulatory approaches were then tried (and, for the most part, discarded) to the application of anti-trust laws, resulting in a shift to more price competitive markets and the development of managed care to, currently, a possible

trend toward consumer-directed health care. The role of large employers has also changed as they attempt to control rising employee medical costs and promote the use of Report Cards.

Among the most dramatic changes that have occurred is with regard to medical technology. Advances in imaging technology have improved the physician's ability to diagnose (at an earlier stage of disease) and improve outcomes of surgical procedures. Less invasive surgery has become possible, recovery times are shorter, patients with previously untreatable diseases can now survive, and drug therapy has reduced the need for more expensive treatment methods, improved patients' lifestyles, and increased life expectancy.

Some predictions are relatively easy. The demand for medical services will continue rising as the population ages, incomes increase, people live longer, and new technology increases the benefits of medical treatment. Medical costs are likely to continue rising more rapidly than inflation, primarily driven by increases in emerging medical technology, including the development of genomics. Consequently, medical care will consume an increasing portion of Gross Domestic Product.

More difficult to predict is the effect that rising medical expenditures will have on the ability of federal and state governments to fund Medicare and Medicaid and the reaction of the middle class to devoting an increasing portion of their incomes for medical care.

The safe prediction is that major changes in the financing and delivery of medical services will not occur in the near term.

More difficult to predict are the likely political changes that will be required when the baby boomers start to retire in 2011 and much greater taxes will be needed to fund an increasingly expensive and financially weak Medicare system (and the new prescription drug benefit promised to the aged). At that time, the middle class is likely to be faced with much greater out-of-pocket payments for their medical services, concerned about their access to care, and be required to pay a higher portion of their incomes in taxes to save Medicare. In coming years, rising medical costs and the need for increased taxes to finance Medicare are likely to sharpen the ideological debate over the three basic questions: how much should be spent on medical services, how medical services should be produced, and how should medical services be distributed.

Medical care will continue to be in the forefront of public policy. To participate in that process one must understand and apply the tools of economic analysis.

Medical care is different from other industries. Yet economic analysis is useful in many ways: it offers a perspective by which medical care issues can be viewed and analyzed; the effects of legislation, both current and proposed, affecting the demand and supply sides of the medical markets can be evalu-

ated; and economics can be used to perform such traditional tasks as planning and forecasting that are required in any industry. In addition to its tools—the prediction of changes in prices, quantities, and total expenditures, and the formulation of rules for cost minimization—economics provides a set of criteria for evaluating whether or not various policies achieve greater efficiency and equity in medical care. The application of these tools and criteria should increase our understanding of medical care issues, enable us to separate differences in values from differences in approaches to achieving a given set of values, and provide us with the ability to evaluate the costs and benefits of different choices in medical care.

GLOSSARY

Actual versus list prices—Actual prices are the fees collected or paid for a particular good or service. The difference between actual and list prices are provider discounts, which vary by type of payer.

Actuarially fair insurance—The expected insurance payments (benefits) are equivalent to the premiums paid by beneficiaries (plus a competitive loading charge).

Adverse selection—This occurs when high-risk individuals have more information on their health status than the insurer and are thus able to buy insurance at a premium based on a lower risk group.

Ambulatory surgical center (ASC)—A freestanding outpatient facility that performs certain types of procedures.

American Medical Association (AMA)—A national organization established in 1897 to represent the collective interests of physicians.

Antitrust laws—A body of legislation that promotes competition in the United States economy.

Any Willing Provider laws—Laws that lessen price competition in that they permit the participation of any physician in an insurer's provider panel, thereby negating providers' incentive to compete on price to be included in the panel.

Assignment/participation—An agreement whereby the provider accepts the approved fee from the third-party payer and is not permitted to charge the patient more, except for the appropriate copayment fees.

Balance billing—When the physician collects from the patient, the difference between the third-party payor's approved fee and the physician's fee.

Barriers to entry—Barriers that may be legal, e.g., licensing laws and patents, and/or economic, i.e., economies of scale, that limit entry into an industry.

Benefit/premium ratio—The percentage of the total premium paid out in benefits to each insured group divided by the price of insurance.

Blue Cross/Blue Shield—Non-profit health insurers that provide insurance for hospital (Blue Cross) and physician (Blue Shield) services.

Canadian type health system—A form of national health insurance in which medical services are free to everyone, and the providers are paid by the government. Expenditure limits are used to restrict the growth in medical use and costs.

Capitation incentives—The provider becomes concerned with the coordination of all medical services, providing care in the least costly manner, monitoring the cost of enrollee's hospital use, increasing physician productivity, prescribing less costly drugs, and being innovative in the delivery of medical services. Conversely, the provider has an incentive to reduce use of services and decrease patient access.

Capitation payment—A risk-sharing arrangement in which the provider group receives a predetermined fixed payment per member per month (PMPM) in return for providing all of the contracted services.

Case-mix index—A measure of the relative complexity of the patient mix treated in a given medical care setting.

Certificate of Need (CON) laws—State laws requiring health care providers to receive prior approval from a state agency for capital expenditures exceeding certain predetermined levels. CON laws are an entry barrier.

Charity hypothesis of physician pricing—Physicians charge higher prices to those with higher incomes and thereby claim that they are able to charge lower prices to those with lower incomes.

Coinsurance/Copayment—A fixed percentage of the medical provider's fee made by the insurance beneficiary at the point of service.

Community rating—The insurance premium is the same to all of the insured, regardless of their claims experience or risk group.

Comparable worth-based wages—Wages and salaries are based upon an evaluation of each position, including skill required, effort involved, working conditions, and level of responsibility, rather than by supply and demand conditions for that position.

Competitive markets—The interaction between a large number of buyers and suppliers where no single seller or buyer can influence the market price.

Concentrated interests—When some regulation or legislation has a sufficiently large effect on a group to make it worthwhile for that group to invest resources to either forestall or promote that effect.

Consumer expenditure survey—Conducted as part of the Consumer Price Index, it is a survey of spending patterns for a specified period of time. It consists of two components: an interview survey to determine expenditures on those items (and quantity) that people purchase, and a diary or record-keeping survey in which individuals are asked to record small, frequently purchased items.

Consumer Price Index—Calculated by the Bureau of Labor Statistics, it is used as a measure of the rate of inflation or the rate at which a family's income would have to increase to keep up with rising prices.

Consumer sovereignty—Consumers, rather than health professionals or government, choose the goods and services they can purchase with their incomes.

Cost containment programs—Approaches used to reduce health care costs, such as utilization review and deductibles.

Cost of Treatment Price Index—An index of the price of medical care based upon how the price of a treatment for a particular diagnosis changes over time.

Cost shifting—The belief that providers charge a higher price to privately insured patients because some payers, such as Medicaid or the uninsured, do not pay their full costs.

Cost-effectiveness analysis—Determining which programs and/or inputs are least costly for achieving a given objective.

Criteria for cost minimization—The combination of services and/or inputs used to provide medical care that are both technically and economically efficient.

Declining marginal productivity of health inputs—The additional contribution to output of a health input declines as more of that input is used.

Decreasing marginal utility of wealth—The marginal utility of money decreases as the person's income or wealth increases.

Deductible—Consumers pay a flat dollar amount for medical services before their insurance picks up all or part of the remainder of the price of that service.

Demand shift (or an Increase in Demand)—Changes in factors affecting demand, other than the price of the service.

Derived Demand—Demand for the particular service or input is based on the demand for the service for which it is an input.

Determinants of a firms' demand for employees—Based upon the employees' wage relative to other inputs, their employees' marginal productivity, the demand for the firm's product, and the price at which the firm's product is sold.

Diagnosis-related group (DRG)—A method of reimbursement established under Medicare to pay hospitals based upon a fixed price per admission, according to diagnostic-related groupings.

Diffuse costs—When the burden of a tax or program is spread over a large population and is relatively small per person so that the per person costs of opposing such a burden exceeds the actual size of the burden on the person.

Direct subsidies—Financial aid targeted to a specific group.

Dynamic shortages—Occurs when demand is increasing more rapidly than supply so that an equilibrium price has not yet been established.

Economic shortage—Occurs when the quantity demanded exceeds the quantity supplied at a given price.

Economic efficiency—The optimal rate of output occurs when all marginal benefits equal all marginal costs.

Economic Theory of Government—A theory of legislative and regulatory outcomes that assumes political markets are no different from economic markets in that organized groups seek to further their self interests.

Economies of scale—The relationship between long-run average total cost (LRATC) and size of firm; as firm size increases, LRATC falls, reaches a minimum, and eventually rises. In a competitive market, each firm operates at that size that is at the lowest point on the LRATC curve. For a given size market, the larger the firm size required to achieve the minimum costs of production, the fewer the number of firms that will be able to compete.

Employee Retirement Income Security Act of 1974 (ERISA)—A federal law that applies to employee welfare plans and preempts all state laws with regard to reporting and disclosure policies. Applicable to self-funded plans.

Employer-mandated health insurance—Under this health reform plan all employers are required to provide to medical insurance to their employees.

Equal financial access—A value judgement underlying national health insurance in which the financial barriers to medical care would be the same for all.

Equal treatment for equal needs—A value judgement underlying national health insurance in which everyone should have equal consumption of medical services, regardless of economic or other factors affecting utilization.

Expected utility—It is the weighted sum of the utilities of each outcome, with the weights being the probabilities of each outcome. With regard to the demand for health insurance, expected utility has a linear relationship.

Experience rating—Insurance premiums are based upon the claims experience or risk level, such as age, of each insured group.

Externalities—Occur when an action undertaken by an individual (or firm) has secondary effects on others and that these effects are not taken into account by the normal operations of the price system.

Fee-for-service payment—A method of payment for medical care services in which payment is made for each unit of service provided.

Flexner report—Published in 1910, it was a highly critical report evaluating the medical training of physicians in the United States and Canada. This report led to the restructuring of the education and training of physicians and the eventual closure of many medical schools.

Food and Drug Administration (FDA)—A government agency that regulates entry into the U.S. market of all drugs and relevant medical devices by requiring manufacturing firms to demonstrate that their products are safe and efficacious.

Formulary—A list of prescription drugs reimbursed under a managed care plan.

Foundations for medical care (FMCs)—Non-profit organizations that own plant, property, and equipment associated with medical practice and employ non-physician employees. The foundation, in turn, contracts with the medical group on a mutually exclusive basis to see all of the foundation's patients. The foundation controls the contracts with payers, owns the medical records, and distributes a negotiated share to the medical group.

"Free choice of provider"—Included in the original Medicare and Medicaid legislation, all beneficiaries had to have access to all providers. Precluded closed provider panels and capitated HMOs. This provision is considered by economists to be anti-competitive in that it limits competition; beneficiaries could not choose a closed provider panel in return for lower prices or increased benefits.

Gatekeeper—In many HMOs the primary care physician, or "gatekeeper," is responsible for the administration of the patient's treatment and must coordinate and authorize all medical services, laboratory studies, specialty referrals, and hospitalizations.

Geographic market definition—Used in anti-trust analysis to determine the relevant market in which a health care provider competes. The broader the geographic market, the greater are the number of substitutes available to the purchaser, hence the smaller the market share of merging firms.

Government policy instruments—The use of tax policy, expenditures, and regulation available to government to achieve its policy objectives.

Government policy objectives—According to the Public Interest Theory, government has two policy objectives: improve market efficiency, and improve equity and/or redistribute resources (based on a societal value judgement).

Guaranteed issue—Health insurers have to offer health insurance to those willing to purchase it.

Guaranteed renewal—Requires health insurers to renew all health insurance policies within standard rate bands, thereby precluding insurers from dropping individuals or groups who incur high medical costs.

Health Care Financing Administration (HCFA)—It is part of the U.S. Department of Health and Human Services and is responsible for administering Medicare and the federal aspect of state Medicaid programs.

Health inputs—The resources that are used to produce a specific output referred to as "good health."

HIPAA—Enacted in 1996, the Health Insurance Portability and Accountability Act (HIPAA) removed certain health insurance market imperfections. Included in the legislation was *Guaranteed Issue* whereby health insurers have to offer group health insurance to groups willing to purchase it. *Guaranteed Renewal* requires health insurers to renew all health insurance policies, precluding them from dropping individuals or groups who incur high medical costs. *Portability* enables employees to continue their insurance coverage if they move to another employee group or if they become self employed.

Health maintenance organization (HMO)—A type of managed care plan that offers prepaid comprehensive health care coverage for hospital and physician services, relying on its medical providers to minimize the cost of providing medical services. HMOs contract with or directly employ participating health care providers. Enrollees must pay the full cost of receiving service from non-network providers.

Health manpower surplus—Occurs when physicians (or other health professionals) are earning a below-normal rate of return (price would be below the average total cost curve).

Health production function—Describes the technical relationship between each of the health inputs and their effect (marginal productivity) on health.

HEDIS—The two most commonly accepted measures of health plan and provider performance are based on data from the Health Plan Employer Data Information Set (HEDIS) and the Consumer Assessment of Health Plan Survey (CAHPS). HEDIS measures, such as preventive measures and physician certifications, are gathered from administrative records of health plans and their participating providers. CAHPS data, which measures enrollee satisfaction with participating providers, are based on surveys of health plan enrollees.

HHI Index—(Herfindahl-Hirschman Index)—The measure of concentration used by the Department of Justice in its merger guidelines. This index, by summing the square of each provider's market share, makes it sensitive to both the number of firms and to their relative sizes.

Horizontal merger—When two or more firms from the same market merge to form one firm.

Hospital collusion—Competing hospitals in the same market agree on price, output, and/or wage policies.

Incidence of the payroll tax—The extent to which the payroll tax is borne by employers or employees is determined by the elasticity of demand and supply curves for labor.

Income Contingent Loan Repayment Plans—A student loan program to cover both tuition and living expenses which would be repaid by paying a fixed percentage of their adjusted gross income. The fixed percentage would be based on the amount borrowed.

Indemnity insurance—Medical insurance that pays the provider or the patient a pre-determined amount for the medical service provided.

Independent Provider Association (IPA)—A physician owned and controlled contracting organization comprised of solo and small groups of physicians (on a non-exclusive basis) that enables the physicians to contract with payers on a unified basis.

Indirect subsidies—Financial aid not targeted to a specific group or recipient, available to all users of the subsidized service.

Individual mandate—A proposed national health insurance plan under which individuals are required to buy a minimum level of health insurance. Refundable tax credits are provided to those having incomes below a certain level of income.

Inferior good—An increase in income leads to a decrease in consumption of that good or service.

Infra-marginal externalities—Even though there may be external benefits, the private market produces the optimal quantity (e.g., physicians).

In-kind subsidies—Non-cash subsidies provided to specific beneficiary groups based on the donor's (middle class') preferences.

Insurance premium—Consists of two parts: the expected medical expense of the insured group, and the loading charge which includes administrative expenses and profit.

Integrated Delivery System (IDS)—A health care delivery system that includes or contracts with all the health care providers to provide coordinated medical services to the patient. An IDS also views itself as being responsible for the health status of its enrolled population.

Law of Demand—The lower the price, the greater the quantity demanded.

Law of Supply—The higher the price, the greater is the quantity firms are willing to produce.

Loading charge—That portion of the health insurance premium that is added to the pure (actuarially fair) premium to include administrative expense and profit.

Managed Care Organization (MCO)—An organization that controls medical care costs and quality through utilization management, drug formularies, and profiling participating providers according to their appropriate use of medical services.

Mandated benefits—According to state insurance laws, specific medical services, providers, and/or population groups must be included in health insurance policies.

Marginal benefits—The change in total benefits from purchasing one additional unit.

Marginal contribution of medical care to health—The increase in health status resulting from an additional increment of medical services.

Marginal costs—The change in total costs from producing one additional unit.

Market equilibrium—When the independent actions of buyers and suppliers cause quantity demanded to equal quantity supplied. The result is an equilibrium price and quantity.

Market failure—May occur when there are market imperfections so that price-competitive markets will not produce the optimal amount of output, which is defined as price equaling marginal cost.

Market imperfections—Occur as a result of lack of information by consumers regarding their medical diagnoses, treatment needs, the quality of different providers, and prices charged by different providers. Additional imperfections are tax-free employer-paid health insurance, restrictions on entry and on tasks, and externalities.

Market performance—An indication of the economic efficiency of the market. Economic efficiency occurs when the market price equals marginal cost. When there are no positive or negative externalities, then the resulting rate of output is optimal. The marginal benefit (as indicated by market price) equals the marginal cost of producing that last unit.

Market power—An indication of the degree of monopoly power possessed by the firm. It is measured by the ratio of the firm's price to its marginal cost. The higher the price relative to its cost, the greater the firm's market power.

Market structure—The number of suppliers within the market, which is determined by the extent of economies of scale in relation to the size of the market, and entry barriers usually define the competitiveness of the market.

Medicaid—A health insurance program financed by federal and state governments and administered by the states for qualifying segments of those with low incomes.

Medicaid Risk contracts—A Medicaid managed care program in which an HMO contracts to provide medical services in return for a capitation premium.

Medical Care Price Index—Calculated by the Bureau of Labor Statistics and included as part of the Consumer Price Index, it is used as a measure of the rate of inflation in medical care prices.

Medical group—A group of physicians who coordinate their activities in one or more group facilities and who share common overhead expenses, medical records, and professional, technical and administrative staffs.

Medical loss ratio—The percentage of the total premium paid out in benefits to each insured group. (Also see benefit/premium ratio.)

Medical Savings Accounts (MSA)—A form of national health insurance in which a person can annually contribute, tax free, an amount into their MSA equal to 75 percent of their deductible. The unused portion of the MSA can accumulate over time.

Medicare—A federally sponsored and supervised health insurance plan for the elderly. Part A provides hospital insurance for inpatient care, home health agency visits, hospice and skilled nursing facility. The aged are responsible for a deductible but do not have to pay an annual premium. Part B provides payments for physician services, physician-ordered supplies and services, and outpatient hospital services. Part B is voluntary, and the aged pay an annual premium that is 25 percent of the cost of the program in addition to having to pay a deductible and copayment.

Medicare risk contract—Federally qualified HMOs receive from the government a monthly capitated fee for each enrolled Medicare beneficiary (in addition to the Part B beneficiary premium) and in return provide both Part A and Part B services, plus additional services such as prescription drugs as determined by the HMO. Enrollees using non-HMO participating providers are responsible for the full charges of such providers.

Medigap insurance policies—Privately purchased insurance policy by the elderly to supplement Medicare coverage by covering deductibles and copayments.

Monopolistic competition—A market structure that is characterized by many competing firms, each producing a slightly differentiated product that is a close substitute to the products produced by competing firms.

Monopoly—A market structure in which there is a single seller of a product that has no close substitutes.

Monopoly model of physician pricing—Physicians face a downward-sloping demand curve for their services and set prices according to where marginal revenue equals marginal costs.

Monopsony—A market structure characterized by a single purchaser.

Moral hazard—A situation where the individual alters their behavior when they have acquired insurance. Since insurance lowers the price of medical care, the insured will consume more care than if they had to pay the full price themselves.

Mortality rate—For a given population, it is the ratio of number of individuals who die divided by the average size of the population.

Multihospital system—A system in which a corporation owns, leases, or manages two or more acute care hospitals.

Multipayer system—A system in which reimbursement for medical services is made by multiple third-party payers.

Negative prices—A negative price is when a person or beneficiary group is paid to use a service. When the time and travel costs of a beneficiary group is lowered, e.g., locating facilities closer to the beneficiaries, these may also be considered to be negative prices.

Network Health Maintenance Organization—A type of HMO that signs contracts with a number of group practices to provide medical services.

Non-market care giving—Medical or nursing care that is provided by the patient's spouse or family without pay.

Non-price hospital competition—Hospitals compete on the basis of their facilities and services and the latest technology rather than on price.

Normal good—An increase in income leads to greater consumption.

Normative judgment of a shortage—A non-economic definition of a health manpower shortage. Estimates of such a shortage are based upon a determination of "need" in the population or upon some professional estimate of health manpower requirements.

Not-for-profit—An institution that is not allowed to disburse its profits.

Nurse participation rates—The percentage of trained nurses that are employed.

Oligopoly—A market structure characterized by few firms, with each firm considering the actions of the other firms when making price and output decisions (interdependence among firms).

Omnibus Budget Reconciliation Act of 1989—Congressional passage of this legislation resulted in restructuring of physician reimbursement under the Medicare program.

Opportunity costs—Relevant costs for economic decision-making, they include explicit as well as implicit costs. For example, the opportunity costs of a medical education include the foregone income the student could have earned had they not gone to medical school.

Optimal rate of output—Occurs when the marginal benefit of the last unit equals the price of that unit, which in turn equals the marginal cost of producing the last unit.

Optimization techniques (marginal analysis)—Specify the appropriate criteria to be used when allocating scarce resources so as to minimize the cost of producing a given output or, similarly, maximize output, subject to a budget constraint. For example, costs are minimized when the ratio of the marginal product of each input divided by its cost is equal.

Out-of-pocket price—The amount that the beneficiary must pay after all other payments have been considered by the health plan.

Over-the-counter drug—A drug that is available for public purchase and self-directed use without a prescription.

Patient dumping—A situation where high-cost patients are not admitted to or are discharged early from a hospital because the patient either has no insurance or that the amount reimbursed by the third-party payor will be less than the cost of caring for that patient.

Per diem payments—A method of payment to institutional providers that is based on a fixed daily amount and does not differ according to the level of service provided.

Periodic re-examination—Would require physicians to maintain their qualifications by requiring them to undergo periodic testing for re-licensure.

Physician agency relationships—The physician acts on behalf of the patient. Agency relationships may be perfect or imperfect and method of physician payment, fee-for-service or capitation, would produce different behavioral responses among imperfect physician agents.

Physician control model of the hospital—The hospital's behavior, pricing, cost control, and investments, are expected to be determined according to the medical staff's economic interests.

Physician Hospital Organization (PHO)—An organization where hospitals and their medical staffs develop new types of group practice arrangements that will allow the hospitals to seek contracts from HMOs and other carriers on behalf of physicians and the hospitals together.

Physician market entry barriers—Licensure, graduation from an approved medical school, and continual increases in training times cause the supply of physicians to be smaller than if such barriers did not exist. The ostensible reasons for such barriers, namely, a high-quality work force, could be achieved more directly.

Physician-to-population ratio—The number of physicians per 100,000 population has often been used as an indicator of a shortage or surplus of physicians. These ratios do not consider changes in demands for physicians, increases in physician productivity, nor do differences in these ratios over time indicate the importance, in terms of physician fees, of shortages or surpluses using this approach.

Play or pay—Under this form of national health insurance (also referred to as an employer mandate), employers are required to either provide some basic level of medical insurance to their employees ("play") or pay a certain amount per employee into a government pool that would provide the employee with insurance.

Point-of-service—A plan that allows the beneficiary to select from participating providers (the HMO) or use non-participating providers and pay a high copayment.

Portability—Included as part of health insurance reform that enables the insured to change jobs without losing their insurance or having to be liable for another pre-existing exclusion period.

Pre-existing exclusion—To protect themselves against adverse selection by new enrollees, insurers use a pre-existing exclusion clause that excludes treatment for any or specified illnesses that have been diagnosed within the previous (usually) 12 months.

Preferred Provider Organization (PPO)—An arrangement between a panel of health care providers and purchasers of health care services in which a closed panel of providers agree to supply services to a defined group of patients on a discounted fee-for-service basis. This type of plan offers a limited number of physicians and hospitals, negotiated fee schedules, utilization review, and consumer incentives to use PPO participating providers.

Preferred risk selection—Occurs when insurers receive the same premium for everyone in an insured group and try and attract only those with lower risks whose expected medical costs would be less than the group's average premium.

Prepaid Group Practice (PGP)—A type of practice where the providers are reimbursed a capitated amount per enrollee for a stipulated length of time.

Prescription drug—A drug that can be obtained only with a physician's prescription.

Prestige maximization goal—Not-for-profit providers (hospitals and medical schools) whose pricing and investment behavior is directed to increase the prestige of the institution rather than increase the rate of return on their investments.

Price discrimination—An indication of monopoly power by a provider. The provider is able to charge different purchasers different prices according to the purchaser's elasticity of demand (willingness to pay) for the same or similar service.

Price fixing—Occurs when competing firms agree to set prices to increase profits. The competing firms act like a monopolist in that they use the industry demand curve, which is less price elastic, to establish their prices. Such actions are considered to be a per se violation of the anti-trust laws.

Price of legislation—Is the political support an organized group can offer to legislators, namely campaign contributions, volunteer time, and votes.

Primary Care Physician (PCP)—A physician that coordinates all of the routine medical care needs of an individual. Typically, this type of physician specializes in family practice, internal medicine, pediatrics, or obstetrics/gynecology.

Process measures of quality—A type of quality assessment that evaluates process of care by measuring the specific way in which care is provided or, with respect to health manpower, their training requirements.

Producer legislation—May be categorized into five types: Demand-Increasing, Secure the Highest Method of Payment, Reduce the Price and/or Increase the Quantity of Complements, Decrease the Availability and/or Increase the Price of Substitutes, and Limit Increases in Supply.

Product market definition—Used in anti-trust cases to determine whether the product or service in question has close substitutes, which depends on the willingness of purchasers to use other services if their relative prices change. The closer the substitutes, the smaller is the market share of the product being examined.

Production possibilities curve—Shows the different combinations (trade-off) of two different goods or outputs that can be produced with a fixed amount of resources.

Professional licensure—A prerequisite that requires health professionals, such as physicians, who want to practice to obtain a license from the government.

Profit maximizing model of hospital behavior—Not-for-profit hospitals act as though they tried to maximize profits by setting price at that point on their demand curve where marginal revenue equals marginal cost. Further, such hospitals would invest so as to receive the highest rate of return on their assets. Any "profits" generated would be internally invested rather than paid out to shareholders.

Prospective payment—A method of payment for medical services in which providers are paid based on a predetermined rate for the services rendered regardless of the actual costs of care incurred. Medicare uses a prospective payment system for hospital care based on a fixed price per hospital admission (by diagnosis).

Public interest theory of government—Assumes that legislation is enacted to serve the public interest. The two basic objectives of government according to this theory are to improve market efficiency and, based on a societal value judgement, redistribute income.

Pure premium—Is the expected claims experience for an insured group, exclusive of the loading charge. As described in the text, the pure premium for an individual is calculated by multiplying the size of the loss by the probability the loss will occur.

QALYs—Quality-adjusted life years, which is the time spent in a health state (for a particular disease with specific symptom severity) multiplied by the utility score of that state.

Rate of return to a professional education—Is calculated by estimating the costs of an investment in a medical education, including both explicit and implicit (opportunity) costs and the expected higher financial returns as a result of that investment. More precisely, the internal rate of return is that discount rate which, when applied to the future earnings stream, will make its present value equal to the cost of the investment in a medical education.

Rational behavior—Assumes that the decision-maker chooses that course of action offering the highest ratio of marginal benefits to marginal costs.

Redistribution—Is based on society's value judgment that those with higher incomes should be taxed to provide for those with lower incomes.

Refundable tax credits—A proposal for national health insurance under which individuals are given a tax credit to purchase health insurance. The tax credit may be income related, i.e., declining at higher levels of income. Persons whose tax credit exceeded their tax liabilities would receive a refund for the difference. For those with little or no tax liability, the tax credit is essentially a voucher for a health plan.

Regressive taxes—When those with lower incomes pay a higher portion of their income for that tax than do those with higher incomes.

Report cards—Standardized data representing both process and outcome measures of quality and is collected by independent organizations to enable purchasers to make more informed choices of health plans and their participating providers.

Resource-based relative value scale (RBRVS)—The current Medicare fee-for-service payment system for physicians, initiated in 1992, under which each physician service is assigned a relative value based on the presumed resource costs of performing that service. The relative value for each service is then multiplied by a conversion factor (in dollars) to arrive at the physician's fee.

Risk-adjusted premiums—The employer adjusts the insurance premium to reflect the risk levels of the employees enrolled with different insurers.

Risk aversion—Preferring an assured outcome to a more risky alternative.

Risk pool—Represents a population group that is defined by its expected claim experience.

Risk selection—Occurs when insurers attempt to attract a more favorable risk group than the average risk group, which was the basis for the group's premium (preferred risk selection). Similarly, enrollees may seek to join a health plan at a premium that reflects a lower level of risk than their own (adverse selection).

"Rule of reason"—Used in anti-trust cases to determine whether the anti-competitive harm caused by a particular activity (e.g., merger) exceeds the procompetitive benefits of not permitting the particular activity.

Scarce resources—A basic assumption underlying economic analysis that there are insufficient resources, i.e., time or money, to satisfy all wants.

Second opinions—A utilization review approach in which decisions to initiate a medical intervention are typically reviewed by two physicians.

Self funding self-insurance—A health care program in which employers fund benefit plans from their own resources without purchasing insurance. Self-funded plans may be self-administered, or the employer may contract with an outside administrator for an administrative service only (ASO) arrangement. Employers who self-fund can limit their liability via stop-loss insurance.

Shadow pricing—A practice previously engaged in by HMOs to set their premiums just below those charged by traditional insurers.

Sherman Antitrust Act—Antitrust legislation established in 1890 to prevent anti-competitive behavior.

Shift in supply—Caused by changes in input prices and/or a technology which would change the marginal productivity of inputs.

Single payer—A form of national health insurance in which a single third-party payer, usually government, pays the health care providers and the entire population has free choice of all providers at zero (or little) out-of-pocket expense.

Skilled Nursing Facility (SNF)—A long-term care facility that provides inpatient skilled nursing care and rehabilitation services.

Specialty HMOs—A type of HMO that offers one or more limited health care benefits, such as pharmacy, vision, and dental.

Specialty PPOs—A type of PPO that offers one or more limited health care services or benefits, such as anesthesia, vision, and dental services.

Staff-model health maintenance organization—A type of HMO that hires salaried physicians to provide health care services on an exclusive basis to the HMO's enrollees.

Static economic shortage—A situation in which demand exceeds supply at the market price. May occur because price is set below the equilibrium level by government or because of barriers to entry. In the case of entry barriers, the market price or wage is greater than if entry were permitted; the effect is to cause those in the industry to earn excess profits, which is an indication of a long-run shortage.

Stop-loss insurance—Insurance coverage providing protection from losses resulting from claims greater than a specific dollar amount (equivalent to a large deductible).

Structural quality measures—Measures of the quality of care that focus on the context of the environment within which medical services are provided. At the institutional level these measures can include facility licensure, compliance with health and safety codes, and medical staff appointments.

Sunk costs—Costs that have already been incurred and should be ignored for economic decision-making.

Supplier-induced demand—When physicians modify their diagnosis and treatment to favorably affect their own economic wellbeing.

Supply and demand analysis—Used for predicting new equilibrium situations; for example, predicting the effect of a change in demand for a service or in its cost of production on the price and quantity of that service.

Surplus—When the quantity supplied exceeds the quantity demanded at the market price. With respect to health professionals, a surplus occurs when the profession, on average, earns a below-normal rate of return.

Survivor Analysis—An approach for estimating economies of scale by examining the size distribution of firms in an industry to determine which size of firms become more numerous.

Target income hypothesis—A model of supplier-induced demand that assumes physicians will induce demand only to the extent they will achieve a target income, which is determined by the local income distribution, particularly with respect to the relative incomes of other physicians and professionals in the area.

Task licensure—Task or specific purpose licenses would recognize that physicians are not always qualified to do all the tasks for which they are licensed to perform. Task licensure would ensure that only those qualified for a particular task would be permitted to perform that task.

Tax Equity and Fiscal Responsibility Act of 1982 (TEFRA)—Legislation that set limits on Medicare reimbursements on per-case basis for hospital costs (DRGs) and limited the annual rates of increase in DRG payments.

Tax-exempt employer-paid health insurance—Health insurance purchased by the employer on behalf of their employees is not considered to be taxable income to the employee. By lowering the price of insurance, the quantity demanded is increased (as well as its comprehensiveness). The major beneficiaries are those who are in higher income tax brackets.

Technical efficiency—The inputs used in a production function produce the maximum output for a given time period.

Tertiary care—This type of care includes the most complex services such as transplantation, open heart surgery, and burn treatment, provided in inpatient hospital settings.

Third-party administrator (TPA)—An independent entity that provides administrative services such as the processing of claims to a company that self insures. A TPA does not underwrite the risk.

Third-party payer—An organization, such as an HMO, insurance company, or government agency, that pays for all or part of the insured's medical services.

Triple option health plan—A type of health plan in which employees may choose from an HMO, PPO, or indemnity plan, depending on how much they are willing to contribute.

Uncompensated care—Services rendered by the provider without reimbursement, as in the case of charity care and bad debts.

Universal coverage—When the entire population is eligible for medical services or health insurance.

Usual, customary, and reasonable fees (UCR)—A method of reimbursement in which the fee is 'usual' in that physician's office, 'customary' in that community, and 'reasonable' in terms of the distribution of all physician charges for that service in the community.

Utility maximizing model of hospital behavior—The non-profit hospital's pricing and investment policies are assumed to be undertaken for the purpose of maximizing the utility of the hospital's decision makers, namely, the management and trustees of the hospital. These decision-makers prefer a large, high quality, prestigious institution.

Utilization Review Organization (URO)—An organization that conducts utilization reviews to determine whether specific health care service(s) are medically necessary and delivered at an appropriate cost and quality. These organizations provide their services to various health plans, employers, and insurers.

Vacancy rates—The percentage of a hospital's budgeted registered nursing positions that are unfilled.

Value judgment of minimum provision—A value judgement underlying national health insurance in which all persons should receive a minimum quantity of medical services.

Vertical Integration—The organization of a delivery system that provides an entire range of services, to include inpatient care, ambulatory care clinics, outpatient surgery, and home care.

Vertical merger—A merger between two firms that have a supplier-buyer relationship.

Virtual integration—The organization of a delivery system which relies upon contractual relationships rather than complete ownership to provide all medical services required by the patient.

Voluntary performance standard—An expenditure target adopted by the Medicare program to limit the rate of increase in its expenditures for physician's services.

Welfare criteria—Economics relies on a set of welfare criteria to determine whether someone is made better or worse off as a result of a policy change.

INDEX